Wound, Ostomy and Continence Nurses Society™

Core Curriculum

CONTINENCE
MANAGEMENT

EDITED BY

Dorothy B. Doughty, MN, RN, CWOCN, FAAN
WOC Nurse Clinician
Emory University Hospital
Atlanta, Georgia

Katherine N. Moore, PhD, RN
Professor, Faculty of Nursing
University of Alberta
Edmonton, Alberta, Canada

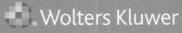 **Wolters Kluwer**

Philadelphia · Baltimore · New York · London
Buenos Aires · Hong Kong · Sydney · Tokyo

 Wound
Ostomy and
Continence
Nurses
Society®

Executive Editor: Shannon W. Magee
Senior Product Development Editor: Emilie Moyer
Editorial Assistant: Kathryn Leyendecker
Senior Marketing Manager: Mark Wiragh
Senior Production Project Manager: Cynthia Rudy
Design Coordinator: Teresa Mallon
Manufacturing Coordinator: Kathleen Brown
Prepress Vendor: Quad/Graphics

10 9 8 7 6 5 4 3

Printed in the United States of America

Cataloging-in-Publication Data available on request from the Publisher.
ISBN: 978-1-4511-9441-8

LWW.com

CONTRIBUTORS

Laurie L. Callan, MSN, ARNP, FNP, CWOCN
Family Nurse Practitioner; Wound, Ostomy, Continence
  Consultant
Whiteside County Health Department
Rock Falls, Illinois
Mercy Medical Center, Wound Center
Clinton, Iowa

Michael Clark, DrNP, MSN, CRNP, DCC
Director, Doctor of Nursing Practice Program—
  Adult-Gerontology Primary Care Track
Rutgers School of Nursing—Camden
Camden, New Jersey

Tamara Dickinson, BSN, CURN, CCCN, BCB-PMD
Senior Research Nurse in Continence and Voiding
  Dysfunction
Department of Urology
UT Southwestern Medical Center
Dallas, Texas

Dorothy B. Doughty, MN, RN, CWOCN, FAAN
WOC Nurse Clinician
Emory University Hospital
Atlanta, Georgia

Marcus John Drake, MA, DM, FRCS(Urol)
Senior Lecturer in Urology
School of Clinical Sciences, University of Bristol
Bristol, United Kingdom

Sandra Engberg, PhD, RN, CRNP, FAAN
Professor and Associate Dean for Graduate Clinical
  Education
University of Pittsburgh School of Nursing
Pittsburgh, Pennsylvania

Mandy Fader, RN, PhD
Professor of Continence Technology
Associate Dean (Research)
University of Southampton
Southampton, England

Lynette Franklin, MSN, APRN-BC, CWOCN-AP
Instructor
Nell Hodgson Woodruff School of Nursing
Emory University
Atlanta, Georgia

William Gibson, MBChB, MRCP(UK)
Clinical Research Fellow, Division of Geriatric Medicine
University of Alberta
Edmonton, Alberta, Canada

**Mikel Gray, PhD, FNP, PNP, CUNP, CCCN, FAANP,
  FAAN**
Professor of Nursing
Department of Urology and School of Nursing
University of Virginia
Charlottesville, Virginia

Claire Jungyoun Han, MSN, RN
Doctoral Student
School of Nursing
University of Washington
Seattle, Washington

Margaret Heitkemper, PhD, RN, FAAN
Professor and Chair
Department of Biobehavioral Nursing and Health
  Systems
University of Washington
Seattle, Washington

Anne Jinbo, PhD, MPH, CWOCN, CPNP
Nurse Practitioner
Hawaii Wound, Ostomy and Continence Center
Honolulu, Hawaii

Darcie Kiddoo, MD, FRCSC, MPH
Associate Professor, Pediatric Urology
Department of Surgery
University of Alberta
Edmonton, Alberta, Canada

Katherine N. Moore, PhD, RN
Professor, Faculty of Nursing
University of Alberta
Edmonton, Alberta, Canada

Kelly Kruse Nelles, RN, MS, APRN-BC
Clinical Associate Professor
University of Wisconsin—Madison School
    of Nursing
Madison, Wisconsin

Mary H. Palmer, PhD, RNC
Professor and Helen W. & Thomas L. Umphlet
    Distinguished Professor in Aging
School of Nursing
The University of North Carolina at Chapel Hill
Chapel Hill, North Carolina

**Shiv Kumar Pandian, MBBS, MS, MD, FRCS(Ed),
    FRCS(Urol)**
Senior Clinical Fellow in Urology
Bristol Urological Institute
Bristol, United Kingdom

Joanne P. Robinson, PhD, RN, GCNS-BC, FAAN
Dean and Professor
Rutgers School of Nursing-Camden
Camden, New Jersey

JoAnn Ermer-Seltun, MS, RN, ARNP, FNP-BC, CWOCN
Co-Director and Faculty, webWOC Nursing Education
    Program
Minneapolis, Minnesota
Mercy Medical Center Advanced Wound Center &
    Continence Clinic
Bladder Control Solutions, LLC
Mason City, Iowa

Susan E. Steele, PhD, RN, CWOCN
Associate Professor, School of Nursing
Georgia College
Milledgeville, Georgia

Adrian Wagg, MB, BS, FRCP, FRCP(E), FHEA, (MD)
Professor of Healthy Aging and Division Director
Division of Geriatric Medicine, Department of Medicine
University of Alberta
Edmonton, Alberta, Canada

Mary H. Wilde, RN, PhD
Associate Professor, School of Nursing
University of Rochester
Rochester, New York

Midge Willson, BSN, MSN, CWOCN
Manager of Clinical Education
Hollister Incorporated
Libertyville, Illinois

FOREWORD

It is an honor to be invited to write the foreword to the *Wound, Ostomy and Continence Nurses Society™ Core Curricula*. Having served 22 years as a Wound, Ostomy and Continence (WOC) Nursing Program Director, I can attest as to how valuable a resource these books will be to students, faculty, preceptors, and all clinicians caring for people with wounds, ostomies, and incontinence.

Terms currently popular in health care refer to patient-centered and patient-focused care. For those of you entering the wonderful WOC nursing specialty, know this: the patient has always been the focus of WOC nursing! In fact, our specialty grew from a need identified by patients themselves. As colorectal and urologic surgeries advanced, so did the number of people living with ostomies. In 1958, Akron, Ohio native Norma N. Gill joined her surgeon, Rupert B. Turnbull, Jr., MD, in founding what was then coined by Dr. Turnbull as enterostomal therapy (ET).

Beginning in 1948, when she was a 28-year-old mother of two young children, Norma began a long odyssey battling mucosal ulcerative colitis. She manifested all the gastrointestinal symptoms, including massive bouts of bloody diarrhea associated with this disease, along with many of the extraintestinal manifestations, such as uveitis, iritis, and extensive pyoderma gangrenosum on her face, chest, abdomen, and legs. During a brief remission in 1951, much to the amazement of Norma and her husband Ted, she became pregnant. The pregnancy was fraught with complications, the need for numerous blood transfusions, and fear for the lives of both mother and child throughout. Despite all of these life-threatening occurrences, in June 1952, Norma gave birth to a healthy baby girl. The complications continued after her baby's birth, and Norma's response to treatment was spotty at best. In October 1954, she was admitted to the Cleveland Clinic, and there her life was saved and history forever changed. Dr. Turnbull operated to remove Norma's colon and create an ileostomy. Her postoperative course after ileostomy was rocky, and she had to undergo some additional operations to remove her rectum and have plastic surgery performed on her face.

Despite all of this, Norma began to feel better—incredibly better. As she was resuming her role as a wife and mother, she felt the need, as we now say, to "pay it forward." Norma wanted to help others who were facing the same challenges she had endured and emerged stronger than she had been before her illness. Her journey began with the Akron physicians and hospital she had come to know well during her illness. Norma started from scratch and cobbled together an inventory of the limited equipment available at the time. Soon she had many referrals from the surgeons and knew she had found her calling. In 1958, during an appointment with Dr. Turnbull, she told him what she was doing in Akron to help people with new ostomies and fistulae. He was impressed and called her a couple of months later to offer her a job at the Cleveland Clinic.

August 1958 is when the seeds for the modern specialty of WOC nursing were planted. It was not long before the word was out, and surgeons began requesting that their staff come to train with Norma and Dr. Turnbull. The R.B. Turnbull, Jr. School of Enterostomal Therapy (now WOC Nursing) was established. After her long work day in Cleveland, Norma would return to Akron and see patients in hospitals there before heading home to her family and doing it all again the next day.

There was a child in an Akron hospital who always remembered her first encounter with Norma. Here was a woman who commanded respect. The surgeon, head nurse, and staff nurses, as well as the girl's mom, crowded around the bed as Norma taught the proper way to care for a new ileal conduit. That child grew up well adjusted to her new stoma, and thanks to a great family and the one and only Norma Gill, that child grew up to be me! The baby who was predicted never to be born to Norma and Ted is Sally Gill-Thompson—one of my best friends and a famous ET practitioner in her own right.

After establishment of the formal program in Cleveland, other ET schools soon opened, and graduates from the United States and abroad spread the word across the globe. Professional organizations were established, and admission criteria became more stringent as health care became more complex. ET nurses became well respected for their skills and experience caring for people with complex ostomies and fistulae. It was a natural extension of our practice to embrace wound and continence care, and with a painful good-bye to our ET designation in the 1990s, we became known as WOC nurses to better reflect our practice. As you embark on your studies of WOC nursing, take time to reflect and appreciate the wonderful legacy you are continuing with your specialty practice.

Norma will be watching.

Paula Erwin-Toth, MSN, RN, CWOCN, CNS, FAAN

PREFACE

We are proud to support both wound, ostomy and continence (WOC) nursing education and WOC nursing practice with this evidence-based *Continence Management* textbook, one of a set of three generously funded by the Wound, Ostomy and Continence Nurses Society (WOCN®) to form the *Wound, Ostomy and Continence Nurses Society™ Core Curriculum*. The continence field is growing, new research is informing practice, and practice is shifting with the new evidence. In this book, we address the fundamentals and the advances in both urinary and fecal incontinence in adults and children. The separate urinary and fecal sections begin with basic physiology and pathophysiology; subsequent chapters integrate pharmacology into chapters and case studies, discuss the many complexities of conservative management of urinary and fecal incontinence, and highlight the unique aspects of care for the older patient. There is considerable emphasis on basic and advanced assessment. The fecal section includes an in-depth discussion of normal bowel function and defecation, followed by chapters on motility disorders, fecal incontinence, and bowel dysfunction in the pediatric population.

Unique features of this continence management book are chapters dedicated to the appropriate use of containment devices, absorptive products, and indwelling catheters. To assist the WOC nursing student, each chapter begins with curriculum objectives addressed in the specific chapter and a topic outline to give the reader a quick overview of the chapter content. Throughout each chapter, clinical pearls are embedded to highlight key "take home" messages; and multiple illustrations, tables, and boxes facilitate understanding. Finally, there are questions and answers at the end of each chapter to support the individual's self-assessment of knowledge. Our goal was to present to both the novice and the advanced practitioner a set of logically progressive chapters, thoroughly researched and current on a pervasive problem in the United States.

The chapters are written by expert clinicians—"by continence clinicians, for continence clinicians." As editors, we wish to express our gratitude to the staff at Wolters Kluwer—Lisa Marshall, Emilie Moyer, and others behind the scenes who facilitated the organization and spearheaded the necessary planning to bring this series to publication. Throughout, Nicolette Zuecca, Executive Vice President of WOCN, kept us on track and enhanced the process. Finally, we express our sincere thanks to our extremely knowledgeable and committed contributors, and we thank each of them for saying "yes" to our request!

ACKNOWLEDGMENTS

The Wound, Ostomy and Continence Nurses Society™ (WOCN®) wishes to thank all of the clinical experts who munificently shared their time and expertise to create this textbook. The Society would like to especially acknowledge the consulting editors, Dorothy Doughty and Katherine Moore, for their inspiration, knowledge, and unwavering commitment to the development of this resource and to the field of wound, ostomy and continence nursing.

WOCN would like to acknowledge Hollister Incorporated for providing a commercially supported educational grant for the development of this textbook.

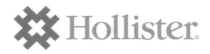

CONTENTS

Voiding Physiology

Dorothy B. Doughty

The lower urinary tract (bladder, urethra, and sphincter) is responsible for storage and elimination of urine, with normal function characterized by cyclical filling and emptying. The ability to delay voiding until a time and place that is socially acceptable and the ability to empty the bladder effectively are important to quality of life for children past the age of toilet training, adolescents, and adults. Normal voiding and urinary continence are dependent on normal bladder and sphincter function, neural control, and intact cognition.

Voiding dysfunction and urinary incontinence are common disorders that have a major impact on quality of life; voiding dysfunction and neurogenic bladder dysfunction can also potentially affect upper tract function and overall health. In order to understand the pathology of voiding dysfunction and the various types of urinary incontinence, it is critical to understand normal function. That is the focus of this chapter.

Structures and Functions Critical to Normal Voiding and Continence

The individual with normal lower urinary tract function never really thinks about the components of bladder control and effective voiding. The average adult with normal function voids approximately six to eight times daily (every 3 to 4 hours) (Zderic & Chacko, 2012). He/she is able to sense bladder filling, delay voiding if necessary (even if the bladder is quite full), and initiate voiding when a socially acceptable time and place are found. The individual with normal lower urinary tract function can also initiate urination even when there is very little urine in the bladder and no "need to void" should this be necessary (e.g., when a urine sample is requested) (Eastham & Gillespie, 2013). These abilities are supported by an anatomically intact lower urinary tract (bladder, urethra, and sphincter) and pelvic floor, an intact and functional neural control system (brain, spinal cord, and nerve pathways), and intact cognition (Yoshimura et al., 2014). The structure and function of each of these structures will be discussed, followed by a brief discussion of changes in function across the life span.

Lower Urinary Tract and Pelvic Floor

Bladder

The bladder has two critical and repetitive functions: to stretch and store moderate volumes of urine at low pressures and to contract effectively to empty. The ability to distend with urine while maintaining low intravesical pressures is a property known as compliance and is important both to preservation of upper tract (renal) health and

to normal voiding intervals and quality of life (Smith et al., 2012; Wyndaele et al., 2011). Maintenance of low filling pressures is essential to renal health because it permits continued delivery of urine from the kidneys to the bladder; once the intravesical pressure rises to a level greater than that exerted by the low-pressure ureters, delivery of urine ceases and there is resulting back pressure on the kidneys, which can eventually result in hydronephrosis. In addition, a rapid rise in intravesical pressure with low volumes of urine is associated with intense urgency in the patient who has normal sensation (because the bladder feels and acts "full" when there is a marked increase in intravesical pressure).

It is also important for the bladder to mount a strong and sustained contraction to effectively empty the urine. A weakly contractile bladder is associated with significant volumes of retained urine, which causes increased urinary frequency and urgency, nocturia, and increased risk of UTI.

The bladder is a hollow organ very well designed for alternate storage and expulsion of urine (Fig. 1-1). It has three layers (urothelium, lamina propria, and detrusor), each of which plays an important role in bladder filling, sensory inputs to the central nervous system regarding state of filling, and effective emptying (Andersson & McCloskey, 2014; Daly et al., 2011; Eastham & Gillespie, 2013).

Urothelium

The urothelium (inner lining of the bladder, composed primarily of transitional cell epithelium) was previously conceptualized as a passive layer that primarily provided separation between the bladder wall and the constituents of the urine. However, it is now recognized that there are a number of ion channels and receptors located in the urothelial layer that detect mechanical, thermal, and chemical stimuli; in response to these stimuli, the urothelium secretes signaling molecules (such as ATP, ACh, and NO) that provide input to the brain regarding bladder filling and messaging to the bladder muscle that help to modulate relaxation and contractility (Birder et al., 2012; Gonzalez et al., 2014). For example, nitric oxide (NO) released by the urothelium may contribute to normal bladder filling via two mechanisms: (1) There is evidence that NO modulates and down-regulates activation of sensory pathways signaling bladder filling; and (2) NO is known to contribute to detrusor muscle relaxation. There is also evidence that activation of stretch receptors in the bladder wall causes release of ATP by the urothelium, which

Urinary Bladder, Anterior View
A. Female

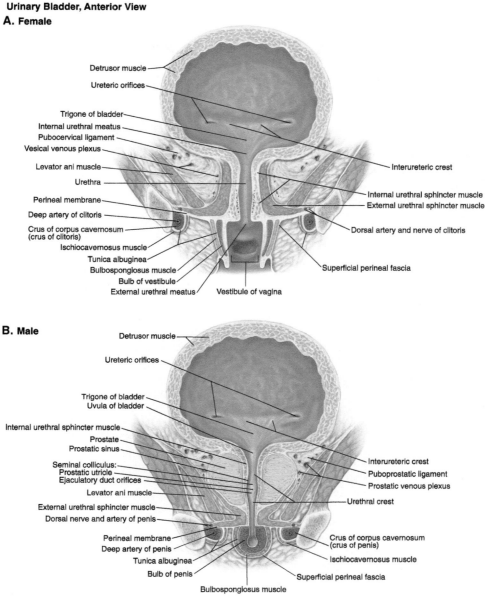

Detrusor muscle
Ureteric orifices
Trigone of bladder
Internal urethral meatus
Pubocervical ligament
Vesical venous plexus
Levator ani muscle
Urethra
Perineal membrane
Deep artery of clitoris
Crus of corpus cavernosum (crus of clitoris)
Ischiocavernosus muscle
Tunica albuginea
Bulbospongiosus muscle
Bulb of vestibule
External urethral meatus
Vestibule of vagina
Interureteric crest
Internal urethral sphincter muscle
External urethral sphincter muscle
Dorsal artery and nerve of clitoris
Superficial perineal fascia

B. Male

Detrusor muscle
Ureteric orifices
Trigone of bladder
Uvula of bladder
Internal urethral sphincter muscle
Prostate
Prostatic sinus
Seminal colliculus:
Prostatic utricle
Ejaculatory duct orifices
Levator ani muscle
External urethral sphincter muscle
Dorsal nerve and artery of penis
Perineal membrane
Deep artery of penis
Tunica albuginea
Bulb of penis
Bulbospongiosus muscle
Interureteric crest
Puboprostatic ligament
Prostatic venous plexus
Urethral crest
Crus of corpus cavernosum (crus of penis)
Ischiocavernosus muscle
Superficial perineal fascia

FIGURE 1-1. **A, B.** Female and male bladders.

stimulates the sensory pathways signaling bladder filling. Finally, emerging evidence suggests that, in the "normal" bladder, there is a balance between release of NO and ATP and that the ATP/NO ratio is one factor determining the frequency of bladder contractions (Daly et al., 2011).

CLINICAL PEARL

The bladder is lined with urothelium, which was previously thought to be a passive layer separating the bladder wall from the constituents of the urine; it is now recognized that the urothelium secretes signaling molecules that provide input to the brain regarding bladder filling and input to the bladder that modulates relaxation and contractility.

The surface of the urothelium is covered with a protective layer (glycosaminoglycans or mucin) that is thought to limit adherence of bacteria and penetration by irritants. Damage to this layer might permit penetration by noxious substances, bacterial adherence and infection, and/or abnormal release of inflammatory molecules by the urothelium, resulting in symptoms such as pain, urgency, and frequency (Birder, 2013).

Lamina Propria
The *lamina propria* is also known as the suburothelium and is the layer lying between the urothelium and the detrusor; it includes interstitial cells, fibroblasts, blood vessels, and both afferent and efferent nerves. This layer is thought to contribute to normal bladder distensibility (compliance)

by maintaining a balance between Type III and Type I collagen (25% and 75%, respectively) and by production of the elastic fibers that allow the bladder to return to its normal shape following emptying (Andersson & McCloskey, 2014). Recent studies suggest that the lamina propria may also contribute to modulation and signaling related to bladder filling and contractility (Andersson & McCloskey, 2014; Gonzalez et al., 2014).

Detrusor

The *detrusor* is the smooth muscle of the bladder and is comprised of bundles of long slender muscle cells surrounded by an extracellular matrix. The smooth muscle cells of the bladder are known as single unit smooth muscle, meaning that the ratio between muscle cells and nerve endings is almost 1:1; this rich innervation provides high-level neural control of bladder contractility (Yoshimura & Chancellor, 2012). The smooth muscle cells of the bladder have length and tension properties that permit them to stretch slowly without inducing a contraction until emptying is initiated voluntarily or until capacity has been reached. In the event of rapid stretch (e.g., rapid bladder filling due to diuresis or rapid filling during cystometrogram), the muscle cells respond initially with a marked increase in tension that dissipates before a detrusor contraction is produced; this phenomenon is known as the stress relaxation response and is dependent in part on normal viscoelastic properties of the detrusor muscle and extracellular matrix (collagen). Excessive stretch on the detrusor muscle cells, as occurs with marked overdistention of the bladder, results in irreversible changes in the muscle; this explains why inadequate management of acute urinary retention can result in chronic urinary retention (Wyndaele et al., 2011; Zderic & Chacko, 2012).

Detrusor contraction occurs in response to parasympathetic stimulation and is normally characterized by a contraction of sufficient force and duration to expel all or most of the urine; normal contractility is dependent both on normal innervation and normal contractility (Osman et al., 2014; Zderic & Chacko, 2012).

CLINICAL PEARL

The inner layer of the bladder (detrusor muscle) is comprised of smooth muscle cells with length and tension properties that permit them to stretch slowly without inducing a contraction until emptying is initiated voluntarily or until capacity has been reached.

In addition to the myocytes (muscle cells), the detrusor contains stretch receptors that signal bladder filling. Further, there is some evidence for a motor–sensory system within the bladder that may increase sensory awareness of the need to void. Specifically, there are data suggesting that, as the bladder becomes progressively more distended with urine, there is increasing low-level muscle activity (localized low amplitude contractions, or "twitches," in the muscle); these low amplitude contractions in response to stretch do not produce voiding, but are thought to contribute to the afferent "noise" produced by the distending bladder that signals the central nervous system regarding the need to void (Eastham & Gillespie, 2013).

CLINICAL PEARL

The detrusor also contains stretch receptors that signal bladder filling.

Urethra and Urethral Sphincter Mechanism

The urethra serves as a conduit for elimination of urine from the bladder (and for semen in men) and plays an important role in both effective bladder emptying and in maintenance of continence. Normally, the urethra functions synergistically with the bladder; during the storage cycle, the urethra remains closed to maintain continence (even during periods of increased abdominal pressure), and during voiding, the urethra funnels and opens to permit unobstructed flow. Normal function is dependent on structural integrity of the bladder neck, urethral sphincter mechanism, and pelvic floor as well as intact neural structures, pathways, and activity.

CLINICAL PEARL

Normally, the urethra functions synergistically with the bladder; during the storage phase, the urethra maintains closure, and during the emptying phase, the urethral funnels and opens to permit unobstructed flow.

Anatomic Features

Anatomically, the urethra is short and straight in women, averaging 4.0 cm (2.5 to 5.0 cm), and long and curved in men, averaging 20 cm (15.0 to 25.0 cm) (Figs. 1-2 and 1-3). The greater urethral length and curvature in men provides increased urethral resistance, and this anatomic difference between men and women is thought to be one factor contributing to the increased risk of incontinence among women (Neveus & Sillen, 2013; Porth, 2011). The male urethra can be subdivided into three sections: the prostatic urethra (the section surrounded by the prostate gland), the membranous urethra (the section involving the voluntary sphincter mechanism), and the penile urethra. The urethra is composed of two layers of smooth muscle lined with epithelium; the smooth muscle maintains a level of tonic contraction that helps to maintain urethral closure during the filling cycle (Sadananda et al., 2011).

Additional support for continence is provided by a rich vascular plexus that is located in the subepithelial layer. This network of vessels acts as a fluid-filled sponge that provides compressive support to the urethra, which seems to be particularly important to continence in women

Medial section

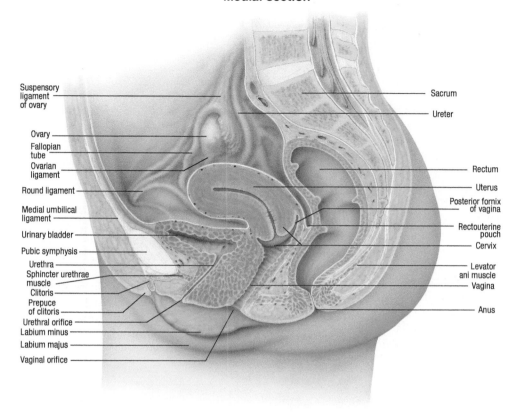

Suspensory ligament of ovary

Ovary
Fallopian tube
Ovarian ligament
Round ligament
Medial umbilical ligament
Urinary bladder
Pubic symphysis
Urethra
Sphincter urethrae muscle
Clitoris
Prepuce of clitoris
Urethral orifice
Labium minus
Labium majus
Vaginal orifice

Sacrum
Ureter
Rectum
Uterus
Posterior fornix of vagina
Rectouterine pouch
Cervix
Levator ani muscle
Vagina
Anus

FIGURE 1-2. Female urethra.

(Mannella et al., 2013; Sadananda et al., 2011). The passive support provided by the prostate gland is another contributing factor to continence in the male, though late in life, prostatic hypertrophy may result in outlet obstruction and urinary retention (Gibson & Wagg, 2014). Finally, in women, anatomic support for continence is provided by coaptation of the urethral walls, which helps to maintain urethral closure and to resist leakage; coaptation is dependent on soft moist urethral tissue and may be adversely affected by estrogen deficiency.

> **CLINICAL PEARL**
>
> Anatomic features of the male urethra contributing to continence include the greater length and curvatures, which increases resistance, and support provided by the prostate gland. In women, the suburethral vascular plexus and coaptation of the urethral walls seems to play an important role.

Smooth Muscle (also known as *internal sphincter*)
The bladder neck is comprised of smooth muscle innervated by the autonomic nervous system and controlled by descending nerve pathways from the pontine micturition center (PMC); the internal sphincter is tonically contracted throughout the filling phase and provides primary support for continence. As noted, neural control of

the bladder neck and detrusor muscle assures synergistic response of the bladder and its outlet. Specifically, during the storage phase, sympathetic pathways are activated; sympathetic stimulation of the alpha-adrenergic receptors in the smooth muscle of the bladder neck causes increased urethral tone, while sympathetic stimulation of the beta-adrenergic receptors in the bladder wall causes detrusor relaxation. Conversely, during voiding, sympathetic stimulation to the bladder neck and detrusor is turned "off," causing relaxation of the bladder outlet, and parasympathetic stimulation of cholinergic/muscarinic receptors in the bladder wall causes detrusor contraction.

There is evidence that the smooth muscle of the bladder neck is more highly developed in the male than in the female. There is also evidence that interstitial cells interspersed throughout the smooth muscle of the bladder neck may function as "pacemakers" to promote contractility and maintain urethral closure during the filling cycle and that there is direct input from the pontine storage center (PSC) to the bladder neck promoting closure (Sadananda et al., 2011).

> **CLINICAL PEARL**
>
> The "internal sphincter" is comprised of smooth muscle fibers within the bladder neck, which are innervated by the autonomic nervous system and controlled by the pons.

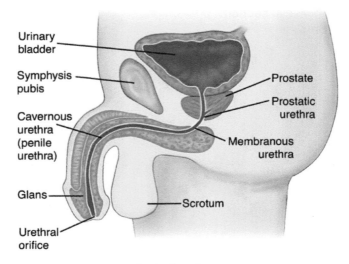

Sagittal section

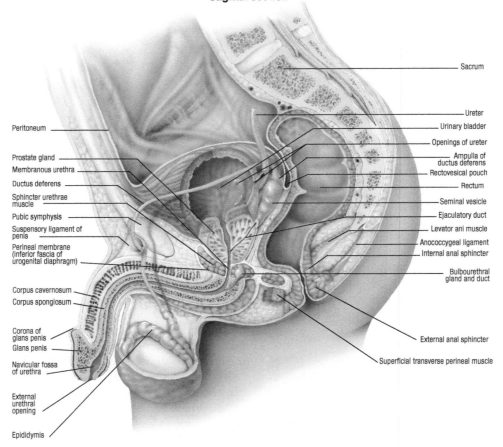

FIGURE 1-3.   Male urethra.

Striated Muscle

The voluntary sphincter (also known as the external sphincter or rhabdosphincter) is located just distal to the prostate gland in men (at the level of the membranous urethra) and at approximately midurethra in women. In men, the rhabdosphincter is one omega-shaped muscle; in women, it is more semicircular in shape and consists of three separate but connected muscles (sphincter urethrae, compressor urethrae, and sphincter urethrovaginalis) that work together to support, compress, and elongate the urethra (Hinata & Murakami, 2014; Jung et al., 2012). The voluntary sphincter is innervated by branches of the pudendal nerve; voluntary contraction significantly increases urethral closure pressure and helps to prevent leakage during periods of increased intra-abdominal pressure.

Pelvic Floor

The pelvic floor is a complex network of fascia, ligaments, and muscles that support the pelvic organs and oppose downward displacement. The levator ani is the primary component of the pelvic floor and is comprised of three different but connected muscles: (1) pubococcygeus muscle, the central and major muscle, which extends from the symphysis pubis to the coccyx; (2) puborectalis, which forms a sling behind the anorectal junction; and (3) the ileococcygeus, a smaller muscle that lies superior to the pubococcygeus (Fig. 1-4). The muscles are covered by fascia, which condenses into ligaments that attach the pelvic organs to the bony pelvis (Mannella et al., 2013).

Role in Continence

A healthy pelvic floor has sometimes been compared to a trampoline; when increased intra-abdominal pressure pushes pelvic organs caudally, the pelvic floor normally provides counterpressure and sufficient support to maintain the organs (vagina, bladder, and urethra) in their normal positions. This is important because there is some evidence that loss of normal intrapelvic position compromises function of the striated sphincter; urethral "hypermobility" (distal displacement of the urethra in response to increased intra-abdominal pressure) is thought to be one factor contributing to stress incontinence in women (Bauer & Huebner, 2013). Pelvic floor support is enabled by the fact that there are connections between the pelvic floor and striated sphincter muscles, so contraction of the striated sphincter also causes contraction of the pelvic floor muscles. This means that pelvic muscle exercise programs strengthen both the striated sphincter and the pelvic floor muscles, thus providing improved support for pelvic organs in addition to increasing sphincter muscle contractility and endurance (McLean et al., 2013).

Fast-Twitch versus Slow-Twitch Muscle Fibers

The pelvic floor muscles are comprised of approximately 2/3 slow-twitch fibers and 1/3 fast-twitch fibers. Slow-twitch fibers provide sustained tonic contraction

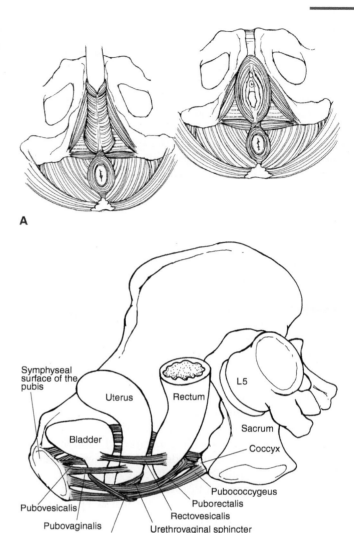

A

Symphyseal surface of the pubis

Uterus

Rectum

L5

Bladder

Sacrum

Coccyx

Pubovesicalis

Pubococcygeus

Puborectalis

Rectovesicalis

Pubovaginalis

Urethrovaginal sphincter

Compressor urethra

B

FIGURE 1-4. A. Pelvic floor, male and female. **B.** Medial view pelvic floor muscles.

and improve baseline support for pelvic organs, while fast-twitch fibers provide rapid strong contractions that prevent leakage during periods of increased abdominal pressure (Marques et al., 2010). Pelvic muscle exercise programs are generally designed to strengthen both slow-twitch and fast-twitch fibers and thus to improve both continence at rest and continence during activities that increase stress on the continence mechanism (Madill et al., 2013; Marques et al., 2010).

Guarding Reflex

The guarding reflex helps to maintain continence by progressively increasing outlet resistance in response to bladder filling. There appear to be at least two pathways involved in the guarding reflex: (1) As the bladder distends with urine, stretch receptors in the bladder wall are activated, and these receptors send signals regarding bladder filling to the sacral cord; this activates the pudendal nerve (in addition to sending messages regarding bladder filling to the brain). The pudendal nerve then activates efferent pathways to the external sphincter that act on nicotinic receptors in the external sphincter muscle to increase outlet resistance. (2) In addition, afferent signals from the distending bladder activate a pathway from the sacral cord to the thoracolumbar cord; this causes increased sympathetic stimulation of the bladder neck and bladder, which results in increased bladder neck tone and detrusor relaxation (Chancellor & Yoshimura, 2004).

> **CLINICAL PEARL**
>
> The guarding reflex helps to maintain continence by progressively increasing outlet resistance in response to bladder filling.

Support for Voiding

In addition to maintaining closure during the filling cycle and thereby preventing incontinence, the normal urethra funnels and opens to provide unobstructed emptying during voiding. There is some evidence that afferent nerves in the urethra may contribute to effective bladder emptying by sensing flow rates and providing feedback that maintains the detrusor contraction as long as flow rates remain high (Osman et al., 2014).

Neural Control

As noted, the bladder and its outlet constantly cycle between filling and emptying, with synergistic activity during each phase (bladder relaxation and sphincter contraction during filling, followed by bladder contraction and sphincter relaxation during emptying). This coordinated and cyclical activity requires complex interaction among multiple signaling pathways and neurologic centers, in addition to an intact lower urinary tract (Sadananda et al., 2011; Scemons, 2013). The primary centers include the cerebral cortex and midbrain; the pons; the sympathetic outflow tracts located in the thoracolumbar cord; the parasympathetic outflow tracts and Onuf's nucleus, both of which are located in the sacral cord; and the signaling neurons in the urothelium and detrusor (Andersson & McCloskey, 2014; Birder, 2013; Daly et al., 2011; Sadananda et al., 2011; Yoshimura et al., 2014) (Fig. 1-5).

Cerebral Cortex and Midbrain

The actual switch between bladder filling (storage) and bladder emptying (voiding) is controlled by midbrain structures (particularly the periaqueductal gray, or PAG)

and the PMC; however, *decision making* regarding voiding (social continence) is the responsibility of higher cortical centers, specifically the prefrontal cortex. The decision regarding voiding is based on sensory input regarding bladder filling as well as environmental input and can involve delay of voiding despite a very full bladder (until an appropriate time and place can be found), or can involve volitional initiation of voiding in the absence of any urgency to void, such as the decision to void "prophylactically" before beginning a long car trip (Eastham & Gillespie, 2013; Sadananda et al., 2011). The primary centers involved in processing signals regarding bladder filling include the periaqueductal gray, the insula, the locus coeruleus, the anterior cingulate gyrus, and the prefrontal cortex. This information is then relayed to the decision-making center.

Functional neuroimaging suggests the following sequence of events: (1) the PAG processes sensory input regarding bladder filling and relays the information to the hypothalamus, insula, anterior cingulate gyrus, and lateral prefrontal cortex; (2) the information is then transmitted from these centers to the medial prefrontal cortex, which maintains inhibitory control of the PAG; (3) the medial prefrontal cortex makes a decision regarding whether or not to void; (4) if the decision is *not* to void, inhibition of the PAG is maintained and voiding is delayed; and (5) when the decision is made to void, inhibitory control of the PAG is withdrawn and the PAG then activates the PMC (Barrington's nucleus) to initiate coordinated voiding (Benarroch, 2010; Eastham & Gillespie, 2013; Sadananda et al., 2011).

> **CLINICAL PEARL**
>
> The actual switch between bladder filling and bladder emptying is provided by the midbrain structures (e.g., periaqueductal gray and pons); however, *decision making* regarding voiding is the responsibility of the prefrontal cortex.

Pons

The pons has two areas involved with continence and voiding: the pontine micturition center (PMC or Barrington's nucleus) and the PSC (Valentino et al., 2011). The PMC is responsible for assuring that both the bladder neck (internal sphincter) and rhabdosphincter (external sphincter) are relaxed before the bladder contracts, in order to provide unobstructed voiding. When activated, the PMC sends input to the cord that inhibits sympathetic stimulation of the bladder neck and innervation of the external sphincter via Onuf's nucleus (thus causing both internal and external sphincter relaxation) and activates the parasympathetic pathways causing detrusor contraction (Benarroch, 2010). When the PSC is activated, there is direct stimulation of pathways causing continued contraction of the striated sphincter via Onuf's nucleus (Valentino et al., 2011).

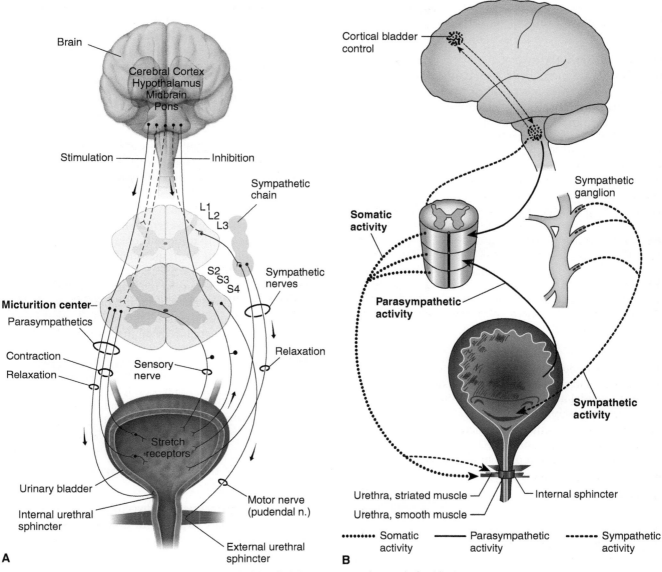

FIGURE 1-5. A, B: Neural control of voiding.

Spinal Cord and Nerve Pathways

The spinal cord and its pathways are essential to continence and to normal voiding, because these structures comprise the communication center of the controlled voiding system, transmitting messages from the bladder and sphincter to the brain and brain stem, and from the brain and brain stem to the bladder and sphincter. Thus, any disruption in the spinal cord causes loss of continence and disruption in effective coordinated voiding, a condition known as neurogenic bladder (David & Steward, 2010) (see also Chapter 7).

Sympathetic Pathways

As explained earlier, sympathetic stimulation activates alpha-adrenergic receptors in the bladder neck (via neurotransmitters such as norepinephrine) to produce increased tone and resistance and also activates beta-adrenergic receptors in the bladder wall to cause detrusor relaxation. Thus, sympathetic pathways are active during the storage phase and quiescent during voiding. Sympathetic pathways exit the cord at the thoracolumbar level (T10–L2).

Parasympathetic Pathways

In contrast, parasympathetic stimulation causes bladder contraction and reflex relaxation of the bladder neck; the primary neurotransmitter is acetylcholine, which mediates contraction via muscarinic receptors (M2 and M3) in the bladder wall. In addition to its direct effects on detrusor contractility, acetylcholine is thought to affect sensory awareness of bladder filling (Sellers & Chess-Williams, 2012). Parasympathetic pathways are active during voiding and quiescent during filling. Parasympathetic pathways exit the cord at S2–S4.

> **CLINICAL PEARL**
>
> Sympathetic pathways are active during the storage phase, causing bladder neck contraction and detrusor relaxation; parasympathetic pathways are active during voiding, causing reflex relaxation of the bladder neck and detrusor contraction.

Pudendal Nerve (Onuf's Nucleus)

The striated sphincter is under voluntary control, via a collection of cells in the sacral cord known as Onuf's nucleus and the pudendal nerve. The cells of Onuf's nucleus appear to receive direct input from the PSC; activation provides contraction of the striated sphincter via the pudendal nerve, which exits the cord at S2–S4 (Sadananda et al., 2011). (As noted, inhibition of Onuf's nucleus via the PMC causes striated sphincter relaxation.)

> **CLINICAL PEARL**
>
> The striated sphincter and pelvic floor are under voluntary control (pudendal nerve).

Signaling Neurons in the Detrusor and Urothelium

As previously discussed, the urothelium and detrusor contain a number of receptors that respond to progressive bladder distention. The gradual increase in intravesical pressures that accompanies bladder filling activates thinly myelinated fibers that send increasingly strong signals of bladder filling along autonomic nerve pathways to the cord; from the cord, they are transmitted to the brain, where there is a gradual increase in awareness that prompts decision making regarding when and where to void (Daly et al., 2011; Sadananda et al., 2011). Studies of normal subjects revealed that bladder filling is perceived as "tingling" or "pressure" and that awareness proceeds along the following continuum: no sensation, weak awareness, stronger awareness, weak need to void, stronger need to void, and absolute need to void (Eastham & Gillespie,

2013; Heeringa et al., 2011). Extreme distention may also activate C fibers, which transmit signals of severe discomfort and pain; C fibers are also activated by noxious substances in the urine or inflammation of the bladder wall (Birder, 2013; Gonzalez et al., 2014).

Intact Cognition

Bladder control is dependent in part on normal cognitive function. The individual must be able to accurately interpret messages related to bladder filling, determine or locate a socially appropriate place to void, move to that location, and remove clothing in order to permit voiding (Gibson & Wagg, 2014). While the controlled voiding process is "automatic" for most individuals, it is in fact a complex process governed at each step by the central nervous system. This is reflected by the fact that incontinence is common among individuals with cognitive impairment, such as those who are sedated and those with advanced dementia. These individuals tend to void whenever the bladder reaches a certain point of filling, regardless of time and place. Incontinence due to cognitive impairment is labeled "functional incontinence" and is discussed in detail in Chapter 10.

> **CLINICAL PEARL**
>
> While the controlled voiding process is "automatic" for most individuals, it is in fact a complex process governed at each step by the central nervous system.

Summary of Normal Lower Urinary Tract Function

The lower urinary tract cycles between "storage" and "emptying" via a complex sequence of events controlled by a myriad of signaling molecules and nerve pathways.

Storage Phase

During storage, the sympathetic pathways are active and the parasympathetic pathways are quiescent. Sympathetic stimulation of the alpha-adrenergic receptors in the bladder neck and proximal urethra maintains bladder neck closure, and sympathetic stimulation of the beta-adrenergic receptors in the bladder wall maintains bladder relaxation. The slow-twitch fibers in the pelvic floor muscles maintain resting tone, and direct input from the PSC to Onuf's nucleus (in the sacral cord) maintains closure of the external sphincter via pudendal nerve innervation.

Progressive filling of the bladder activates stretch receptors in the bladder wall and release of signaling molecules by the urothelium that provide progressively stronger messages to the midbrain (via the cord) regarding bladder filling. Microcontractions of the detrusor muscle may also contribute to signaling regarding bladder filling. This progressive filling also activates the guarding reflex (i.e., activation of pathways that increase tone within the bladder neck and the voluntary sphincter via sympathetic stimulation and pudendal nerve stimulation, respectively). The guarding reflex assures that urethral resistance increases in proportion to the demands placed by a progressively distending bladder and increasing intravesical pressures.

Messages regarding bladder filling are integrated by the midbrain, primarily the PAG; these synthesized messages are forwarded to the medial prefrontal cortex, which maintains inhibitory control of the PAG and where decision making regarding when and where to void takes place. If the decision is made to defer voiding, inhibitory control of the PAG is maintained, as is sympathetic input to the bladder and bladder neck and pudendal nerve input to the voluntary sphincter.

Emptying Phase (Micturition)

If the decision is made to initiate voiding, inhibitory control of the PAG is released; the PAG then directs the PMC to mediate coordinated voiding (sphincter relaxation prior to detrusor contraction). The PMC inactivates sympathetic pathways and the pathways controlling Onuf's nucleus, thus causing relaxation of the internal and external sphincters; the PMC also activates the parasympathetic pathways, thus causing detrusor contraction via acetylcholine stimulation of muscarinic receptors.

Changes across the Lifespan

There are a number of changes that occur in lower urinary tract structure and function across the life span that impact on continence and the ability to empty the bladder effectively; these changes will be discussed briefly in this chapter and in more depth in Chapters 10 and 11.

Infants and Toddlers

Lower urinary tract development and urine production begin early in fetal life, at about 4 to 6 weeks gestation; by the 12th week of gestation, the three-layered structure of the bladder wall is evident, and by 16 weeks, the bladder exhibits limited reservoir capacity. During infancy, bladder function is characterized by lack of coordination between the bladder and sphincter and by interrupted voiding (two separate voids during a 5- to 10-minute period). For many years, it was thought that voiding in infants was a simple spinal reflex; however, recent studies suggest involvement of the CNS, based on evidence of varying degrees of arousal preceding voiding. When the child has matured to the level where she/he recognizes bladder filling and can control bladder emptying, toilet training is appropriate. Once the child has established voluntary control of voiding, the loss of coordination between bladder and sphincter disappears and the filling emptying cycle characteristic of adult bladder function is established (Neveus & Sillen, 2013). For most children, daytime continence is established first, followed by nighttime control; girls typically achieve continence at an earlier age than boys (Bauer & Huebner, 2013).

Middle-Aged Adults

Data indicate that lower urinary tract symptoms (LUTS) begin to manifest during the 4th decade of life in both sexes; among women, storage symptoms are more common, while voiding symptoms are more common among men. For both men and women, LUTS are associated with negative impact on quality of life, resulting in anxiety and depression. For women, symptoms associated with increased anxiety include nocturia, urgency, stress incontinence, leakage during sexual activity, weak stream, and split stream; symptoms associated with increased anxiety in men include nocturia, urgency, incomplete emptying, and bladder pain. Among women, stress incontinence, urgency, and weak stream are associated with depression; symptoms associated with depression in men include frequency and incomplete emptying (Bauer & Huebner, 2013).

Elderly

Urinary incontinence and voiding dysfunction are prevalent conditions among the elderly, affecting about 25% to 50% of women and about 21% of men (Clemens, 2013; DuBeau, 2013). The prevalence of urinary incontinence and voiding dysfunction is due in part to changes in bladder function and sphincter function and in part to increasing comorbid conditions and use of pharmacologic agents that can adversely affect bladder and sphincter function. However, it is important to realize that urinary incontinence and voiding dysfunction are not inevitable consequences of aging; it is also important to realize that most elderly men and women can be effectively treated.

Changes in Bladder Function

Aging is associated with increased collagen content in the bladder wall, which reduces elasticity and bladder capacity and also adversely affects contractility. There is also a reduction in M3 receptors and a loss of caveolae (specialized areas in the muscle cell that affect bladder smooth muscle contractility), which may further reduce contractility. Reduced contractility results in less effective emptying and higher postvoid residual volumes, and the combination of reduced bladder capacity and higher postvoid residuals can produce urinary frequency, a common complaint among older adults (Gibson & Wagg, 2014; Lowalekar et al., 2012). In addition, older adults report less ability to inhibit bladder contractions, which may be due in part to failure of CNS centers or to increased presence of white matter hyperdensities (Gibson & Wagg, 2014). When one considers the fact that many elderly individuals have reduced mobility, changes in bladder function and CNS function that cause increased urinary frequency and urgency place them at significant risk for leakage.

> **CLINICAL PEARL**
>
> Aging is associated with reduced bladder capacity and contractility, which results in higher postvoid residuals and increased urinary frequency.

Changes in Sphincter Function

Changes in sphincter function and in bladder outlet resistance are due in part to hormonal changes resulting in benign prostatic enlargement in men (and increased risk of voiding dysfunction) and to estrogen loss in women. Estrogen deficiency is known to adversely affect urethral coaptation and to increase the risk for storage symptoms such as urgency and frequency; in addition, estrogen affects the synthesis of collagen and muscle in the lower urinary tract and may influence neurologic control of voiding (Mannella et al., 2013).

Comorbid Conditions and Impact of Pharmacologic Agents

Perhaps, the greatest impact of aging on bladder and sphincter function relates to the increasing number of comorbid conditions and the pharmacologic agents used for control of those conditions. Many commonly used pharmaceuticals can adversely affect bladder function, including diuretics, antihypertensives, alpha-adrenergic agonists and antagonists, angiotensin-converting enzyme (ACE) inhibitors, and drugs with anticholinergic effects (e.g., antipsychotics and antidepressants). Thus, effective management of the older individual with urinary incontinence or voiding dysfunction must involve a holistic approach that includes management of comorbid conditions and a careful review of all medications being taken.

> **CLINICAL PEARL**
>
> Factors contributing to bladder dysfunction in the elderly include hormonal changes and the increasing number of comorbid conditions and pharmacologic agents used to control those conditions.

Conclusion

Urinary continence and effective emptying require an intact lower urinary tract (bladder, sphincter, and pelvic floor), normal neural innervation and control, and normal cognitive function. Neural control involves the cortex, midbrain, pons, and spinal cord pathways; the storage phase of the voiding cycle is primarily mediated by sympathetic inputs, while the voiding phase is primarily mediated by parasympathetic stimulation. Any neurologic lesion at any

level can adversely affect bladder control and the ability to empty effectively. There are a number of changes in bladder and sphincter function associated with aging that can increase the risk of incontinence or impaired emptying; however, urinary incontinence and voiding dysfunction are never "normal" findings.

REFERENCES

Andersson, K-. E., & McCloskey, K. (2014). Lamina propria: The functional center of the bladder? *Neurourology & Urodynamics, 33,* 9–16.

Bauer, R., & Huebner, W. (2013). Gender differences in bladder control: From babies to elderly. *World Journal of Urology, 31,* 1081–1085.

Benarroch, E. (2010). Neural control of the bladder: Recent advances and neurologic implications. *Neurology, 75*(20), 1839–1846.

Birder, L. (2013). Nervous network for lower urinary tract function. *International Journal of Urology, 20,* 4–12.

Birder, L., Ruggieri, M., Takeda, M., et al. (2012). How does the urothelium affect bladder function in health and disease: ICI-RS 2011. *Neurourology and Urodynamics, 31*(3), 293–299.

Chancellor, M., & Yoshimura, N. (2004). Neurophysiology of stress incontinence. *Reviews in Urology, 6*(Suppl 3), S19–S28.

Clemens, J. (2013). Urinary incontinence in men. *Up to Date.* Retrieved from http://www.uptodate.com (Context Link).

Daly, D., Collins, V., Chapple, C., et al. (2011). The afferent system and its role in lower urinary tract dysfunction. *Current Opinion in Urology, 21,* 268–274.

David, B., & Steward, O. (2010). Deficits in bladder function following spinal cord injury vary depending on level of injury. *Experimental Neurourology, 226,* 128–135.

DuBeau, C. (2013). Epidemiology, risk factors, and pathogenesis of urinary incontinence. *Up to Date.* Retrieved from http://www.uptodate.com (Context Link).

Eastham, J., & Gillespie, J. (2013). The concept of peripheral modulation of bladder sensation. *Organogenesis, 9*(3), 224–233.

Gibson, W., & Wagg, A. (2014). New horizons: Urinary incontinence in older people. *Age and Ageing, 43,* 157–163.

Gonzalez, E., Merrill, L., & Vizzard, M. (2014). Bladder sensory physiology: Neuroactive compounds and receptors, sensory transducers, and target-derived growth factors as targets to improve function. *American Journal of Physiology–Regulatory, Integrative and Comparative Physiology, 306,* R869–R878.

Heeringa, R., deWachter, S., van Kerrebroeck, P., et al. (2011). Normal bladder sensations in healthy volunteers: A focus group investigation. *Neurourology and Urodynamics, 30*(7), 1350–1355.

Hinata, H., & Murakami, G. (2014). The urethral rhabdosphincter, levator ani muscle, and perineal membrane: A review. *Bio Med Research International,* Volume 2014, Article id. 906921. Retrieved from http://dx.doi.org/10.1155/2014/906921

Jung, J., Ahn, H., & Huh, Y. (2012). Clinical and functional anatomy of the urethral sphincters. *International Neurourology Journal, 16*(3), 102–106.

Lowalekar, S., Cristofaro, V., Radisavljevic, Z., et al. (2012). Loss of bladder smooth muscle caveolae in the aging bladder. *Neurourology and Urodynamics, 31*(4), 586–592.

Madill, S., Pontbriand-Drolet, S., Tang, A., et al. (2013). Effects of PFM rehabilitation on PFM function and morphology in older women. *Neurourology and Urodynamics, 32*(8), 1086–1095.

Mannella, P., Palla, G., Bellini, M., et al. (2013). The female pelvic floor through midlife and aging. *Maturitas, 76,* 230–234.

Marques, A., Stothers, L., & Macnab, A. (2010). The status of pelvic floor muscle training for women. *Canadian Urological Association Journal, 4*(6), 419–424.

McLean, L., Varette, K., Gentilcore-Saulnier, E., et al. (2013). Pelvic floor muscle training in women with stress urinary incontinence causes hypertrophy of the urethral sphincters and reduces bladder neck mobility during coughing. *Neurourology and Urodynamics, 32*(8), 1096–1102.

Neveus, T., & Sillen, U. (2013). Lower urinary tract function in childhood: Normal development and common functional disturbances. *Acta physiologica (Oxford, England), 207,* 85–92.

Osman, N., Chapple, C., Abrams, P., et al. (2014). Detrusor underactivity and the underactive bladder: A new clinical entity? A review of current terminology, definitions, epidemiology, aetiology, and diagnosis. *European Urology, 65,* 389–398.

Porth C. (2011). *Essentials of pathophysiology* (3rd ed.). Philadelphia, PA: Lippincott Williams & Wilkins.

Sadananda, P., Vahabi, B., & Drake, M. (2011). Bladder outlet physiology in the context of LUT dysfunction. *Neurourology and Urodynamics, 30*(5), 708–713.

Scemons, D. (2013). Urinary incontinence in adults. *Nursing, 43*(11), 52–60.

Sellers, D., & Chess-Williams, R. (2012). Muscarinic agonists and antagonists: Effects on the urinary bladder. *Handbook of Experimental Pharmacology, 208,* 375–400.

Smith, P., Deangelis, A., & Kuchel, G. (2012). Evidence of central neuromodulation of bladder compliance during filling phase. *Neurourology and Urodynamics, 31*(1), 30–35.

Valentino, R., Wood, S., Wein, A., et al. (2011). The bladder-brain connection: Putative role of corticotropin-releasing factor. *Nature Reviews Urology, 8,* 19–28.

Wyndaele, J., Gammie, A., Bruschini, H., et al. (2011). Bladder compliance: What does it represent, can it be measured, and is it clinically relevant? *Neurourology and Urodynamics, 30,* 714–722.

Yoshimura, N., & Chancellor, M. (2012). Physiology and pharmacology of the urinary bladder and urethra. In A. J. Wein, L. R. Kavoussi, A. C. Novick, et al. (Eds.), *Campbell-Walsh urology* (10th ed., pp. 1786–1853). St Louis, MO: Elsevier.

Yoshimura, N., Miyazato, M, Kitta, T., et al. (2014) Central nervous system targets for the treatment of bladder dysfunction. *Neurourology and Urodynamics, 33,* 59–66.

Zderic, S., & Chacko, S. (2012). Alterations in the contractile phenotype of the bladder: Lessons for understanding physiological and pathological remodeling of smooth muscle. *Journal of Cellular and Molecular Medicine, 16*(2), 203–217.

QUESTIONS

1. The continence nurse is assessing bladder compliance in an older adult. Which of the following accurately describes this property of the urinary tract system?
   A. The ability to delay voiding until a socially acceptable time and place are found
   B. The ability of the bladder to distend with urine while maintaining low intravesical pressures
   C. The ability of the bladder to contract with sufficient force and duration to expel all or most of stored urine
   D. Detrusor relaxation in response to beta-adrenergic stimulation

2. Which layer of the bladder secretes signaling molecules that provide input to the brain regarding bladder filling and messaging to the bladder muscle that help to modulate relaxation and contractility?
   A. Urothelium
   B. Trigone
   C. Propria
   D. Detrusor

3. The lamina propria contributes to normal bladder distensibility by maintaining the balance between Type III and Type I collagen and:
   A. Secreting signaling molecules that provide input to the brain regarding bladder filling
   B. Secreting signaling molecules that provide input to the brain regarding the need to void
   C. Allowing smooth muscle cells to stretch slowly without inducing a contraction until emptying is initiated
   D. Producing elastic fibers that allow the bladder to return to normal shape after voiding

4. Which of the following describes the main function of the urethra?
   A. Serving as a conduit for elimination of urine from the bladder
   B. Providing stretch receptors that signal bladder filling
   C. Preventing leakage during periods of increased intra-abdominal pressure
   D. Supporting the pelvic organs in normal anatomic position

5. Which anatomic feature of the male urethra predominately contributes to the maintenance of continence?
   A. Rich suburethral vascular plexus
   B. Coaptation of the urethral walls
   C. Greater length and curvature
   D. Prostatic hypertrophy

6. A continence nurse recommends pelvic muscle exercises for a female patient experiencing stress incontinence. What anatomical structure is strengthened by these exercises?
   A. Internal sphincter
   B. External sphincter
   C. Detrusor muscle
   D. Urethra

7. What mechanism is involved in the guarding reflex function that helps to maintain continence?
   A. Increased detrusor contractility in response to increased abdominal pressure
   B. Closing of the urethra during the storage phase
   C. Support of the pelvic organs in normal anatomic position
   D. Progressive increase in outlet resistance in response to bladder filling

8. Which structure controls the actual switch between bladder filling (storage) and bladder emptying (voiding)?
   A. Midbrain
   B. Prefrontal cortex
   C. Spinal cord
   D. Neuronal pathways

9. Which structure is responsible for assuring that both the bladder neck (internal sphincter) and rhabdosphincter (external sphincter) are relaxed before the bladder contracts, in order to provide unobstructed voiding?
   A. Periaqueductal gray (PAG)
   B. Onuf's nucleus
   C. Pontine micturition center (PMC)
   D. Sympathetic pathways

10. A continence nurse assessing elderly patients in a nursing home takes into consideration age-related changes in the urinary system, such as:
    A. Lower postvoid residuals
    B. Reduced bladder contractility
    C. Increased bladder capacity
    D. Decreased urinary frequency

ANSWERS: 1.**B**, 2.**A**, 3.**D**, 4.**A**, 5.**C**, 6.**B**, 7.**D**, 8.**A**, 9.**C**, 10.**B**

CHAPTER 2

Overview of Urinary Incontinence and Voiding Dysfunction

Dorothy B. Doughty and Katherine N. Moore

OBJECTIVES

1. Discuss the impact of incontinence and implications for WOC nurses and other health care providers.
2. Describe reversible factors contributing to incontinence and implications for assessment and management.
3. Define the term "lower urinary tract symptoms" (LUTS), and differentiate among storage symptoms, voiding symptoms, and postvoiding symptoms.
4. Synthesize assessment data to determine type of incontinence/voiding dysfunction and goals for management.
5. Discuss current thinking regarding the difference between "functional factors contributing to incontinence" and "functional incontinence" and implications for management.

Topic Outline

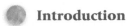

Introduction

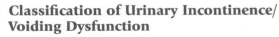

Classification of Urinary Incontinence/ Voiding Dysfunction

Introduction

As explained in Chapter 1, the lower urinary tract is responsible for alternately storing and then emptying urine; normal function is characterized by the ability to store 300 to 500 mL of urine at low intravesical pressures and to delay voiding until a socially convenient time and place and by the ability to empty the bladder completely during voiding, with minimal postvoid urine volumes. Alterations in the ability to store urine effectively and to control the time and place for voiding result in *urinary incontinence*, and altered ability to empty urine effectively results in *voiding dysfunction* and *urinary retention*. Both of these conditions negatively impact on quality of life; some forms of voiding dysfunction and urinary retention are also associated with increased risk for upper tract (kidney) damage.

CLINICAL PEARL

Alterations in the ability to store urine effectively and to control the time and place for voiding result in *urinary incontinence,* and altered ability to empty urine effectively results in *voiding dysfunction* and *urinary retention.*

Urinary incontinence (UI) is a common problem, affecting up to 43% of community-dwelling adults and up to 70% of those in long-term care (Gorina et al., 2014). UI is also costly; according to 2000 data, $19.5 billion is spent annually on management of UI, with 50% to 75% of the money being spent on management (absorptive products, etc.) and only 25% to 50% spent on diagnosis and correction of the underlying problem (Hu et al., 2004). This disproportionate expenditure on management products as opposed to diagnostic studies and corrective therapies may be due in part to the wideheld perception that UI is a normal part of aging and that "nothing can be done." In addition to the fiscal costs, UI is costly to the individual, adversely affecting quality of life and causing significant psychological distress (e.g., anxiety and embarrassment); in addition, UI increases the risk of falls and skin breakdown (Gorina et al., 2014).

This chapter provides a brief overview of the various types of urinary incontinence and voiding dysfunction; the pathology, presentation, assessment, and management of each type are discussed in greater depth in subsequent chapters.

Classification of Urinary Incontinence/Voiding Dysfunction

Urinary incontinence (UI) is the complaint of any involuntary leakage of urine (Abrams et al., 2002). During the interview, the health care professional should ask about specific factors relating to the symptom of UI such as type, frequency, severity, precipitating factors, social impact, effect on hygiene, effect on quality of life, coping strategies such as pads, frequent toileting, or social isolation, goals for management/treatment, and previous investigations/treatments (Abrams et al., 2002).

Urinary incontinence may be classified as either *acute/transient* or *chronic.*

Acute/Transient UI

Transient UI is generally defined as newly occurring UI of relatively sudden onset; it typically lasts <6 months and is the result of reversible factors. By definition, transient UI is usually curable and the focus of management is on

correction of the etiologic factors. There are several mnemonics designed to help clinicians remember the potentially reversible causes of UI, including TOILETED, DRIP, and DIAPPERS (Dowling-Castronovo & Specht 2009; Wound, Ostomy, and Continence Nurses Society, 2007). TOILETED is considered by many to be the preferred mnemonic due to the negative connotations of "diapers" and "drip" in relation to adults with urinary leakage.

CLINICAL PEARL

Transient UI is caused by reversible factors and is usually curable. A mnemonic commonly used to help clinicians remember to assess for and manage reversible factors is TOILETED (thin dry urethral epithelium; obstruction; infection; limited mobility; emotional/psychological issues; therapeutic medications; endocrine disorders; delirium).

T: Thin, Dry Vaginal and Urethral Epithelium (Atrophic Urethritis or Vaginitis)

As explained in Chapter 1, continence in the female is at least partially dependent on normal coaptation of the urethral walls, which is affected by the softness and stickiness of the urethral tissue. Estrogen deficiency is associated with thinning and drying of the urethral tissues, which reduces coaptation and also contributes to the symptoms of urinary urgency and frequency; in addition, atrophic urethritis has been associated with increased incidence of recurrent UTIs in elderly women in long-term care settings. Therefore, postmenopausal women presenting with symptoms of urinary leakage or with recurrent UTIs should be carefully evaluated for evidence of atrophic urethritis (manifest by inflamed hypertrophic urethral meatus) and should be considered for a trial of topical estrogen therapy (Wound, Ostomy, and Continence Nurses Society, 2007).

O: Obstruction (Stool Impaction/Constipation)

The bladder and rectum share the limited space available in the bony pelvis; thus, chronic rectal distention can adversely affect bladder function. Specifically, chronic rectal distention can compromise bladder filling and can exacerbate symptoms of overactive bladder (OAB) (urgency, frequency, and low voided volumes). Severe rectal distention (as may occur with fecal impaction) can also cause bladder outlet obstruction and urinary retention. Assessment of bowel function and interventions to eliminate retained stool and to restore effective bowel elimination patterns are therefore important responsibilities for the continence nurse (Wound, Ostomy, and Continence Nurses Society, 2007).

I: Infection

Urinary tract infection causes inflammation of the bladder wall and urethra, which, in the continent individual, results in urinary urgency, frequency, and dysuria. For the individual with preexisting issues with urgency and frequency, and for the individual with mobility issues, UTI can overwhelm the continence system, resulting in urinary leakage. In addition, infectious processes such as UTI can cause acute alteration in mental status among elders with any degree of preexisting dementia; UTI in these individuals may manifest as sudden onset of incontinence accompanied by acute worsening of mental and functional status (Wound, Ostomy, and Continence Nurses Society, 2007).

L: Limited Mobility (Restricted Mobility)

Continence depends on cognitive awareness of the need to void, normal function of the bladder and sphincters, and the ability to move to an appropriate place (and to manipulate clothing in preparation for voiding) in a timely manner. Any condition that reduces the individual's ability to get to a toilet or suitable alternative (e.g., dependency on ambulatory aids such as walkers) and/or to remove his or her clothing in preparation for voiding (e.g., arthritis) can contribute to incontinence. This is particularly problematic for elderly individuals, who may have less ability to control urgency and to delay voiding due to changes in the central nervous system (CNS). The combination of reduced ability to manage urgency and to delay voiding, and increased time required to get to the toilet and prepare for voiding may combine to produce incontinence, even though the individual retains cognitive function and basic bladder control. Simple measures such as clothing alterations, use of bedside commodes and urinals, and scheduled voiding may be all that is needed to restore continence for these individuals (Wound, Ostomy, and Continence Nurses Society, 2007).

E: Emotional Issues (Psychological, Depression)

There is some evidence that the neurotransmitters that are typically depleted in individuals with clinical depression (e.g., norepinephrine) play an important role in sphincter function and that individuals with clinical depression are at higher risk for incontinence. In addition, severe depression may alter the individual's motivation and ability to manage urinary symptoms. Conversely, incontinent episodes may cause worsening of any existing depression. Thus, the continence nurse must be alert to any indicators of depression and must refer these individuals for treatment (Wound, Ostomy, and Continence Nurses Society, 2007).

T: Therapeutic Medications (Pharmacologic)

Medications are common contributing (exacerbating) factors for both storage disorders (incontinence) and emptying disorders (retention). For example, diuretics may cause sudden production of large volumes of urine, which may precipitate incontinence in the individual with OAB or mobility issues. Conversely, any medication with anticholinergic properties may compromise bladder contractility and precipitate or worsen urinary retention; medications with alpha-adrenergic properties can also cause or worsen retention, because they increase urethral resistance.

The impact of medications is of particular concern with older individuals and those with multiple comorbid conditions, because they may be taking multiple medications, any or all of which could affect the lower urinary tract. As a result, a careful medication history (to include prescription, over-the-counter, and herbal agents) is recommended for all individuals with urinary tract dysfunction; the pharmacist can frequently be of assistance in evaluating an individual's medications for potential adverse effects on bladder and sphincter function. The continence nurse must then collaborate with the patient and the prescribing providers to determine whether any changes in prescribed medications are warranted (Wound, Ostomy, and Continence Nurses Society, 2007).

E: Endocrine Disorders

Endocrine disorders, such as diabetes mellitus with hyperglycemia, can compromise continence by causing production of excessive volumes of urine that can overwhelm the bladder and sphincter, producing sudden urgency and, in some cases, leakage. Diabetes insipidus is another endocrine disorder resulting in production of abnormally high volumes of dilute urine that can contribute to incontinence. The history for a person with incontinence must always include queries regarding other comorbid conditions, with specific focus on endocrine disorders, and management must include measures to normalize endocrine function and urinary output (Wound, Ostomy, and Continence Nurses Society, 2007).

D: Delirium

As noted in Chapter 1, intact cognition is essential to continence; the individual must be able to recognize bladder filling, make appropriate decisions regarding when and where to void, and then move to an appropriate location for voiding. Thus, any condition that adversely affects cognition places the individual at risk for incontinence. It is important for the continence nurse to differentiate between dementia, which is an irreversible decline in cognition, and delirium, which by definition is transient; the nurse must also be aware that delirium can be superimposed on dementia, causing a sudden but reversible worsening of cognitive impairment. Delirium may be caused by an infectious process (in the person with preexisting cognitive impairment), the adverse effects of medications, or electrolyte or chemical imbalance. Implications for the continence nurse include routine assessment of cognitive status and of any recent change in cognition and prompt attention to correction of factors causing cognitive impairment (Wound, Ostomy, and Continence Nurses Society, 2007).

If untreated, transient UI may become established (chronic) UI. In addition, reversible factors are frequently contributing factors to some types of chronic incontinence; thus, continence nurses should assess all incontinent individuals for transient conditions contributing to incontinence; when present, treatment of these factors is a critical "first step" in management of the incontinence.

Chronic UI

Urinary incontinence that lasts more than 6 months despite correction of reversible factors is known as *chronic incontinence*; the most common forms of chronic incontinence are stress, urge, and mixed incontinence. A brief description of each type is provided here, with in-depth discussion provided in subsequent chapters of this core curriculum.

Stress UI

Stress incontinence is defined as "the complaint of involuntary leakage on effort or exertion or on sneezing or coughing." Stress incontinence is also sometimes known as "activity-associated incontinence" because the leakage is associated with activities that increase intra-abdominal pressure (jumping, straining, lifting, coughing, sneezing, laughing, etc.). Stress incontinence occurs as a result of *sphincter dysfunction*; the sphincter muscles are unable to maintain urethral closure during activities that cause an increase in abdominal and bladder pressure (Delancey, 2010). As a result, urine is forced through the partially open urethra.

The volume of urinary leakage varies, depending on the weakness of the sphincter; while leakage is typically low volume, a very weak sphincter may allow higher volume leakage. In addition, a very weak sphincter may permit leakage with relatively low levels of abdominal/bladder pressure; for example, some patients report leakage simply with standing. It is important to realize that stress incontinence occurs *in the absence of any urgency to void*; this is a significant finding because the lack of urgency means that the bladder is not contracting and is not contributing to the leakage.

Stress incontinence is much more common in women, because the female urethra is short and straight and therefore provides less resistance than the male urethra, which is long and curved. In addition, the supporting pelvic floor muscles and ligaments are at risk for damage related to vaginal delivery and/or chronic straining or coughing. However, clinically significant stress incontinence frequently does not become manifest until later in life, when the aging process causes sufficient additional weakness to compromise sphincter function during periods of increased abdominal/bladder pressure. Fortunately, routine pelvic muscle exercises can help to maintain sufficient sphincter and pelvic muscle strength to prevent stress incontinence.

Stress incontinence can also occur in men who require radical prostatectomy, because this surgical procedure involves removal of the prostatic urethra with anastomosis of the distal urethra to the bladder neck. In addition to causing some reduction in urethral length and baseline resistance, radical prostatectomy can result in damage to the voluntary sphincter, which is located just distal to the prostate gland (Robinson et al., 2009) (see Chapter 8).

Stress incontinence is usually diagnosed on the basis of the history and physical exam, which reveals leakage with activity in the absence of urgency, leakage with strong cough, and weak pelvic floor muscles. Definitive diagnosis requires measurement of urethral pressures via placement of catheters with pressure-sensitive transducers.

The first step in management is typically instruction in pelvic muscle exercises, which serves to reverse or reduce the weakness that permits leakage to occur. Refractory or severe stress incontinence may best be managed with surgery; procedures for stress incontinence are designed to provide anatomic support for the sphincter and/or some degree of urethral compression. In women, pessaries may also be used to provide support and compression. Chapter 9 provides in-depth discussion of stress UI in women.

Urge UI

Urge incontinence is the complaint of involuntary leakage accompanied by or immediately preceded by a strong urge to void. Urgency may occur with or without incontinence and is called OAB, urge syndrome, or urgency–frequency syndrome. OAB is the most frequently used term.

As indicated by the term "overactive bladder," urgency and urge incontinence are due to abnormal sensitivity and/or contractility of the bladder. Patients with this condition may present with primary complaints of urgency and frequency but no leakage (sometimes known as "dry OAB") or may complain of urgency and frequency that sometimes results in leakage (OAB with urge incontinence, or "wet OAB"). Not surprisingly, men are more likely to present with dry OAB and women are more likely to present with wet OAB.

The specific cause of OAB and urge incontinence is not known, though there are a number of theories including altered levels of neurotransmitters, up-regulation of sensory fibers signaling bladder fullness, CNS pathology causing impaired ability to inhibit bladder contractions, and changes in the aging detrusor that render the bladder more vulnerable to inappropriate contractions. While the specific cause of OAB is not well defined, the clinical presentation is clear: abnormal urinary frequency, intense urgency that cannot easily be ignored, nocturia, and possibly leakage associated with a strong urge to void (Abrams et al., 2002; Haylen et al., 2010).

As is true of stress incontinence, the "diagnosis" of OAB with/without urge incontinence is based on a thorough history and physical and supported by a bladder chart. Classic findings include the triad of abnormal frequency (>8 voids in 24 hours), intense urgency, and nocturia; patients with urge incontinence report leakage associated with urgency and typically occurring on the way to the bathroom. Low volume voids are another common feature. Objective documentation of OAB and urge incontinence requires urodynamic studies; a catheter with a pressure-sensitive transducer is placed into the bladder and the bladder is slowly filled. OAB and urge incontinence are confirmed by a sudden onset of urgency at low filling volume accompanied by an involuntary bladder contraction and leakage.

Management of OAB is initially focused on elimination of reversible factors that contribute to bladder irritability, such as chronic constipation, atrophic urethritis, and urinary tract infection. Caffeinated and carbonated fluid may serve as irritant factors for some patients; thus, a trial period of reduced intake may be advised. Behavioral strategies to improve bladder control have been shown to be effective for many patients and represent a safe and noninvasive early intervention: patients are taught to manage urgency with pelvic muscle contractions, controlled breathing, avoidance of sudden activity, and distraction. Once the patient learns these basic "urge inhibition" strategies, he/she can be instructed in a "bladder-retraining" program (gradual lengthening of the voiding interval with use of behavioral strategies to manage urgency). Additional treatment options include anticholinergic (antimuscarinic) medications and neuromodulation therapies. See Chapter 5 for more information on OAB and urge incontinence.

> **CLINICAL PEARL**
>
> Management of urge incontinence usually begins with behavioral therapies (elimination of suspected bladder "irritants" and patient re-education: urge suppression strategies and bladder retraining); anticholinergic medications and neuromodulation are additional therapies used for severe or nonresponsive cases.

Mixed UI

Mixed incontinence is the complaint of involuntary leakage associated with urgency and also with exertion, effort, sneezing or coughing. Patients with mixed UI have both sphincter dysfunction and bladder overactivity and therefore present with complaints of leakage associated with urgency as well as leakage associated with activity. Management requires interventions to improve pelvic muscle strength and sphincter function as well as measures to reduce bladder irritability and to improve bladder control.

> **CLINICAL PEARL**
>
> "Mixed UI" refers to a combination of stress UI and urge UI; these patients require dual therapy programs to improve sphincter function and to reduce bladder overactivity.

UI Due to Functional Impairment

"Functional incontinence" is caused by factors outside the urinary tract that compromise the individual's ability to respond appropriately to signals of bladder filling. The two most common types of functional impairments involve mobility and cognitive function. Patients with significant mobility impairments are frequently dependent on others for assistance with toileting and may require significantly greater time to reach the toilet and prepare for voiding; incontinence occurs when they do not get the assistance they need or are unable to reach the toilet in a timely manner. Patients with cognitive impairments frequently do not recognize the sensation of bladder filling or cannot remember the steps involved in toileting; in these individuals, voiding occurs in response to bladder filling as opposed to being a conscious and controlled act. Functional issues may be the *primary etiologic factor* for the incontinence (e.g., incontinence in the individual with advanced dementia); in this case, the incontinence is sometimes labeled "functional incontinence." Functional issues may also be a contributing factor to other types of incontinence, such as mobility issues contributing to incontinence in the individual with OAB (Wound, Ostomy, and Continence Nurses Society, 2007).

There are no objective tests for functional incontinence; diagnosis is based on patient history and physical exam and on simple tests such as the "get up and go" test for mobility and the mini-mental status exam or clock-drawing test for cognitive function.

> **CLINICAL PEARL**
>
> Functional factors such as cognitive impairment and mobility impairment may be either causative or contributing factors for UI; thus, all patients should be assessed for cognitive status and mobility.

Management of functional incontinence and functional issues is dependent on the specific functional impairment; for the patient with impaired mobility, management may involve use of a bedside commode, a raised toilet seat, physical therapy and occupational therapy consults for assistive devices, and/or modifications in clothing to facilitate toileting. For the patient with cognitive impairment, management begins with a toileting trial to determine responsiveness to a toileting program. Patients who are able to respond to toileting cues are placed on a scheduled toileting or prompted voiding program, augmented by appropriate absorptive products. See Chapter 10 for further information.

Extraurethral Incontinence

Extraurethral incontinence is defined as urinary leakage through channels other than the urethra. This is most commonly due to a vesicovaginal fistula, which involves an abnormal opening between the bladder and the vagina that permits free flow of urine from the bladder into the vagina (and an almost constant flow of urine from the vagina). Vesicovaginal fistulas are common in the developing world, due to obstructed labor and obstetric trauma (Ayaz et al., 2012); in the US, these fistulas are uncommon but occasionally occur as a result of radical gynecologic procedures and/or pelvic radiation therapy.

Diagnosis is suggested by the constant leakage of urine and the absence of any associated symptomatology, such as urgency; diagnosis is confirmed by radiologic studies, and management involves either surgical correction or use of absorptive products in conjunction with indwelling catheters to divert the urine (see Chapter 9). In children, continuous urinary leakage is most commonly due to an ectopic ureter that drains into the vagina or the urethra; management involves surgical reimplantation of the ureter.

Voiding Dysfunction

The various forms of urinary incontinence all relate to problems with storage of urine; in contrast, voiding dysfunction is the term used to denote problems with urine elimination.

Retention, or incomplete bladder emptying, may be caused by two types of problems: (1) obstruction at the level of the bladder neck or urethra (e.g., incomplete emptying caused by prostate enlargement or urethral stricture) or (2) ineffective bladder contractions (e.g., neurologic conditions such as multiple sclerosis or long-standing diabetes).

Retention can be complete, in which case the patient is totally unable to eliminate urine, or partial, in which case the patient partially but incompletely empties the bladder. "Acute retention is defined as a painful, palpable, or percussible bladder, when the patient is unable to pass any urine." Chronic retention, on the other hand, "is a nonpainful bladder, which remains palpable or percussible after the patient has passed urine." Such patients may also experience urinary leakage (Abrams et al., 2002).

The patient with chronic retention typically reports a weak urinary stream and prolonged time required to void and may complain of a sensation of incomplete emptying.

The patient may also report recurrent urinary tract infections. Physical exam reveals bladder distention, which is confirmed by a postvoid residual test. Urodynamic studies are typically required to determine whether the problem is due to urethral obstruction or to ineffective bladder contractions; urodynamic studies allow the clinician to correlate the strength of the bladder contraction with the urinary flow rate (Abrams et al., 2002).

CLINICAL PEARL

Voiding dysfunction indicates impaired ability to empty the bladder effectively and may be caused by bladder outlet obstruction or by reduced contractility of the detrusor muscle; management depends on the underlying cause.

Management of urinary retention depends on the cause; obstruction can usually be eliminated through medical surgical intervention, while management of ineffective bladder contractions typically requires intermittent catheterization or insertion of an indwelling catheter.

Chapter 6 provides details on urinary retention.

Neurogenic Bladder

Neurogenic bladder dysfunction refers to lower urinary tract dysfunction caused by disturbance of the neurologic control mechanisms; it is thus only diagnosed in the presence of neurologic pathology, most commonly a lesion between the sacral cord and the brain. Common specific etiologic factors include spinal cord injury or multiple sclerosis (MS) lesions (Stöhrer et al., 1999).

Patients with neurogenic bladder dysfunction typically lack sensory awareness of bladder filling, are unable to voluntarily initiate voiding, and have no control over the urinary sphincter, because there is a loss of communication between the cortex and brain stem and the bladder and sphincter. In the absence of voluntary control of voiding, the bladder empties by a reflex arc triggered by bladder filling. However, patients with neurogenic bladder dysfunction are at risk for a serious complication known as detrusor sphincter dyssynergia; this denotes failure of sphincter relaxation in response to detrusor contraction and is associated with significant risk of upper tract dysfunction.

CLINICAL PEARL

Neurogenic bladder refers to loss of normal neural control of bladder and sphincter function; it is usually caused by a spinal cord lesion and results in impaired sensory awareness of bladder filling, inability to consistently initiate voiding on a voluntary basis, loss of sphincter control, and possibly loss of "coordinated voiding."

Diagnosis of neurogenic bladder is suggested by reports of urinary leakage or voiding dysfunction in a patient with a known neurologic diagnosis and is confirmed by urodynamic studies. Urodynamic studies are an essential element of workup for these patients since it is critical to determine the presence or absence of detrusor sphincter dyssynergia.

Management most commonly involves intermittent catheterization to assure complete emptying and to prevent leakage; selected patients with minimal or no detrusor sphincter dyssynergia may elect management with containment products (such as external catheter to bedside drainage bag). Indwelling catheters have been used in the past for management of these individuals but are associated with unacceptably high complication rates; therefore, their use is generally limited to short-term management or patients who cannot be effectively managed with other interventions.

Chapter 7 provides a comprehensive overview of etiology and management.

Assessment and Diagnosis: Overview

The evaluation of an individual with urinary incontinence or voiding dysfunction begins with a thorough assessment of the presenting signs and symptoms. Signs are objective indicators that can be observed by the health care professional, for example, leaking when coughing, cystocele with straining, bladder distention, or high postvoid residual volumes. Symptoms are the individual's experience of a problem such as pain or the sensation of incomplete emptying; symptoms are subjective and qualitative in nature. Additional qualitative and quantitative data can be obtained via bladder diaries, pad tests, and quality of life questionnaires.

Lower Urinary Tract Symptoms

LUTS can be categorized as

- Storage symptoms
- Voiding symptoms
- Postvoiding symptoms (Abrams et al., 2002)

Storage LUTS

These symptoms, as the name suggests, are indicators of problems related to the storage phase of the voiding cycle and are common among individuals with urinary incontinence and irritative bladder disorders. Storage LUTS include frequency, urgency, dysuria (pain on voiding), nocturia, nocturnal polyuria, and urinary leakage associated with urgency or activity or both (symptoms of OAB with urge incontinence, stress incontinence, or mixed stress–urge incontinence).

Voiding LUTS

In contrast to storage LUTS, voiding LUTS suggest problems with bladder emptying and include hesitancy, poor and/or intermittent stream, straining to void, and terminal dribble. These symptoms are common among individuals with some degree of voiding dysfunction and urinary retention. Voiding symptoms in men are most likely to be caused by bladder outlet obstruction related to prostatism; in women, outlet obstruction and voiding symptoms may be caused by severe cystocele or pelvic organ prolapse. These symptoms may also be caused by a poorly contractile detrusor, which can occur in individuals with long-standing diabetes or other conditions affecting detrusor innervation.

Postvoiding LUTS

Individuals with voiding dysfunction and urinary retention may also report postvoiding LUTS, which include postvoid dribbling and the sensation of incomplete emptying.

CLINICAL PEARL

Diagnostic workup for the individual with UI or voiding dysfunction begins with a careful exploration of presenting signs and symptoms, followed by an appropriately focused history and physical and limited diagnostics (bladder chart, urinalysis, postvoid residual if indicated); serum studies and urodynamics may be required for the individual with complex or nonresponsive conditions.

Diagnostic Workup

Definitive determination of the type of incontinence or voiding dysfunction begins with a careful review of symptomatology, followed by a careful history, focused physical examination, and limited diagnostic studies (e.g., bladder diary, urinalysis, and postvoid residual urine measurement). Individuals with complex problems may require advanced assessment including urodynamic studies and possibly serum and radiologic studies. Chapter 3 provides in-depth review of the components of primary assessment for the individual with incontinence or voiding dysfunction, and Chapter 4 provides in-depth information on advanced assessment techniques such as urodynamics.

General Principles of Management

Management of urinary incontinence or voiding dysfunction has two major goals: (1) prevention of any upper tract damage or deterioration and (2) enhanced quality of life for the individual and/or caregivers. If the individual presents with a condition that creates a threat to the kidneys (e.g., high-pressure chronic retention), the primary goal is to reduce the high intravesical pressures in order to restore normal urinary drainage from the kidneys to the bladder; this typically involves medical–surgical interventions to eliminate bladder outlet obstruction (see Chapter 6).

CLINICAL PEARL

Management for the patient with UI or voiding dysfunction is focused on prevention of upper tract distress and measures to optimize the patient's and/or caregiver's quality of life. Behavioral strategies are considered first-line therapy for most individuals; pharmacologic therapy and surgical intervention are usually reserved for patients with complex or refractory conditions.

However, for most individuals, the focus is on eliminating, minimizing, and/or effectively managing the problem with urinary leakage or voiding dysfunction in order to improve quality of life. In general, behavioral strategies are considered first-line interventions; pharmacologic and/or surgical interventions are typically recommended for individuals with inadequate response to behavioral therapies. However, the treatment plan must always be established based on the goals and priorities of the patient (and/or caregiver). For example, the patient who presents with signs and symptoms of OAB and urgency incontinence is typically managed initially with behavioral strategies (elimination of potential bladder irritants, instruction in urge suppression strategies, and bladder retraining); however, anticholinergic medications may be added to the initial management plan for the individual with severe urgency or the patient who requests medication. Similarly, pelvic floor rehabilitation is typically recommended as initial therapy for the individual with stress incontinence caused by weak sphincter and pelvic floor muscles; however, the individual who requests evaluation for surgical intervention should be referred appropriately *in addition to* receiving education about pelvic floor muscle exercises and their importance as adjunct therapy. The individual with functional incontinence due to significant cognitive impairment who is cared for by a family member may be managed with a toileting program and adjunct absorbent products or with absorbent products alone; the choice is up to the caregiver.

Conclusion

Urinary incontinence and voiding dysfunction are common problems that typically have a profound impact on quality of life and may also place the individual at risk for physical complications. Workup begins with a thorough exploration of presenting signs and symptoms and with assessment for and correction of any reversible factors commonly associated with bladder dysfunction. This should be followed by an appropriately focused history and physical examination; individuals with complex conditions may also require advanced assessment including urodynamic studies. Management is directed toward two major goals: protection of the upper tracts (in selected situations where the voiding dysfunction creates upper

tract distress) and enhancement of the individual's quality of life. Behavioral strategies are usually considered "first-line" therapy; pharmacologic and surgical interventions are usually reserved for individuals who fail to respond adequately to behavioral therapy. However, medical and surgical intervention may be first-line therapy in selected situations, due to the complexity or severity of the problem or the patient or caregiver's preferences.

REFERENCES

Abrams, P., Cardozo, L., Fall, M., et al.; Standardisation Subcommittee of the International Continence Society. (2002). The standardization of terminology in lower urinary tract dysfunction: Report form the standardization sub-committee of the International Continence Society. *Neurololology & Urodynamics, 21*(2), 162–178.

Ayaz, A., unNisa, R., Anwar, S., et al. (2012). Vesicovaginal and rectovaginal Fistulas: 12 year results of surgical treatment. *Journal of Ayub Medical College Abbottabad, 24*(3–4), 25–27.

Delancey, J. (2010). Why do women have stress urinary incontinence? *Neurourology & Urodynamics, 29*(Suppl 1), S13–S17.

Dowling-Castronovo, A., & Specht, J. K. (2009). Assessment of transient urinary incontinence in older adults. *American Journal of Nursing, 109*(2), 62–71.

Gorina, Y., Schappert, S., Bercovitz, A., et al. (2014). Prevalence of incontinence among older Americans. *Vital Health Statistics. Series 3, # 36*. Washington, DC: National Center for Health Statistics, Department of Health and Human Services.

Haylen, B. T., de Ridder, D., Freeman, R. M., et al. (2010). An International Urogynecological Association (IUGA)/International Continence Society (ICS) joint report on the terminology for female pelvic floor dysfunction. *Neurourology and Urodynamics, 29*(1), 4–20.

Hu, T., Wagner, T., Bentkorn, J., et al. (2004). Costs of urinary incontinence and overactive bladder in the United States: A comparative study. *Urology, 63*(3), 461–465.

Robinson, J., Weiss, R., Avi-Itshak, T., et al. (2009). Pilot testing of a theory-based pelvic floor training intervention for radical prostate patients. *Neurololology & Urodynamics, 28*(7), 682–683.

Stöhrer, M., Goepel, M., Kondo, A., et al. (1999). The standardization of terminology in neurogenic lower urinary tract dysfunction with suggestions for diagnostic procedures. *Neurourology and Urodynamics, 18*(2), 139–158.

Wound, Ostomy, and Continence Nurses Society. (2007). *Reversible causes of urinary incontinence: A guide for clinicians*. Mt. Laurel, NJ: Wound, Ostomy and Continence Nurses Society.

QUESTIONS

1. The continence nurse is assessing an 80-year-old female patient who complains that she is unable to get to a bathroom in time when she feels the need to urinate. What is the term for this urinary alteration?
   A. Urinary retention
   B. Voiding dysfunction
   C. Urinary incontinence
   D. Postvoiding LUTS

2. What is the main characteristic of acute/transient urinary incontinence (UI) that distinguishes it from chronic UI?
   A. It mainly occurs in the evening hours and overnight.
   B. It is short term and usually curable.
   C. It is caused by irreversible factors.
   D. It comes and goes over a long period of time.

3. The continence nurse is using the mnemonic TOILETED to assess a patient for reversible factors causing urinary incontinence (UI). Which of the following describes one of these factors?
   A. O = Obstruction
   B. L = LUTS
   C. T = Time frame
   D. D = diabetes

4. For which of the following conditions associated with urinary incontinence (UI) might the continence nurse recommend a trial of topical estrogen therapy?
   A. Atrophic urethritis
   B. Dementia
   C. Urinary infection
   D. Endocrine disorders

5. An elderly patient is prescribed an anticholinergic medication to treat depression. For what adverse side effect affecting urinary continence would the continence nurse monitor this patient?
   A. Sudden production of large volumes of urine precipitating incontinence
   B. Depression altering motivation to manage urinary symptoms
   C. Increased urethral resistance worsening urinary retention
   D. Compromise in bladder contractility worsening urinary retention

6. A 65-year-old female patient is diagnosed with urge incontinence. What is the usual cause of this urinary disorder?
   A. Weak pelvic floor
   B. Bladder (detrusor) overactivity
   C. Weak sphincter muscles
   D. Cognitive impairment

7. The continence nurse is assessing a patient with multiple sclerosis for urinary dysfunction. For which of the following voiding dysfunctions is this patient at risk?
   A. Obstruction of the bladder neck
   B. Obstruction of the urethra
   C. Ineffective bladder contractions
   D. Pelvic floor dysfunction

8. What therapeutic measure might the continence nurse recommend for a patient with chronic urinary retention related to ineffective bladder contractions?
   A. Instruction in intermittent catheterization
   B. Surgical intervention
   C. Pharmacologic intervention
   D. Interventions to improve pelvic muscle strength

9. Which of the following is the usual cause of neurogenic bladder?
   A. Spinal cord lesion
   B. Dementia
   C. Brain tumor
   D. Diabetes

10. The continence nurse is assessing a patient diagnosed with storage lower urinary tract symptoms (LUTS). Which of the following is a common symptom of this urinary alteration?
    A. Intermittent stream
    B. Straining to void
    C. Terminal dribble
    D. Frequency

ANSWERS: 1.**C**, 2.**B**, 3.**A**, 4.**A**, 5.**D**, 6.**B**, 7.**C**, 8.**A**, 9.**A**, 10.**D**

CHAPTER 3

Primary Assessment of Patients with Urinary Incontinence and Voiding Dysfunction

Kelly Kruse Nelles

OBJECTIVES

1. Identify goals for the assessment of the individual with urinary incontinence.
2. Describe data to be gathered during the patient interview and the significance of these data to accurate diagnosis.
3. Describe key elements of a focused physical examination for the patient with urinary incontinence or voiding dysfunction to include interpretation of findings.
4. Describe data provided by a bladder chart and the importance of a completed bladder chart to assessment and management of the patient with urinary incontinence.
5. Utilize data gathered during the interview and physical assessment to determine appropriate laboratory testing for the patient with urinary incontinence or voiding dysfunction.
6. Synthesize assessment data to determine type of incontinence/voiding dysfunction and goals for management.

Topic Outline

 Assessment Goals

 Key Principles Underlying Accurate Assessment
Review of Onset and Duration of the Problem
   Stress UI
   Urge UI
   Mixed UI
   Functional UI
   Neurogenic UI
   Voiding Dysfunction
Key Elements of Continence Assessment

 Health History/Interview Guidelines
Chief Complaint
   Symptoms
   Impact on Quality of Life
   Goals for Treatment
Medical/Surgical History and Related Review of Systems
   General Assessment/Review of Constitutional Symptoms
   Cardiovascular System
   Respiratory System
   Endocrine System
   Gastrointestinal System
   Genitourinary System
   Obstetric/Gynecologic System
   Skin
   Musculoskeletal System
   Neurologic System
   Cognitive and Psychological Status
Medication Profile
Social History
Nutritional Assessment
Environmental and Functional Assessment
   Environmental Assessment
   Functional Assessment

 Bladder Diary

 Focused Physical Examination
General Assessment
Mental Status
Musculoskeletal Examination
Neurologic Examination
Skin Assessment
Abdominal Examination
Genitourinary Examination in Men

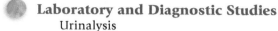
A comprehensive and accurate assessment of the individual with urinary incontinence or voiding dysfunction is the foundation for effective management. This chapter addresses primary assessment strategies; advanced diagnostic tests such as urodynamic studies are addressed in Chapter 4.

Assessment Goals

The goals of primary assessment are to

1. Screen for and identify conditions that mandate further evaluation and/or referral
2. Determine the type(s) of urinary incontinence
3. Determine the goals for treatment

> **CLINICAL PEARL**
>
> The goals of primary (initial) assessment of the individual with urinary incontinence or voiding dysfunction are to identify conditions that require further evaluation or medical/surgical intervention, determine the specific type of incontinence or voiding dysfunction, and determine the individual's goals for treatment.

Key Principles Underlying Accurate Assessment

Accurate diagnosis and management of urinary incontinence (UI) and voiding dysfunction is based on the data obtained through a tailored urologic assessment. The continence nurse uses basic and advanced health assessment skills to perform a focused health history and physical assessment and obtains appropriate laboratory and diagnostic studies as indicated.

As discussed in Chapter 1, *Voiding Physiology*, and Chapter 2, *Introductory Concepts*, continence and voiding dysfunction symptoms are usually caused by a disruption in anatomical, physiological, psychological, and/or neurologic function. Continence requires an intact lower urinary tract, the cognitive ability to recognize the urge to void, and the functional ability to get to the bathroom to use the toilet or commode. In addition, the patient must be motivated to maintain continence and have an environment that supports that process (Jirovec et al., 1988). When performing a health history, it is important for the nurse to remember these concepts and to assess urologic function in relation to the person's medical and surgical history; social history and health habits; neurologic, cognitive, and psychological function; gastrointestinal and bowel function; and obstetric/gynecologic history in women and genitourinary/prostate history in men. In addition, when assessing an older individual, the continence nurse should be alert to changes associated with aging that can affect continence and voiding, for example, reduced bladder capacity, benign prostatic hypertrophy (BPH) in men, and loss of estrogen in postmenopausal women (Bradway & Yetman, 2002).

> **CLINICAL PEARL**
>
> When assessing an older individual, the continence nurse should be alert to changes associated with aging that can affect continence and voiding, for example, reduced bladder capacity, BPH in men, and estrogen deficiency in women.

Review of Onset and Duration of the Problem

When obtaining the history of a person with UI or voiding dysfunction, it is important to ask specific questions regarding the onset and duration of the problem, in order to differentiate between transient and established problems. Transient UI or voiding dysfunction is considered acute and generally reversible, while established UI or voiding dysfunction is described as chronic or persistent (Newman & Wein, 2009). Established UI or voiding dysfunction may develop either suddenly or gradually, and initial onset may be associated with an acute illness, hospitalization, or a sudden change in environment or daily routine (Palmer, 1996). Types of established UI and voiding dysfunction include stress, urge, mixed, neurogenic, and functional incontinence and urinary retention; the continence nurse should ask questions and conduct testing to determine the specific type of incontinence or voiding dysfunction affecting this individual.

> **CLINICAL PEARL**
>
> The continence nurse should ask questions and conduct testing to determine the specific type of incontinence or voiding dysfunction affecting this individual.

Stress UI

Stress UI is characterized by an involuntary loss of urine associated with an increase in intra-abdominal pressure (e.g., position change, cough, sneezing). Urine loss usually occurs in small amounts and is observable on physical examination during a cough test. Stress UI is more common in women although it also occurs in some men postprostatectomy.

Urge UI

Urge incontinence is described as an involuntary loss of urine associated with a strong urge to void. Persons with urge UI (UUI) often report they are unable to hold their urine and leak on the way to the bathroom; they typically report frequency and nocturia as well as urgency. Individuals may also report symptoms of urgency, frequency, and nocturia without urine loss; this is characteristic of the syndrome of overactive bladder or OAB. UUI and OAB become more prevalent with aging and put older adults at risk for sleep disruption and falls (Bolz et al., 2012).

Mixed UI

Mixed incontinence is the term used to denote a combination of stress and urge UI; these individuals experience involuntary loss of urine associated with increased intra-abdominal pressure and also experience leakage associated with urgency and frequency (Jayasekara, 2009).

Functional UI

Functional incontinence is caused by conditions outside the urinary tract itself that cause leakage, such as cognitive impairment and/or mobility impairment; these individuals may be unaware of the leakage or may report leakage that occurs because they are unable to get out of the bed or chair and to the bathroom.

Neurogenic UI

Neurogenic bladder is caused by a neurologic lesion (such as a spinal cord injury or multiple sclerosis) that disrupts the neurologic pathways that provide voluntary control of voiding; these individuals typically are unable to sense bladder filling and unable to voluntarily initiate voiding. In addition, they are at risk for detrusor–sphincter dyssynergia, which means loss of coordination between the detrusor and the sphincter; failure of the sphincter to relax during a bladder contraction places the person at high risk for impaired emptying and ureteral reflux. These individuals require referral for advanced assessment including urodynamic studies.

Voiding Dysfunction

Voiding dysfunction (also known as retention) is characterized by difficulty emptying the bladder and may be either acute or chronic. Acute onset retention is usually characterized by total inability to void and severe pain and requires emergent intervention. In contrast, chronic retention is characterized by bladder distention and by symptoms of dribbling, urinary hesitancy, and an uncomfortable sensation of fullness or pressure in the lower abdomen; some individuals also experience leakage that may or may not be associated with urgency. Voiding dysfunction requires further workup to determine the underlying cause, which is usually either outlet obstruction (e.g., retention associated with BPH) or hypocontractility of the detrusor muscle (Jayasekara, 2009; Moore, 2006).

Differentiating the type of UI or voiding dysfunction is essential in determining the management plan and goals of treatment and, as previously stated, is based on a careful history and focused assessment (DuBeau et al., 2010).

Key Elements of Continence Assessment

Critical components of a comprehensive assessment include (1) focused health history; (2) focused physical examination; (3) appropriate selection of laboratory and diagnostic tests; and (4) a synthesis of the data collected to determine the type of UI and/or voiding dysfunction and to develop an individualized management plan.

CLINICAL PEARL

Critical components of a continence assessment include a focused health history and physical exam, appropriate selected laboratory tests, and synthesis of the data to determine the type of UI/voiding dysfunction and to develop an appropriate management plan.

Health History/Interview Guidelines

The history is the most critical element of the comprehensive assessment; it includes an in-depth review of the chief complaint; discussion of the impact of the problem on the individual's quality of life and their goals and expectations for treatment; and a focused review of systems and medication profile.

Chief Complaint

The interview begins with a discussion of the problem(s) prompting the individual to seek care, the impact of those symptoms on quality of life, and the individual's goals for treatment.

Symptoms

Individuals may present with a variety of incontinence or voiding dysfunction symptoms, including storage symptoms (involuntary loss of urine, urgency, frequency, nocturia, or enuresis), voiding symptoms (difficulty starting the stream, poor or intermittent stream, straining to void), or postvoiding symptoms (postvoid leaking or dribbling and/or a sensation of pressure or incomplete bladder emptying). Each symptom should be fully investigated, including the onset, duration, frequency with which the symptom occurs, precipitating factors, and symptom severity. Questions regarding current management of symptoms and previous treatments and effectiveness are also important; the answers provide insight into the individual's understanding of the problem, access to resources, and self-efficacy.

CLINICAL PEARL

Questions regarding current management of symptoms and previous treatments and effectiveness provide insight into the individual's understanding of the problem, access to resources, and self-efficacy.

Impact on Quality of Life

Validated tools can be beneficial in assessing health-related quality of life and symptom distress related to UI and voiding dysfunction (Dowling-Castronovo & Spiro, 2013).

The Urinary Distress Inventory-6 (UDI-6) and the Incontinence Impact Questionnaire-7 (IIQ-7) are shortened versions of the original UDI and IIQ and are appropriate for assessing established UI. The UDI-6 describes a set of six UI symptoms and asks individuals to identify the degree of distress related to each symptom over the past 3 months. The IIQ-7 consists of seven questions specific to accidental urine loss and asks individuals to rate the effect on activities, relationships, and feelings using a rating scale from 0 to 3. While tested predominately in community-dwelling women, IIQ-7 has also been validated in men (Moore & Jensen, 2000), correlates strongly with the original long versions, and may be useful as part of the general assessment (Dowling-Castronovo & Spiro, 2013; Lemack & Zimmern, 1999; Shumaker et al., 1994; Uebersax et al., 1995; Van der Vaart, et al., 2003). The Male Urogenital Distress Inventory (MUDI) and the Male Urinary Symptoms Impact Questionnaire (MUSIQ), variations of the UDI and IIQ specific to males, are also reliable in measuring health-related quality of life for men with UI or voiding dysfunction (Dowling-Castronovo & Spiro, 2013; Robinson & Shea, 2002) (Table 3-1).

Goals for Treatment

An initial step in the assessment is to establish the individual's goals and expectations for the visit and for management of the problem, while the nurse gathers objective data and considers appropriate strategies. It is critical to understand expectations and previous experiences as these can strongly influence care going forward. Patient-centered continence care involves partnering with the individual to discuss potential goals and outcomes and working together to develop an individualized plan of care. This process involves discussion of the individual's motivation and ability to self-manage as well as explaining possible treatment and management options and prioritizing continence-related concerns. While UI is not always reversible, appropriate management and support can always improve outcomes.

Medical/Surgical History and Related Review of Systems

Obtaining a pertinent medical and surgical history and accurate review of systems allows the continence nurse to identify health conditions that may directly impact continence status and/or contribute to voiding dysfunction.

CLINICAL PEARL

Obtaining a pertinent medical and surgical history and review of systems allows the continence nurse to identify health conditions that may impact on continence status and/or contribute to voiding dysfunction.

General Assessment/Review of Constitutional Symptoms

The nurse should begin by assessing for *general constitutional* symptoms that would affect ability and motivation to toilet, such as fatigue, weakness, depression, and

TABLE 3-1 Validated Assessment Tools

Assessment	Instrument
Symptoms and health-related quality of life	Urinary Distress Inventory-6 (UDI-6) and the Incontinence Impact Questionnaire-7 (IIQ-7). Access online at http://consultgerirn.org/uploads/File/trythis/try_this_11_2.pdf International Prostate Symptom Score (IPSS). Access online at http://www.baus.org.uk/Resources/BAUS/Documents/PDF%20Documents/Patient%20information/IPSS.pdf
Activities of daily living/function	Katz Index of Independence of Activities of Daily Living (ADL). Access online at http://consultgerirn.org/uploads/File/trythis/try_this_2.pdf The Lawton Instrumental Activities of Daily Living (IADL) Scale. Access online at http://consultgerirn.org/uploads/File/trythis/try_this_23.pdf
Cognitive assessment	Mental status assessment of older adults: The Mini-Cog. Access online at http://consultgerirn.org/uploads/File/trythis/try_this_3.pdf
Depression	The Geriatric Depression Scale (GDS). Access online at http://consultgerirn.org/uploads/File/trythis/try_this_4.pdf Patient Health Questionnaire (PHQ-9). Access online at http://www.integration.samhsa.gov/images/res/PHQ%20-%20Questions.pdf
Risk of falls	Fall Risk Assessment in Older Adults: The Hendrich II Fall Risk Model. Access online at http://consultgerirn.org/uploads/File/trythis/try_this_8.pdf Assessment of Fear of Falling in Older Adults: The Falls Efficacy Scale-International (FES-1). Access online at http://consultgerirn.org/uploads/File/trythis/try_this_29.pdf
Medication	AGS Beers Criteria for Potentially Inappropriate Medication Use in Older Adults. Access online at http://www.americangeriatrics.org/files/documents/beers/PrintableBeersPocketCard.pdf
Mobility	Get Up and Go Test. Access online at https://www.healthcare.uiowa.edu/igec/tools/mobility/getUpAndGo.pdf

confusion. Sensory impairments, specifically alterations in vision and hearing, may negatively affect the individual's ability to find the bathroom and to respond appropriately to caregiver instructions regarding toileting.

Cardiovascular System

Cardiovascular issues, especially hypotension, heart failure, and arrhythmias, place the individual at risk for dizziness, weakness, and falls; peripheral dependent edema is an indicator of impaired perfusion and third spacing and is typically associated with increased nocturnal urine production, nocturia, and increased risk of falls. In addition, diuretics are commonly used to treat heart failure, and the marked increase in urine production is frequently associated with urinary urgency and frequency. In hypertensive patients with peripheral edema, symptoms of urinary urgency and transient UI can also result from diuresis (Gray & Moore, 2009).

Respiratory System

It is also important to identify *respiratory* conditions resulting in acute or chronic coughing, which increases intra-abdominal pressure and can cause or contribute to episodes of stress UI. The nurse should ask about nicotine use; smoking contributes to chronic cough, which increases the risk of UI, and nicotine has been shown to act as a bladder irritant in some individuals, which increases the risk of frequency and urgency (Moore et al., 2013). A well-known side effect of ACE inhibitors is chronic cough; thus, these medications increase the risk for UI. An acute upper respiratory infection can cause severe coughing that results in transient stress incontinence; the stress incontinence will resolve when the URI resolves. In contrast, coughing related to chronic obstructive pulmonary disease is an example of a chronic condition associated with increased risk of UI that is not spontaneously reversible. Effective management of this patient would involve measures to control cough; assessing readiness to quit smoking and offering assistance to do so is an appropriate role for the continence nurse.

> **CLINICAL PEARL**
>
> Smoking contributes to chronic cough, which increases the risk of UI, and nicotine has been shown to be a bladder irritant in some individuals, increasing the risk of urgency and frequency.

Endocrine System

Metabolic conditions such as diabetes and obesity are risk factors for bladder dysfunction and incontinence; this is significant since these conditions are increasingly prevalent (Shamliyan et al., 2007; Subak et al., 2009). Poorly controlled DM results in hyperglycemia and polyuria, which increases the risk for urgency, frequency, and urge UI; in addition, longstanding DM can cause autonomic neuropathy (diabetic cystopathy) and chronic urinary retention (Gray & Moore, 2009). Truncal obesity is associated

with increased intra-abdominal pressure, which increases the risk for episodes of stress UI. Thus, education and support for weight reduction can be an important strategy for improving continence.

> **CLINICAL PEARL**
>
> Metabolic conditions such as diabetes and obesity are risk factors for bladder dysfunction and incontinence. Support for weight reduction can be an important strategy for improving continence.

Gastrointestinal System

Gastrointestinal problems are common contributing factors to UI and voiding dysfunction; thus, assessment of bowel history (to include surgical procedures) and current bowel function and control is a critical element of the assessment. Conditions such as acute or chronic diarrhea and diarrhea-predominant irritable bowel syndrome are risk factors for fecal urgency and fecal incontinence and will be addressed further in Chapter 15. Constipation is associated with increased urinary urgency and frequency, due to the effects of a full rectum and sigmoid on bladder filling and detrusor irritability. Severe constipation and fecal impaction can cause urethral compression and bladder outlet obstruction, which causes or exacerbates urinary retention; this is sometimes the cause of worsening retention in a male with mild retention due to BPH. Finally, fecal incontinence may be indicative of a neurologic lesion affecting the sacral nerve pathways; these individuals would also be at risk for UI and/or voiding dysfunction (Gray & Moore, 2009).

> **CLINICAL PEARL**
>
> Constipation is associated with urgency and frequency, due to the effects of a full rectosigmoid on bladder filling and detrusor instability; impaction can cause urethral obstruction and bladder outlet obstruction.

Genitourinary System

When assessing a male with UI or voiding dysfunction, the *genitourinary* (GU) history is of critical importance and should include questions regarding UI episodes, urinary tract infections (UTIs), BPH, prostatitis, any urologic surgical procedures, and history of bladder/kidney stones. A clear understanding of the person's GU history may provide insight into factors contributing to current symptoms and into appropriate management, that is, interventions to mitigate symptoms and to reduce the risk for recurrence. For example, finding that the person has been diagnosed with BPH and has had problems with retention in the past provides the foundation for education and counseling regarding current symptom management and measures to prevent recurrent episodes (such as assuring appropriate bowel management and avoidance of medications that could increase outlet resistance or reduce detrusor contractility).

Such measures will help to prevent episodes of acute retention, which increase the risk for UTIs, upper urinary tract damage, bladder and renal calculi, and eventual renal insufficiency (Gray & Moore, 2009). Similarly, prostatitis is known to contribute to irritative voiding symptoms including urge UI, and treatment of prostate cancer with radical prostatectomy and radiation therapy increases the risk for UI and voiding problems (Gray & Moore, 2009; Shamliyan et al., 2007). Symptoms can be assessed using the International Prostate Symptom Score (IPSS). This validated tool consists of eight questions with the first seven designed to measure irritative and obstructive symptoms, while the eighth captures the degree to which symptoms are bothersome and negatively affect quality of life (BAUS).

CLINICAL PEARL

A history of BPH and retention should prompt education regarding prevention of constipation and avoidance of medications that reduce bladder contractility or increase the risk of bladder outlet obstruction (e.g., anticholinergics and alpha-adrenergic agonists).

Obstetric/Gynecologic System

In women, the obstetric and gynecologic history should include information regarding pregnancies, deliveries, and menopausal status as well as any gynecologic or urologic surgical procedures. The number of pregnancies, type of delivery (vaginal vs. C-section), and use of episiotomy are factors known to affect UI risk (Shamliyan et al., 2007). Multiple deliveries, episiotomy, breech delivery, and traumatic deliveries involving perineal tears have all been shown in various studies to increase the risk of pelvic floor denervation and stress UI (Gray & Moore, 2009).

In women who are still menstruating, it is helpful to obtain a menstrual history including use of contraception and specific methods; recent data indicate that some progestin-only contraceptives (i.e., Depo-Provera) can contribute to estrogen depletion and can therefore increase the risk for UI (Schulling & Likis, 2013). For women who are no longer menstruating, determining the age and type of menopause (i.e., natural vs. medically or surgically induced) is useful as bladder problems often begin or become more noticeable around the time of menopause. Gathering information about current or previous hormone replacement therapy and any indicators of urogenital atrophy (e.g., dyspareunia, itching, irritation, vaginal dryness or pain, urinary urgency and frequency, and dysuria) is critical since atrophic changes are thought to contribute to both SUI and UUI and are generally reversible with topical estrogen therapy (Greenblum et al., 2008; Kinsberg et al., 2009; Lekan-Rutledge, 2004; North American Menopause Society, 2012; Schulling & Likis, 2013). Irritative bladder symptoms or urge UI may occur in women with endometriosis or vaginitis; thus, the nurse should ask about any history of endometriosis and any symptoms of vaginitis

(i.e., vaginal discharge, odor, or itching) (Gray & Moore, 2009). The woman should be asked about pelvic pressure or pain, history of pelvic organ prolapse, prior pelvic procedures, and any sensation of a vaginal "bulge," because pelvic organ prolapse increases the risk of stress UI and UTI; in addition, severe prolapse can result in significant urinary retention (Gray & Moore, 2009; Shamliyan et al., 2007).

CLINICAL PEARL

Information about current or past hormone replacement therapy and indicators of urogenital atrophy is critical since atrophic changes are thought to contribute to both stress incontinence and urge incontinence and are generally reversible with topical estrogen therapy.

Skin

The patient with atypical alterations in perineal skin integrity should be asked about systemic dermatologic conditions such as dermatitis, eczema, and psoriasis, because these conditions can recur in the urogenital area with similar symptoms.

Musculoskeletal System

Some musculoskeletal problems can contribute to alterations in function and mobility that impact continence status (Offermans et al., 2009; Shamliyan et al., 2007). Arthritis (either osteo- or rheumatoid arthritis) and/or back problems including spinal stenosis should be identified as these conditions impact on dexterity and clothing management, sensory awareness of bladder filling, and overall mobility and ability to toilet safely. In many individuals, motivation to toilet is impacted by chronic pain and fatigue due to musculoskeletal disorders; this increases the risk for functional UI (Gray, 2006).

CLINICAL PEARL

In many individuals, motivation to toilet is impacted by chronic pain and fatigue due to musculoskeletal disorders.

Neurologic System

Neurologic conditions are an essential area of investigation. In addition to affecting overall function and mobility, neurologic conditions and lesions can adversely affect neural control of voiding. For example, CVA (stroke) and Parkinson's disease are associated with increased risk of urge UI due to impaired ability to inhibit voiding (Gray & Moore, 2009; Shamliyan et al., 2007). Spinal cord disorders resulting in paralysis (e.g., spinal cord injury and progressive multiple sclerosis of the spinal cord) are associated with neurogenic bladder, increased risk of reflux and upper tract damage, and/or urinary retention (Gray & Moore, 2009). Clinicians should also ask about surgeries of the spine, since these procedures can result in denervation injuries that profoundly affect bladder function and continence. Both musculoskeletal and neurologic alterations can contribute to alterations in functional status, which should be fully assessed on physical examination.

Cognitive and Psychological Status

Cognitive and psychological alterations including dementia and depression have a significant impact on the ability and motivation to toilet and are risk factors for functional UI. Delirium is a reversible alteration in mental status that is associated with acute or transient UI, while dementia is a generally irreversible deterioration in cognitive function that contributes to progressively more severe functional incontinence. Psychiatric disorders may also increase the risk for UI or voiding dysfunction, due to impact on motivation to toilet and to the medications used for treatment. For example, the medications used to treat anxiety, schizophrenia, and other psychiatric conditions increase the risk for urinary retention due to their anticholinergic properties. Depression is common and underdiagnosed in the elderly and in individuals with cognitive impairment, and depression increases the risk for UI; thus, the nurse needs to be alert to indicators of depression in these individuals. In addition, many persons with UI are reluctant to seek health care due to embarrassment or fear of stigma; they often attempt to self-manage their symptoms by limiting or avoiding social activities, which increases their risk of social isolation and depression (Diokno et al., 2000; DuBeau et al., 2006). Therefore, accurate screening and assessing for both depression and cognitive impairment is an important part of the continence assessment.

The nurse may find validated tools beneficial in assessing for these conditions. The Mini-Cog is a brief assessment tool designed to identify dementia and cognitive changes. Easy to administer, this 3-minute tool assesses cognitive function, memory, language comprehension, visual–motor skills, and executive function. The Mini-Cog is appropriate for older adults and can be used in all health care settings to track cognitive changes over time (Doerflinger, 2013). The Geriatric Depression Scale is used in community, acute, and long-term care settings to screen for depression among the elderly, including those with mild to moderate cognitive impairment (Greenberg, 2012). The Patient Health Questionnaire-9 (PHQ-9) is another short and easily administered tool designed to screen and monitor depressive symptoms over time. It is most commonly used in adults, but there is also an adolescent version. Table 3-1 lists several of the most commonly used assessment tools.

CLINICAL PEARL

Dementia and depression are risk factors for functional incontinence.

Medication Profile

Medications are known to affect bladder function and continence; therefore, the interview must include queries regarding all over-the-counter, herbal, and prescription medications with current dosages, administration routes, and frequency of use. Each medication should be assessed for efficacy and side effects, with particular attention to the elderly and those persons using multiple medications. The *2012 American Geriatrics Society Updated Beers Criteria for Potentially Inappropriate Medication Use in Older Adults* is an important medication reconciliation resource for the continence nurse who is working with older adults. This safety tool provides an in-depth review of all medication categories and the potential side effects and contraindications for use in older adults (Molony & Greenberg, 2013) (Table 3-1). The pharmacist can also provide invaluable assistance in evaluating the individual's medications for potential interactions and for potential adverse effects on bladder function and continence.

There are multiple medications that have the potential to impact continence status; some are more likely to contribute to UI and voiding dysfunction than others. For example, diuretics increase urinary output and are associated with increased urinary frequency, urgency, and risk of urge UI; therefore, the clinician should be alert to initiation of a diuretic or an increase in dosing. α-adrenergic blockers (alpha blockers) are associated with increased risk of stress incontinence (due to reduced urethral tone); the chronic cough associated with ACE inhibitors also increases the risk for stress incontinence. Many medications cause drowsiness or sedation, which can compromise sensory awareness of bladder filling and the ability to respond to toileting cues and can therefore result in functional and/or transient UI as well as risk of falls. Risk of urinary retention is increased with the use of calcium channel blockers, β-adrenergic agonists (beta-blockers), anticholinergic medications, antispasmodics, antidepressants, antipsychotics, sedative/hypnotics, and narcotic analgesics. Decongestants are sympathomimetic agents that increase urethral resistance and therefore increase the risk for retention in men with prostate enlargement; they are therefore considered contraindicated in this group (Bolz et al., 2012; Gray & Moore, 2009). All patients on sedating or anticholinergic medications should be monitored for side effects (e.g., confusion, cognitive changes, dry mouth, constipation) as these interfere with function and increase fall risk. The nurse should consult/refer for adjustment of medications when there are identified concerns regarding safety, efficacy, or duplicative medications.

CLINICAL PEARL

Multiple medications have the potential to impact on continence and voiding; the pharmacist can be invaluable in assessing an individual's medications for potential adverse effects on bladder and sphincter function.

Social History

The social history provides the continence nurse an opportunity to examine additional contributing factors to UI, voiding dysfunction, and quality of life. Asking about *primary or significant relationship* status and the impact of the continence or bladder problem on the relationship is important. Issues surrounding sexuality, social isolation, and sleep disruption should be explored along with the willingness and ability of the significant other to provide emotional support and/or assistance when considering the management plan. Determining the person's *occupation* may provide insight into other contributing factors. For example, individuals with jobs that require heavy lifting are at increased risk for stress UI. Others may work in jobs that limit opportunities for toileting and may have to postpone voiding until a scheduled break (e.g., factory line worker, teacher); this may increase the risk for urge UI or for retention.

Asking about *exercise and activity* level provides insight into alterations in quality of life and/or activities associated with risk of UI. For example, high-impact physical activities correlate to increased risk of leaking and stress UI. Reduced mobility and a sedentary lifestyle may contribute to a loss of core strength that makes it difficult for the individual to get up from a chair or the toilet. In addition, these alterations may contribute to a loss of pelvic floor muscle tone, which increases the likelihood for pelvic floor relaxation and urine loss consistent with stress UI.

Nutritional Assessment

A brief nutritional assessment can be useful in determining special dietary considerations and the presence of any swallowing difficulties that could impact the management plan. A brief 24-hour dietary recall can provide a snapshot of usual food and fluid intake, to include usual intake of dietary fiber and the pattern, types, and amounts of fluids ingested. The use and number of beverages consumed daily that contain caffeine, artificial sweeteners (e.g., NutraSweet, aspartame), or alcohol should be assessed, and the relationship between their use and an increase in bladder symptoms should be explored (Gray, 2006). Lifestyle changes that include reducing or eliminating these types of beverages can be beneficial in reducing symptoms of urgency and frequency in some individuals (Newman & Wein, 2009). Dietary review and bladder diary may reveal excessive fluid intake, and further assessment is indicated to determine the reasons for the high volume intake; poorly controlled or undiagnosed diabetes mellitus and deliberate use of water intake to control appetite and reduce food intake are two common reasons that would require very different management approaches (Gray, 2006).

> **CLINICAL PEARL**
>
> The use and number of beverages consumed daily that contain caffeine, alcohol, or artificial sweeteners should be assessed.

While excessive fluid intake can be an issue for some individuals, voluntary restriction is more common as many persons with UI limit their fluid intake in an attempt to manage their incontinence. While understandable, it is important for the nurse to be able to emphasize the benefits of adequate fluid intake. Specifically, excessive fluid restriction results in highly concentrated urine that may increase irritative bladder symptoms (e.g., urgency and frequency), UTI risk, and constipation. For the elderly, dehydration can contribute to transient changes in cognitive status. A bladder record that includes fluid intake and voided amounts is helpful in gathering objective data to correlate fluid intake with voiding frequency, irritative symptoms, and UI. In providing patient and education, the nurse should be aware that most adults need about 1,500 mL of fluid per day (or 30 mL/kg).

Environmental and Functional Assessment

Environmental assessment should include toilet availability and safety issues, while functional assessment focuses on the ability of the individual to independently perform toileting and related activities of daily living (ADL).

Environmental Assessment

During the patient interview, the nurse should identify the setting where the person lives (e.g., home, assisted living, nursing home) and the support needed to toilet successfully. The nurse should ask specifically about toileting regimes, bathroom accessibility, and available assistive devices (e.g., urinal, raised toilet seat, grab bars, bedside commode or bedpan) and should be alert to safety issues, such as obstacles in the path to the toilet, poor lighting, ambulatory instability, and footwear with slick soles. Conducting the evaluation in the person's residence allows the nurse to assess the environment first hand and to identify barriers to continence. Cleanliness and presence of urine odor should be assessed as well as accessibility of laundry facilities; this helps assure appropriate recommendations related to reusable versus disposable absorptive products.

Determining the sleeping situation (i.e., where they sleep and presence of a sleeping partner) is helpful, as some persons opt to sleep in a bed while others choose other alternatives due to various health problems (e.g., a recliner). In either situation, the person's ability to get up to toilet and the potential benefit of assistive devices should be assessed. Protective bed coverings and use of absorptive products should be explored. Types of products used, frequency of use, hygiene, and appropriate disposal of used products should be reviewed. Availability and responsiveness of caregivers is also important as is the presence of community resources and family support, particularly for the elderly and those with disability (Gray, 2006).

Functional Assessment

The functional assessment should be conducted at the same time as the environmental assessment and should focus on the level of independence and assistance needed to carry out ADL. This is another area where the use of validated tools can be helpful. The Katz Index of Independence of ADL and the Lawton Instrumental Activities of Daily Living (IADL) Scale are two such tools. The Katz ADL assesses independence in six areas, with yes/no answers to questions about bathing, dressing, toileting, transferring, continence, and feeding. A score of 6 indicates fully independent function, 4 indicates moderate functional impairment, and 2 or less correlates with severe functional impairment. This tool can be used with adults in a variety of care settings and can capture baseline function as well as changes over time (Shelkey & Wallace, 2012).

The Lawton IADL assesses independent living skills that are considered more complex than those assessed with the Katz Index of ADLs. This tool may be used for both men and women and assesses ability to use the telephone, shop, prepare food, complete housekeeping chores and laundry, manage transportation, manage medications, and handle finances. It is useful for identifying current function and for reflecting functional changes over time. Persons are scored on a scale of 0 (lowest function) to 8 (highest function, independent) for activities in each category. The tool can be used in clinic, community, and hospital settings but is not applicable for institutionalized adults (Graf, 2013) (Table 3-1).

Assessing both environment and functional status as part of the focused health history not only provides an opportunity to identify barriers to continence but also identifies safety issues that include fall risk. Many older adults are at risk for falling on the way to the bathroom, and this risk increases in the presence of bladder symptoms (e.g., urgency, leaking of urine) and accompanying alterations in function and mobility (Brown et al., 2000; Morris & Wagg, 2007). The Hendrich II Fall Risk Model and the Falls Efficacy Scale-International (FES-I) are two validated tools for identifying fall risk in older adults (Greenberg 2011; Hendrich, 2013). Originally tested in the acute care setting, the Hendrich II Fall Risk Model has demonstrated validity and has been adapted for use across a variety of settings. Advantages of this tool are that it is short, includes assessment of risk related to medications, and includes the "Get Up and Go" test. The "Get Up and Go" test is a short assessment designed to test an individual's ability to safely rise from a chair, an essential function for safe toileting and fall prevention (Mathias et al., 1986). This tool also helps the nurse to identify specific areas of risk and to design and implement interventions that address those areas (Hendrich, 2013).

The FES-I is designed to assess fear of falling; while it does not specifically ask about continence or toileting, it does assess related areas of function and may provide additional insight regarding persons at risk for depression and social isolation. The short tool asks about fall concern related to social and daily activities and uses a Likert scale (1 = not at all, 4 = very concerned) to measure concern (Greenberg, 2011).

CLINICAL PEARL

Assessment of the individual's environment and functional status permits identification of barriers to continence as well as safety issues such as fall risk.

Bladder Diary

The bladder record or diary is an important tool in gathering objective data related to voiding patterns, fluid intake, and incontinence. When possible, this should be included as a routine part of the assessment. In persons with cognitive impairment who are not able to complete the diary, a caregiver may complete a "modified" diary if she/he is willing to do so. (A "modified" diary typically involves hourly documentation as to wet or dry status, which provides insight into voiding frequency and is helpful in developing an individualized toileting schedule. The caregiver may also elect to take the person to the bathroom every 2 hours and provide verbal cues to void; the caregiver should then record the individual's response. This also provides very helpful information as to whether or not the person is likely to benefit from a toileting program.)

Many variations on bladder diaries exist, ranging from very basic to quite detailed. Bladder diaries can also be tailored to a variety of settings. It can be helpful for the continence nurse to have several different types of bladder diaries available for use and to select the specific tool depending on care setting and the symptoms to be monitored.

All bladder diaries require the willingness of the individual or caregiver to complete them. In the simplest of bladder records, the person simply documents the time of each voluntary voiding episode and each episode of leakage. More involved diaries also capture fluid intake, activities or symptoms surrounding the loss of urine (e.g., lifting, urgency), and the amount of urine lost (e.g., minimal urine loss = several drops or wet spot on underwear, moderate urine loss = several teaspoons or tablespoons of urine, large urine loss = several ounces soaking clothing or saturating a large pad or absorbent brief) (Gray, 2006).

CLINICAL PEARL

Bladder diaries provide important objective data regarding voiding frequency, fluid intake, and incontinence.

Bladder diaries can be completed for varying lengths of time with 1- to 14-day diaries shown to produce reliable results with or without intensive instruction (Gray, 2006). Since it is difficult for many persons or caregivers to collect data for an extended time, the nurse should realize that diaries maintained for 1 to 3 days produce valuable information (Gray, 2006). To increase the likelihood of completion, it is important for the nurse to explain the purpose of the bladder record, how the information collected will be used, and strategies for ensuring completion (e.g., place record near the toilet or at the bedside, or download an electronic diary to one's phone).

All bladder diaries provide data regarding voiding frequency and frequency of leakage episodes and therefore help to quantify the severity of the leakage. More complex diaries provide insight as to type of incontinence and the potential role of fluid intake; for example, leakage that is always associated with activity is indicative of stress incontinence, and normal voided volumes associated with urgency in a person with daily fluid intake of 4 liters suggest that the problem relates to volume of intake and not to bladder dysfunction.

> **CLINICAL PEARL**
>
> The caregiver can complete a modified bladder diary for the person with cognitive impairment; data to be gathered would include "wet/dry" status on an hourly basis, response to q2-hour toileting attempts, and fluid intake.

Focused Physical Examination

During the interview, the continence nurse has the opportunity to observe the individual and begins to collect objective data that are part of the focused physical examination. For example, the nurse assesses general appearance, gait, dexterity, and mobility when meeting the individual and throughout the interview as well as general demeanor, cognition, and affect. As stated, validated tools can be used throughout the interview to provide quantifiable objective data regarding cognition, presence or absence of depression, and functional status.

The interview also provides time and opportunity for establishment of the nurse–patient relationship. This relationship enhances patient comfort during the physical exam and is further developed by a respectful and sensitive approach to the examination. Specifically, the nurse should ask permission to examine the person, explain the examination process, assist with positioning and draping, and convey consistent respect for the individual's privacy and the sensitive nature of the examination. As the nurse moves from one part of the examination to the next, the patient should be informed of the next steps in the examination and permission sought to continue.

General Assessment

In addition to the observations and interactions described in the previous paragraph, general assessment includes an overall impression of the client's state of health. This general assessment is documented, for example, healthy-appearing adult and frail-appearing older adult. Vital signs including height and weight are included in the general assessment.

Mental Status

The purpose of the mental status examination is to assess the individual's cognitive status and functional ability, including ability to respond appropriately to information and instruction. Physical appearance, appropriateness of dress, facial expression, and body posture are all indicators of mental function. Orientation to person, place, and time is an important indicator of memory and cognition.

Emotional affect and alertness should also be assessed. As discussed previously, when there are any concerns as to cognitive status or depression, a validated tool should be used for objective assessment and documentation.

> **CLINICAL PEARL**
>
> When there are concerns regarding cognitive status or depression, a validated tool should be used for objective assessment and documentation.

Musculoskeletal Examination

Observation and assessment of dexterity, gait, and mobility are important components of the examination in relation to continence. Dexterity includes the ability of an individual to manage their own clothing and toileting hygiene. Gait and mobility include the individual's ability to walk to the bathroom with reasonable speed and to transfer to the toilet independently versus walking or moving slowly, needing assistance of one or two persons, or being totally dependent on caregivers for mobility. Observation for any visible abnormalities in the extremities and palpation for detection of edema are also important. Many continence clinicians measure the time required by an elderly patient with UI to get to the bathroom, manage clothing, and sit on the toilet (Gray, 2006). The continence nurse can often provide recommendations that facilitate clothing management (e.g., suspenders instead of belts, elastic waist pants rather than zippers) and safe toileting (e.g., urinal or bedside commode, grab bar, or elevated toilet seat).

Neurologic Examination

Along with assessment of mobility, dexterity, and cognition, the back, buttocks, and lower extremities may be assessed for signs of neurologic lesions such as spina bifida occulta. For example, if there are any concerns regarding neurologic function, the back should be inspected for indicators of spinal dysraphism (e.g., lipomatous area, hairy tuft, or skin tag near the lumbosacral spinal area) (Gray, 2006). When indicated, the buttocks should be inspected for asymmetry or signs of muscle atrophy, and the lower extremities and feet can be assessed for atrophy or other obvious signs of neurologic abnormality (Gray, 2006). If there is ambulatory instability, the clinician should assess for diminished or absent position sense, which is associated with increased fall risk. Additional components of the neurologic examination are included in the examination of the perineum, genitalia, and rectum when indicated.

Skin Assessment

Skin temperature, turgor, and condition are the main components of this examination. Temperature and turgor reflect hydration, which is of great importance. In addition, general skin assessment includes inspection for significant bruising or lesions. Perineal skin assessment is the main focus; the nurse should assess for redness and denudement consistent with incontinence-associated dermatitis (IAD) and for a maculopapular rash with distinct satellite lesions, consistent with candidiasis. Both are common findings in persons with persistent urinary leakage and individuals managed with containment devices; individuals with combined urinary and fecal incontinence are even higher risk for skin damage. Skin changes range in severity; mild IAD is characterized by erythema that may be more intense in skin folds, while advanced IAD is characterized by extensive erosion with or without candidiasis (Doughty et al., 2012; Gray, 2006).

Abdominal Examination

Inspection of the abdomen begins with general observation for symmetry, obvious distension or masses, and skin abnormalities; any pathologic findings should prompt referral for further evaluation (e.g., evidence of hernia or mass, areas of intense erythema, and induration suggestive of abscess). *Auscultation* of bowel sounds should be performed if there are any concerns regarding obstruction or ileus, but is not routinely indicated for the individual with UI. *Percussion* is utilized to detect fluid, gaseous distention, stool retention, and masses. The entire abdomen should be lightly percussed with tympany expected throughout most of the abdomen due to the presence of gas in the large and small bowel. Solid masses will produce a dull percussion note as will a distended bladder (Jarvis, 2011).

To assess for bladder distention, the nurse percusses from the xiphoid to the symphysis, noting any change in percussion note; a distended bladder is usually visible and percussible in a thin individual but may be difficult to appreciate in an obese person. In a relatively thin person, percussion can be used to define the outline of the distended bladder. Evidence of bladder distention mandates measurement of postvoid residual (PVR) urine volume, either by catheterization or ultrasound. Percussion along the length of the colon is helpful in determining the presence or absence of retained stool (fecal loading). As stated, the percussion note along the colon is normally tympanic, due to presence of gas; however, the percussion note over areas of retained stool is dull. Evidence of fecal loading should prompt initiation of a bowel cleansing regimen and bowel management program. Light and deep *palpation* may be performed to assess for hypersensitivity, muscle spasticity, liver or spleen enlargement, and masses. The bladder is not normally palpable on examination unless it is distended with urine, in which case it is felt as a smooth, round, somewhat tense mass.

CLINICAL PEARL

The abdominal examination should include percussion to assess for bladder distention and/or fecal loading.

Genitourinary Examination in Men

A thorough inspection of the external genitalia and perineal skin should be respectfully performed assessing for skin integrity. *Examination of the penis* includes observation of the absence or presence of the foreskin (circumcised vs. uncircumcised). The foreskin when present should be easily retractable with the glans and urethra easily visualized. The condition of phimosis should be considered when the foreskin is not easily retractable or is difficult to return to normal position. The urethra should be midline on the glans and patent with intact skin integrity. Urethral discharge, redness, or irritation should be further investigated. The presence of urethral stricture or hypospadias requires further assessment to rule out voiding dysfunction and urinary retention. (Hypospadias is a congenital condition in which the opening of the urethra is located on the underside of the penis rather than on the glans.)

In older men, atrophic changes, including penile retraction, may be evident. The *scrotum* should be inspected for areas of diffuse or localized redness, excoriations, or ulcerations. It is appropriate for continence nurses to perform a *testicular examination* assessing for symmetry, masses, swelling, or tenderness. Any positive findings should be referred for further evaluation. In individuals with a previous history of infections, the advanced practice nurse (APN) may expand the examination by palpating the epididymis in each testicle. Previous infections may present as fibrosis or scarring and can be a contributing factor in individuals with long-standing detrusor–sphincter dyssynergia or prostatitis resulting in bladder outlet obstruction (Gray, 2006).

Genitourinary Examination in Women

The examination begins with inspection of the external genitalia. Hair pattern, skin condition of the perineum (e.g., presence of lesions, scars, rashes, erythema, discharge, or discoloration), and size and shape of the labia majora are observed. Diminished size of the clitoris and labia majora is consistent with aging and hypoestrogenic effects. Tissues that are pale, thin, dry, or fissured are indicative of significant atrophic changes due to estrogen deficiency. Palpation of the area includes separation of the labia majora to inspect and palpate the labia minora. Atrophic changes include diminution in size of the labia and, in some cases, fusion of the tissues. The urethral meatus should be inspected for relaxation or gaping, redness, or discharge. In some cases, urinary leakage may be readily observable when the woman bears down or changes position; this signifies major sphincter dysfunction. Atrophic changes may include a urethral caruncle, a cherry red protruding (prolapsed) urethral meatus. The introitus to the vagina should be assessed for narrowing, erythema, adhesions, and stenosis.

The woman should be asked to bear down, and the nurse should observe for an observable bulge or protrusion of tissue that extends to the introitus or beyond; this is indicative of pelvic organ prolapse (addressed in detail in Chapter 9). The vaginal and vulvar tissues may be tender or sensitive due to irritation or dryness caused by a decline in estrogen levels. Vaginal discharge is generally not present in postmenopausal women and should be investigated further if observed. A change in vaginal discharge, odor, and itching should be further investigated in all sexually active women regardless of age as vaginitis and/or sexually transmitted infections can contribute to irritative bladder symptoms (Robinson & Cardozo, 2011; Schulling & Likis, 2013).

CLINICAL PEARL

Pelvic examination in women should include assessment for atrophic changes (thinning and drying of the vaginal mucosa, urethral caruncle), pelvic organ prolapse, and pelvic muscle strength and endurance.

Digital vaginal examination is done to assess pelvic muscle tone and sensation; the advanced practice continence nurse also conducts a bimanual examination to evaluate pelvic organ structures. The nurse gently inserts one or two gloved fingers into the vagina and asks the woman if she is able to feel the presence of the finger in the vagina. The woman is then asked to contract the vaginal muscles around the examiner's finger as if trying to stop her urine stream or keep from passing gas. This allows the nurse to determine the individual's ability to identify, isolate, contract, and relax the pelvic floor muscles. In addition, the nurse can observe for use of accessory muscles (such as abdominal and buttocks muscles) and the presence of hypertonus or muscle spasm. Pelvic muscle tone, accessory muscle use, and muscle hypertonus/spasm can all be scored using the Oxford grading system, an internationally accepted muscle grading system (Laycock, 1994; Messelink, et al., 2005) (Box 3-1). This assessment of pelvic muscle strength provides an excellent opportunity for the nurse to teach and provide feedback regarding the performance of pelvic muscle exercises. The digital vaginal examination also presents an opportunity to further palpate for pelvic organ prolapse. With one to two fingers in the vagina, the nurse can ask the woman to bear down and can palpate for any descent of the bladder (cystocele), uterus (uterine prolapse), or rectum (rectocele) into the vaginal vault. When these structural changes are identified, the woman should be referred for further evaluation.

All nurses providing continence assessment should be able to provide inspection and palpation of the external genitalia and vagina including pelvic muscle tone (Box 3-1). The APN has additional health assessment skills that include the vaginal speculum and pelvic examination. It is important for APNs performing this part of the examination to be competent in pelvic examination in order to ensure accuracy and to reduce the risk of

BOX 3-1. Pelvic Floor Muscle Assessment

Scale for Grading Digital Evaluation of Pelvic Muscle Strength

(Check one) _____ Vaginal Examination _____ Rectal Exam

Scale	Grade	Description
None	0	No discernable muscle contraction, pressure, and/or displacement of examiner's finger
Flicker	1/5	Trace but instant contraction <1 second, very slight compression of examiner's finger
Weak	2/5	Weak contraction or pressure with or without elevation/lifting of examiner's finger, held for >1 second but <3 seconds
Moderate	3/5	Moderate contraction or compression of examiner's finger with or without elevation/lifting of finger, held for at least 4 to 6 seconds, repeated 3 times
Firm	4/5	Firm contraction with good compression of examiner's finger with elevation/lifting of finger toward the pubic bone, held for at least 7 to 9 seconds, repeated 4 to 5 times
Strong	5/5	Unmistakable strong contraction and grip of examiner's finger with posterior elevation/lifting of finger, held at least 10 seconds, repeated 4 to 5 times

Use of Accessory Muscle Groups

Abdominal	_____ Yes	_____ No
Gluteal	_____ Yes	_____ No
Thigh/Abductor	_____ Yes	_____ No

Evaluation During Examination—Muscle Hypertonus/Spasm

0	No pressure or pain
1	Comfortable pressure
2	Uncomfortable pressure
3	Moderate pain that interferes with muscle contraction
4	Severe pain; patient unable to perform muscle contraction because of pain

Based on Oxford Grading System (Laycock, 1994; Messelink et al., 2005).

inadvertent pain with speculum insertion. The speculum examination is used to visualize the vaginal tissues and the cervix, and the size and type of speculum should be selected based on clinical presentation of the vagina. For example, in multiparous women or obese women, the larger Graves speculum will likely allow for better visualization, while nulliparous or postmenopausal women will tolerate the smaller and narrower Pederson or pediatric speculum.

Following insertion of the speculum into the vagina, the vaginal tissue is assessed for rugae, color, moisture, and flexibility. An absence of vaginal rugae and the presence of tissue thinning and dryness are all consistent with vaginal atrophy due to estrogen deficiency. The cervix may or may not be present depending on surgical history; if present, paleness and retraction into the pelvic floor are also common findings consistent with atrophy and hypoestrogenism. The vaginal pH can be determined by touching litmus paper to the lower third of the vaginal wall; an alkaline pH in postmenopausal women is consistent with estrogen deficiency. If obtaining a vaginal culture, the swab is taken from the posterior vaginal vault. With the speculum closed or using just the posterior blade, the clinician should apply pressure to the posterior wall of the vagina and should then ask the woman to bear down; bulging of the anterior wall may be an indicator of urethral hypermobility and/or cystocele. The diagnosis of stress UI is supported by an observable loss of urine during the maneuver. The APN can then gently rotate the position of the speculum blade so that it is now stabilizing the anterior vaginal wall. The woman should again be asked to bear down while the nurse observes for bulging of the posterior vaginal wall consistent with rectocele.

Throughout both procedures, descent of the cervix into the vaginal vault may be observed and can be more specifically assessed by placing the speculum blades in the distal vaginal vault and asking the woman to bear down (Gray, 2006; Laycock, 1994; Messelink, et al., 2005; Schulling & Likis, 2013). The Baden-Walker system is a five-point grading system for pelvic organ prolapse that is in widespread use and is summarized in Table 3-2 (Newman & Wein, 2009).

Following removal of the speculum, the bimanual examination is performed to assess the internal pelvic organs. With the first two fingers of the dominant hand inserted into the vagina and the nondominant hand positioned on the abdomen, the presence or absence of pelvic organs should be discerned. Uterine position, size, shape, and consistency should be assessed. The presence of uterine position in relation to the bladder should be determined as uterine enlargement or displacement can put pressure on the bladder, thus affecting voiding. The adnexae should be assessed for palpable masses, fullness, or tenderness with a rectal–vaginal examination completing the examination.

Rectal Examination

The rectal examination is an essential component of the continence assessment for men as it is the only approach to evaluate pelvic muscle strength; it is also essential for women with coexisting fecal incontinence. For women with UI but no issues with fecal incontinence, it is not as critical but does provide the opportunity to more fully assess for anal sphincter/pelvic muscle strength, masses, and the presence of stool impaction (Gray, 2006). In addition, inspection of the perianal skin may reveal the presence of external hemorrhoids and anal fissures as well as anal irritation or skin changes. Determination of perineal sensation in relation to light touch as well as differentiation of sharp and dull stimuli can be included when there is concern regarding altered neurologic function. Inspection of the anus for prolapse, gaping, or incomplete closure is important in identifying issues related to bowel evacuation and is usually indicative of neurologic dysfunction. The presence of the bulbocavernosus reflex (BCR) indicates intact neurologic pathways between the motor neurons in the sacral spinal cord and the pelvic muscles. The BCR can be assessed on digital rectal examination (DRE) or through anal observation. In both situations, the reflex is stimulated by gently tapping the clitoris in women or squeezing the glans of the penis in men. On DRE, contraction is felt, whereas on anal observation, the contraction or "wink" is visualized.

The BCR, while helpful, is a somewhat limited test in that it only tests gross neurologic function. For persons with diminished or absent BCR, this finding may or may not be significant in relation to urinary problems. Gray (2006) recommends that further assessment of neurologic denervation be pursued when additional indicators of neurologic deficits are identified. For example, women with neurologic voiding dysfunction who also have chronic constipation or fecal incontinence and vaginal dryness or dyspareunia not explained by estrogen deficiency should be evaluated for perineal denervation. In men, voiding dysfunction, constipation or fecal incontinence, and erectile or ejaculatory dysfunction are representative of neurologic deficits. In both situations, referral for further neurologic consultation and multichannel urodynamics testing may be indicated (Gray, 2006).

Grade	Amount of Prolapse
0	No prolapse
1	Prolapse descends or bulges halfway down to the hymen/vaginal opening
2	Descent of the prolapse to the hymen/vaginal opening
3	Prolapse protrudes halfway from the hymen/vaginal opening.
4	Maximal descent: the vagina with the vaginal vault and uterus protrudes completely outside the body without a Valsalva maneuver Procidentia: the most severe form of prolapse

TABLE 3-2 **Baden-Walker Five-Point System for Grading Pelvic Organ Prolapse**

Adapted from Newman, D. K. (2009). *Managing and treating urinary incontinence* (2nd ed.). Baltimore, MD: Health Professions Press.

The DRE can be used to test pelvic floor muscle tone in men and in women who are unable to tolerate a vaginal examination. With a single gloved finger inserted into the rectum, the person is asked to contract their rectal muscles around the examiner's finger. The same Oxford grading system can be used to assess pelvic muscle tone on rectal examination (Box 3-1). For men, DRE also provides an opportunity to identify the presence and consistency of stool in the rectum and to assess the prostate for size, consistency, and symmetry. The presence of tenderness or pain on palpation of the prostate raises concerns about prostatitis. Symmetric enlargement of the prostate is consistent with BPH, while asymmetric enlargement is characteristic of cancer (Jarvis, 2011). The consistency of the prostate is normally rubbery; therefore, a boggy, firm, or hardened prostate warrants further evaluation. Prostate examination is generally considered the purview of the APN.

🔵 Laboratory and Diagnostic Studies

Urinalysis

A urinalysis is an important component of continence evaluation in those individuals who are exhibiting symptoms of voiding dysfunction and UTI. Urinalysis can be conducted using urine dipstick or microscopic analysis and is best obtained midstream or clean catch to decrease the likelihood of bacterial contamination. In those individuals who are unable to perform perineal hygiene or obtain a clean catch urine specimen, sterile straight catheterization is an alternative. For best results, the urine should be tested within 2 hours following its collection (Jarvis, 2011).

Components of the UA include specific gravity, pH, glucose, nitrites and leukocytes, hemoglobin, and protein. Specific gravity provides an indicator of the kidneys' ability to concentrate urine. The test is reported as the ratio of the weight of the urine tested to the weight of water. Low specific gravity can be related to excessive fluid intake or to renal tubular dysfunction associated with some metabolic conditions (e.g., diabetes insipidus), while an elevated specific gravity may reflect inadequate fluid intake. The pH of freshly voided urine is normally acidic; alkaline urine is associated with some bacterial UTIs. The presence of glucose is not a normal finding; when glucose is present on UA, the individual should be evaluated for uncontrolled or undiagnosed diabetes mellitus. Nitrites and leukocytes in general should be absent; however, among older adults living in community or institutional settings (e.g., assisted living, nursing homes), there is an increased likelihood for these indicators to be present.

Positive nitrites and leukocytes without urinary symptoms are consistent with asymptomatic bacteriuria (ASB), which does not require treatment (Benton et al., 2006; Nicolle et al., 2005). Microscopic analysis should be performed in those individuals in whom symptoms of UTI are present. Hemoglobin should also be negative; positive hemoglobin is consistent with hematuria and infection and should be further evaluated. Negative protein is a normal finding but may be positive when leukocytes are also present. Proteinuria that persists after treatment of infection may be indicative of renal disease, and the individual should be referred for further evaluation.

Urine Culture and Sensitivity

This test is done when the UA findings are consistent with UTI and the patient has symptoms of UTI. Urine in the bladder is normally sterile; when bacteria are present, the urine can be cultured and monitored for bacterial growth. Little to no growth is considered a negative culture, while bacterial growth is microscopically and chemically analyzed to determine the amount and type(s) of bacteria as well as the organisms' sensitivity or resistance to antibiotics that could be used for treatment. Reassessment of UTI symptoms is important after completion of treatment to determine if treatment has been effective. Unresolved symptoms require further workup to determine whether they are caused by persistent UTI or by another type of pathology.

Postvoid Residual Volume

PVR should be measured on anyone at risk for incomplete bladder emptying or urinary retention. Indicators for PVR measurement include the following: signs and symptoms of incomplete emptying (bladder distention on physical exam; sensation of incomplete emptying; urinary hesitancy; straining to void; intermittent or poor stream; postvoid dribbling); history of voiding dysfunction/urinary retention; recurrent UTIs; known or suspected BPH; evidence of pelvic organ prolapse; neurologic conditions; spinal or endocrine disorders; and stool impaction. Antidepressants, antipsychotics, sedatives and hypnotics, alpha-adrenergic agonists, anticholinergics, and calcium channel blockers also increase the risk of urinary retention, and patients taking one or more of these medications should be considered for PVR evaluation (Gray & Moore, 2009).

PVR can be obtained by the use of ultrasound or catheterization and should be done as soon as possible after voiding. Catheterization done by an experienced clinician can be inexpensive and accurate; however, there is a slight risk of UTI associated with the procedure and some individuals experience varying degrees of discomfort (Bolz et al., 2012; Gray, 2006; Gray & Moore, 2009). Ultrasound is more expensive; however, it is less invasive and presents minimal risk of infection or discomfort. Both ultrasound and catheterization are considered accurate PVR methods. There is no clear consensus on a specific PVR volume that signifies urinary retention; however, comparison of the voided amount to the PVR is important in obtaining a clear picture regarding completeness of bladder emptying. In general, PVRs of 50 to 100mL are considered on the low end of abnormal; typically, these individuals are managed with monitoring and conservative strategies to improve bladder emptying. PVRs that exceed 250 mL are considered significant, and those above 350 mL increase the risk for upper urinary tract dilatation and renal insufficiency (Gray, 2006; Kelly, 2004).

CLINICAL PEARL

PVR > 250 mL is considered significant; PVR >350 mL increases the risk for upper tract dilatation and renal damage.

Serum Studies

There are instances when serum studies are indicated as part of the continence assessment. These studies most commonly include BUN (blood, urea, nitrogen) and creatinine, electrolytes, complete blood count (CBC), fasting blood sugar (FBS), and hemoglobin A1c. Often, the chemistry panel will include all of these measures including the estimated glomerular filtration rate (eGFR). Together, these studies provide a snapshot of overall renal and endocrine function. BUN and creatinine should be monitored for elevation caused by medications, metabolic disorders, or voiding dysfunction related to outlet obstruction (e.g., BPH). If upper urinary tract distress is suspected (e.g., recurring pyelonephritis, renal insufficiency), urology consultation is indicated (Gray, 2006). An electrolyte panel may be needed when low specific gravity is noted on UA, there are concerns related to dehydration, or a change in cognition is observed. The CBC provides an overall measurement of white and red blood cell activity. FBS and Hgb A1c are helpful in understanding the individual's blood sugar control at present and retrospectively over the past 3 months, which is essential since elevated and uncontrolled blood sugars play a significant role in voiding dysfunction as well as the development of neuropathy and urinary retention.

The eGFR is helpful in determining how well the kidneys are functioning and is estimated using the individual's creatinine level as well as gender, age, race, and weight. Medications, chronic illness, and upper urinary tract dysfunction can all contribute to an elevation in eGFR; thus, this value should be monitored in these patients. In addition, the eGFR is used to monitor the progression of chronic kidney disease over time and is used to guide decision making surrounding treatment (National Kidney Foundation, Inc., 2011; Table 3-3).

TABLE 3-3 Glomerular Filtration Rates and Kidney Disease

Stage	Description	GFR (mL/min/1.73 m²)
	At risk	90–120 (with CKD symptoms)
1	Kidney damage with normal or elevated GFR	≥90
2	Kidney damage with mildly reduced GFR	60–89
3	Moderately reduced GFR	30–59
4	Severely reduced GFR	15–29
5	Kidney failure (ESRD)	<15 (or dialysis)

GFR, Glomerular filtration rate.
Source: National Kidney Foundation.

Data Synthesis: Pulling It All Together

Once the key elements of the continence assessment have been completed, the next step is for the nurse to determine the diagnosis using data collected from the focused history, physical, bladder diary, and laboratory tests. Type(s) of UI and related voiding dysfunction should be identified along with factors that could worsen symptoms or interfere with treatment and management. These findings should be reviewed with the individual and the goals of care prioritized in joint discussion. Based on input from the patient, an individualized plan of care should be developed that includes treatment and management options as well as the goals for care. Patient education should be provided along with support for any needed lifestyle and health behavior changes. With the patient's permission, it may be helpful to include family members and/or caregivers in this process as well. Recommendations for monitoring and follow-up should be determined, and referrals for further consultation should be made. Communication with the patient, the family, the primary provider, and other members of the health care team completes the assessment process. Mutually agreed-upon goals should be included in the overall plan of care.

Conclusion

Continence nurses are in prime positions to assess UI and voiding dysfunction and to develop plans of care that treat and manage symptoms, reduce risk, and improve overall quality of life. Critical elements of assessment include a patient history and review of systems, focused physical examination, completion and assessment of a bladder diary, and selected diagnostic procedures (e.g., UA and PVR). A comprehensive assessment provides the data needed to determine the type of incontinence or voiding dysfunction and appropriate treatment options or to identify the need for referrals for additional workup or for medical–surgical intervention.

REFERENCES

American Geriatrics Society 2012 Beers Criteria Update Expert Panel. (2012). American Geriatrics Society updated Beers Criteria for potentially inappropriate medication use in older adults. *Annals of Long-Term Care: Clinical Care and Aging, 20*(3), 9–10.

Benton, T., Young, R., & Leeper, S. (2006). Asymptomatic bacteriuria in the nursing home. *Annals of Long-Term Care: Clinical Care and Aging, 14*(7), 17–22.

Bolz, M., Capezuti, E., Fulmer, T., et al. (2012). *Evidence-based geriatric nursing protocols for best practice* (4th ed.). New York, NY: Springer Publishing Co.

Bradway, C., & Yetman, G. (2002). Genitourinary problems. In V. T. Cotter & N. E. Strumpf (Eds.), *Advanced practice nursing with older adults: Clinical guidelines* (pp. 83–102). New York, NY: McGraw-Hill.

British Association of Urological Surgeons (BAUS). *International Prostate Symptom Score (IPPS)*. http://www.baus.org.uk/Resources/BAUS/Documents/PDF%20Documents/Patient%20information/IPSS.pdf

Brown, J. S., Vittinghoff, E., Wyman, J. F., et al. (2000). Urinary incontinence: Does it increase risk for falls and fractures? *Journal of the American Geriatrics Society, 48,* 721–725.

Diokno, A., Burgio, E., Arnold, P., et al. (2000). Epidemiology and natural history of urinary incontinence. *International Urogynecology Journal, 11,* 301–319.

Doerflinger, D. (2013). Mental status assessment of older adults: The Mini-Cog. *Try this: Best practices in nursing care of older adults.* The Hartford Foundation. http://consultgerirn.org/uploads/File/trythis/try_this_3.pdf

Doughty, D., Junkin, J., Kurz, P., et al. (2012). Incontinence-associated dermatitis consensus statements, evidence-based guidelines for prevention and treatment, and current challenges. *Journal of Wound, Ostomy & Continence Nursing, 39*(3), 303–315.

Dowling-Castronovo, A., & Spiro, E. (2013). Urinary incontinence assessment in older adults: Part II—Established urinary incontinence. *Best practices in geriatric nursing: The Hartford Institute for Geriatric Nursing, 11*:2. http://consultgerirn.org/uploads/File/trythis/try_this_11_2.pdf

DuBeau, C., Kuchel, G., Johnson, T., et al. (2010). Incontinence in the frail elderly: Report from the 4th International Consultation on Incontinence. *Neurology and Urodynamics, 29*(1), 165–178.

DuBeau, C., Simon, S., & Morris, J. N. (2006). The effect of urinary incontinence on quality of life in older nursing home residents. *Journal of the American Geriatrics Society, 54*(9), 1325–1333.

Graf, C. (2013). The Lawton Instrumental Activities of Daily Living (IADL) Scale. *Try this: Best practices in nursing care of older adults.* The Hartford Foundation. http://consultgerirn.org/uploads/File/trythis/try_this_23.pdf

Gray, M. (2006). Assessment of the patient with urinary incontinence or voiding dysfunction. In D. Doughty (Ed.), *Urinary and fecal incontinence: Current management concepts* (3rd ed.). St. Louis, MO: Mosby Elsevier.

Gray, M., & Moore, K. N. (2009). Urinary incontinence. In M. Gray & K. N. Moore (Eds.), *Urologic disorders: Adult and pediatric care.* (pp. 119–159). St. Louis, MO: Mosby Elsevier.

Greenberg, S. (2011). Assessment of fear of falling in older adults: The Falls Efficacy Scale-International (FES-1). *Try this: Best practices in nursing care of older adults.* The Hartford Foundation. http://consultgerirn.org/uploads/File/trythis/try_this_29.pdf

Greenberg, S. (2012). The Geriatric Depression Scale (GDS). *Try this: Best practices in nursing care of older adults.* The Hartford Foundation. http://consultgerirn.org/uploads/File/trythis/try_this_4.pdf

Greenblum, C., Greenblum, J., & Neff, D. (2008). Vaginal estrogen use in menopause: Is it safe? *American Journal for Nurse Practitioners, 13*(9), 26–34.

Hendrich, A. (2013). Fall risk assessment in older adults: The Hendrich II Fall Risk Model. *Try this: Best practices in nursing care of older adults.* The Hartford Foundation. http://consultgerirn.org/uploads/File/trythis/try_this_8.pdf

Jarvis, C. (2011). *Physical examination and health assessment* (6th ed.). W.B. Saunders.

Jayasekara, R. (2009). Urinary incontinence: Evaluation. *JBI database evid summaries,* Publication ES-610.

Jirovec, M., Brink, C., & Wells, T. (1988). Nursing assessment in the inpatient geriatric population. *The Nursing Clinics of North America, 23*(1), 219–230.

Kelly, C. (2004). Evaluation of voiding dysfunction and measurement of bladder volume. *Reviews in Urology, 6*(Supp1), 532–537.

Kinsberg, S. A., Kellogg, S., & Krychman, M. (2009). Treating dyspareunia caused by vaginal atrophy: A review of treatment options using vaginal estrogen therapy. *International Journal of Women's Health, 1,* 105–111.

Laycock, J. (1994). Clinical evaluation of the pelvic floor. In B. Schussler, J. Laycock, P. Norton, et al. (Eds.), *Pelvic floor re-education: Principles and practice* (pp. 42–48). London, UK: Springer-Verlag.

Lekan-Rutledge, D. (2004). Urinary incontinence strategies for frail elderly women. *Urologic Nursing, 24*(4), 281–301.

Lemack, G., & Zimmern, P. (1999). Predictability of urodynamic findings based on the Urogenital Distress Inventory-6 questionnaire. *Urology, 54*(3), 461–466.

Mathias, S., Nayak, U. S. L., & Isaacs, B. (1986). Balance in elderly patients: The "get-up and go" test. *Archives of Physical Medicine and Rehabilitation, 67,* 387–389.

Messelink, B., Benson, T., Berghamans, B., et al. (2005). Standardization of terminology of pelvic floor muscle function and dysfunction: Report from the pelvic floor clinical assessment group of the International Continence Society. *Neurourology Urodynamics, 24,* 374–380.

Molony, S., & Greenberg, S. (2013). The 2012 American Geriatrics Society updated Beers Criteria for potentially inappropriate medication use in older adult. *Try this: Best practices in nursing care of older adults.* The Hartford Foundation. Access tool online at: http://consultgerirn.org/uploads/File/trythis/try_this_16.pdf

Moore, K. N. (2006). Urinary retention. In D. Doughty (Ed.), *Urinary and fecal incontinence: Current management concepts* (3rd ed.). St. Louis, MO: Mosby Elsevier.

Moore, K. N., Dumoulin, C., Bradley, C., et al. (2013). Adult conservative management. In P. H. Abrams, L. Cardoza, A. E. Khoury, et al., (Eds.), *5th International Consultation on Incontinence* (5th ed., pp. 1–200). London, UK: European Association of Urology. ISBN: 978-9953-493-21-3.

Moore, K. N., & Jensen, L. (2000). Testing of the Incontinence Impact Questionnaire (IIQ-7) with men after radical prostatectomy. *Journal of Wound, Ostomy, & Continence Nursing, 27*(6), 304–312.

Morris, V., & Wagg, A. (2007). Lower urinary tract symptoms, incontinence and falls in elderly people: Time for an intervention study. *International Journal of Clinical Practice, 61,* 320–323.

National Kidney Foundation, Inc. (2011). *Frequently asked questions about GFR estimates.* http://www.kidney.org/professionals/kls/pdf/12-10-4004_KBB_FAQs_AboutGFR-1.pdf

Newman, D., & Wein, A. (2009). *Managing and treating incontinence* (2nd ed.). Baltimore, MD: Health Professionals Press.

Nicolle, L., Bradley, S., Colgan, R., et al. (2005). Infectious Disease Society of America guidelines for diagnosis and treatment of asymptomatic bacteriuria in adults. *Clinical Infectious Diseases, 40*(5), 643.

North American Menopause Society. (2012). The 2012 Hormone therapy position statement of The North American Menopause Society. (2012). *Menopause: The Journal of the North American Menopause Society, 19*(3), 257–271. doi: 10.1097/gme.0b013e31824b970a. http://www.menopause.org/docs/default-document-library/psht12.pdf

Offermans, M., du Moulin, M., Hamers, J., et al. (2009). Prevalence of urinary incontinence and associated risk factors in nursing home residents: A systematic review. *Neurourology and Urodynamics,* 28(4), 288–294.

Palmer, M. (1996). *Urinary incontinence assessment and promotion.* Gaithersburg, MD: Aspen.

Robinson, D., & Cardozo, L. (2011). Estrogens and the lower urinary tract. *Neurology and Urodynamics,* 30, 754–757.

Robinson, J. P., & Shea, J. A. (2002). Development and testing of a measure of health-related quality of life for men with urinary incontinence. *Journal of the American Geriatrics Society, 50*(5), 935–945.

SAMHSA-HRSA Center for Integrated Health Solutions, *Depression screening tools.* Substance Abuse and Mental Health Services Administration and the U.S. Department of Health and Human Services. http://www.integration.samhsa.gov/clinical-practice/screening-tools#depression. Accessed November 15, 2014.

Schulling, K. D., & Likis, F. E. (2013). *Women's gynecologic health* (2nd ed.). Burlington, MA: Jones & Bartlett Learning.

Shamliyan, T., Wyman, J., Bliss, D., et al. (2007). Prevention of urinary and fecal incontinence in adults. *Evidence Report/Technology Assessment (Full Rep),* (161), 1–379.

Shelkey, M., & Wallace, V. (2012). Katz index of independence of activities of daily living (ADL). *Try this: Best practice in nursing care of older adults.* The Hartford Foundation. http://consultgerirn.org/uploads/File/trythis/try_this_2.pdf

Shumaker, S. A., Wyman, J. F., Uebersax, J. S., et al. (1994). Health related quality of life measures for women with urinary incontinence: The Incontinence Impact Questionnaire and the Urogenital Distress Inventory. *Quality of Life Research, 3,* 291–306.

Subak, L., Richter, H., & Hunskaar, S. (2009). Obesity and urinary incontinence: Epidemiology and clinical research update. *The Journal of Urology, 182*(6 Suppl), S2–S7.

Uebersax, J. S., Wyman, J. F., Shumaker, S. A., et al. (1995). Short forms to assess life quality and symptom distress for urinary incontinence in women: The Incontinence Impact Questionnaire and the Urogenital Distress Inventory. *Neurology and Urodynamics, 14,* 131–139.

Van der Vaart, C. H., De Leeuw, J. R. J., Roovers, J.-P., et al. (2003). Measuring health-related quality of life in women with urogenital dysfunction: The Urogenital Distress Inventory and Incontinence Impact Questionnaire revisited. *Neurology and Urodynamics, 22,* 97–104.

QUESTIONS

1. A continence nurse is assessing older adults in a long-term care facility for urinary incontinence. What age-related change places this population at greater risk for this condition?
   A. Increased bladder capacity
   B. Benign prostatic hypertrophy in men
   C. Increased estrogen production in women
   D. Decreased will to remain continent

2. Which condition would the continence nurse document as transient urinary incontinence as opposed to established urinary incontinence?
   A. Stress UI (leakage with activity)
   B. Urge UI (leakage associated with urgency)
   C. Mixed UI (leakage associated with both activity and urgency)
   D. New-onset incontinence in a patient with UTI

3. A patient tells a continence nurse that he is unable to hold his urine and leaks on the way to the bathroom. What type of incontinence would the nurse suspect?
   A. Urge UI
   B. Stress UI
   C. Neurogenic UI
   D. Mixed UI

4. Which patient would the continence nurse consider at high risk for detrusor–sphincter dyssynergia?
   A. A patient with stress UI
   B. A patient with acute diarrhea
   C. A patient with neurogenic UI
   D. A patient with diabetes mellitus

5. Which medical condition would the continence nurse recognize as placing the patient at risk for urinary retention?
   A. Fecal impaction
   B. Newly diagnosed diabetes mellitus
   C. Truncal obesity
   D. Hypertension

6. The continence nurse is performing an abdominal examination of a patient with urinary incontinence. Which assessment technique would the nurse use to detect fluid, gaseous distention, stool retention, and masses?
   A. Inspection
   B. Auscultation
   C. Palpation
   D. Percussion

7. The continence nurse is performing a genitourinary examination of a 68-year-old female who is experiencing stress UI. Which finding is *not* an expected age-related condition?
   A. Diminished size of the clitoris
   B. Observable bulge extending to the introitus or beyond
   C. Tissues that are pale, thin, and/or dry
   D. Lack of vaginal discharge

8. A continence nurse examining a female patient for pelvic muscle strength documents the following findings: trace but instant contraction <1 second, very slight compression of examiner's finger. What grade would the nurse document?
   A. 0
   B. 1/5
   C. 2/5
   D. 4/5

9. The continence nurse conducting a genitourinary examination of a female patient documents: "Grade 3 pelvic organ prolapse." Which findings are indicative of this grading?
   A. The prolapse descends or bulges halfway down to the hymen/vaginal opening.
   B. Descent of the prolapse to the hymen/vaginal opening.
   C. Prolapse protrudes halfway from the hymen/vaginal opening.
   D. Maximum descent; the vagina with the vaginal vault and uterus protrudes completely outside the body without a Valsalva maneuver.

10. Which test finding indicates to the continence nurse the possibility of inadequate fluid intake in a patient?
   A. Elevated specific gravity
   B. Bacteria present in the urine
   C. Postvoid residual volume exceeding 250mL
   D. Nitrites and leukocytes present in the urine

ANSWERS: 1.**B**, 2.**D**, 3.**A**, 4.**C**, 5.**A**, 6.**D**, 7.**B**, 8.**B**, 9.**C**, 10.**A**

Advanced Assessment of the Patient with Urinary Incontinence and Voiding Dysfunction

Tamara Dickinson

OBJECTIVES

1. Identify goals for assessment of the individual with urinary incontinence.
2. Describe data provided by a bladder chart and the importance of a completed bladder chart for assessment and management of the patient with urinary incontinence.
3. Utilize data gathered during the interview and physical assessment to determine appropriate laboratory testing for the patient with urinary incontinence.
4. Describe indications for urodynamic testing and basic interpretation of urodynamic findings.

Topic Outline

Evaluation and management of lower urinary tract dysfunction requires a carefully obtained history and a thorough physical exam. Even with carefully honed patient interview skills and physical assessment skills, the clinical diagnosis may be unclear, and more advanced assessment may be required. Advanced assessment may include laboratory studies, endoscopic procedures, radiologic evaluation, or urodynamic studies (Chapple et al., 2009). Urodynamic studies are of particular value in evaluation of lower urinary tract function and will be the focus of this chapter.

The goal of urodynamics is to reproduce the patient's symptoms to provide a clear clinical diagnosis. Urodynamic testing evaluates the filling and voiding phases of the micturition cycle and provides information regarding the functionality of the lower urinary tract, specifically the bladder's ability to store urine at low pressures and to empty effectively, and the sphincter's ability to maintain closure during filling and to open for voiding.

BOX 4-1.

AUA/SUFU Guideline Summary

Stress urinary incontinence/prolapse: Assess urethral function, postvoid residual, and occult urinary incontinence in the presence of high-grade prolapse.

Overactive bladder, urge urinary incontinence, mixed urinary incontinence: Assess for evidence of altered compliance and evidence of bladder outlet obstruction (BOO).

Neurogenic bladder: Assess postvoid residual and perform multichannel urodynamics including pressure flow studies and electromyography as part of a baseline evaluation (with or without symptoms), when symptoms change and when there is concern of upper tract compromise.

Lower urinary tract symptoms: Assess postvoid residual and uroflowmetry initially and during routine follow-up, and assess pressure flow studies for evidence of obstruction when invasive treatments are considered.

Data from Winters et al. (2012).

TABLE 4-1 **Urodynamic Tests**

Urodynamics Component	Description
Uroflowmetry	The noninvasive measurement of the flow of urine over time
Simple cystometrogram	The measurement of bladder pressure (Pves) in response to being filled
Complex cystometrogram	The measurement of bladder pressure (Pves) and estimated abdominal pressure (Pabd) to estimate detrusor pressure (Pdet)
Pressure flow study	The measurement of Pves, Pabd, and Pdet while voiding to assess pressure and flow relationships
Valsalva leak point pressure	The measurement of the amount of abdominal force needed to cause leakage across the urethral sphincter
Electromyography	Study of pelvic floor muscle activity during filling and voiding
Urethral pressure profile	Study measuring pressures and landmarks along the length of the urethra

 ## Indications

Urodynamic testing is invasive and relatively expensive in the United States, and the quality of the studies is dependent in large part on the skill of the urodynamicist; thus, there should be clear clinical indications for its use (Schäfer et al., 2002). The specific indications for urodynamic testing remain controversial; therefore, representatives of the American Urological Association (AUA) and the Society of Urodynamics, Female Pelvic Medicine and Urogenital Reconstruction (SUFU) reviewed the literature and developed guidelines to assist clinicians in determining which patients should undergo urodynamic testing (Box 4-1) (Winters et al., 2012).

CLINICAL PEARL

The goal of urodynamics is to reproduce the patient's symptoms to provide a clear clinical diagnosis.

Overview and Description

Urodynamics is a broad term that comprises several different tests of lower urinary tract function and that, taken together, create a picture of its functional status. Conventional urodynamic testing is performed in a clinical setting; the test involves filling the bladder in an artificial and retrograde manner (Abrams et al., 2003) and then having the patient void while bladder pressures and urinary flow are measured. The specific tests included in urodynamic testing are described in Table 4-1.

A patient who is to undergo urodynamic testing should be given written information about what will occur during the test. Specifically, the patient should know that a small catheter will be placed into the bladder and a small balloon-tipped tube will be placed into the rectum to measure pressures within the bladder and the abdomen and that the bladder will be slowly filled and then he/she will be asked to urinate into a special commode. (A sample patient fact sheet to explain urodynamic testing is available at https://suna.org/download/members/urodynamics.pdf). The patient should be assured that usually the test is not painful and should be instructed to arrive with a comfortably full bladder. Urodynamic testing should not be a traumatic event for the patient; the clinician should be skilled at providing a calming environment. This is critical not only because it minimizes stress for the patient but also because it impacts significantly on the accuracy of the test results. Postprocedure, patients may experience mild dysuria and possibly some mild hematuria and should be encouraged to push fluids.

Testing should not be performed in the presence of a urinary tract infection, because the results of the test will not be accurate; therefore, screening for infection should be done prior to the procedure. It is controversial whether or not periprocedural antibiotics should be used and there is a lack of concrete evidence either "pro" or "con" (Gurbuz et al., 2013; Onur et al., 2004).

CLINICAL PEARL

Urodynamic testing should not be a traumatic event for the patient; the clinician should be skilled at providing a calming environment.

Uroflowmetry

Uroflowmetry involves measurement of the rate of urine flow over time and is measured in milliliters/second. It is noninvasive and is often used as an initial screening tool for lower urinary tract (voiding) dysfunction (Schäfer et al., 2002). Patients are instructed to arrive with a comfortably full bladder, if they are able. The patient urinates into a commode with a funnel that utilizes a weight and force sensing transducer or a rotating disk style sensor to measure the rate of urine flow. The patient should be given adequate privacy and instructions about the uroflow commode and should be asked to void as normally as possible. Once the patient voids into the uroflow commode, a bladder scanner can be used to obtain a noninvasive postvoid residual volume; the combination of uroflow and postvoid residual provides a complete screening assessment of the emptying phase of the micturition cycle. These tests can also be used to evaluate the response to treatment of urinary retention, either medical or surgical.

Normal uroflowmetry should be a bell-shaped curve. Abnormal uroflowmetry manifests as intermittent or uneven bursts of flow, or a low velocity flat flow rate; however, the clinician must remember that abnormal results can also be the result of low voided volumes. This is the reason for preparing patients for the test by instructing them to come to the clinic with a full bladder. Figure 4-1A depicts a normal voiding pattern, and Figure 4-1B indicates a uroflow from a patient with probable voiding dysfunction (e.g., BOO). The area under each curve represents the volume of urine voided.

An abnormal uroflow such as that in Figure 4-1B suggests problems with bladder emptying, but it does not provide enough information to determine the clinical cause, that is, reduced bladder contractility versus BOO (Schäfer et al., 2002). Consistently low voided volumes and low flow rates can be indicative of decreased detrusor contractility, increased outlet resistance, overactive detrusor, or a combination of these factors, and further urodynamic testing is indicated to confirm the diagnosis (Hanno et al., 2007). Obstruction that is constrictive such as a urethral stricture typically creates a plateau pattern, whereas obstruction caused by prostatic hypertrophy usually creates a compressed pattern that tapers off at the end (Schäfer et al., 2002) (Figs. 4-2 and 4-3). However, these patterns may also be produced by a weak detrusor contraction. Intermittent bursts of flow can be caused by detrusor sphincter dyssynergia (as may be seen in the patient with

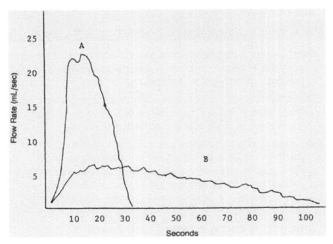

FIGURE 4-1. Urinary flow studies. **A.** Normal voiding. **B.** Obstructed voiding. The area under each curve represents the volume.

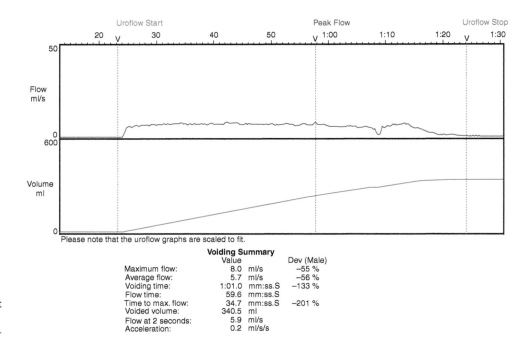

Please note that the uroflow graphs are scaled to fit.

Voiding Summary

	Value		Dev (Male)
Maximum flow:	8.0	ml/s	−55 %
Average flow:	5.7	ml/s	−56 %
Voiding time:	1:01.0	mm:ss.S	−133 %
Flow time:	59.6	mm:ss.S	
Time to max. flow:	34.7	mm:ss.S	−201 %
Voided volume:	340.5	ml	
Flow at 2 seconds:	5.9	ml/s	
Acceleration:	0.2	ml/s/s	

FIGURE 4-2. Obstruction that is constrictive, such as a stricture, typically creates a plateau pattern.

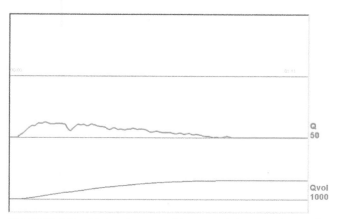

FIGURE 4-3. Obstruction caused by prostatic hypertrophy usually creates a compressed pattern that tapers off at the end of the void.

a neurologic condition), pelvic floor dysfunction in the absence of a neurologic condition, or abdominal straining. Box 4-2 lists the uroflowmetry data points.

CLINICAL PEARL

Abnormal uroflow may be the result of obstruction or poor detrusor contractility but may also be due to low voided volume. Patient preparation includes instruction on attending the appointment with a full bladder.

BOX 4-2.

Uroflowmetry Data Points

Maximum Flow Rate (Q_{max}): Maximum measured flow rate 30–35 mL/s for women; 25 mL/s in men under 40 and 15 mL/s in men over 60 years of age

Average Flow Rate: Voided volume divided by flow time. Normal values vary depending on age and sex (Wein et al., 2012). In men, urine flow declines with age. Women have less change with age:

- Ages 4–7
  - The average flow rate for both males and females is 10 mL/s.
- Ages 8–13
  - The average flow rate for males is 12 mL/s.
  - The average flow rate for females is 15 mL/s.
- Ages 14–45
  - The average flow rate for males is 21 mL/s.
  - The average flow rate for females is 18 mL/s.
- Ages 46–65
  - The average flow rate for males is 12 mL/s.
  - The average flow rate for females is 18 mL/s.
- Ages 66–80
  - The average flow rate for males is 9 mL/s.
  - The average flow rate for females is 18 mL/s.

Time to Maximum Flow: Time from onset of measurable flow to the maximum flow rate

Flow Time: Time that measureable flow occurs

Voided Volume: Total volume voided

 Filling Cystometry

Filling cystometry evaluates the filling phase of the micturition cycle and begins when filling is initiated and lasts until the urodynamicist gives the patient permission to void (Schäfer et al., 2002). Data gathered include bladder capacity, sensory awareness of bladder filling, bladder wall compliance (the ability to stretch and store at low volumes), and the presence or absence of overactive bladder contractions (Schäfer et al., 2002).

Simple versus Complex Cystometry

There are two types of filling cystometry, simple and complex. Simple cystometry is accomplished by placing a small dual lumen catheter into the bladder specifically designed for urodynamic testing; the catheter is equipped with a pressure transducer that permits measurement of bladder pressures throughout bladder filling. The pressures measured reflect both intra-abdominal events (such as coughing) that increase pressures within the bladder and changes in bladder pressures caused by bladder wall stiffness or by detrusor contractions. Because there is no way to differentiate between pressure changes caused by forces outside the bladder wall and those resulting from bladder contractions or bladder wall stiffness, simple cystometry is considered inaccurate and is rarely performed (Chapple et al., 2009).

Complex filling cystometry involves measurement of both intravesical and intra-abdominal pressures; the pressure-sensitive catheter in the bladder measures bladder pressures (Pves), and a pressure-sensitive catheter placed into the rectum measures abdominal pressures (Pabd). The computer then subtracts the abdominal pressures from the bladder pressures, and the subtracted pressure (Pdet) represents the pressures exerted by the detrusor muscle and bladder wall. Complex cystometry is currently considered the gold standard because it provides for differentiation between abdominal pressures and bladder wall pressures. Figure 4-4 provides an illustration of how the urodynamic parameters are monitored.

CLINICAL PEARL

In contrast to simple cystometry, complex filling cystometry involves measurement of both intravesical and intra-abdominal pressures and provides a more accurate representation of bladder filling and emptying.

Cystometry Technology

Many catheter and transducer technologies have entered the urodynamics marketplace over the years. Currently, there are three primary types. These include water-filled manometry system catheters with an external pressure

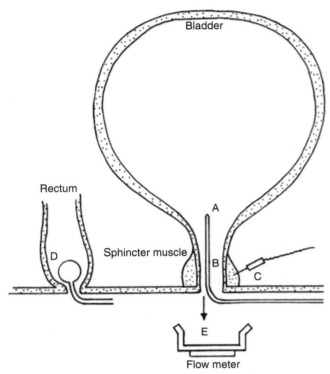

FIGURE 4-4. Urodynamics setup. Simultaneous monitoring of various urodynamics parameters is shown. Intravesical pressure minus intra-abdominal pressure will produce the detrusor pressure (Pdet). **A.** Intravesical pressure, Pves. **B.** Urethral sphincter pressure, Pur. **C.** Urethral sphincter electromyography. **D.** Intra-abdominal pressure, Pabd. **E.** Urine flow rate.

transducer (Figs. 4-5 and 4-6), catheter-mounted transducers (microtip, Fig. 4-7), and the newest air-charged catheter technology (Schäfer et al., 2002). Air-charged catheters have been marketed as easier to use, but many argue that the results are not comparable to those of water-filled manometry catheters, which are the gold standard according to the International Continence Society (Schäfer et al., 2002). A recent study demonstrated significant variation in pressure measurements obtained simultaneously by the different catheter systems (Digesu et al., 2014).

After the catheters are placed in the bladder and rectum, all pressures are zeroed to atmospheric pressure. The patient should be asked to cough to assure accurate transmission of intra-abdominal pressures, and baseline resting pressures should be obtained prior to the start of filling.

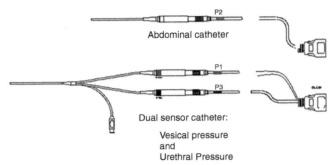

FIGURE 4-6. Examples of electronic urodynamic catheters.

The bladder is then filled with sterile water or saline, and the patient is asked to inform the urodynamicist of sensations throughout the filling cycle.

Data Provided by Filling Cystometry. As noted, filling cystometry provides data regarding bladder capacity, sensory awareness of bladder filling, detrusor stability, and bladder wall compliance.

Bladder Capacity
Cystometric bladder capacity differs from the patient's functional capacity, which is obtained from a voiding diary or frequency/volume chart. The cystometric capacity is the volume in the bladder at the end of filling cystometry (Abrams et al., 2003). This includes any residual urine as well as the filling solution (Abrams et al., 2003). A normal adult bladder can be filled to approximately 500 mL before a strong desire to void is felt. The determination of normal bladder capacity in children is based on the following formula (Chapple et al., 2009):

$$\text{Age}(\text{years}) \times 30 + 30 = \text{bladder capacity in mL}$$

Abnormally low capacity can be caused by chronic detrusor overactivity (DO), irritative disorders such as interstitial cystitis, or long-term indwelling catheter use resulting in a small contracted bladder. Neurologic conditions causing loss of sensory awareness of bladder filling can lead to abnormally high capacity, as can chronic distention (e.g., the patient with diabetic cystopathy).

Sensory Awareness of Bladder Filling
Definitions related to sensory awareness of bladder filling are listed in Table 4-2. There are no data to support specific volumes at which the individual should report first sensation or first desire to void; strong desire to void normally occurs at about 500 mL, as noted (Chapple et al., 2009).

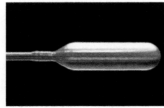

FIGURE 4-5. Examples of water-filled manometry catheters.

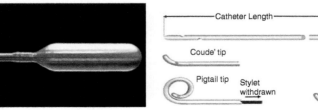

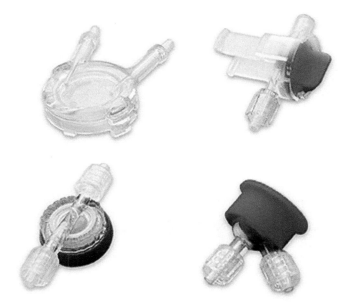

FIGURE 4-7. Examples of transducers that are used with water-filled catheters.

Increased bladder sensation occurs when, during filling, the patient experiences an early desire to void that is persistent, with or without urgency. This abnormally heightened awareness of bladder filling is typically seen in patients with overactive bladder, pelvic floor dysfunction, or interstitial cystitis. Reduced bladder sensation means that the desire to void is felt later in the filling phase than expected, but does occur, as opposed to absent bladder sensation, which indicates that the individual is completely unaware of bladder filling and does not experience the urge to void (Abrams et al., 2003). Diminished or absent awareness of bladder filling is usually seen in patients with chronic overdistention, diabetes, or lower motor neuron lesions.

TABLE 4-2 Sensations of Bladder Filling During Urodynamic Testing

Sensation	Definition
First sensation	When he/she first becomes aware of filling
First desire	When he/she would urinate at the next appropriate time, but it can be delayed
Strong desire	Continuing desire to void but without a fear of leaking
Urgency	Sudden strong desire to void
Maximum cystometric capacity	When the patient feels they can no longer delay voiding

Data from Abrams et al. (2003).

Bladder capacity and sensation are closely related. For example, the sensation of fullness reflects the volume of urine the individual is able to hold comfortably, and the volume associated with the sensation of being unable to delay voiding is considered maximum cystometric bladder capacity. Pain during filling is an abnormal sensation.

CLINICAL PEARL

Heightened awareness of bladder filling is typically seen in patients with overactive bladder, pelvic floor dysfunction, or interstitial cystitis. Reduced bladder sensation or absent awareness of bladder filling is usually seen in patients with chronic overdistention, diabetes, or lower motor neuron lesions.

Detrusor Stability

Stability of the detrusor refers to the absence or presence of involuntary detrusor contractions. During filling, the bladder should remain relaxed and there should be no contractile activity even if the urodynamicist employs provocative maneuvers such as asking the patient to cough or putting the patient's hand in water (Abrams et al., 2003). Absence of contractile activity is normal and indicative of a stable detrusor muscle. Any involuntary contractions of the detrusor are considered abnormal and are termed DO (Chapple et al., 2009). These involuntary contractions may be *phasic* (Fig. 4-8) or *terminal* (Fig. 4-9); phasic contractions occur during filling and may or may not result in urinary leakage, while terminal detrusor contractions typically result in complete loss of bladder volume and thereby terminate the study. When unstable bladder contractions cause urinary leakage, the condition is labeled detrusor overactivity incontinence (DOI), which may be neurogenic or idiopathic in origin (Abrams et al., 2003).

Figure 4-8 tracing shows phasic increases in Pves and Pdet. Since Pabd has no activity, the phasic contractions are the detrusor. The increase in EMG activity is likely a guarding reflex.

CLINICAL PEARL

When unstable bladder contractions cause urinary leakage, the condition is labeled detrusor overactivity incontinence (DOI), which may be neurogenic or idiopathic in origin.

The slow rise in both Pves and Pdet reflect an increase in intra-abdominal pressure with a Valsalva maneuver to assess for urodynamic stress in continence (Fig. 4-9).

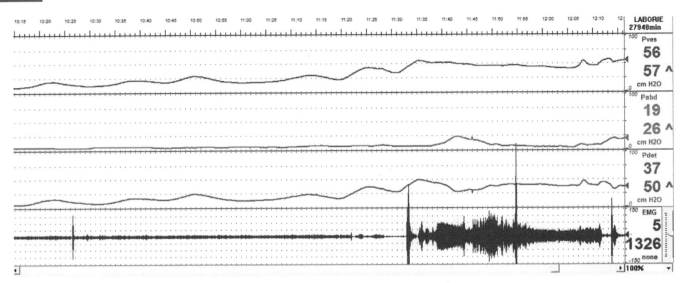

FIGURE 4-8. Phasic contractions occur during filling.

Bladder Wall Compliance

Bladder wall compliance describes the bladder's ability to stretch and to maintain low pressures throughout the filling cycle (Abrams et al., 2003; Chapple et al., 2009). The formula for determining bladder compliance is

$$\text{Compliance}\left(mL \,/\, cm \, H_2O\right)$$
$$= \text{change in volume}\left(\Delta V\right)$$
$$/\, \text{change in detrusor pressure}\left(\Delta Pdet\right)$$

The ICS recommends use of the following points for calculation of bladder compliance: the detrusor pressure at the point when filling begins and detrusor pressure at capacity or just before any detrusor contraction. Using the formula above, normal bladder compliance is >30 to 40 mL/cm H_2O; this means that the pressures within the bladder wall rise only 1 cm H_2O for every 30 to 40 mL of urine. The urodynamic tracing of a poorly compliant bladder would show a steady steep rise in bladder pressure, often with small infused volumes. When leakage occurs in association with poor bladder compliance, the pressure when the leakage occurs is called the detrusor leak point pressure (LPP). Poor compliance can be caused by long-standing obstruction, which may result from pelvic organ prolapse, an enlarged prostate, or neurogenic bladder with detrusor–sphincteric dyssynergia. A poorly compliant bladder with high filling pressures (i.e., ≥40 cm H_2O change from baseline) creates resistance to the inflow of urine and places the individual at great risk for upper tract damage (Chapple et al., 2009).

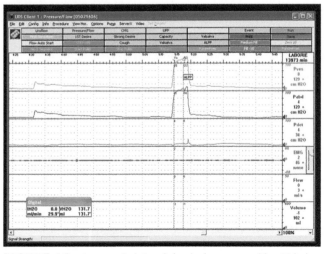

FIGURE 4-9. Increase in intra-abdominal pressure with a Valsalva maneuver to assess for SUI.

> **CLINICAL PEARL**
>
> Normal bladder compliance is > 30 to 40 mL/cm H_2O; this means that the pressures within the bladder wall rise only 1 cm H_2O for every 30 to 40 mL of urine; hostile bladder pressures (low compliance) can result in upper tract damage.

Figure 4-10 shows a slow, steady steep rise in Pves and Pdet pressures in response to filling. The elongated trabeculated bladder shape is typical of obstructive neurological disease, particularly lower motor neuron lesions. The compliance change is >40 cm H_2O, which is considered a *hostile bladder pressure* (Dickinson, 2007).

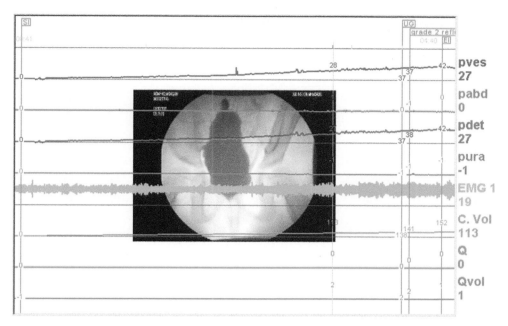

pves	27
pabd	0
pdet	27
pura	-1
EMG 1	19
C. Vol	113
Q	0
Qvol	1

FIGURE 4-10. A slow steady steep rise in Pves and Pdet in response to filling. Bladder is elongated and trabeculated typical of obstructive neurologic disease. Compliance change is >40 cm H₂O, which is considered a hostile bladder.

Pressure Flow Studies

When cystometric capacity is reached (i.e., when the patient states he/she can no longer delay voiding), permission to void is given. This begins the voiding phase of urodynamics, which is known as a pressure flow study. The patient voids into the uroflow commode with the pressure-sensitive catheter still in place in the bladder; thus, the pressure flow study allows for simultaneous measurement of urine flow and pressures generated by detrusor muscle contraction.

Urine Flow Pattern

The flow is defined as either continuous or intermittent, and a continuous flow pattern is further defined as smooth or fluctuating (Abrams et al., 2003). A pressure flow study is essential in assessing incomplete bladder emptying, because it provides the answer to the following question: *Is the bladder contracting effectively and working hard to pass urine through a bladder outlet obstruction, or is the detrusor contraction inadequate?* (Chapple et al., 2009).

Uroflow measurements have been discussed previously, and the data provided are listed in Box 4-2. Maximum flow rates should be 30 to 35 mL/s in women, over 25 mL/s in men under 40 years of age, and over 15 mL/s in men over 60 years of age (Chapple et al., 2009).

Detrusor Contraction Strength

The pressure flow study provides data regarding the strength of detrusor contraction in addition to data regarding urinary flow (Box 4-3). A normal bladder should empty fully with a maximum detrusor pressure of 25 to 50 cm H₂O.

Normal detrusor function involves a voluntary sustained contraction that results in continuous flow of urine and that empties the bladder over a normal time span. Detrusor underactivity is manifested by a poorly sustained contraction and a prolonged flow of urine, while BOO is characterized by high voiding pressures and low flow rates as seen in Figure 4-11. An acontractile detrusor typically has a pressure-flow pattern consistent with Valsalva voiding, as illustrated in Figure 4-12. An explosive flow pattern with high maximum flow rates and low pressures likely indicates very little outlet resistance and may be seen in patients with stress urinary incontinence or postprostatectomy incontinence.

In Figure 4-11, the patient is voluntarily voiding. Pves and Pdet pressures begin to rise, quite some time before flow is initiated. EMG remains quiet during voiding, signaling normal sphincter relaxation and a synergic voiding event. Flow is very slow and poor despite a very high-pressure contraction (so high that it bleeds into the next pressure channel on the tracing). This is consistent with BOO.

BOX 4-3. Pressure Measurements during Urodynamic Testing

Opening pressure: Pressure immediately before the detrusor contraction

Opening time: Time from the rise in detrusor pressure to the start of urine flow

Maximum pressure: Maximum pressure measured during voiding

Pressure at maximum flow: Pressure measured at Q_{max}

Closing pressure: Pressure at the end of urine flow

Data from Abrams et al. (2003).

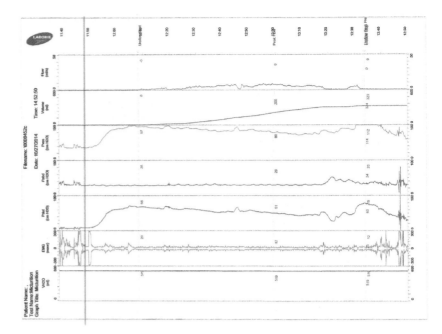

FIGURE 4-11. Example of BOO with very slow flow and high-pressure detrusor contraction.

This patient was an elderly male with an enlarged prostate, but the same pattern could be seen in a female with significant pelvic organ prolapse or following a surgical procedure for stress incontinence that resulted in excessive urethral resistance.

CLINICAL PEARL

The pressure flow study provides data regarding the strength of detrusor contraction in addition to data regarding urinary flow. A normal bladder should empty fully with a maximum detrusor pressure of 25 to 50 cm H_2O.

In Figure 4-12, there is no contraction of the detrusor. The Pves and Pabd pressures mimic each other, indicating that the increase in pressure is due to abdominal muscle contraction as opposed to bladder contraction (a Valsalva voiding event). The increase in EMG activity can also be consistent with Valsalva voiding. The flow pattern is intermittent, reflecting bursts of urine flow coinciding with Valsalva.

Electromyography

Historically performed using needle electrodes, most electromyogram (EMG) studies are now done with surface electrodes, similar to those used for EKG. Surface electrodes record the total electrical output from the pelvic floor muscles (Chapple et al., 2009). During the filling phase, it is normal to see a slight increase in EMG activity; this is known as the "guarding reflex." During voiding, the pelvic floor muscles should relax, producing little or no EMG activity. Increased

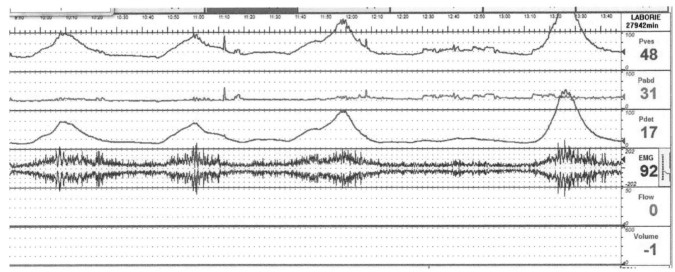

FIGURE 4-12. Phasic detrusor sphincter dyssynergia; EMG rises with each detrusor contraction causing obstruction at the urethral sphincter and impeding bladder emptying. Increase in Pves and Pdet mimic each other. EMG activity increases as Pdet rises in an attempt to empty the bladder.

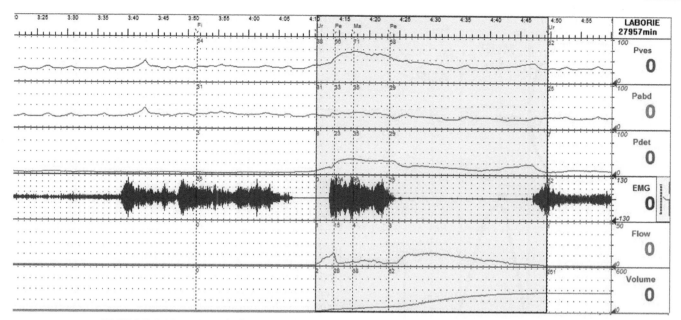

FIGURE 4-13. Pves and Pdet pressures rise and at the same time EMG activity increases (rather than relaxing as is normal) and results in bladder neck obstruction and obstructed voiding.

EMG activity during voiding is abnormal. If it is continual, it may be due to dysfunctional voiding, detrusor sphincter dyssynergia, or Valsalva artifact (apparent increase in sphincter activity during Valsalva voiding caused by use of surface electrodes to measure pelvic floor activity, as opposed to use of needle electrodes that measure actual sphincteric activity).

Dysfunctional voiding or pelvic floor dysfunction is manifested by an intermittent flow pattern, intermittent detrusor contractions, and increased EMG activity during voiding in neurologically normal individuals. Dysfunctional voiding can be a learned behavior or can be due to pelvic floor muscle dysfunction. Pelvic floor dysfunction is characterized by high tone or spasm of the pelvic floor musculature, which can result in various lower urinary tract symptoms. The same pattern in those with a neurologic diagnosis is called detrusor sphincter dyssynergia (Abrams et al., 2003) (Fig. 4-13). This is commonly seen in patients with certain spinal cord injuries and in multiple sclerosis and occurs when the sphincter fails to relax during the emptying phase due to loss of normal neural control.

CLINICAL PEARL

During voiding, the pelvic floor muscles should relax, producing little or no EMG activity. Increased EMG activity during voiding is abnormal. If it is continual, it may be due to dysfunctional voiding, detrusor sphincter dyssynergia, or Valsalva artifact.

In Figure 4-13, Pves and Pdet pressures rise during a voiding event, whether voiding is voluntary or involuntary. At the same time, the EMG activity increases significantly, thus resulting in BOO and obstructed voiding. This places the patient at risk for incomplete emptying, urinary tract infections, and vesicoureteral reflux.

Urethral Pressure Profiles

A urethral pressure profile (UPP) provides a graphic representation of the pressures along the entire length of the urethra (Abrams et al., 2003). Urethral pressures can be measured at rest, during stress maneuvers (cough, strain), or during voiding. The UPP is obtained by utilizing a pulling apparatus or withdrawal unit to precisely and steadily withdraw a pressure-sensitive catheter through the urethra (Fig. 4-14). A resting UPP provides data regarding urethral resistance during the filling cycle; it is thought that a low

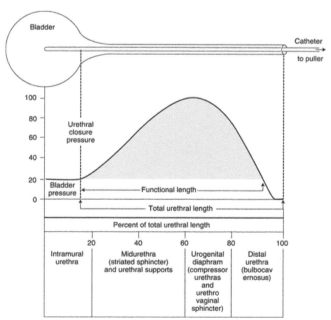

FIGURE 4-14. Correlation of mid-urethral anatomy with urodynamic anatomy (EMG).

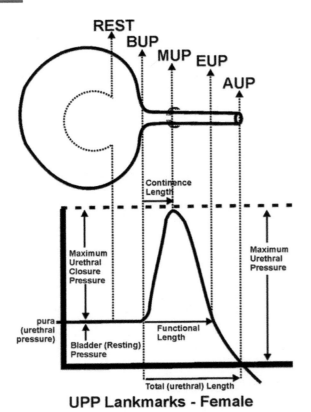

UPP Lankmarks - Female

FIGURE 4-15. Urethral pressure profile data points. REST, resting pressure; BUP, baseline urethral pressure; MUP, maximum urethral pressure; EUP, end urethral pressure; AUP, atmospheric urethral pressure.

maximum urethral closure pressure (Fig. 4-15) is associated with low outlet resistance and may help to confirm a diagnosis of stress urinary incontinence. The resting UPP is the most common measurement in clinical practice. In more advanced urodynamic hands, a voiding UPP may be used to indicate the site and pressure relationship of a urethral obstruction (Chapple et al., 2009).

Abdominal Leak Point Pressure

In the early 1990s, clinicians and urodynamicists began to look for alternatives to UPP studies. There was a need to identify patients with intrinsic sphincter deficiency who needed surgical procedures that would provide increased urethral resistance and who would *not* benefit from procedures designed simply to support the bladder neck. It was thought that the UPP, although correlated with poor urethral function, was cumbersome and not easily reproducible (Dickinson, 2007). This led to the development of the abdominal LPP study, which measures the level of intra-abdominal pressure required to push urine across a (partially) closed sphincter.

The abdominal LPP is assessed during the course of the filling cystometry; the patient is placed in the upright position (seated or standing) and is asked to perform coughing and straining maneuvers at certain standardized bladder volumes (Fig. 4-16). The abdominal LPP is easily reproducible and quantifies the ability of the urethra to resist increases in abdominal pressure. In Figure 4-16, the

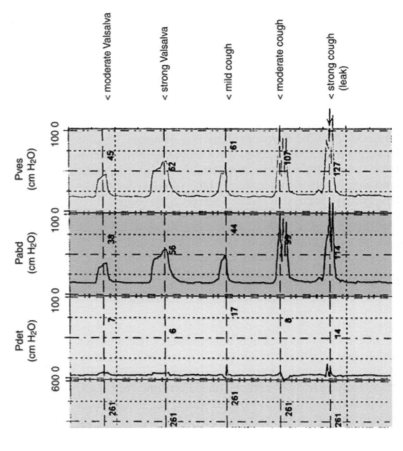

FIGURE 4-16. The abdominal leak point pressure (LPP) is 114 cm H_2O (the abdominal pressure at which the patient leaked urine).

abdominal LPP is 114 cm H$_2$O (the abdominal pressure at which the patient leaked urine).

 ## Video Urodynamics

Video urodynamic testing involves filling cystometry utilizing contrast medium and simultaneous use of fluoroscopic evaluation. The addition of radiology equipment is quite costly, and many offices do not have this capability. So when is video urodynamic testing recommended? Those with known or suspected neurologic disorders may benefit from the more complex video urodynamic investigation. Complex cases involving lower urinary tract symptoms not responding to medical therapy, suspected primary bladder neck obstruction, suspected or known pelvic floor dysfunction, and/or failure of previous operative procedures may also benefit from video urodynamics (Chapple et al., 2009; Winters et al., 2012). Video urodynamics permit assessment of vesicoureteral reflux in an individual with neurologic disease and can also be used to identify the level of urethral obstruction.

CLINICAL PEARL

Video urodynamics is usually reserved for complex cases: those with known or suspected neurologic disorders; when lower urinary tract symptoms have not responded to medical therapy; if primary bladder neck obstruction is suspected; if pelvic floor dysfunction is known or suspected; and/or when previous operative procedures have failed.

 ## Further Diagnostics

In evaluation of lower urinary tract dysfunction, urinalysis for evaluation of hematuria, proteinuria, glucose, and infection is considered standard (Rosenberg et al., 2013) and is addressed in Chapter 3 (Primary Assessment). Abnormal findings should prompt further testing or referral. Measurement of postvoid residual either by bladder scan or catheterization is indicated whenever there are concerns about the patient's ability to empty effectively. Renal ultrasound can provide a noninvasive means of evaluating for hydronephrosis and stones (Hanno et al., 2007). Cystoscopy not only permits evaluation of the bladder mucosa for malignancy, stones, or foreign bodies but also provides visual confirmation of trabeculation (caused by overwork of the detrusor), bladder neck

abnormalities, and presence or absence of bladder diverticulum. Patients should be referred for these additional studies whenever there are concerns about renal function or bladder complications. Laboratory studies may also be needed to assess for renal damage.

Conclusion

Urodynamic testing is considered an advanced assessment reserved for patients with complex histories or for those who have not responded to initial treatment. It provides a graphic picture of bladder and sphincter function and, combined with patient history and presenting symptoms, can be very helpful in identifying the cause of voiding or pelvic floor dysfunction.

REFERENCES

Abrams, P., Cardozo, L., Fall, M., et al. (2003). The standardisation of terminology in lower urinary tract function: Report from the standardisation sub-committee of the International Continence Society. *Urology, 61*, 37–49. doi:10.1016/S0090-4295(02)02243-4.

Chapple, C. R., MacDiarmid, S. A., & Patel, A. (2009). *Urodynamics made easy* (3rd ed.). Edinburgh, UK: Elsevier Churchill Livingstone.

Dickinson, T. (2007). Demystifying leak point pressures: The valuable tool for functional assessment. *Urologic Nursing, 27*(2), 128–132. Retrieved June 29, 2014, from http://eds.b.ebscohost.com.libproxy.usouthal.edu/ehost/pdfviewer/pdfviewer?vid=9&sid=48b26921-909e-4477-82d5-8203b6afbdd1%40sessionmgr114&hid=109

Digesu, G. A., Derpapas, A., Robshaw, P., et al. (2014). Are measurements of water-filled and air-charged catheters the same in urodynamics? *International Urogynecology Journal, 25*, 123–130. doi:10.1007/s00192-013-2182-z.

Gürbuz, C., Güner, B., Gökhan, A., et al. (2013). Are prophylactic antibiotics necessary for urodynamic study? *Kaohsiung Journal of Medical Sciences, 29*, 325–329. Dx.doi.org/10.1016/j.kjms.2012.06.001.

Hanno, P. M., Malkowicz, S. B., & Wein, A. J. (2007). *Penn Clinical Manual of Urology*. Philadelphia, PA: Saunders Elsevier.

Onur, R., Özden, M., Orhan, I., et al. (2004). Incidence of bacteraemia after urodynamic study. *Journal of Hospital Infection, 57*, 241–244. doi:10.1016/j.jhin.2004.03.025.

Rosenberg, M. T., Staskin, D., Riley, J., et al. (2013). The evaluation and treatment of prostate related LUTS in the primary care setting: The next STEP. *Current Urology Report, 14*, 595–605. doi:10.1007/s11934-013-0371-4.

Schäfer, W., Abrams, P., Liao, L., et al. (2002). Good urodynamic practices: Uroflowmetry, filling cystometry and pressure-flow studies. *Neurourology and Urodynamics, 21*, 261–274. doi:10.1002/nau.10066.

Wein, A. J., Kavoussi, L. R., Novick, A. C., et al. (2012). Urodynamic and video-urodynamic evaluation of the lower urinary tract. In A. J. Wein, L. R. Kavoussi, A. C. Novick, et al. (Eds.), *Campbell-Walsh urology* (Chapter 62, pp. 1847–1870). Philadelphia, PA: Elsevier/Saunders.

Winters, J. C., Dmochowski, R. R., Goldman, H. B., et al. (2012). Urodynamic studies in adults: AUA/SUFU guideline. *Journal of Urology, 188*, 2464–2472. doi:10.1016/j.juro.2012.09.081.

QUESTIONS

1. A continence nurse orders urodynamic testing for a patient with urinary incontinence. Which statement accurately describes an aspect of this type of testing?
   A. Urodynamic testing evaluates the filling and voiding phases of the micturition cycle.
   B. Urodynamic testing provides information regarding the functionality of the upper urinary tract.
   C. Urodynamic testing is noninvasive and relatively inexpensive in the United States.
   D. Urodynamic testing can be used to detect the presence of a urinary tract infection or hematuria.

2. Which of the following describes normal uroflowmetry results?
   A. Low velocity flat flow rate
   B. Intermittent burst of flow
   C. Plateau pattern of flow
   D. Bell-shaped curve of flow

3. The continence nurse records test results for a patient experiencing incontinence and notes the following data: bladder capacity, sensory awareness of bladder filling, detrusor stability, and bladder wall compliance. Which test provides this information?
   A. Electromyogram
   B. Filling cystometry
   C. Pressure flow study
   D. Urethral pressure profile

4. What is the major advantage of using complex cystometry as opposed to simple cystometry?
   A. It provides for differentiation between abdominal pressures and bladder wall pressure.
   B. It is noninvasive and is often used as an initial screening tool for lower urinary tract (voiding) dysfunction.
   C. It determines if the bladder is contracting effectively or if the detrusor contraction is inadequate.
   D. It provides data regarding the strength of detrusor contraction in addition to data regarding urinary flow.

5. Which catheter used for performing filling cystometry is considered to be the gold standard according to the International Continence Society?
   A. Air-charged catheters
   B. Catheter-mounted transducers
   C. Water-filled manometry system catheters
   D. Suprapubic urinary catheter

6. The continence nurse is assessing the bladder capacity of a child who is 12 years old. What is the normal capacity in milliliters for this patient?
   A. 300 mL
   B. 360 mL
   C. 390 mL
   D. 430 mL

7. Which patient would the continence nurse place at higher risk for reduced bladder sensation?
   A. A patient with overactive bladder
   B. A patient with pelvic floor dysfunction
   C. A patient with interstitial cystitis
   D. A patient with diabetes

8. Which condition occurring during filling is indicative of a normal, stable detrusor muscle?
   A. Absence of bladder sensation
   B. Absence of contractile activity
   C. Phasic contractions of the detrusor
   D. High filling pressures

9. The continence nurse records bladder compliance in a patient as 40 mL/cm H_2O. What does this information signify?
   A. High potential for upper tract damage.
   B. High potential for lower tract damage.
   C. Risk for pelvic floor dysfunction.
   D. This is a normal bladder compliance result.

10. A continence nurse is performing the pressure flow study involved in urodynamic testing. What condition does this test assess?
    A. Sensory awareness of bladder filling
    B. Bladder wall compliance
    C. Bladder emptying
    D. Bladder capacity

11. Which condition is indicative of normal voiding patterns tested by electromyogram?
    A. Intermittent flow pattern
    B. Tensing of the pelvic floor muscles increasing EMG activity during voiding
    C. Dramatic increase in EMG activity during filling phase
    D. Little or no EMG activity during voiding

12. Which urodynamic testing provides the most accurate assessment of the ability of the urethral sphincter to resist increases in abdominal pressure such as cough or straining?
    A. Urethral pressure profile
    B. Abdominal leak point pressure
    C. Video urodynamics
    D. Pressure flow study

ANSWERS: 1.**A**, 2.**D**, 3.**B**, 4.**A**, 5.**C**, 6.**C**, 7.**D**, 8.**B**, 9.**D**, 10.**C**, 11.**D**, 12.**B**

CHAPTER 5

Overactive Bladder/Urgency UI
Pathology, Presentation, Diagnosis, and Management

William Gibson and Adrian Wagg

OBJECTIVES

1. Explain how bladder and sphincter functions change with aging and how these changes affect voiding patterns and continence.

2. Describe current theories regarding the etiology and pathology of overactive bladder with/without urgency incontinence.

3. Describe indications and guidelines for each of the following: urge suppression strategies; bladder retraining; anticholinergic medications; topical estrogen; percutaneous tibial nerve stimulation and sacral nerve stimulation (neuromodulation).

Topic Outline

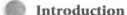
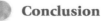

Introduction

Overactive bladder (OAB) is a clinically defined symptom complex that consists of urinary urgency, with or without urgency incontinence, usually with increased daytime frequency and nocturia in the absence of urinary tract infection or other obvious pathology (Abrams et al., 2009). The single defining symptom, said to drive the others, is urinary *urgency*, a sudden, overwhelming desire to pass urine that is difficult to defer (Haylen et al., 2010) and often accompanied by fear of leakage. This is different from the normal *urge* to void, the physiological sensation that can be deferred until it is convenient to do so.

> **CLINICAL PEARL**
>
> OAB is a symptom complex involving urgency (with or without urgency incontinence), frequency, and nocturia in the absence of UTI or other obvious pathology.

OAB is a clinical diagnosis, made on the basis of a detailed history, and is not reliant on invasive tests such as multichannel cystometry. OAB with urgency incontinence denotes the symptoms of OAB associated with urinary leakage; the leakage is the result of involuntary bladder (detrusor) contractions. Not all individuals with OAB have objectively documented involuntary detrusor contractions; indeed, only approximately 60% of people with clinical OAB will have demonstrable detrusor overactivity (DO), the observation of involuntary detrusor contractions during filling cystometry. Furthermore, 36% of people with DO on filling cystometry *do not* have symptomatic OAB (Hashim & Abrams, 2006). Lower urinary tract symptoms (LUTS), of which urinary frequency, nocturia, and urinary urgency are the most prevalent, are common in the general population.

Prevalence and Incidence

In the EPIC (European Prospective Investigation into Cancer and Nutrition) study of adults over 40, based upon a structured telephone interview of over 19,000 people from four European countries and Canada, 19.1% (95% CI: 17.5 to 20.7) of community dwelling men and 18.3% (16.9 to 19.6) of women over the age of 60 years indicated that they had urinary urgency, and 2.5% (1.9 to 3.1) of men and 2.5% (1.9 to 3.0) of women indicated that they had urgency incontinence (Irwin et al., 2006). Similarly, a population-based survey of 5,204 adults in the United States, the National Overactive BLadder Evaluation (NOBLE) study, found an overall prevalence of OAB of 16% in men and 16.9% in women; prevalence increased with age (Stewart et al., 2003). More recent reports from longitudinal studies in cohorts of men and women have illustrated the age-related increase in LUTS over time, including urgency and urgency incontinence. In the study of women, 2,911 women responded to a self-administered postal questionnaire in 1991, and 1,408 of

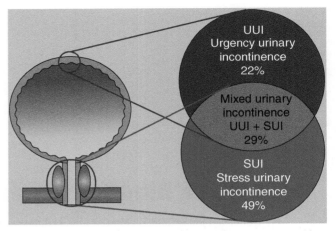

FIGURE 5-1. Definition and classification of UI. UUI occurs with a strong sudden and uncontrollable desire to urinate as a result of involuntary detrusor contractions; overactive bladder is defined by the symptom of urgency with or without urgency incontinence; SUI is involuntary leakage on effort or exertion or on sneezing or coughing, as a result of insufficient urethral closure pressure.

these women replied to the same survey in 2007. Over that time, the prevalence of urinary incontinence (UI), OAB, and nocturia increased by 13%, 9%, and 20%, respectively. The proportion of women with OAB and urgency incontinence increased from 6% to 16% (Wennberg et al., 2009). In the study of men (Malmsten et al., 2010), 7,763 responded to a self-completed postal questionnaire in 1992, and 3,257 responded to the same survey in 2009. In a similar fashion to the women, prevalence of UI and OAB increased from 4.5% to 10.5% and from 15.6% to 44.4%, respectively.

Thus, it is clear that OAB symptoms are prevalent in both men and women, especially in those in the older age range. Figure 5-1 shows the proportion of urgency and stress urinary incontinence in women; Figure 5-2 reflects the spectrum of OAB and illustrates that it often coexists with stress urinary incontinence (SUI), the condition termed *mixed urinary incontinence*. Note that overactive

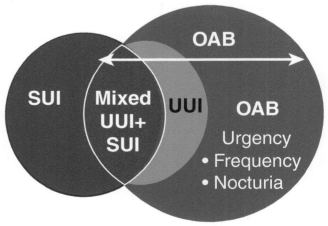

FIGURE 5-2. Spectrum of OAB.

bladder is defined by the symptom of urgency with or without urinary incontinence (UUI), usually with frequency and nocturia.

Pathology

Following the development of urinary continence in the second or third year of life, micturition should only occur at a time and in a place of one's own choosing, when it is convenient and socially acceptable to do so. The bladder has only two modes—storage and voiding. The switch between the two is under conscious control. The brain receives sensory information generated by both the urothelium and detrusor muscle via the pudendal, hypogastric, and pelvic nerves. Afferent signals from the bladder may arise from the urothelium, the detrusor muscle, or both (Fig. 5-3).

Urothelial Hypothesis

The urothelium is not, as previously thought, merely a passive barrier separating urine from person. It is a highly active organ, responding to stretch and to substances in the urine by expressing numerous signaling molecules including acetyl choline (ACh), nitric oxide, prostaglandins, and adenosine triphosphate (ATP); the multiple receptors in the urothelium include alpha A_1 and β_3 adrenoreceptors, muscarinic (principally M_2) (Bschleipfer et al., 2007) and nicotinic (Beckel & Birder, 2012) receptors, and purinergic (Rapp et al., 2005), cannabinoid (Tyagi et al., 2009), and vallinoid receptors (Birder & Andersson, 2013).

The urothelium is innervated by afferent and autonomic efferent nerves, and as such the urothelium can be thought of as a "first responder" to mechanical and noxious stimulation associated with bladder filling. In addition, there is a suburothelial layer of myofibroblasts that may respond to ATP produced by the urothelium, and the detrusor muscle itself has stretch receptors. Thus, the urothelium, suburothelial layer, and detrusor act as a sensory organ that provides information to the brain on the fullness of the bladder and communicates the need to void. In overactive bladder, there is evidence that this system is dysfunctional. For example, in vitro urothelium taken from overactive bladders releases three times the

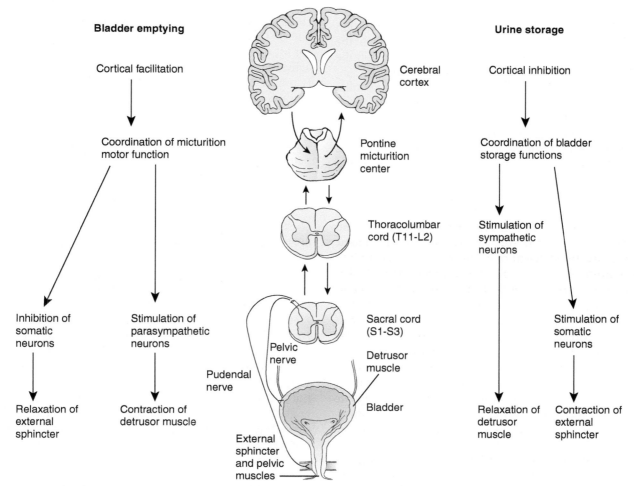

FIGURE 5-3. Pathways and central nervous system centers involved in the control of bladder emptying (*left*) and storage (*right*) functions. Efferent pathways for micturition (*left*) and urine storage (*right*) also are shown.

amount of ATP released from normal urothelium when exposed to capsaicin (Birder et al., 2013).

CLINICAL PEARL

The exact pathology leading to OAB and urgency incontinence is not clearly defined; theories include abnormal sensory input regarding bladder filling and/or abnormalities in detrusor muscle function.

Myogenic Hypothesis

There is also evidence that the detrusor muscle itself is abnormal in overactive bladder. In several species, including humans, the detrusor muscle produces spontaneous microcontractions, the amplitude of which increases with increasing bladder volume (Coolsaet, 1985). The physiological role, if any, of these contractions is unknown, and they are not detectable by standard urodynamic measurement (Chacko et al., 2014). There is evidence that these contractions are exaggerated in DO; isolated strips of detrusor taken from patients with urodynamically proven DO demonstrate higher levels of intracellular calcium, greater oscillations in the levels of calcium, and more spontaneously active cells than normal bladder (Sui et al., 2009).

Alterations in regulation of contractile protein function have also been implicated in the pathogenesis of DO. In the presence of bladder outlet obstruction, proteins within the detrusor muscle undergo chemical changes that increase contractile strength (Su et al., 2003); it is conceivable that similar processes are involved in idiopathic DO. Denervation is frequently observed in detrusor muscle biopsies from overactive bladders, and it has been proposed that partial denervation of detrusor myocytes leads to increased coupling between cells and therefore increased excitability (Mills et al., 2000). This may lead to the spread throughout the detrusor of contractions normally limited to isolated parts of the bladder, which could be interpreted as an urgent desire to void.

These two models of OAB are termed the urothelial and myogenic hypotheses, respectively. The reality is likely to be that they are both important in the generation of urgency.

The sensation of needing to void is processed by numerous areas of the brain, including the pons (Barrington's nucleus), periaqueductal gray matter, hypothalamus, and the medial frontal cortex (Fowler et al., 2008). These areas allow an individual to assess the need to void and the convenience and social acceptability of voiding. In children with primary nocturnal enuresis, there is evidence of underdevelopment of continence-related areas, in particular the thalamus, the frontal lobe, the anterior cingulate cortex, and the insula (Lei et al., 2012); in older adults, age-related changes to the brain are associated with overactive bladder symptoms (Tadic et al., 2010).

OAB may therefore arise from an increase in afferent signals from the bladder to the brain, from a failure of the brain to correctly handle these signals and control the bladder, or from both.

OAB Risk factors

Risk factors that have been identified in several studies include

- Increasing age
- Obesity
- Lifestyle
- Diet
- Urinary outflow obstruction
- Childhood continence issues
- Pregnancy
- Ethnicity

Age

Age is a key risk factor as the prevalence of all LUTS rises with age (Irwin et al., 2006), and numerous studies, both cross-sectional (Hannestad et al., 2000; Irwin et al., 2006) and longitudinal (Irwin et al., 2010), support this statement. Numerous changes occur in the bladder in association with aging. These include increased collagen content, changes to gap junctions, increased space between myocytes, and changes in the sensitivity of sensory afferents (Siroky, 2004). ATP-dependent detrusor contractions rise with age, whereas cholinergic-dependent contractions decline (Yoshida et al., 2004). There is also a reduction in the number of detrusor M_3 receptors (Mansfield et al., 2005). Additionally, the aging brain is less able to suppress the sensation of urgency (Griffiths et al., 2009). The presence of white matter hyperintensities in the brain is associated with LUTS in older adults (Kuchel et al., 2009), and there is a correlation between vascular risk factors such as hypertension and hypercholesterolemia and incontinence (Ponholzer et al., 2006). OAB, particularly in the elderly, may be considered as a neurological as much as a urological disease.

Obesity

Obesity is a strong risk factor for UI, although the effect is greater for SUI than OAB (Subak et al., 2009).

Lifestyle Factors and Diet

Contrary to popular belief, there is no consistent association between consumption of tea or coffee with OAB (Tettamanti et al., 2011), although "high" caffeine intake (over 400 mg/day) has been shown to correlate with DO (Arya et al., 2000), and a relationship between the consumption of "diet" soft drinks and OAB has been demonstrated (Cartwright et al., 2007). There is also a reported but inconsistent association with smoking (Dallosso et al., 2003; Maserejian et al., 2012; Tahtinen et al., 2011) as well as other diet and lifestyle factors and OAB. In a model tracking incidence of OAB over a period of 3 years, low physical exercise levels and a high-carbohydrate diet, in conjunction with obesity and diabetes, were associated with doubling of the risk for developing OAB (McGrother et al., 2012).

Urinary Outflow Obstruction

There also appears to be a relationship between bladder outflow obstruction (BOO) and DO (see also Chapter 6, Urinary Retention). Spontaneous detrusor contractions are associated with BOO in animal models (Su et al., 2003), and BOO causes detrusor hypertrophy and hyperactivity (Zhang et al., 2004). In humans, there is a reported association between BOO and DO; the relief of BOO with prostatectomy has been shown to reduce DO. The histological detrusor denervation associated with BOO appears to improve after prostatectomy, and DO can be induced by surgical treatment for SUI, if the procedure results in some degree of bladder outlet obstruction (Brading & Turner, 1994).

Childhood Continence Issues

Childhood continence problems, including urgency and enuresis, are also strong risk factors for the development of OAB in adult life; children who wet the bed are more than twice as likely to have OAB as adults than those who do not (Fitzgerald et al., 2006).

Pregnancy

Symptoms of urinary urgency are also common during pregnancy, with increasing prevalence as pregnancy progresses (Liang et al., 2012).

Ethnicity

There is mixed evidence for the influence of ethnicity. The multinational EpiLUTS study suggested a higher prevalence in Hispanic and African American men but no differences in women (Coyne et al., 2009), and studies in hospital populations have found no differences in prevalence between different ethnic groups (Finkelstein et al., 2008). A Swedish twin study suggested genetic influences on UI, frequency, and nocturia but not on the development of OAB (Wennberg et al., 2011).

Evaluation/Clinical Presentation

Up to half of people with significant LUTS will never present to health care professionals (Irwin et al., 2008; Shaw et al., 2001). LUTS, particularly incontinence, are associated with high levels of embarrassment, not just of wetness and odor but also of embarrassment related to going to the toilet frequently, fear of being seen to be "unclean" or being mocked and, in men, a fear of being thought to be impotent (Elstad et al., 2010). Patients also fail to seek help because they believe that incontinence is a normal part of aging, an unavoidable consequence of childbirth, or that UI and LUTS are untreatable (Shaw et al., 2001).

As such, it is imperative that health care professionals specifically ask people at risk of LUTS/UI if they have any bladder problems; this includes older people, women postchildbirth, and those with neurological disease such as multiple sclerosis.

Clinical Symptoms

The classic triad of symptoms associated with OAB are urgency, frequency, and nocturia.

Urgency

The hallmark symptom of OAB is *urinary urgency*. Patients report a sudden sensation of needing to empty their bladder, which they struggle to suppress; they are unable to delay voiding until a socially convenient time. This sensation is often accompanied by the fear of leaking urine or by actual incontinence. Individuals often report increased daytime frequency; some of these findings reflect adaptive behaviors, such as "going frequently, just in case" in an attempt to avoid symptoms and unplanned toilet visits. The volume of urine passed is usually relatively small, often as little as 50 to 75 mL because of the frequency of voiding, but typically results in complete bladder emptying.

> **CLINICAL PEARL**
>
> The hallmark symptom of OAB is urgency, the inability to delay voiding until a socially acceptable time.

Frequency

It is generally accepted that urinary *frequency* becomes bothersome if it occurs more than 13 times per day, although this has not been formally evaluated in research trials, which use a diurnal frequency of eight as a defining criterion. Moreover, frequency of voiding is subjective, and for some people, every 2 hours is interpreted as "frequency." In all cases, bladder diaries are invaluable as a baseline assessment tool.

Nocturia

The complaint of waking at night one or more times to void is a particularly bothersome symptom. It is important to differentiate true nocturia, where the desire to void causes the person to wake, from waking for another reason and deciding to visit the toilet. Most people will accept nocturia once per night, but waking twice or more is associated with increasing levels of bother (Bing et al., 2006).

The symptom associated with most bother has been reported variably as UI during sexual intercourse (Coyne et al., 2009), urgency incontinence (Liberman et al., 2001), or urinary urgency (Coyne et al., 2004), depending on the study and the framing of the question.

> **CLINICAL PEARL**
>
> The most bothersome symptom associated with OAB varies and includes urinary incontinence during intercourse, urgency incontinence, and urinary urgency.

Other Symptoms

As well as urgency, frequency, and nocturia, patients with OAB will often report symptoms such as toilet mapping, where they will make a conscious effort to know the locations of facilities when out in public, and latch-key (or garage door) incontinence, which is the sensation of a sudden onset of urgency at the point of putting the key in the door when arriving home. Other anecdotal exacerbating factors to explore are cold weather, running water, and psychological stress.

History

As already mentioned, the diagnosis of overactive bladder is a clinical one and is not reliant on any diagnostic tests. The National Institute of Clinical Excellence (NICE) issued guidelines in 2013, which state "history taking is regarded as the cornerstone of assessment of UI" (NICE, 2013).

At the end of the initial assessment, a diagnosis of the type and cause of UI and its impact on the patient should be made without needing further investigation.

The history should cover the following:

- General health
- Fluid intake amounts and types, particularly carbonated and caffeinated drinks
- Diet
- Smoking habits
- A detailed obstetric history including number and mode of delivery or deliveries
- All prescribed and over-the-counter medications taken
- Medical conditions that predispose to incontinence (Table 5-1), which should be treated, if possible, to ameliorate the impact on continence status

TABLE 5-1 Associated Conditions Affecting Continence Status

Condition	Impact	Mitigating Factors
Diabetes mellitus	Poor control can cause polyuria and precipitate or exacerbate incontinence; also associated with increased likelihood of urgency incontinence and diabetic neuropathic bladder	Better control of diabetes can reduce osmotic diuresis and associated polyuria and improve incontinence
Degenerative joint disease	Can impair mobility and precipitate UUI	Optimal pharmacologic and nonpharmacologic pain management can improve mobility and toileting ability
Chronic pulmonary disease	Associated cough can cause SUI	Cough suppression can reduce stress incontinence and cough-induced UUI
Congestive heart failure Lower extremity venous insufficiency	Redistribution of edema when lying flat increases nighttime urine production and can contribute to nocturia and UI	Optimizing pharmacologic management of congestive heart failure, sodium restriction, support stockings, leg elevation, and a late-afternoon dose of a rapid-acting diuretic may reduce nocturnal polyuria and associated nocturia and nighttime UI
Sleep apnea	May increase nighttime urine production by increasing production of atrial natriuretic peptide	Diagnosis and treatment of sleep apnea, usually with continuous positive airway pressure devices, may improve the condition and reduce nocturnal polyuria and associated nocturia and UI
Stroke	Can precipitate urgency and less often retention; also impairs mobility	UI after an acute stroke often resolves with rehabilitation; persistent UI should be further evaluated Regular toileting assistance essential for those with persistent mobility impairment
Parkinson's disease	Associated with UUI; also causes impaired mobility and cognition in late stages	Optimizing management may improve mobility and improve UI. Regular toileting assistance is essential for those with mobility and cognitive impairment in late-stage disease
Normal pressure hydrocephalus	Presents with UI, along with gait and cognitive impairments	Patients presenting with all three symptoms should be considered for brain imaging to rule out this condition, as it may improve with a ventricular–peritoneal shunt
Dementia (Alzheimer's, multi-infarct, others)	Associated with UUI; impaired cognition and apraxia interfere with toileting and hygiene	Regular toileting assistance essential for those with mobility and cognitive impairment in late stages
Depression	May impair motivation to be continent; may also be a consequence of incontinence	Optimizing pharmacologic and nonpharmacologic management of depression may improve UI

Adapted from Wagg, A., Gibson, W., Johnson, T, III., et al. (2014b). Urinary incontinence in frail elderly persons: Report from the 5th International Consultation on Incontinence. *Neurourology and Urodynamics*, Epub ahead of print.

- Bowel regularity/constipation, which can exacerbate OAB symptoms, and UI and fecal incontinence (FI) frequently coexist
- The individual's beliefs about the cause of the problem, impact on quality of life, and his or her goals for treatment

The impact of UI on a person's quality of life is extremely variable. There is little correlation between severity and impact (Barentsen et al., 2012), but there is evidence that urgency incontinence leads to greater detriment in life quality than stress incontinence, perhaps due to its unpredictability (Shaw, 2001). An assessment should therefore be made of the impact of an individual's symptoms on their quality of life, to allow the formulation of realistic and acceptable goals of treatment.

CLINICAL PEARL

The impact of UI on quality of life is extremely variable, and there is little correlation between severity of UI and impact on QoL.

Continence-specific aspects that need to be covered in detail include

- Daytime and nighttime frequency and intensity of symptoms (bladder diary, Fig. 5-4)
- Urgency
- The length of time they can "hold on," and any symptoms of stress incontinence
- Coping strategies

An enquiry should be made about strategies used to cope with urine loss as well as over-the-counter products for UI, many of which are perceived as expensive. A study on willingness to pay for a treatment for UI in Sweden found that people would be prepared to pay up to an eighth of their net income to reduce UI episodes by half, when given a hypothetical model (Johannesson et al., 1997). Having UI is costly, with direct and indirect annual costs per person of around $900 in a 2006 US study (Subak et al., 2006). In the United Kingdom, the total annual NHS cost of UI in community-dwelling adults was £536 (2000 prices), with total costs borne by individuals of an additional £207. Women spent much more than men (Turner et al., 2004). A European study in 2005 found the average annual out-of-pocket expenses to be between €359 and €655 (approximately US $480 to $900) (Papanicolaou et al., 2005). Many patients with UI improvise, using things such as sanitary towels, wadded toilet tissue, or towels cut in pieces to absorb urine. (See Chapter 12 for details on the many continence products available.)

Consideration should also be given to the fact that successful toileting relies not just on the ability to control urgency, but also on being able to locate and get to the toilet, and undress and redress. Therefore, when relevant, the clinician should assess mobility, cognition, visual impairment and functional impairment, with the goal of intervening to address modifiable associated factors.

Number of pads changed today ___1___
Type of pad used ___Maxi pad___

	Urinate in toilet (time and amount)		Accident (time)	Activity during accident	Fluid intake (time, type, amount)
To Bed	2200	240 cc			1 glass water
	0300	660 cc	0300	Leak on way to bathroom	
	0500	540 cc	0500	Preparing to urinate	
Up For Day	0700	150 cc			16 oz coffee 1 cup water
	0845	35 cc			
	1145	160 cc			
	1200				16 oz lemonade
	1540	60 cc			
	1800	100 cc			2 glasses wine 2 cups water
	1940	60 cc			16 oz diet coke 1 glass water

FIGURE 5-4. Voiding diary (also called bladder chart). Daytime frequency is seven. The patient has nocturia (gets up to void two times during sleeping hours) and also has nocturnal polyuria (an increased proportion of the 24-hour output occurs at night; note that nighttime urine output excludes the last void before sleep but includes the first void of the morning). She has urge incontinence, likely caused by the relatively larger bladder volumes voided at night, which in turn may be related to her greater fluid, caffeine, and alcohol consumption in the evening.

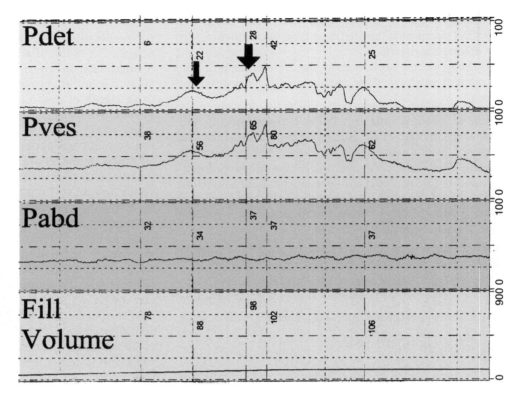

FIGURE 5-5. Detrusor overactivity on filling cystometrography. The patient begins to sense urgency, accompanied by an unstable bladder contraction, when 88 mL of water are instilled into the bladder. The detrusor pressure rises, and when 96 mL of water are instilled, she leaks. Pabd, abdominal pressure; Pdet, detrusor pressure; Pves, vesical pressure.

Physical Examination

- Abdominal exam (checking for scars, distended bladder, fecal loading)
- Perineal examination (perineal skin status, health of vaginal mucosa, evidence of prolapse)
- Evaluation of pelvic floor muscle strength and the ability to perform a pelvic floor contraction
- Rectal examination if constipation or poor rectal tone is suspected

In people who experience urgency incontinence, a quantification of the frequency, circumstance, and volume of urine lost should be made. The clinician should ask about situations and factors that aggravate OAB symptoms, such as caffeine intake, stressful situations, or hearing running water.

Baseline Tests

- Standard urinalysis with urine dip if there is a history or symptoms of UTI, diabetes, or hematuria
- Postvoid residual urine if incomplete emptying suspected

Urodynamics

Urodynamic testing is seldom necessary in the initial assessment of OAB and is usually reserved for individuals with neurologic conditions, those with a complex history such as prior surgery, or those who have not responded to treatment.

Figure 5-5 shows a typical urodynamic pattern for an individual with OAB and DO resulting in urgency incontinence. (See also Chapter 4, Advanced Assessment [Urodynamics].)

CLINICAL PEARL

Urodynamic testing is not usually indicated for individuals with OAB, unless there is an associated neurologic condition, prior surgery for UI, or failure to respond to treatment.

Management Options

Many national and international guidelines for the management of UI have been published, including those by the American Urological Association (Gormley et al., 2012), the European Association of Urology (Thuroff et al., 2011), the National Institute of Clinical and Healthcare Excellence in the United Kingdom (NICE, 2010; 2013), and the Canadian Urological Association (Bettez et al., 2012).

Conservative Treatment

Conservative treatment of OAB includes lifestyle interventions such as weight loss, reduction in caffeine intake, reduction/cessation of smoking, treatment of constipation, and fluid management. While these are all healthy lifestyle choices, there is very little research to support these recommendations as being of particular benefit in the treatment of OAB (Moore et al., 2013). Other noninvasive approaches include bladder training and electrical stimulation therapy. For cases of pelvic floor weakness or mixed UI, pelvic floor muscle therapy may be helpful, especially in combination with bladder training.

> **CLINICAL PEARL**
>
> Lifestyle interventions such as weight loss, reduction in caffeine intake, smoking cessation, and constipation management are commonly recommended, though there is little objective research to prove effectiveness.

General Measures

Once a diagnosis of OAB is reached, the first step is to consider and treat any coexisting medical conditions or functional impairments that may be contributing to the overall symptom load. Bowel function should be normalized to avoid constipation.

Weight Loss

In common with most conditions, patients who are obese should be tactfully encouraged to attain a lower BMI, and those who smoke strongly encouraged to stop, although, again, there are no intervention trials to support this practice in the treatment of OAB.

Caffeine Reduction

It is common practice to advise a reduction in the intake of caffeinated drinks in patients who experience urgency. There has been one randomized controlled trial of caffeine reduction, which compared bladder training with caffeine reduction to bladder training alone in men; these investigators found that a reduction of caffeine intake to below 100 mg/day was associated with statistically significant reductions in episodes of urgency and urgency incontinence (Bryant et al., 2002). Another small trial ($n = 11$) in which participants were randomized to decaffeinated versus caffeinated coffee also found a significant improvement in urgency and frequency and improved scores on the ICI-Q OAB questionnaire (Wells et al., 2014). Although these studies are small, there is a suggestion that for some individuals, caffeine reduction may assist in symptom resolution.

Smoking Cessation

In a comprehensive review of the literature on smoking and the relationship to LUTS (Moore et al., 2013), smokers were more likely to report UI than nonsmokers in some studies (5 studies), but not others (3 studies). The review authors noted that during the postpartum period, smokers may have an increased risk of UI compared to nonsmokers, after adjusting for age, parity, type of delivery, and prepregnancy BMI; they also noted that the risk for incontinence was higher among women smokers after adjusting for perimenopausal status, BMI, diabetes, and ethnicity. There were no recent studies addressing the question of smoking and LUTS and no studies evaluating the effects of quitting on continence status. However, current data suggest that smoking increases the risk of more severe UI. Given the health benefits of smoking cessation, it is reasonable to discuss this with an individual. It is important to remember, however, that most people have tried to quit many times and may resent "advice" about quitting (Moore et al., 2013).

Fluid Intake

It is generally held that fluid intake should be around 2 L/day. There is a widespread belief that concentrated urine is irritating to the urothelium and worsens OAB symptoms, although there is no supporting evidence for this. Overhydration predictably leads to polyuria and therefore increased urinary frequency. However, analysis of the Nurses' Health Study cohort found no link between fluid intake and the development of incontinence (Townsend et al., 2011). In a study of older adults in hospital, older people with DO were found to drink less than those without, possibly as a result of voluntary fluid restriction, and there was a strong correlation between increased fluid intake and increased frequency of micturition (Griffiths et al., 1993).

There is a paucity of high-quality evidence to support fluid intake changes as treatment for UUI. A small trial (Dowd et al., 1996) suggested that increasing fluid intake reduced episodes of UUI, but adherence to the study protocol was poor. A trial of medication alone versus medication and lifestyle interventions (including general advice on fluid intake and specific advice to reduce fluid intake for those who habitually drank more than 2.1 L/day) found no additional benefit of lifestyle intervention and little impact of specific advice on drinking habits (Zimmern et al., 2010).

Constipation

The effect of regulating bowel function on UI has not been well studied, the data that exist are old, and to date, there are no intervention trials that address the effect of resolving constipation on UI (Moore et al., 2013). In a small observational study, 30% of women with SUI and 61% of women with uterovaginal prolapse reported straining at stool as a young adult, compared to 4% of women without urogynecological symptoms (Spence-Jones et al., 1994). In a large population-based study of 1,154 women over age 60 years, those with UI were slightly more likely to report constipation than those who were continent of urine (31.6% vs. 24.7%) (Diokno & Bromberg, 1990). After adjusting for demographic and obstetric confounders, women who reported straining at stool were more likely to report SUI and urgency (Alling-Møller et al., 2000).

It has been suggested that straining and pudendal nerve function may be related, but more research is required to explore this relationship. It should be stressed that, although "lifestyle" interventions are common practice in the initial treatment of OAB, there is very little high-quality evidence to support their use. However, as they are low cost and low risk and are general recommendations for healthy living, there is little to be lost through their adoption.

Urgency Suppression/Bladder Training

Patients can be taught techniques to override the sensation of urgency, allowing them to delay voiding until convenient. Several methods have been described, including rapid pelvic floor contraction at the onset of urgency, sitting on a hard surface, and distraction techniques.

Bladder drill, also known as bladder training or bladder retraining, is a self-guided method of increasing the time between onset of urge to void and the actual time of voiding. Although it requires significant patient enthusiasm and engagement, bladder training has been shown to be effective in reducing urgency and urge incontinence episodes (Roe et al., 2007b).

Figure 5-6 provides an example of a patient teaching brochure that can be used for bladder training.

> **CLINICAL PEARL**
>
> Urgency suppression and bladder training (bladder drill) have been proven to be effective in management of OAB and/or urgency incontinence.

Toileting Programs for Frail Elders

Behavioral interventions have been especially designed for frail older people with cognitive and physical impairments. Because they have no side effects, they have been the mainstay of UI treatment in frail older people (Roe et al., 2007b). The technique with the most evidence for its use is *prompted voiding*. Subjects are prompted to use the toilet and encouraged with social reward when successfully toileted. This technique increases patient requests for toileting and self-initiated toileting and decreases the number of UI episodes (Palmer, 2005). A 3-day trial during which the number of incontinent episodes is reduced by at least 20% should be considered successful. The second commonly used technique, *habit retraining*, requires identification of the incontinent person's individual toileting pattern and UI episodes, usually by means of a bladder diary. A toileting schedule is then devised to preempt them (Palmer, 2004; Roe et al., 2007a). *Timed voiding* involves toileting at fixed intervals, such as every 3 hours. There is no patient education, reinforcement of desirable behaviors, or attempt to reestablish normal voiding patterns (Ostaszkiewicz et al., 2005).

Functional Intervention Training

This program incorporates musculoskeletal strengthening exercises into toileting routines by nursing home care aides or nursing assistants (Schnelle et al., 1995).

There is increasing evidence for the effectiveness of physical exercise as an intervention for UI in populations in diverse settings. In a Veterans nursing home population in the United States, the combination of individualized prompted voiding and functionally oriented endurance and strength-training exercises (offered four times per day, 5 days per week, for 8 weeks) delivered by trained research staff was effective in significantly reducing UI (Ouslander et al., 2005). An intervention that provided exercise and incontinence care every 2 hours from 8:00 AM to 4:30 PM (total of 4 daily care episodes) for 5 days a week over 32 weeks in a nursing home population was also found to be effective in significantly reducing incontinence (Bates-Jensen et al., 2003). Similarly, a study of walking exercise for 30 minutes per day in a small group of cognitively impaired residents over 4 weeks resulted in a significant reduction in daytime incontinence episodes and an increase in gait speed and stamina (Jirovec, 1991). In community-dwelling older people, a 30-minute evening walk proved effective in reducing nocturia, while also improving daytime urinary frequency, blood pressure, body weight, body fat ratio, triglycerides, total cholesterol, and sleep quality (Sugaya et al., 2007).

Cognitive and functional impairment, common in frail elderly people, may preclude the use of some of these interventions. Additionally, the context in which care is provided needs to be considered (Booth et al., 2009; Dingwall, 2008; Wright et al., 2007). Many of these interventions are time consuming and need staff engagement for effective delivery (Vinsnes et al., 2007). Although pelvic floor muscle rehabilitation has not been studied extensively in frail older people, age and frailty alone should not preclude their use in appropriate patients with sufficient cognition to participate. The research supporting the above interventions is older, and little recent examination of these strategies has occurred. With an ever-increasing aging population and increasing prevalence of OAB, there is a major need for research in this area.

> **CLINICAL PEARL**
>
> There is increasing evidence that physical exercise programs can be beneficial in the treatment of UI in diverse care settings.

Topical Estrogens

The application of topical estrogens, in the form of cream, as a pessary, or vaginal ring, is commonly used as a treatment for OAB in postmenopausal women. It is known that estrogen has a major role in the function of the female urogenital tract and well recognized that urogenital atrophy can lead to dysuria. There is some, limited, evidence that topical estrogens are of benefit in OAB without urogenital atrophy, although data are conflicting and there is no definitive role (Robinson et al., 2014).

Introduction

Around 6 million people in Canada have a bladder control problem, and can affect men and women of any age.

Despite being so common, bladder difficulties are often hidden. As a result, many people do not get the help they need and they suffer in silence.

This pamphlet contains useful and practical advice about bladder retraining, a simple technique that can help people who have an urgent need to go to the washroom.

Bladder urgency is also called **over-active bladder**.

Overactive bladder

Many bladder problems are caused by an overactive bladder:

- A sudden urge to go to the washroom (**urgency**)
- Unable to hold the urgency and reach the toilet in time (**urgency incontinence**)
- Needing to go very often - (**frequency**)
- Getting up during the night (**nocturia**)
- Wetting the bed at night (**nocturnal enuresis**)

These problems are caused when the bladder is very sensitive, or the bladder muscle squeezes when it shouldn't—even when you want to hold on.

How the bladder works

The bladder is made of muscle. It is positioned in the lower part of the tummy just behind the pubic bone.

In between visits to the washroom the bladder relaxes and fills up. When you go to the washroom the bladder squeezes and urine comes out through a tube called the urethra.

The pelvic floor is made of layers of muscle, which support the bladder and bowel. The pelvic floor also helps to stop leaks from the bladder and bowel.

The urethral sphincter is a circular muscle that goes around the urethra. The sphincter muscle normally squeezes as the bladder is filling up—it creates a seal so urine can't leak out. When you go to the toilet, the sphincter muscle relaxes and lets the urine flow.

Bladder retraining

Many people with urgency will get into the habit of going to the toilet too often—trying to make sure they are never "caught short".

This can make the problem of urgency worse. The bladder gets used to holding less urine, so it becomes even more sensitive. See our pamphlet **"Healthy Bladder Habits"**.

Bladder retraining is a method that helps the bladder hold more urine and allows you to hold on for longer.

Keep a record of when you pass urine and how much you drink for at least three days. You can ask for one of our bladder diaries to help you.

Gradually increase the amount of time between visits to the wash-room. When you get the urge to pass water, hold on for a bit—just a minute or two to start with.

Try to hold on a little bit longer each time you feel the urge to go, the urge often stops if you hold on when you feel the first urge to go. Your goal is to be able to wait for 3 to 4 hours between emptying your bladder.

Bladder retraining takes time and determination. Improvement does not happen overnight, but it can be very successful.

Urgency Suppression

If you have trouble reaching the bathroom before you start losing urine, try this:

When you get the urge to urinate:

- Stop and stay still, sit down if you can
- Squeeze your pelvic floor muscles (**ask your health professional about pelvic floor exercises**) quickly 3 to 5 times; repeat as needed
- Try sitting on a hard surface; some people find that sitting on a rolled up towel can help with trying to hold on
- Relax the rest of your body and take a deep breath
- Concentrate on suppressing the urge
- Distract yourself to get your mind on something else
- Wait until the urge subsides, then walk to the washroom at a normal pace

Other Sources of Information

There are a number of other organizations which can help you manage your bladder problem. Some of their contact details are below.

Many have websites which you might like to view and read for useful information. If you are unsure about the type of information you want, please ask the doctor or nurse in the clinic.

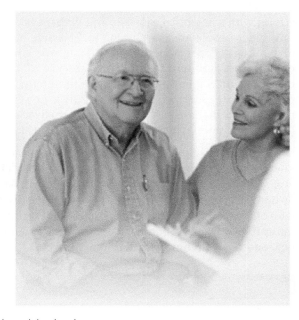

FIGURE 5-6. Example of a bladder training brochure.

Pharmacologic Treatment

Should conservative management fail, then a pharmacological approach should be considered.

Antimuscarinics

For many years, the mainstay of drug therapy for overactive bladder has been the bladder antimuscarinics, including darifenacin, fesoterodine, imidafenacin (Japan), oxybutynin, propiverine (non-US), solifenacin, tolterodine, and trospium chloride. These agents block activation of the muscarinic receptors in the urothelium and detrusor, thereby reducing the sensation of urgency and increasing bladder storage capacity. Although effective, long-term adherence to treatment is poor, with discontinuation rates of up to 80% after 12 months' treatment (Wagg et al., 2012). Common side effects include xerostomia (dry mouth) and constipation. Some of the bladder antimuscarinics, particularly oxybutynin, have been shown to cause cognitive impairment in older people, and its use in the elderly is therefore not recommended (Gibson et al., 2014).

In contrast to oxybutynin, darifenacin, trospium, solifenacin, and tolterodine have much lower central nervous system (CNS) concentrations, as they do not cross the blood–brain barrier (BBB) well, and some (5-hydroxymethyl tolterodine, the active metabolite of both tolterodine and fesoterodine, darifenacin, and trospium) are actively removed from the CNS by the permeability glycoprotein (P-GP) system, further lowering CNS levels and the potential for related adverse effects. The BBB becomes more permeable with increasing age and in association with some other diseases, and perhaps because of this, older people are more prone to CNS side effects of many drugs (Popescu et al., 2009). Thus, one advantage of the newer antimuscarinics is the absence of deleterious effects on cognition, at least in the short term, in cognitively intact older persons (Wagg, 2012); however, the newer agents do have similar rates of other adverse effects (such as xerostomia) as the older drugs (Buser et al., 2012).

Mirabegron

Mirabegron, a β_3 agonist, was introduced in 2012 (Sacco et al., 2014) and has shown to be an effective option for OAB in both young and older people, with significantly lower rates of dry mouth. The side effect profile avoids typical antimuscarinic side effects but includes a concern about either new-onset or worsening hypertension (Wagg et al., 2014a).

CLINICAL PEARL

Pharmacologic therapy should be considered for any patient for whom conservative therapy provides insufficient improvement; the major types of medications include antimuscarinics, mirabegron, and Botox.

Botox

OnabotulinumtoxinA (Botox), one of the subtypes of the neurotoxin produced by the bacterium *Clostridium*

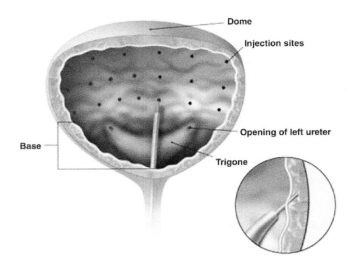

FIGURE 5-7. Example of an injection template for botulinum, with 20 injections and sparing of the trigone and dome.

botulinum, is a potent inhibitor of acetylcholine release from the motor axon (Proft, 2009). It has been shown to be of value in the treatment of refractory overactive bladder, leading to increased bladder capacity, decreased intravesical pressure, and reduced incontinence episodes (Kuo & Kuo, 2013). Treatment involves injection of botulinum toxin into the suburothelium via a cystoscope and can be performed as an outpatient procedure under local anesthesia. It has been shown to be safe in older people, although there is an increased risk of large postvoid residual and treatment failure compared to younger patients (Liao & Kuo, 2013). Figure 5-7 shows Botox injection patterns.

Neuromodulation

Neuromodulation is a therapeutic modality that uses electrical signals to alter the involuntary reflexes of the lower urinary tract, thus inhibiting the voiding reflex, reducing involuntary detrusor contractions, and assisting patients to regain voluntary control of micturition. The exact mode of action is still unclear (Leng & Chancellor, 2005). There are two commonly used approaches to neuromodulation.

Percutaneous Tibial Nerve Stimulation

Percutaneous tibial nerve stimulation (PTNS) uses needle electrodes placed through the skin of the lower leg at the ankle; and pulsed low-current electrical signals are then used to stimulate the posterior tibial nerve for a period of time (usually 30 minutes) once weekly for a variable number of weeks (usually 10 to 12). A blinded trial of PTNS versus sham treatment found that 55% of those treated had moderate or marked improvements in their OAB symptoms, compared to 20% in the sham group (Peters et al., 2010). Further research with PTNS is needed to compare the benefit of lifestyle adjustments, bladder training, and/or PTNS.

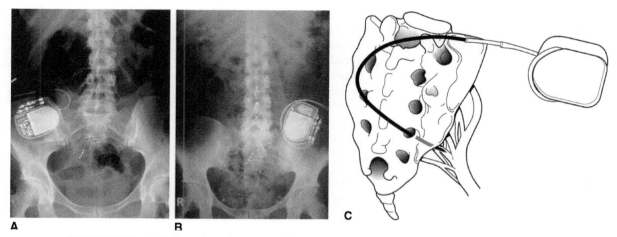

FIGURE 5-8. **A.** Unilateral sacral neuromodulation. **B.** Bilateral sacral neuromodulation. **C.** Illustration showing sacral neuromodulation.

Sacral Nerve Stimulation

Sacral neuromodulation uses an implantable electrode placed in a sacral foramen, commonly S3 (Fig. 5-8). Although effective, with reported success rates of 70% and cure rates of 20% for incontinence and 33% cure for urinary urgency, around 40% of patients will require reintervention, most commonly for lead migration or infection (Peeters et al., 2014). It is normal practice to first use a temporary system and, should a bladder diary show benefit (>50% symptom resolution) during a trial period of 2 weeks, a permanent device is implanted, usually under the skin of the buttock.

CLINICAL PEARL

Neuromodulation has been shown to be effective in management of OAB refractory to other therapies; options include "Percutaneous Tibial Nerve Stimulation" and "Sacral Nerve Stimulation."

Augmentation Cystoplasty

When all else has failed, augmentation cystoplasty can be considered (Fig. 5-9). This is a surgical procedure, performed either open or laparoscopically, that uses a length of small intestine to enlarge the bladder and

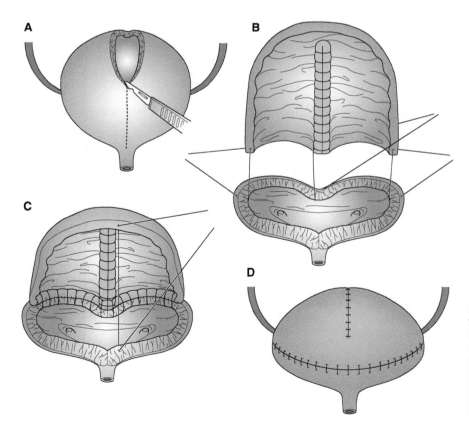

FIGURE 5-9. Bladder augmentation with an intestinal segment. **A.** The bladder is opened as a "clam shell." **B.** The intestinal segment is detubularized by longitudinal incision along the antimesenteric border. A cup-patch is fashioned by suturing one edge of the resultant rectangle to itself. **C.** The cup-patch is sutured to the remnant bladder plate. **D.** Final appearance.

increase bladder capacity. Although effective in reducing OAB symptoms, the procedure carries not only the operative risks but also postprocedure risks of UTI, with rates between 4% and 46% depending on definition and study method. Perforation of the augmented bladder is reported, occurring in between 6% and 9% of cases, and can be fatal (Reyblat & Ginsberg, 2010). Reliance on intermittent self-catheterization is extremely common, with between 26% and 100% of patients needing to self-catheterize; however, reliance on self-catheterization is much less common in patients undergoing augmentation cystoplasty for idiopathic OAB as compared to those with neurogenic bladder or postradiotherapy cystitis (Veeratterapillay et al., 2013). An inability to self-catheterize is a contraindication to cystoplasty.

Conclusion

Overactive bladder is a common and potentially debilitating condition, which is underreported and undertreated. It can usually be diagnosed on the basis of a detailed history and examination, without the need for invasive testing. The recent development of newer pharmaceutical treatments has improved the options for patients, and there are also options when these fail or are inappropriate. The understanding of the function and dysfunction of the urothelium, detrusor, and brain is increasing, providing new and hopefully more effective treatment options.

REFERENCES

Abrams, P., Artibani, W., Cardozo, L., et al.; & International Continence Society. (2009). Reviewing the ICS 2002 terminology report: The ongoing debate. *Neurourology and Urodynamics, 28,* 287.

Alling-Møller, L., Lose, G., & Jørgensen, T. (2000). Risk factors for urinary tract symptoms in women 40 to 60 years of age. *Obstetrics and Gynecology, 96*(3), 446–451.

Arya, L. A., Myers, D. L., & Jackson, N. D. (2000). Dietary caffeine intake and the risk for detrusor instability: A case–control study. *Obstetrics and Gynecology, 96,* 85–89.

Barentsen, J. A., Visser, E., Hofstetter, H., et al. (2012). Severity, not type, is the main predictor of decreased quality of life in elderly women with urinary incontinence: A population-based study as part of a randomized controlled trial in primary care. *Health QualityLife Outcomes, 10,* 153. doi:10.1186/1477-7525-10-153.

Bates-Jensen, B. M., Alessi, C. A., Al-Samarrai, N. R., et al. (2003). The effects of an exercise and incontinence intervention on skin health outcomes in nursing home residents. *Journal of the American Geriatric Society, 51,* 348–355.

Beckel, J. M., & Birder, L. A. (2012). Differential expression and function of nicotinic acetylcholine receptors in the urinary bladder epithelium of the rat. *Journal of Physiology, 590,* 1465–1480.

Bettez, M., Tu L. M., Carlson, K., et al. (2012). 2012 update: Guidelines for adult urinary incontinence collaborative consensus document for the Canadian Urological Association. *Canadian Urological Association Journal, 6,* 354–363.

Bing, M. H., Møller, L. A., Jennum, P., et al. (2006). Prevalence and bother of nocturia, and causes of sleep interruption in a Danish population of men and women aged 60–80 years. *BJU International, 98,* 599–604.

Birder, L., & Andersson, K. E. (2013). Urothelial signaling. *Physiological Reviews, 93,* 653–680.

Birder, L. A., Wolf-Johnston, A. S., Sun, Y., et al. (2013). Alteration in TRPV1 and Muscarinic (M3) receptor expression and function in idiopathic overactive bladder urothelial cells. *Acta Physiologica (Oxford, England), 207,* 123–129.

Booth, J., Kumlien, S., & Zang, Y. (2009). Promoting urinary continence with older people: Key issues for nurses. *International Journal of Older People Nursing, 4,* 63–69.

Brading, A. F., & Turner, W. H. (1994). The unstable bladder: Towards a common mechanism. *British Journal of Urology, 73,* 3–8.

Bryant, C. M., Dowell, C. J., & Fairbrother, G. (2002). Caffeine reduction education to improve urinary symptoms. *British Journal of Nursing, 11,* 560–565.

Bschleipfer, T., Schukowski, K., Weidner, W., et al. (2007). Expression and distribution of cholinergic receptors in the human urothelium. *Life Sciences, 80,* 2303–2307.

Buser, N., Ivic, S., Kessler, T. M., et al. (2012). Efficacy and adverse events of antimuscarinics for treating overactive bladder: Network meta-analyses. *European Urology, 62,* 1040–1060.

Cartwright, R., Srikrishna, S., Cardozo, L., et al. (2007). Does Diet Coke cause overactive bladder? A 4-way crossover trial, investigating the effect of carbonated soft drinks on overactive bladder symptoms in normal volunteers. *Annual Meeting of the International Continence Society* (Abstract 19), Rotterdam. http://www.ics.org/Abstracts/Publish/45/000019.pdf

Chacko, S., Cortes, E., Drake, M. J., et al. (2014). Does altered myogenic activity contribute to OAB symptoms from detrusor overactivity? ICI-RS 2013. *Neurourology and Urodynamics, 33,* 577–580.

Coolsaet, B. (1985). Bladder compliance and detrusor activity during the collection phase. *Neurourology and Urodynamics, 4,* 263–273.

Coyne, K. S., Payne, C., Bhattacharyya, S. K., et al. (2004). The impact of urinary urgency and frequency on health-related quality of life in overactive bladder: Results from a national community survey. *Value Health, 7,* 455–463.

Coyne, K. S., Sexton, C. C., Thompson, C. L., et al. (2009). The prevalence of lower urinary tract symptoms (LUTS) in the USA, the UK and Sweden: Results from the Epidemiology of LUTS (EpiLUTS) study. *BJU International, 104,* 352–360.

Dallosso, H. M., McGrother, C. W., Matthews, R. J., et al.; Leicestershire MRC Incontinence Study Group. (2003). The association of diet and other lifestyle factors with overactive bladder and stress incontinence: A longitudinal study in women. *BJU International, 92,* 69–77.

Dingwall, L. (2008). Promoting effective continence care for older people: A literature review. *British Journal of Nursing, 17,* 166–172.

Diokno, A. C., Brock B. M., Herzog, A. R., et al. (1990). Medical correlates of urinary incontinence in the elderly. *Urology, 36*(2), 129–138.

Dowd, T. T., Campbell, J. M., & Jones, J. A. (1996). Fluid intake and urinary incontinence in older community-dwelling women. *Journal of Community Health Nursing, 13,* 179–186.

Elstad, E. A., Taubenberger, S. P., Botelho, E. M., et al. (2010). Beyond incontinence: The stigma of other urinary symptoms. *Journal of Advanced Nursing, 66,* 2460–2470.

Finkelstein, K., Glosner, S., Sanchez, R. J., et al. (2008). Prevalence of probable overactive bladder in a private obstetrics and gynecology group practice. *Current Medical Research and Opinion, 24,* 1083–1090.

Fitzgerald, M. P., Thom, D. H., Wassel-Fyr, C., et al.; Reproductive Risks For Incontinence Study At Kaiser Research, Group. (2006). Childhood urinary symptoms predict adult overactive bladder symptoms. *Journal of Urology, 175,* 989–993.

Fowler, C. J., Griffiths, D., & de Groat, W. C. (2008). The neural control of micturition. *Nature Reviews Neuroscience, 9,* 453–466.

Gibson, W., Athanasopoulos, A., Goldman, H. B., et al. (2014). Are we short-changing the elderly when it comes to the pharmacological treatment of urgency urinary incontinence? *International Journal of Clinical Practice, 68*(9), 1165–1173. doi: 10.1111/ijcp.12447.

Gormley, E. A., Lightner, D. J., Burgio, K. L., et al. (2012). Diagnosis and treatment of overactive bladder (non-neurogenic) in adults: AUA/SUFU guideline. *Journal of Urology, 188*, 2455–2463.

Griffiths, D. J., Mccracken, P. N., Harrison, G. M., et al. (1993). Relationship of fluid intake to voluntary micturition and urinary incontinence in geriatric patients. *Neurourology and Urodynamics, 12*, 1–7.

Griffiths, D. J., Tadic, S. D., Schaefer, W., et al. (2009). Cerebral control of the lower urinary tract: How age-related changes might predispose to urge incontinence. *NeuroImage, 47*, 981–986.

Hannestad, Y. S., Rortveit, G., Sandvik, H., et al. (2000). A community-based epidemiological survey of female urinary incontinence: The Norwegian EPINCONT study. Epidemiology of Incontinence in the County of Nord-Trondelag. *Journal of Clinical Epidemiology, 53*, 1150–1157.

Hashim, H., & Abrams, P. (2006). Is the bladder a reliable witness for predicting detrusor overactivity? *Journal of Urology, 175*, 191–194; discussion 194–5.

Haylen, B. T., De Ridder, D., Freeman, R. M., et al.; International Continence Society. (2010). An International Urogynecological Association (IUGA)/International Continence Society (ICS) joint report on the terminology for female pelvic floor dysfunction. *Neurourology and Urodynamics, 29*, 4–20.

Irwin, D. E., Milsom, I., Chancellor, M. B., et al. (2010). Dynamic progression of overactive bladder and urinary incontinence symptoms: A systematic review. *European Urology, 58*, 532–543.

Irwin, D. E., Milsom, I., Hunskaar, S., et al. (2006). Population-based survey of urinary incontinence, overactive bladder, and other lower urinary tract symptoms in five countries: Results of the EPIC study. *European Urology, 50*, 1306–1314; discussion 1314–1315.

Irwin, D. E., Milsom, I., Kopp, Z., et al. (2008). Symptom bother and health care-seeking behavior among individuals with overactive bladder. *European Urology, 53*, 1029–1037.

Jirovec, M. M. (1991). The impact of daily exercise on the mobility, balance and urine control of cognitively impaired nursing home residents. *International Journal of Nursing Studies, 28*, 145–151.

Johannesson, M., O'Conor, R. M., Kobelt-Nguyen, G., et al. (1997). Willingness to pay for reduced incontinence symptoms. *British Journal of Urology, 80*, 557–562.

Kuchel, G. A., Moscufo, N., Guttmann, C. R., et al. (2009). Localization of brain white matter hyperintensities and urinary incontinence in community-dwelling older adults. *The Journals of Gerontology. Series A, Biological Sciences and Medical Sciences, 64*, 902–909.

Kuo, Y. C., & Kuo, H. C. (2013). Botulinum toxin injection for lower urinary tract dysfunction. *International Journal of Urology, 20*, 40–55.

Lei, D., Ma, J., Shen, X., et al. (2012). Changes in the brain microstructure of children with primary monosymptomatic nocturnal enuresis: A diffusion tensor imaging study. *PLOS One, 7*, e31023. doi: 10.1371/journal.pone.0031023.

Leng, W. W., & Chancellor, M. B. (2005). How sacral nerve stimulation neuromodulation works. *Urologic Clinics of North America, 32*, 11–18.

Liang, C. C., Chang, S. D., Lin, S. J., et al. (2012). Lower urinary tract symptoms in primiparous women before and during pregnancy. *Archives of Gynecology and Obstetrics, 285*, 1205–1210.

Liao, C. H. & Kuo, H. C. (2013). Increased risk of large post-void residual urine and decreased long-term success rate after intravesical onabotulinumtoxinA injection for refractory idiopathic detrusor overactivity. *Journal of Urology, 189*, 1804–1810.

Liberman, J. N., Hunt, T. L., Stewart, W. F., et al. (2001). Health-related quality of life among adults with symptoms of overactive bladder: Results from a U.S. community-based survey. *Urology, 57*, 1044–1050.

Malmsten, U. G., Molander, U., Peeker, R., et al. (2010). Urinary incontinence, overactive bladder, and other lower urinary tract symptoms: A longitudinal population-based survey in men aged 45–103 years. *European Urology, 58*(1), 149–156.

Mansfield, K. J., Liu, L., Mitchelson, F. J., et al. (2005). Muscarinic receptor subtypes in human bladder detrusor and mucosa, studied by radioligand binding and quantitative competitive RT-PCR: Changes in ageing. *British Journal of Pharmacology, 144*, 1089–1099.

Maserejian, N. N., Kupelian, V., Miyasato, G., et al. (2012). Are physical activity, smoking and alcohol consumption associated with lower urinary tract symptoms in men or women? Results from a population based observational study. *Journal of Urology, 188*, 490–495.

McGrother, C. W., Donaldson, M. M., Thompson, J., et al. (2012). Etiology of overactive bladder: A diet and lifestyle model for diabetes and obesity in older women. *Neurourology and Urodynamics, 31*, 487–495.

Mills, I. W., Greenland, J. E., Mcmurray, G., et al. (2000). Studies of the pathophysiology of idiopathic detrusor instability: The physiological properties of the detrusor smooth muscle and its pattern of innervation. *Journal of Urology, 163*, 646–651.

Moore, K. N., Dumoulin, C., Bradley, C., et al. (2013). Adult conservative management. In P. Abrams, L. Cardozo, S. Khoury, et al. (Eds.), Incontinence (5th ed., pp. 1101–1227). The Netherlands: European Association of Urology.

National Institute for Health and Care Excellence (NICE). (2010). CG97 Lower urinary tract symptoms: The management of lower urinary tract symptoms in men [Online]. Retrieved from www.nice.org.uk/guidance/cg97/chapter/introduction

National Institute for Health and Care Excellence (NICE). (2013). CG171 Urinary Incontinence in Women [Online]. Retrieved from http://guidance.nice.org.uk/CG171/NICEGuidance/pdf/English

Ostaszkiewicz, J., Johnston, L., & Roe, B. (2005). Timed voiding for the management of urinary incontinence in adults. *Journal of Urology, 173*, 1262–1263.

Ouslander, J. G., Griffiths, P., Mcconnell, E., et al. (2005). Functional Incidental Training: Applicability and feasibility in the Veterans Affairs nursing home patient population. *Journal of the American Medical Directors Association, 6*, 121–127.

Palmer, M. H. (2004). Use of health behavior change theories to guide urinary incontinence research. *Nursing Research, 53*, S49–S55.

Palmer, M. H. (2005). Effectiveness of prompted voiding for incontinent nursing home residents. In B. M. Melnyk & E Fineout-Overholt. (Eds.), *Evidence-based practice in nursing & healthcare: A guide to the best practice*. Philadelphia, PA: Lippincott Williams & Wilkins.

Papanicolaou, S., Pons, M. E., Hampel, C., et al. (2005). Medical resource utilisation and cost of care for women seeking treatment for urinary incontinence in an outpatient setting. Examples from three countries participating in the PURE study. *Maturitas, 52*(Suppl 2), S35–S47.

Peeters, K., Sahai, A., De Ridder, D., et al. (2014). Long-term follow-up of sacral neuromodulation for lower urinary tract dysfunction. *BJU International, 113*, 789–794.

Peters, K. M., Carrico, D. J., Perez-Marrero, R. A., et al. (2010). Randomized trial of percutaneous tibial nerve stimulation versus Sham efficacy in the treatment of overactive bladder syndrome: Results from the SUmiT trial. *Journal of Urology, 183*, 1438–1443.

Ponholzer, A., Temml, C., Wehrberger, C., et al. (2006). The association between vascular risk factors and lower urinary tract symptoms in both sexes. *European Urology, 50*, 581–586.

Popescu, B. O., Toescu, E. C., Popescu, L. M., et al. (2009). Blood-brain barrier alterations in ageing and dementia. *Jounal of the Neurological Sciences, 283*, 99–106.

Proft, T. (2009). *Microbial toxins: Current research and future trends.* Norfolk, UK: Caister Academic Press.

Rapp, D. E., Lyon, M. B., Bales, G. T., et al. (2005). A role for the P2X receptor in urinary tract physiology and in the pathophysiology of urinary dysfunction. *European Urology, 48,* 303–308.

Reyblat, P., & Ginsberg, D. A. (2010). Augmentation enterocystoplasty in overactive bladder: Is there still a role? *Current Urology Reports, 11,* 432–439.

Robinson, D., Cardozo, L., Milsom, I., et al. (2014). Oestrogens and overactive bladder. *Neurourol Urodyn, 33*(7), 1086–1091. doi:10.1002/nau.22464.

Roe, B., Milne, J., Ostaszkiewicz, J., et al. (2007a). Systematic reviews of bladder training and voiding programmes in adults: A synopsis of findings on theory and methods using metastudy techniques. *Journal of Advanced Nursing, 57,* 3–14.

Roe, B., Ostaszkiewicz, J., Milne, J., et al. (2007b). Systematic reviews of bladder training and voiding programmes in adults: A synopsis of findings from data analysis and outcomes using metastudy techniques. *Journal of Advanced Nursing, 57,* 15–31.

Sacco, E., Bientinesi, R., Tienforti, D., et al. (2014). Discovery history and clinical development of mirabegron for the treatment of overactive bladder and urinary incontinence. *Expert Opinion on Drug Discovery, 9,* 433–448.

Schnelle, J. F., Macrae, P. G., Ouslander, J. G., et al. (1995). Functional Incidental Training, mobility performance, and incontinence care with nursing home residents. *Journal of the American Geriatric Society, 43,* 1356–1362.

Shaw, C. (2001). A review of the psychosocial predictors of help-seeking behaviour and impact on quality of life in people with urinary incontinence. *Journal of Clinical Nursing, 10,* 15–24.

Shaw, C., Tansey, R., Jackson, C., et al. (2001). Barriers to help seeking in people with urinary symptoms. *Family Practice, 18,* 48–52.

Siroky, M. B. (2004). The aging bladder. *Reviews in Urology, 6*(Suppl 1), S3–S7.

Spence-Jones C., Kamm M. A., Henry M. M., et al. (1994). Bowel dysfunction: A pathogenic factor in ureterovaginal prolapse and urinary stress incontinence. *British Journal of Obstetrics and Gynecology, 101*(2), 147–152.

Stewart, W. F., Van Rooyen, J. B., Cundiff, G. W., et al. (2003). Prevalence and burden of overactive bladder in the United States. *World Journal of Urology, 20,* 327–336.

Su, X., Stein, R., Stanton, M. C., et al. (2003). Effect of partial outlet obstruction on rabbit urinary bladder smooth muscle function. *American Journal of Physiology: Renal Physiology, 284,* F644–F652.

Subak, L. L., Brown, J. S., Kraus, S. R., et al.; Diagnostic Aspects Of Incontinence Study Group. (2006). The "costs" of urinary incontinence for women. *Obstetrics and Gynecology, 107,* 908–916.

Subak, L. L., Richter, H. E., & Hunskaar, S. (2009). Obesity and urinary incontinence: Epidemiology and clinical research update. *Journal of Urology, 182,* S2–S7.

Sugaya, K., Nishijima, S., Owan, T., et al. (2007). Effects of walking exercise on nocturia in the elderly. *Biomedical Research, 28,* 101–105.

Sui, G., Fry, C. H., Malone-Lee, J., et al. (2009). Aberrant Ca^{2+} oscillations in smooth muscle cells from overactive human bladders. *Cell Calcium, 45,* 456–464.

Tadic, S., Griffiths, D., Murrin, A., et al. (2010). Structural damage of brain's white matter affects brain-bladder control in older women with urgency incontinence. *Joint Annual Meeting of the International Continence Society, ICS and International Urogynecological Association, IUGA Toronto, ON Canada, 29,* 1109–1110. http://www.ics.org/Abstracts/Publish/105/000211.pdf

Tahtinen, R. M., Auvinen, A., Cartwright, R., et al. (2011). Smoking and bladder symptoms in women. *Obstetrics and Gynecology, 118,* 643–648.

Tettamanti, G., Altman, D., Pedersen, N. L., et al. (2011). Effects of coffee and tea consumption on urinary incontinence in female twins. *BJOG : An International Journal of Obstetrics and Gynaecology, 118,* 806–813.

Thuroff, J. W., Abrams, P., Andersson, K. E., et al. (2011). EAU guidelines on urinary incontinence. *European Urology, 59,* 387–400.

Townsend, M. K., Jura, Y. H., Curhan, G. C., et al. (2011). Fluid intake and risk of stress, urgency, and mixed urinary incontinence. *American Journal of Obstetrics and Gynecology, 205*(73), e1–e6.

Turner, D. A., Shaw, C., McGrother, C. W., et al. (2004). The cost of clinically significant urinary storage symptoms for community dwelling adults in the UK. *BJU International, 93,* 1246–1252.

Tyagi, V., Philips, B. J., Su, R., et al. (2009). Differential expression of functional cannabinoid receptors in human bladder detrusor and urothelium. *Journal of Urology, 181,* 1932–1938.

Veeratterapillay, R., Thorpe, A. C., & Harding, C. (2013). Augmentation cystoplasty: Contemporary indications, techniques and complications. *Indian Journal of Urology, 29,* 322–327.

Vinsnes, A. G., Harkless, G. E., & Nyronning, S. (2007). Unit-based intervention to improve urinary incontinence in frail elderly. *Nordic Journal of Nursing Research & Clinical Studies, 27,* 53.

Wagg, A. (2012). The cognitive burden of anticholinerigics in the elderly—implications for the treatment of overactive bladder. *European Urological Reviews, 7*(1), 42–49.

Wagg, A., Cardozo, L., Nitti, V. W., et al. (2014a). The efficacy and tolerability of the beta3-adrenoceptor agonist mirabegron for the treatment of symptoms of overactive bladder in older patients. *Age and Ageing, 43*(5), 666–675. doi.org/10.1093/ageing/afu017.

Wagg, A., Compion, G., Fahey, A., et al. (2012). Persistence with prescribed antimuscarinic therapy for overactive bladder: A UK experience. *BJU International, 110,* 1767–1774.

Wagg, A., Gibson, W., Johnson, T, III., et al. (2014b). Urinary incontinence in frail elderly persons: Report from the 5th International Consultation on Incontinence. *Neurourology and Urodynamics,* Epub ahead of print.

Wells, M. J., Jamieson, K., Markham, T. C. W., et al. (2014). The effect of caffeinated versus decaffeinated drinks on overactive bladder: A double-blind, randomized, crossover study. *Journal of Wound Ostomy & Continence Nursing, 41*(4), 371–378. doi: 10.1097/WON.0000000000000040.

Wennberg, A. L., Altman, D., Lundholm, C., et al. (2011). Genetic influences are important for most but not all lower urinary tract symptoms: A population-based survey in a cohort of adult Swedish twins. *European Urology, 59,* 1032–1038.

Wennberg, A. L., Molander, U., Fall, M., et al. (2009). A longitudinal population-based survey of urinary incontinence, overactive bladder, and other lower urinary tract symptoms in women. *European Urology, 55*(4), 783–791.

Wright, J., Mccormack, B., Coffey, A., et al. (2007). Evaluating the context within which continence care is provided in rehabilitation units for older people. *International Journal of Older People Nursing, 2,* 9–19.

Yoshida, M., Miyamae, K., Iwashita, H., et al. (2004). Management of detrusor dysfunction in the elderly: Changes in acetylcholine and adenosine triphosphate release during aging. *Urology, 63,* 17–23.

Zhang, E. Y., Stein, R., Chang, S., et al. (2004). Smooth muscle hypertrophy following partial bladder outlet obstruction is associated with overexpression of non-muscle caldesmon. *American Journal of Pathology, 164,* 601–612.

Zimmern, P., Litman, H. J., Mueller, E., et al. (2010). Effect of fluid management on fluid intake and urge incontinence in a trial for overactive bladder in women. *BJU International, 105,* 1680–1685.

QUESTIONS

1. A continence nurse is counseling a female patient diagnosed with overactive bladder (OAB). What would the nurse state is the defining symptom of this condition?
   A. Urinary retention
   B. Urinary urgency
   C. Stress urinary incontinence
   D. Urinary tract infection

2. Which condition found in isolated strips of detrusor taken from patients with urodynamically proven DO indicates the existence of overactive bladder?
   A. Lower levels of intracellular calcium
   B. Chemical changes in protein function that reduce contractile strength
   C. Greater oscillations in the levels of calcium
   D. Fewer spontaneously active cells than normal bladder

3. The continence nurse is counseling a 65-year-old male patient who has been diagnosed with overactive bladder. He states that his doctor mentioned medications that might be helpful for his condition. Which of the following categories of drugs is considered first-line pharmacologic therapy?
   A. Muscle relaxants
   B. Serotonin reuptake inhibitors
   C. Anticholinergics
   D. Tricyclic antidepressants

4. The continence nurse is teaching a patient about proven risk factors that may double the risk for developing overactive bladder. One of these factors is:
   A. High caffeine intake
   B. High physical activity level
   C. Diet high in protein/low in carbohydrates
   D. Obesity or diabetes

5. For which patient with urinary urgency would the continence nurse include a recommendation for urodynamic testing to be performed to diagnose overactive bladder?
   A. A patient with a history of childhood enuresis
   B. A patient with a neurologic condition such as Parkinson's disease
   C. A patient who has frequency and nocturia in addition to urgency
   D. A patient who is a smoker

6. A continence nurse is teaching a patient diagnosed with overactive bladder the techniques of bladder training. Which teaching point accurately describes this technique?
   A. Performing slow pelvic floor contraction at the onset of urgency
   B. Sitting on a soft surface
   C. Increasing the time between onset of urge to void and actual time of voiding
   D. Limiting the amount of fluid intake during the day

7. The continence nurse is caring for frail older people who have urinary incontinence. Which behavioral intervention is a mainstay of UI treatment in this population?
   A. Prompted voiding
   B. Pelvic floor rehabilitation
   C. Double voiding
   D. Use of absorptive products

8. The continence nurse is explaining the technique of functional intervention training to a nursing home resident who is experiencing urinary incontinence. Which element combined with toileting routines comprises this method?
   A. Pharmacological treatment
   B. Restricted fluid intake
   C. Pelvic floor muscle rehabilitation
   D. Musculoskeletal strengthening exercises

9. For which patient would a continence nurse recommend the use of a topical estrogen for overactive bladder?
   A. A 78-year-old male with prostate cancer
   B. A 38-year-old pregnant woman
   C. A postmenopausal woman
   D. A 45-year-old male with diabetes

10. Which pharmaceutical agent has been shown to be of value in the treatment of *refractory* overactive bladder, leading to increased bladder capacity, decreased intravesical pressure, and reduced incontinence episodes?
    A. Oxybutynin
    B. Mirabegron
    C. OnabotulinumtoxinA
    D. Tolterodine

11. Which of the following has been shown to provide positive outcomes for many patients with OAB who "fail" pharmacologic therapy?
    A. Surgical denervation of the bladder
    B. Indwelling catheter
    C. Neuromodulation
    D. Urodynamics

ANSWERS: 1.**B**, 2.**C**, 3.**C**, 4.**D**, 5.**B**, 6.**C**, 7.**A**, 8.**D**, 9.**C**, 10.**C**, 11.**C**

CHAPTER 6

Retention of Urine

Shiv Kumar Pandian and Marcus John Drake

OBJECTIVES

1. Describe the etiology and pathology of urinary retention to include the potential impact on upper tract function.

2. Explain the significance and methodology for distinguishing between retention caused by impaired detrusor contractility and retention caused by outlet obstruction.

3. Describe indications, mechanisms of action, and points to be included in patient education for each of the following: alpha-adrenergic antagonists; double voiding/scheduled voiding; clean intermittent catheterization; and indwelling catheter.

Topical Outline

Introduction

As discussed in Chapter 2, urinary incontinence is one type of lower urinary tract problem and refers to unintentional leakage of urine. In contrast, voiding dysfunction denotes problems emptying the bladder effectively, and difficulty with emptying frequently results in acute or chronic urinary retention. This chapter will focus on the prevalence, incidence, pathology, presentation, and management of urinary retention.

Retention of urine implies the inability to empty the bladder to completion (Kaplan et al., 2008). It is often stressful for patients and may have significant implications for their health. In many cases, it merits immediate catheterization of the bladder to alleviate the patient's distress. Prompt recognition and effective management are essential, as inadequate management may lead to further morbidity and even mortality.

CLINICAL PEARL

Retention is the inability to empty the bladder to completion; it can be classified as acute, chronic, or acute on chronic.

Acute urinary retention (AUR) is defined by the International Continence Society (ICS) as a painful, palpable, or percussable bladder, when the patient is unable to pass any urine (Abrams et al., 2003). The retained volume of urine is usually significantly greater than normal bladder capacity. While this is the classic presentation, the clinician should be aware that bladder pain is not always a presenting complaint and that the bladder is not always palpable or percussable. For example, pain may not be a presenting feature in retention due to prolapsed intervertebral disc, postpartum retention, or retention following regional anesthesia such as an epidural anesthetic. In patients with retention occurring during the immediate postoperative period following abdominal surgery, the bladder may not be painful, palpable, or percussable, due to anterior abdominal wall pain or dressings in the lower abdomen.

Chronic urinary retention (CUR) is defined as a nonpainful bladder that remains palpable or percussable after the patient has passed urine. Such patients may also be incontinent of urine. The ICS no longer recommends the term "overflow incontinence" although this is still commonly used in clinical practice; the term is considered confusing, and there is no convincing definition. If the patient presents with both retention and incontinence, it is better to document a mixed problem involving both chronic urinary retention and urinary incontinence and to specify the type of incontinence once known (e.g., chronic urinary retention and urgency incontinence; chronic urinary retention and nocturnal enuresis; and chronic urinary retention and stress incontinence with cough, laugh, and sneeze). The term chronic retention excludes transient voiding difficulty (e.g., following surgery for stress incontinence) and implies a significant volume of residual urine;

a minimum figure of 300 mL has been quoted (Abrams et al., 2003).

Acute-on-chronic retention implies that a man with a background of CUR presents with an episode of AUR.

CLINICAL PEARL

Acute urinary retention is the total inability to pass urine and requires immediate intervention. Chronic retention is inability to empty the bladder completely and develops slowly over time.

Epidemiology of Urinary Retention

Retention is much more common in men than in women and most of the epidemiologic data referred to in the literature are for AUR; data for CUR are sparse (Kaplan et al., 2008). The reported incidence of AUR in large population-based studies varies from 2.2 to 6.8 per 1,000 men per year (Barry et al., 1997; Cathcart et al., 2006; Jacobsen et al., 1997; Meigs et al., 2001; Verhamme et al., 2005). AUR is rare in younger men; men in their 70s are at five times more risk of AUR than men in their 40s. In one study, it was calculated that as many as 1 in 10 men in their 70s may experience AUR if they survive for a 5-year period (Jacobsen et al., 1997).

Based on the Hospital Episode Statistics (HES) database of the Department of Health, England, 2002–2003, 0.25% (32,162) of hospital consultant episodes were for retention of urine. Of these episodes, 83% required hospital admission, with 75% requiring emergency admission. 86% of episodes involved men and 14% involved women. The mean length of stay in hospitals was 5.3 days, and the mean age of patients hospitalized for retention of urine was 69 years. Only 18% of episodes occurred in 15- to 59-year-olds and 48% occurred in people over the age of 75. Only 7% of hospital consultant episodes for retention of urine were single-day episodes (Armitage, 2011).

The HES database was also used to investigate mortality (Armitage, 2011) after AUR. In 100,067 men with spontaneous AUR, the 1-year mortality was 4.1% in men aged 45 to 54 and 32.8% in those aged 85 and over. In men with spontaneous AUR aged 75 to 84, the most prevalent age group, the 1-year mortality was 12.5% in men without comorbidity and 28.8% in men with comorbidity (Armitage, 2011).

Etiology of Urinary Retention

Causes of retention differ and will be addressed within the context of AUR and chronic retention.

Acute Urinary Retention

Acute urinary retention (AUR) refers to the sudden inability to pass any urine. AUR may be further classified into *precipitated* or *spontaneous* retention (Emberton & Fitzpatrick, 2008; Fitzpatrick & Kirby, 2006; Kaplan et al., 2008).

Precipitated AUR

In precipitated AUR, there is typically a definable triggering event. Of the 344 patients who experienced AUR in

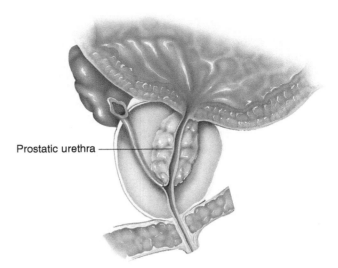

FIGURE 6-1.   Early prostatic hyperplasia showing area of urethral obstruction.

the Dutch epidemiological study (Verhamme, et al., 2005), more than 40% were considered to have had precipitated retention. AUR was preceded by a procedure (surgery, urologic interventions, anesthesia) in 77 cases (22%); in 72 cases (21%), AUR was preceded by a urinary tract infection (UTI), the presence of a neurologic disorder, or treatment with a drug that has been associated with AUR. See Box 6-1 for triggering events for AUR.

Spontaneous AUR

When no triggering event is identified, AUR is considered spontaneous. Spontaneous AUR is most commonly associated with prostatic enlargement due to benign prostatic hyperplasia (BPH) and is indeed considered as a sign of BPH progression (Emberton & Fitzpatrick, 2008; Fitzpatrick & Kirby, 2006; Kaplan et al., 2008). The difference between precipitated and spontaneous retention has treatment implications because BPH-related surgery is less commonly required in cases of precipitated AUR (Emberton & Fitzpatrick, 2008; Kaplan et al., 2008).

CLINICAL PEARL

Acute urinary retention can occur spontaneously (usually as a result of BPH) or can be precipitated by anesthesia, medications, UTI, or a neurologic process.

Role of Benign Prostatic Hypertrophy

BPH is the most common benign neoplasm in men and a major etiological factor in the occurrence of AUR. The term BPH is, however, the source of considerable confusion. It is a histologic diagnosis characterized by the presence of varying degrees of stromal and epithelial hyperplasia. Its prevalence increases with age, with approximately 60% of men in their 50s and 90% of men in their 80s showing evidence of the disease (Berry et al., 1984). BPH may be evident clinically as benign prostatic enlargement (BPE). Due to the relatively inflexible prostatic capsule, cellular proliferation in the periurethral and transitional zones of

the prostate can lead to compression of the urethra and bladder outflow obstruction (BOO; Fig. 6-1). This may result in the clinical manifestations of the disease such as lower urinary tract symptoms (LUTS) and AUR. Nurse practitioners and advanced practice nurses will undertake a digital rectal examination (DRE). Figure 6-2 shows DRE. A lubricated, gloved index finger is inserted to palpate prostate size, shape, sensitivity, and consistency as well as perianal skin integrity, sensation or pain, anal sphincter tone, presence of stool (and consistency), and hemorrhoids or fissures. Any abnormalities are referred to a urologist.

Data from the placebo arm of the Prostate Long-Term Efficacy and Safety Study (PLESS) demonstrated that prostate volume, prostate-specific antigen (PSA) levels, and symptom severity were all predictors of AUR occurrence in patients with BPH (Roehrborn et al., 1999). In

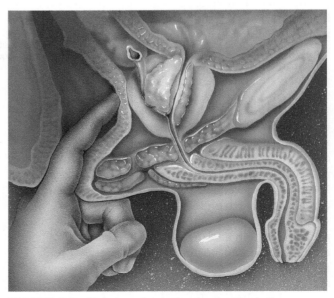

FIGURE 6-2.   Digital rectal exam for abnormalities in the anus, rectum, and prostate.

men with a serum PSA of <1.4 ng/mL, the incidence of AUR increased from 5.6% for those with mild symptoms to 7.7% for those with severe symptoms; in men with a PSA of >1.4 ng/mL, the respective incidences were 7.8% and 10.2%. This was further confirmed by pooled analysis of data from PLESS and three other large prospective randomized controlled trials, each with 2 years follow-up; serum PSA and prostate volume were found to be strong predictors of AUR (Roehrborn et al., 2001). Box 6-2 lists risk factors for AUR.

CLINICAL PEARL

For the patient with BPH, prostate size/volume, PSA levels, and symptom severity are all predictors for development of AUR.

BOX 6-2. **BPH-Related Risk Factors Associated with Spontaneous Acute Urinary Retention**

Prostate volume (>30 to 40 mL)

PSA (>1.4 ng/mL)

Previous episode of AUR

Deteriorating LUTS (worsening of IPPS by ≥4 points)

Lack of response to medical treatment (α-blocker ±5-ARI)

An individual's response to treatment has recently been identified as a predictor of the risk for BPH disease progression and AUR (Armitage & Emberton, 2006). Response is frequently measured by the International Prostate Symptom Score (IPSS), a validated tool used widely to assess effect of treatment (Fig. 6-3). In the Health Professionals

	Not at all 0	Less than 1 time in 5 1	Less than half the time 2	About half the time 3	More than half the time 4	Almost always 5
1. INCOMPLETE EMPTYING Over the last month or so, how often have you had a sensation of not emptying your bladder completely after you finished urinating?	0	1	2	3	4	5
2. FREQUENCY During the last month or so, how often have you had to urinate again <2 hours after you finished urinating?	0	1	2	3	4	5
3. INTERMITTENCY During the last month or so, how often have you stopped and started again several times when you urinated?	0	1	2	3	4	5
4. URGENCY During the last month or so, how often have you found it difficult to postpone urination?	0	1	2	3	4	5
5. WEAK STREAM During the last month or so, how often have you had a weak urinary stream?	0	1	2	3	4	5
6. STRAINING During the last month or so, how often have you had to push or strain to begin urination?	0	1	2	3	4	5
7. SLEEPING During the last month, how many times did you most typically get up to urinate from the time you went to bed at night until the time you got up in the morning?	0	1	2 (times at night)	3	4	5

SCORE: (0-35)_____

The <u>International Prostate Symptom Score (IPSS)</u> uses the same 7 questions as the AUA Symptom Index, but adds a "Disease Specific Quality of Life Question (sometimes referred to as the "bother score") and scored from 0 to 6 points ("delighted" to "terrible").

If you were to spend the rest of your life with your urinary condition just the way it is now, how would you feel about that?

Delighted 0	Pleased 1	Mostly satisfied 2	Mixed 3	Mostly disappointed 4	Unhappy 5	Terrible 6

FIGURE 6-3. International Prostate Symptom Score is also known as the American Urological Association assessment tool. It is a validated tool for assessing voiding dysfunction and the effect on quality of life.

Follow-Up Study, the incidence of AUR was higher in patients whose LUTS had worsened over a 2-year period. Increased severity of an individual LUTS or the overall LUTS score was associated with increased risk of AUR, independent of baseline severity (Meigs et al., 1999). This observation was supported by data from the Alf-One study, in which a prior episode of AUR was the most important predictor of AUR. Worsening of the IPSS by 4 points and a bother score greater than 3 at end point were also predictive (Emberton & Fitzpatrick, 2008).

Pathology of AUR

Several mechanisms have been proposed to explain why AUR occurs, although it is still not very clear. Possible mechanisms include sudden increased resistance to flow of urine due to mechanical obstruction (urethral stricture, clot retention), dynamic obstruction (increased α-adrenergic activity, prostatic inflammation), bladder overdistension (immobility, constipation, drugs inhibiting bladder contractility), and/or neuropathic or metabolic conditions causing impaired bladder contractility (e.g., diabetic cystopathy) (Choong & Emberton, 2000; Emberton & Fitzpatrick, 2008; Fitzpatrick & Kirby, 2006; Kaplan et al., 2008).

Chronic Urinary Retention

CUR is more complex and can be classified as either *high-pressure* chronic retention (HPCR) or *low-pressure* chronic retention (LPCR); the two are distinguished by the detrusor pressure at the end of micturition (i.e., at the start of the next filling phase) (Abrams et al., 1978, 2001; George et al., 1983).

High-Pressure Chronic Retention

BOO is the usual cause for HPCR, so flow rate is generally poor even though detrusor pressure is high. The continually elevated bladder pressure in HPCR, during both the storage and voiding phases of micturition, often results in bilateral hydronephrosis. Figure 6-4 shows hydronephrosis as a result of chronic prostatic obstruction of the lower urinary tract.

Low-Pressure Chronic Retention

Other patients may have large-volume retention caused by a poorly contractile but very compliant bladder; these patients are said to have LPCR and typically exhibit no hydronephrosis or renal failure. Urodynamic studies in these patients show low detrusor pressures, low flow rates, and very large postvoid residual (PVR) volumes. LUTS can be of mild severity in CUR, at least in the early stages. Nocturnal enuresis may be the first symptomatic presentation and may result from a slight reduction in urethral pressure when asleep.

CLINICAL PEARL

Chronic urinary retention can be classified as HPCR (high-pressure chronic retention) and LPCR (low-pressure chronic retention); HPCR creates resistance to delivery of urine from the kidneys and can cause eventual hydronephrosis.

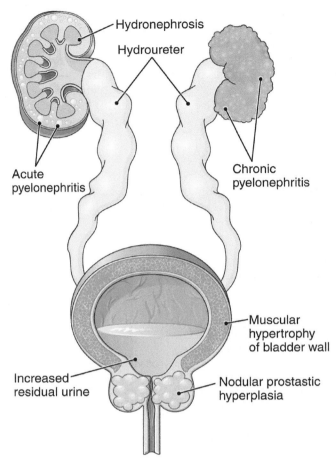

FIGURE 6-4. Consequences of prostatic chronic obstruction of the lower urinary tract. Incomplete emptying of the bladder causes nocturia, urgency, frequency, and loss of control. Ureteral reflux may cause infection and chronic kidney disease.

Less Common Causes of Urinary Retention

There are a number of other processes that can cause urinary retention, though they are relatively uncommon.

Cancer

Malignancies of the urinary tract can cause urinary obstruction, but the process is more gradual and generally indicates a more advanced stage of malignancy. Cancer of the ureters, bladder, prostate, penis, or urethra can gradually obstruct urine output. Cancers often present with hematuria, weight loss, and lower back and/or groin pain.

Retention in Women

Urinary retention in women is much less common but may be caused by pelvic masses (e.g., uterine, ovarian) or pelvic prolapse (cystocele, rectocele, uterine) causing urethral compression, following pelvic surgery, such as surgery to treat stress urinary incontinence, urethral stenosis, or urethral diverticulum. Transient retention may occur as a result of infection or inflammation occurring postpartum or secondary to herpes simplex infection, Bartholin's abscess, acute urethritis, or vulvovaginitis. Fowler's syndrome can also cause retention; this is a condition involving impaired relaxation of the external sphincter that occurs in premenopausal women, often in association with polycystic ovaries.

Bladder Neck Dyssynergia

Bladder neck obstruction/dyssynergia is another functional cause of BOO (rather than a mechanical cause) that is more commonly seen in relatively younger men and rarely reported in women; it is due to failure of the bladder neck muscle fibers (internal sphincter) to relax during voiding. This condition usually occurs *de novo* without any underlying neurological abnormality. Figure 6-5 shows video urodynamics findings typical of detrusor sphincter dyssynergia (DSD) often seen in motor neuron disease such as multiple sclerosis as well as spinal cord injury. DSD can also be behavioral.

Detrusor Underactivity

Nonobstructive causes of retention include detrusor underactivity (hypotonia, atonia) and can occur in both sexes. Specific etiologic factors include underlying neurological disorders (e.g., stroke, multiple sclerosis) or idiopathic detrusor underactivity, which is usually an age-related phenomenon seen in the elderly.

Neurological disease can cause obstruction or retention by impairment of bladder contractility, nonrelaxation of the outlet, or failure of coordination between bladder contraction and sphincter/pelvic floor relaxation, depending on the precise level of the neurological deficit(s).

Retention in Children

AUR is rare in children and is usually associated with infection or occurs postoperatively (e.g., circumcision).

Paruresis

Paruresis is the inability to urinate in the presence of others, such as in public toilets; this is also called "shy bladder syndrome," which, in extreme cases, can result in urinary retention.

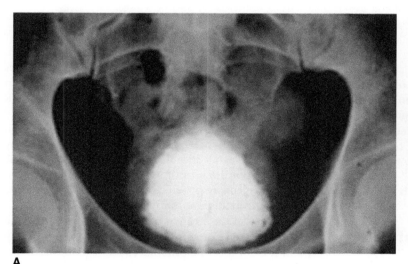

A

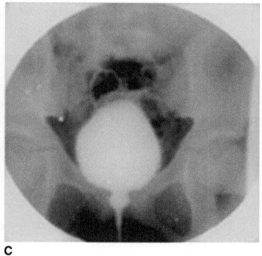

C

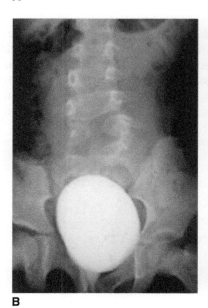

B

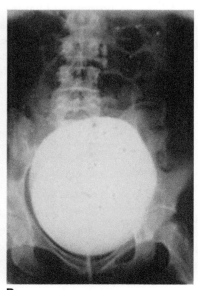

D

FIGURE 6-5. Video urodynamics. **A.** Spastic bladder in a spinal cord injury patient without adequate management, beginning "Christmas tree" shape, trabeculation, and many small diverticula. **B.** Detrusor sphincter dyssynergia in myelodysplasia patient. Note the abnormalities of the spinal column. **C, D.** Bladder acontracility because of overdistension.

TABLE 6-1 Causes of Urinary Retention Based on the Level of the Urinary Tract Involved

	Male	Female
Urethra	Congenital urethral valves Phimosis and/or pinhole meatus Circumcision Obstruction in the urethra caused by stricture, calculus, or tumor STD lesions (gonorrhea commonly causes multiple strictures, leading to a "rosary bead" appearance, whereas chlamydia usually causes a single stricture)	Pelvic prolapse compressing the urethra Urethral stenosis Urethral diverticulum Postsurgery for stress urinary incontinence Postpartum infection/inflammation Genital herpes Bartholin's abscess Acute urethritis/vulvovaginitis
Prostate/bladder neck	Benign prostatic hyperplasia (BPH) Prostate cancer and other pelvic malignancies invading the prostate Acute prostatitis Bladder neck obstruction (dyssynergia, stenosis—iatrogenic scarring following prostate surgery, indwelling catheters)	Fowler's syndrome Pelvic mass compressing/invading bladder neck Bladder neck obstruction (dyssynergia, stenosis—scarring due to indwelling catheters, bladder neck surgery)
Bladder	Detrusor sphincter dyssynergia Neurogenic bladder (commonly pelvic splanchnic nerve damage, cauda equina syndrome, descending cortical fibers lesion, pontine micturition or storage center lesions, demyelinating diseases, or Parkinson's disease)	

Medication

Medications with anticholinergic properties can cause retention due to reduced contraction strength of the detrusor. In an individual at risk for AUR, ingestion of medications with anticholinergic or alpha-adrenergic agonist properties may precipitate AUR. Psychoactive substances can cause retention due to enhanced outlet resistance; drugs in this category include stimulants such as MDMA (ecstasy) and other amphetamines.

Common causes of urinary retention in both men and women are listed in Table 6-1.

Pathology and Pathogenesis of Urinary Retention

Five different factors have been implicated in the pathogenesis of urinary retention (Choong & Emberton, 2000; Emberton & Fitzpatrick, 2008; Fitzpatrick & Kirby, 2006; Mishra et al., 2007; Tuncel et al., 2005). They are:

- Prostatic infarction
- α-Adrenergic activity
- Decrease in the prostatic stromal–epithelial ratio
- Neurotransmitter modulation
- Prostatic inflammation (Box 6-3)

Spiro et al. (1974) found evidence of infarction (caused by infection, instrumentation, and/or thrombosis) in 85% of prostatectomy specimens obtained from patients with AUR, but in only 3% of the transurethral resection of the prostate (TURP) specimens obtained from patients with LUTS alone. Of course, catheterization is a confounding factor in this situation. It is hypothesized that prostatic infarction affects smooth muscle relaxation or increases

urethral pressure due to contained swelling. However, infarction is a controversial theory; Anjum and colleagues found no significant difference in the rate of infarction between men who did and those who did not have AUR (Anjum et al., 1998).

Some cases of AUR have been postulated to result from a rise in the prostatic intraurethral pressure caused by increased α-adrenergic stimulation; the increased adrenergic stimulation could result from stress, cold weather, sympathomimetic agents (e.g., selected cold remedies), prostatic infarction, prostatitis, and/or bladder overdistension.

A decrease in the stromal to epithelial ratio within the prostate has been noted in AUR. This decrease may partly explain the effect of the pharmaceutical agent finasteride, which may act mainly on the epithelial component of the prostate and has been reported to reduce the risk of retention (McConnell et al., 1998).

There is evidence of increased incidence of histologic prostatic inflammation in men with AUR compared to men with LUTS alone (Armitage & Emberton, 2005; Tuncel et al., 2005). This finding is further supported by evidence suggesting that such prostatic inflammation

BOX 6-3. Factors Implicated in the Pathogenesis of Urinary Retention

Prostatic infarction
Increased α-adrenergic activity
Decrease in the prostatic stromal–epithelial ratio
Reduction in nonadrenergic noncholinergic neurotransmitters
Prostatic inflammation

may also be a predictor of BPH progression (Mishra et al., 2007). In addition, the Medical Therapy of Prostatic Symptoms (MTOPS) study showed prostatic inflammation in biopsy specimens. Overall, during the 4.5 years follow-up, patients with prostatic inflammation were significantly more likely to develop AUR. In the presence of inflammation, 5.6% went on to develop AUR compared to none of the patients with no prostatic inflammation (Armitage & Emberton, 2005; Roehrborn et al., 2001).

Complications of Urinary Retention

Urinary retention is typically treated in a hospital, and the more quickly one seeks treatment, the fewer the complications. Long-term complications associated with obstruction of the urinary tract and urinary retention include:

- Vesical calculi (bladder stones)
- Atrophy or hypertrophy of the detrusor muscle
- Hydronephrosis
- Chronic renal failure
- Diverticula (formation of pouches) in the bladder wall
- Urinary tract infection

Obstructive Uropathy

It is now well established that lower urinary tract dysfunction may adversely affect the upper urinary tract. Furthermore, since the effects may be asymptomatic, ongoing impact through nondiagnosis can lead to severe dysfunction. HPCR of urine is a good human model to exemplify the physiological changes that occur synchronously within the lower and upper tracts (George, 1999).

Prostatism and Obstructive Uropathy

The three-stage theory of prostatism purported that BOO caused by an enlarged prostate led to hypertophy and trabeculation (cord-like thickening into the bladder lumen; Fig. 6-6) of the bladder wall. Further progression was hypothesized to result in sacculation and diverticulum formation. Untreated disease was believed to lead, in due course, to failure of the valve-like function of the vesicoureteric junctions, resulting in ureteric dilation and hydronephrosis, the precursor to renal failure. The final element of the process was bladder "decompensation," when the bladder became excessively capacious and relatively insensitive. "Overflow incontinence" was then said to occur (George, 1999).

However, this progressive model has never been proven or indeed modeled. It is also hard to envisage how a hypertrophic, trabeculated bladder would transition to a thinwalled, overdistended organ. In 1951, Wallace looked at the

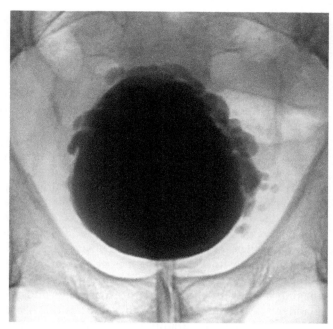

FIGURE 6-6. Bladder wall thickening. Contrast cystogram demonstrates markedly trabeculated bladder with multiple small outpouchings consistent with multiple diverticula. These findings are commonly seen with chronic bladder outlet obstruction.

association between the type of prostate enlargement and the associated structure of the upper urinary tract, finding a clearer association between bladder neck hypertrophy and hydronephrosis, which was not seen with enlargement of the lateral lobes (Wallace, 1951). Accordingly, the range of structural changes seen, in both the lower and upper urinary tract, may reflect the specific nature of outlet changes, rather than a progressive transition.

To understand the pathogenesis of HPCR, it is necessary to appreciate the comparatively small amount of time spent overall in the voiding phase of the micturition cycle. Voiding time is <1% of the overall cycle, which indicates that upper tract consequences of HPCR more likely reflect the impaired drainage of the ureters during the filling phase (George et al., 1986).

Loss of Bladder Wall Compliance

It appears likely that secondary structural changes in the bladder wall alter the filling-phase properties of the bladder. Of these, the most important is probably the property of "compliance," which is the ability of the normal bladder to change volume considerably with almost no change in pressure. Compliance reflects normal detrusor muscle function, and altered structure of the bladder wall will affect it, especially if there is connective tissue infiltration. If this crucial property is lost, pressure rises with bladder filling and hampers the drainage of the ureters. This is particularly important if the bladder fails to empty completely with voiding, as the consequence will be high bladder pressures almost continuously. Structurally, another influence is the thickening of the bladder wall, which may compress or distort the vesicoureteric junction, impairing the effective drainage of the ureter. It is not clear to what extent either process contributes, but the consequence is potentially the onset of progressive upper tract dilation (George et al., 1983).

Figure 6-7 illustrates a schematic diagram of putative pressure changes in the bladder for someone with HPCR. It shows a poorly compliant bladder, since pressure rises with filling (the pressure rise becoming more pronounced at higher volumes). In this situation, a postvoid residual inevitably means the bladder pressure will always be elevated. Clearly, filling and voiding are volume changes occurring above the postvoid residual. Thus, seemingly normal voiding may be present, but the reality may be very abnormal, with continuous pressure making it hard for the ureters to expel urine into the bladder (George, 1999). From this illustration, it can be surmised that fully draining the bladder (e.g., using intermittent catheterization) would provide at least some time with low bladder pressures (George et al., 1984).

> **CLINICAL PEARL**
>
> Loss of compliance causes high intravesical pressures throughout most of the filling/voiding cycle and is a major risk factor for upper tract damage.

In a normally compliant bladder, the rise in intravesical pressure associated with filling from empty to physiological bladder capacity (typically around 500 mL) is

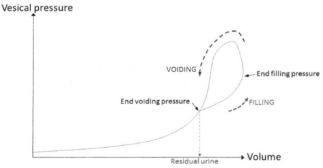

FIGURE 6-7. Pressure–volume relationship in high-pressure chronic retention. Following micturition (end void point), the pressure within the bladder rises as filling takes place from the upper tracts. Eventually, the end fill pressure is reached at which point the patient is experiencing the normal desire to void. A detrusor contraction takes place (over and above the intrinsic pressure within the bladder) and urine is expelled in the usual fashion. At the end of micturition, the pressure returns once again to the end void point, thus completing the pressure "loop."

<5 cm H_2O. Uncomplicated BOO does not affect bladder compliance, so upper tract dilation does not result. Only if there is a poorly compliant bladder is there risk of structural damage to the upper urinary tract and impaired renal function.

An important point to recognize is that reflux (the backward flow of urine from the bladder to the upper urinary tract) is often absent. Thus, the upper tract changes probably reflect impedance to normal flow, rather than direct transmission of bladder pressure to the renal system (George, 1999). The crucial threshold bladder pressure is probably 25 cm H_2O, above which urine flow from the upper tract is substantially impaired (Ghose, 1990; Holden et al., 1984).

Clinical Presentation and Assessment of Retention of Urine

Acute Urinary Retention

AUR is a medical emergency and requires prompt treatment. The lower abdominal pain can be excruciating when urine cannot be expelled. The individual in AUR can develop severe sweating, chest pain, anxiety, and high blood pressure, and there is a risk of precipitating angina or myocardial infarction. Patients with AUR may or may not have a history of previous LUTS. Some of these patients may not report prior LUTS, either because they did not recognize the significance of their symptoms or because they have learned to live with them. In AUR, there is a palpable mass that arises from the pelvis (i.e., the lower border of the mass is not palpable), which is dull on percussion. DRE in men should include assessment of the size and consistency of the prostate, anal sphincter tone, and presence or absence of retained stool. Vaginal examination should include assessment for prolapse or other mass (using a speculum), any tenderness or mass in the vaginal fornices, and bimanual palpation of organs and any pelvic mass. (See Chapter 9 for vaginal examination.) It will be easier for the patient and will be more informative for the clinician if the rectal or vaginal examination is carried out after the patient has been catheterized and the retention has been relieved. Although AUR is primarily a clinical diagnosis, a bladder volume scan will further confirm the diagnosis before catheterization. The volume of urine drained is usually <1 L; if the volume drained is >1 L, it suggests the possibility of an acute-on-chronic retention, particularly if the level of discomfort is moderate rather than severe (Kalejaiye & Speakman, 2009).

Chronic Urinary Retention

CUR occurs when a patient retains a substantial volume of urine in the bladder after each void (Kaplan et al., 2008). Defining a threshold volume for CUR has not been standardized. The finding of persistent residual volumes of >300 mL (some authors suggest >500 mL) after voiding is often used as evidence of CUR; some patients may present with many liters in their bladders (Ghalayini et al., 2005; Kaplan et al., 2008). Patients may be asymptomatic, or they may void little and often, or they may have difficulty with initiating and completing micturition. Other features of CUR include nocturnal enuresis and a painless palpable bladder; at its extreme, there may be symptoms attributable to chronic renal failure (malaise, loss of appetite, anorexia, fatigue) (Ghalayini et al., 2005; Kaplan et al., 2008). In general, previous LUTS are uncommon in patients with CUR (Abrams et al., 1978; George et al., 1983).

Diagnostic Studies

In both types of retention, urinalysis should always be performed and a catheter specimen of urine (CSU) should be sent if there are signs of infection. Urinary infection should be treated with appropriate antibiotics. Blood urea, serum creatinine, electrolytes, and estimated glomerular filtration rate (eGFR) should be checked; this is especially important in HPCR. Renal ultrasound is indicated in patients with high-volume retention and in patients with abnormal renal function. Figure 6-8 is an ultrasound scan postvoiding in a man with CUR and illustrating hydronephrosis and residual urine in the bladder. PSA testing is best avoided during the acute episode, since any instrumentation of the prostate leads to a spurious rise in PSA (Pruthi, 2000). Interpreting the PSA after the acute episode is settled requires recognition that PSA is a nonspecific test that can be elevated in prostate cancer, BPH, and prostatitis. *A TRUS (transrectal ultrasound)-guided biopsy of the prostate can distinguish between these prostate conditions.*

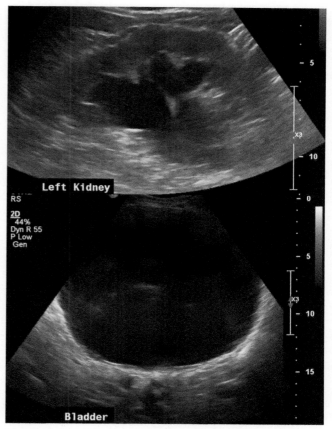

FIGURE 6-8.   Ultrasound scan taken after voiding in a man with chronic retention. The kidney shows hydronephrosis, that is, prominent and swollen collecting system, with loss of the acute angles typical of a normal kidney collecting system. The bladder still contains a considerable volume, which should not be present after voiding.

CLINICAL PEARL

Assessment of the patient with retention should include a urinalysis to assess for infection and BUN, creatinine, and eGFR to rule out renal damage.

When AUR is associated with neurologic symptoms, specific evaluation is required, which may be urgent, since irreversible change can result in some circumstances. New-onset pain in the lumbar spine, numbness in the perianal area (saddle anesthesia), paresthesias, diminished anal sphincter tone, or altered deep tendon reflexes may be indicative. In these circumstances, an urgent neurological referral may be required. An MRI of the lumbar spine should be considered to further assess for possible spinal cord compression or cauda equina syndrome.

Differentiating AUR from other possible diagnoses is not usually difficult, but diverticulitis or a diverticular abscess, perforated or ischemic bowel, and abdominal aortic aneurysm are all recognized as potentially more serious conditions that can inappropriately be referred into hospital as AUR. Urinary retention may occur secondary to many medical conditions; accordingly, the patient should be reexamined soon after catheterization to confirm that the symptoms and signs have resolved. Additionally, any patient with a lower abdominal mass should be considered for catheterization to exclude a distended bladder prior to further examination or investigation (Kalejaiye & Speakman, 2009). Occasionally, an obese patient with anuria or oliguria due to renal failure may mistakenly be thought to be in AUR. A bladder scan can be helpful in this situation. Urodynamics is not a first-line assessment method for etiology of urinary retention but is useful when conservative treatment has failed. Figure 6-9 shows a voiding cystourethrogram (VCUG) of an individual with a trabeculated bladder and dilated posterior urethra typical of mechanical obstruction from an anterior urethral stricture.

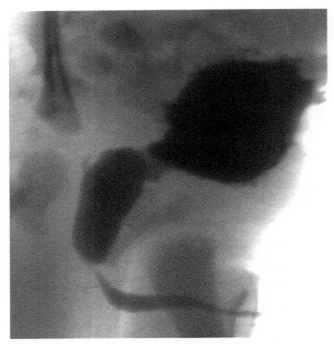

FIGURE 6-9. Voiding cystourethrogram (VCUG). Lateral oblique view of the urinary bladder and urethra during voiding after removal of the urinary catheter shows that the bladder is trabeculated and the posterior urethra is dilated. An abrupt change in caliber of the urethra is present in which the large caliber of the dilated, patent posterior urethra is juxtaposed against that of the small anterior urethra.

Treatment of Urinary Retention

Acute Urinary Retention

Treatment of AUR requires urgent catheterization. Whether patients are catheterized in the community or primary care by a general practitioner, in accident and emergency departments, or in surgical or urology wards depends mainly on local circumstances, as does the decision to admit or send home after catheterization (Bates et al., 2003; Emberton & Fitzpatrick, 2008; Fitzpatrick & Kirby, 2006). Keeping patients in hospital awaiting definitive treatment results in a longer total hospital stay. The urine volume drained in the first 10 to 15 minutes following catheterization must be accurately recorded in the patient's notes to enable a distinction between acute and acute-on-chronic retention. This has important clinical implications. The results of the Alfuzosin in Acute Urinary Retention (ALFAUR) study show a significantly increased risk of failure for trial without catheterization (TWOC) in the elderly (>65 years) and in patients with a drained volume >1 L (Emberton & Fitzpatrick, 2008). In the second part of the study, patients with initially successful TWOC were more likely to have recurrent AUR if their post-TWOC residual volume was high. It has been proposed that these patients should be offered elective transurethral resection of prostate (TURP) at an earlier stage.

> **CLINICAL PEARL**
>
> Treatment of acute urinary retention requires urgent catheterization; the volume drained during the first 10 to 15 minutes should be accurately recorded to help differentiate acute from acute-on-chronic retention.

Chronic Retention

Management of CUR is more complex.

Catheterization

Catheterization is less urgent because the condition is generally less painful or painless. Early catheterization is indicated if renal dysfunction or hydronephrosis is present. Following relief of the obstruction, the majority of individuals have complete recovery of kidney function. However, a few will have marked polyuria (>4 to 5 L/day) after bladder drainage, which effectively restores the ability of each kidney to drain fully. This is termed "postobstructive diuresis." There are several *physiological* and *pathologic* factors that lead to the development of this condition.

Postobstructive Diuresis

Following catheter placement, the volume of urine output can be considerably greater than the postvoid residual volume. This can result from rectification of excess sodium and water retention in patients with HPCR and renal dysfunction, along with an osmotic diuresis that is caused by the accumulation of urea and other nonreabsorbable solutes (Sparks, 2010).

The pathologic factors include

- Decreased tubular reabsorption of sodium secondary to altered expression of proximal and distal renal tubular sodium transporters
- Inability to maximally concentrate urine, secondary to a decreased medullary concentrating gradient (hence impaired response to antidiuretic hormone (ADH))
- Increased tubular transit flow time affecting equilibration of sodium and water
- Increased production of prostaglandins immediately following relief of obstruction (Sparks, 2010)

Sparks warns that those who develop postobstructive diuresis require close monitoring for potentially severe fluid volume deficits and hypokalemia. The nurse must monitor urine output closely; when it is noted that the patient has diuresed to the point of normal output, fluid replacement should be administered as needed to prevent volume contraction in the circulation. Various approaches may be utilized, such as replacing 75% of the urine losses with 0.45% normal saline. The critical point is to monitor the patient closely for any signs of circulating volume depletion. Postobstructive diuresis is usually self-limiting and resolves over several days to a week, once surplus waste products (e.g., urea) are eliminated. Persistent polyuria beyond a week is often due to overzealous volume repletion (Sparks, 2010).

In a small percentage of cases (about 10%), diuresis is excessive and requires careful fluid replacement. Daily weights are helpful in monitoring fluid losses. Maximal excretory urine volumes and electrolyte excretion occur during the first 24 hours. After the first 24 hours, fluid replacement should not strictly follow output, as this would perpetuate the diuresis. Potassium levels, which are often high prior to catheterization, should be monitored and will usually (but not always) fall with the diuresis. Replacement should be guided by electrolyte levels, the patient's oral intake, and presence of comorbid conditions (such as heart disease). Most of the early improvement in the glomerular filtration rate (GFR) is related to tubular recovery, although a late glomerular recovery phase occurs as well (Jones et al., 1989).

Catheterization for CUR is often followed by hematuria; this is caused by renal tract decompression and not usually by the catheter itself. The practice of slow decompression of bladder is unnecessary, and hematuria usually settles after 48 to 72 hours.

Definitive Management of an Obstructive Condition

Even if renal failure settles with catheterization, the patient should not undergo a TWOC (trial without catheterization) until the patient has been evaluated for a definitive procedure such as TURP. In patients with CUR who have normal renal function, it is best to avoid catheterization so as to avoid infection and bladder shrinkage before TURP, but the patients should be listed for early surgery. Patients with LPCR do poorly after TURP, frequently failing to void completely after surgery, even after prolonged periods of catheterization; this is probably due to detrusor changes over time (Bates et al., 2003; Ghalayini et al., 2005). Patients with LPCR should be warned of this possibility prior to consenting them for a TURP. In these patients, clean intermittent self-catheterization (CISC) should be considered as an option prior to and potentially after a TURP (Ghalayini et al., 2005).

CLINICAL PEARL

Patients with low-pressure chronic retention may not do well following TURP and should be informed of this prior to surgery; they may require self-catheterization to empty the bladder.

Catheterization for Urinary Retention

Catheterization for management of urinary retention may be done via the urethral route or via suprapubic placement.

Urethral Catheterization

In urethral catheterization, a latex, polyurethane, or silicone tube is inserted into a patient's bladder via the urethra, to permit continual drainage of urine. Catheterization is typically performed by a health care professional, but patients who require intermittent catheterization (IC) can be taught CISC. Catheterization may involve placement of a catheter that is left in place (indwelling catheter) or "in and out" catheterization. In the case of the latter, the

patient should be monitored; if sent home, they must be given clear options for timely management if they develop evidence of recurrent retention.

A Foley catheter (indwelling urinary catheter) is retained by means of a balloon near the tip that is inflated with sterile water. The balloons typically come in two different sizes: 10 and 30 mL. The larger balloon is generally indicated only for hemostasis following prostatic surgery. A hematuria catheter is a type of Foley catheter used for patients who are retaining blood clots and urine. These are usually three-way catheters (triple lumen). One channel of the catheter is used for the inflow of irrigation fluid (warm normal saline) and another channel for the outflow of the urine and blood from the bladder. The third channel is used to inflate the balloon. Figure 6-10 shows examples of the various catheters available for indwelling catheterization.

An intermittent catheter/Robinson catheter is a flexible catheter used for "in and out" drainage of urine. Unlike the Foley catheter, it has no balloon on its tip and therefore cannot stay in place unaided. These can be noncoated or coated with a hydrophilic film that minimizes urethral irritation.

A coudé catheter is designed with a curved and pointed tip that makes it easier to pass through the curvature of the prostatic urethra. The curved end is designed to negotiate urethral obstruction. When inserting a coudé catheter, the tip of the catheter should face anteriorly (up) so that the rounded tip is able to pass through the urogenital diaphragm.

Catheter diameters are sized by the French (Fr) or "Charrière" (Ch) scale. The sizes range from 10 F (3.3 mm)

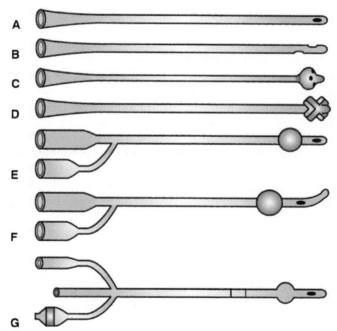

FIGURE 6-10. Various types of commonly used catheters. **A, B.** Simple urethral catheters. **C.** Mushroom or de Pezzer. **D.** Winged tip or Malecot. **E.** Foley with inflated retention balloon. **F.** Foley with coudé tip. **G.** Three-way catheter (in this illustration, the third lumen opens into the urethra to permit irrigation and usually opens at tip for irrigation of the bladder).

to 28 F (9.3 mm). The clinician selects a size large enough to allow free flow of urine, taking into account urine content, including debris, mucous, blood, or clots. Larger catheters, however, are more likely to damage the urethra and bladder neck. If allergies or sensitivities to latex develop, silicone catheters can be substituted, and these are also more suitable for long-term usage. There is some evidence that silver alloy–coated urinary catheters may reduce infections in short-term catheterization (Lederer et al., 2014), but a recent Cochrane review noted that current studies are limited by sample size and heterogeneity and further studies are required if clinicians are to make informed decisions about these products (Jahn et al., 2012).

Catheterization can be complicated in females due to anatomical variations in the perineal structures, which can be caused by obesity, obstetric history, pelvic organ prolapse, or other factors. It is generally accepted that cleaning the area surrounding the urethral meatus with 0.9% sodium chloride solution is sufficient for both male and female patients, as there is no reliable evidence to suggest that the use of antiseptic agents reduces the risk of UTI.

If bladder spasms occur, or there is no urine in the drainage bag, it may indicate blockage of the catheter by blood, thick sediment, or a kink in the catheter or drainage tubing. It is critical that the catheter is well supported, with no tugging on the bladder neck. There are several commercial devices available that provide good support to catheters. Bladder spasms can occur, causing pain and leakage around the catheter. Anticholinergic medications, such as oxybutynin, may help, although most patients eventually adjust to the irritation and the spasms settle down (Hedlund et al., 2001).

Catheterization is a sterile medical procedure undertaken by trained, qualified personnel. Incorrect technique may cause trauma to the urethra or prostate, UTI, or a paraphimosis in the uncircumcised male. Insertion of a catheter may cause pain, particularly for a younger male or one in AUR, so a topical anesthetic such as lidocaine gel 2% is recommended (Garbutt et al., 2008; Siderias et al., 2004). The gel comes in a 5 to 10 mL preloaded syringe with a tip designed for insertion into the meatus. To instill, the clinician should hold the penis firmly and extended, place the tip of the syringe in the meatus, and apply gentle but continuous pressure on the plunger. A gloved finger should be held at the urethral opening for 2 to 3 minutes to allow the anesthetic to take effect. Some topical gels contain chlorhexidine, and potentially serious reactions can occur if this type of gel is used on a patient with chlorhexidine allergy; thus, patients should be routinely queried regarding any allergies prior to use of the anesthetic gel.

A catheter that is left in place for more than a short period of time is generally attached to a drainage bag to collect the urine. This also allows for measurement of urine volume. There are two types of drainage bags: (1) a leg bag, which is a smaller drainage device that attaches by stretch bands to the leg. A leg bag is usually worn during the day, as it fits discreetly under trousers or skirts and is easily emptied into a toilet; and (2) a night bag, which is hung on a hook under the patient's bed. Drainage bags should not be placed on the floor, due to risk of bacterial infection.

Long-term catheterization carries a significant risk of UTI. Other long-term complications include urosepsis, urethral injury leading to stricture, skin breakdown (catheter-induced hypospadias), bladder stones, and hematuria. After many years of catheter use, due to irritation of the bladder mucosa, squamous metaplasia may replace some of the normal urothelium, placing the patient at risk for squamous cell carcinoma of the bladder.

Suprapubic Catheterization

When placement of a urethral catheter is contraindicated or unsuccessful, percutaneous suprapubic urinary bladder catheterization can be performed to relieve urinary retention. Suprapubic catheterization (SPC) placement is absolutely contraindicated in the absence of an easily palpable or ultrasonographically distended urinary bladder (Ramos-Fernandez et al., 2013). Relative contraindications to SPC placement include coagulopathy (until the abnormality is corrected) and previous lower abdominal or pelvic surgery (due to potential bowel adherence to the bladder or anterior abdominal wall). In the latter situation, it is safer for the urologist to perform an open cystostomy. SPC is also relatively contraindicated in pelvic cancer, with or without pelvic radiation, owing to increased risk of adhesions (Harrison et al., 2011). Figure 6-11 shows SPC in a male.

SPC is a painful procedure, even with proper local anesthesia. Patients may require parenteral analgesia, with or without sedation. The currently preferred method for SPC is the Seldinger technique (catheter over needle technique). Informed consent is obtained from the patient or guardian prior to the procedure. The patient is placed in the supine position. The lower abdominal wall is cleaned and shaved if necessary. The distended bladder is palpated and the site of insertion is marked in the midline, roughly 5 cm above the pubic symphysis. Routine use of ultrasonography is recommended by some urologists to verify bladder location, especially in the obese patient, and to ensure that no loops of bowel are present between the abdominal wall and the

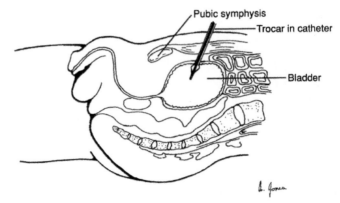

FIGURE 6-11. Technique of suprapubic catheterization by using a trocar with a catheter.

bladder. An antiseptic solution is applied and a local anesthetic agent (1% or 2% lidocaine ±0.25% or 0.5% bupivacaine) is infiltrated at the insertion site. The needle is then advanced through the skin, subcutaneous tissue, rectus sheath, retropubic space, and anterior bladder wall, until urine is seen to enter the syringe. As the needle is advanced, local anesthetic is infiltrated, but regular aspiration is needed to see if blood or other matter enters the syringe, in which case the treatment strategy must be reviewed. A custom-made needle from the SPC kit (e.g., Mediplus) is then passed into the bladder through the anterior abdominal wall and urine is again aspirated to ensure correct needle placement. A small (<0.5 cm) suprapubic incision is made on either side of the needle; the length of the incision needs to be able to accommodate the circumference of the insertion sheath. A guide wire is then passed through the needle into the bladder and the needle removed. A disposable trocar and cannula (made of a peel-away sheath) is passed over the guide wire into the bladder and the guide wire removed. Removal of the trocar will usually result in immediate return of urine from the bladder through the cannula; a suitably sized Foley catheter (usually 12 to 16 Fr) is then quickly placed into the bladder through the cannula, before the bladder empties of urine, and the catheter balloon is inflated (usually with 10 mL of sterile water). The cannula sheath is then easily removed by peeling it away around the catheter. Placing an anchoring skin suture to hold the catheter in place may be considered (Vasdev et al., 2014).

When changing an SPC via an established track, speed is very important. The new catheter should be inserted immediately following removal of the old catheter; an SPC should not be removed unless the practitioner is ready to insert the replacement catheter. Potential complications of SPCs include the following:

- Hematuria (typically transient)
- Cellulitis and abscess formation
- Catheter blockage
- Urinary calculi
- Urinary tract infections
- Dermatitis at the stoma site from urine leak causing chemical irritation
- Urethral leakage in females with stress incontinence

If displacement or malposition is a concern, a cystogram should be performed; if the bladder is not outlined, urgent action should be taken to restore urine drainage and to prevent and manage trauma to affected organs, as bowel perforation and intra-abdominal visceral injuries and peritonitis may occur (Ahmed et al., 2004). Every effort should be made to ensure bladder position with palpation and ultrasonography to prevent or minimize the chance of these complications.

Urethral versus Suprapubic Catheterization

The principal advantages of SPC are reduced urethral irritation and stricture formation, ability to have sexual intercourse in the absence of a urethral catheter, and the ability to provide a trial without catheter by simply clamping the catheter (as opposed to removing the catheter). This is often referred to as "trial of voiding (TOV)"; the SPC is clamped and the patient is allowed to void urine naturally, following which the SPC can be unclamped and the residual volume measured (Horgan et al., 1992). Although it has been suggested that UTI is lower with SPC, in long-term use, there appears to be no difference in UTI rates (Hunter et al., 2013). In classic papers on the use of SPCs, it is noted that patients frequently expressed a preference for SPC, specifically indicating increased comfort and ease of sexual intercourse with an SPC (Abrams et al., 1980; Ahluwalia et al., 2006; Horgan et al., 1992; Ichsan & Hunt, 1987). The latter is often overlooked when deciding on the type of catheter to provide patients but should be routinely considered; the ability to maintain active sexual function is particularly important to some patients.

> **CLINICAL PEARL**
>
> One advantage of an SPC as opposed to urethral catheter is the ability to conduct a "trial of voiding" without removing the catheter; another advantage is the lack of interference with sexual activity.

The ability to provide a TOV without removing the catheter is another major advantage of SPC. A significant number of patients with retention will fail TWOC and will require repeat catheterization, with all the resulting discomfort (Emberton & Fitzpatrick, 2008). The benefits of SPC in AUR have been shown in many studies, and SPC may be regarded as the preferred route of catheterization. Despite this, the Reten-World survey reported that most urologists perform urethral catheterization (>80%), with SPCs inserted only for urethral catheter failures (Emberton & Fitzpatrick, 2008). Additionally, the survey reported similar complication rates for both types of catheters. Surprisingly, there was no difference in asymptomatic bacteriuria, UTI, or urosepsis between the two catheterization approaches. This may be a result of shorter catheterization duration and evolution in catheter types. Urethral catheters were associated with an increased incidence of urinary leakage. Recent advances in SP catheterization method may replace the blind trocar method (Vasdev et al., 2014).

Trial without Catheterization

TWOC is now considered for most patients. It involves catheter removal, typically after 1 to 3 days; patients are allowed to void spontaneously and are monitored for recurrent retention. About 23% to 40% of patients are able to effectively empty the bladder (Emberton & Fitzpatrick, 2008; Fitzpatrick & Kirby, 2006), which enables them to return home without the potential morbidities associated with an *in situ* catheter (Emberton & Fitzpatrick, 2008). TWOC also allows surgery to be delayed to an elective setting or may eliminate the need for surgery (Emberton & Fitzpatrick, 2008; Fitzpatrick & Kirby, 2006).

Factors leading to a better chance of success with TWOC include:

- Younger age (<65 years)
- UTI with no previous voiding LUTS
- Identified precipitating cause (e.g., gross constipation)
- Recent initiation of anticholinergic or sympathomimetic drugs (which should be discontinued for TWOC)
- Drained volume/PVR <1,000 mL

CLINICAL PEARL

Factors increasing the chance of a successful trial without catheter include younger age, identified precipitating cause for the acute urinary retention episodes, recent initiation of anticholinergic or sympathomimetic drugs, or drained volume >1,000 mL.

Conversely, factors leading to a high probability of unsuccessful TWOC include

- Patient age >75 years
- Drained volume >1 L
- Previous LUTS
- Voiding detrusor contraction (on urodynamics) of <35 cm H_2O (Abrams et al., 1980; Emberton & Fitzpatrick, 2008; Fitzpatrick & Kirby, 2006)

The duration of catheterization before TWOC influences the chance of successfully restoring voiding (Choong & Emberton, 2000; Emberton & Fitzpatrick, 2008; Fitzpatrick & Kirby, 2006; Manikandan et al., 2004). In one study, a successful TWOC was achieved in 44% of patients after 1 day of catheterization, in 51% of patients after 2 days, and in 62% of patients after 7 days (Armitage & Emberton, 2006). Patients most likely to benefit from prolonged catheterization were those with PVR/drained volume >1,300 mL (Choong & Emberton, 2000; Emberton & Fitzpatrick, 2008; Fitzpatrick & Kirby, 2006). Catheterization >3 days, however, significantly increased the risk of comorbidities and prolonged hospitalization, which creates a dilemma for health care providers (Armitage & Emberton, 2006; Emberton & Fitzpatrick, 2008). The clinician should be aware that initial success with TWOC does not necessarily mean durability of successful voiding. Half of those for whom initial TWOC is successful will experience recurrent AUR over the next year and 35% undergo surgery within the following 6 months (Emberton & Fitzpatrick, 2008; Fitzpatrick & Kirby, 2006). Patients with PVR > 500 mL, no precipitating factor for AUR, and maximum flow rate <5 mL/s were at increased risk of further retention (Shergill et al., 2008). In the ALFAUR study, most of the patients who required surgery after an initially successful TWOC required surgical intervention for recurrent AUR (Emberton & Fitzpatrick, 2008; Fitzpatrick & Kirby, 2006). This emphasizes the importance of follow-up for patients with risk factors for recurrent AUR, even if they are initially successful with TWOC.

Alpha-Blockers and Trial without Catheter

AUR due to BPH may be associated with an increase in α-adrenergic activity (Fitzpatrick, & Kirby, 2006; McNeill et al., 1999). Inhibition of these receptors by α-blockers may decrease bladder outlet resistance, thereby facilitating normal micturition (Fitzpatrick & Kirby, 2006; McNeill et al., 1999; Zeif & Subramonian, 2009). Alfuzosin 10 mg daily for 2 to 3 days after catheterization almost doubles the likelihood of a successful TWOC, even in patients who are elderly (>65 years) with PVR more than 1,000 mL (Emberton & Fitzpatrick, 2008; Fitzpatrick & Kirby, 2006; McNeill et al., 1999). Furthermore, continued use of alfuzosin significantly reduced the risk of BPH surgery in the first 3 months, but not after 6 months (Emberton & Fitzpatrick, 2008; Fitzpatrick & Kirby, 2006). This allows more patients to return home without a catheter in situ, thereby reducing the subsequent perioperative complications of prostate surgery (McNeill et al., 1999). Patients at risk for recurrent AUR after successful TWOC included those with a high PSA and PVR (Emberton & Fitzpatrick, 2008; Fitzpatrick & Kirby, 2006). The Reten-World survey revealed that 82% of patients received an α1-blocker before catheter removal; TWOC success was greater in those receiving α-blockers, regardless of age (Emberton & Fitzpatrick, 2008).

CLINICAL PEARL

Use of alpha-adrenergic antagonists almost doubles the likelihood of successful trial without catheter.

Hospitalization

The decision regarding whether to admit patients or to send them home is dependent on local resources and preference (Emberton & Fitzpatrick, 2008; Fitzpatrick & Kirby, 2006; McNeill et al., 2004). A UK survey found that most urologists preferred to admit their patients and that presence of abnormal renal function was a consideration (Manikandan, et al., 2004).

Clean Intermittent Self-Catheterization

Clean intermittent self-catheterization (CISC) is an alternative to an indwelling catheter. It is a safe, simple, and well-accepted technique that results in fewer UTIs than indwelling catheterization. There are no external devices, and maintenance of sexual activity is possible. It may also increase the rate of successful spontaneous voiding. CISC can be used instead of an indwelling catheter after an episode of AUR or CUR, or it can be used in patients who fail to void following a prostatectomy. A period of CISC prior to TURP may be useful in patients with LPCR, as it may allow recovery of bladder contractility. For those with spinal cord lesions and neurogenic bladder dysfunction, IC is a standard method for bladder emptying. Patients' quality of life may also be enhanced (Choong & Emberton, 2000; Ghalayini et al., 2005).

Surgical Treatment

Previously, AUR was considered an absolute indication for TURP (Choong & Emberton, 2000; Emberton & Fitzpatrick, 2008; Fitzpatrick & Kirby, 2006). At present, AUR is the indication for prostatectomy in 25% of patients in the United States and in 50% of patients in the United Kingdom. Prostatectomy for AUR is associated with increased morbidity due to infection, perioperative bleeding, and increased transfusion rates and with a threefold increase in mortality. Additionally, a higher percentage of men undergoing TURP for AUR fail to void following surgery, as compared with men undergoing surgery for symptoms but no retention (Choong & Emberton, 2000). Complications of TURP also include retrograde ejaculation, erectile dysfunction, urinary incontinence (1%), TUR syndrome (dilutional hyponatremia due to systemic absorption of the irrigation fluid), urethral stricture, and bladder neck stenosis. Nonetheless, advances in surgical techniques have made TURP a much safer procedure; for example, bipolar diathermy using normal saline as the irrigation fluid appears to be safer than monopolar resection using glycine solution for irrigation. Figure 6-12 provides a schematic illustration of different approaches to prostate surgery.

In men with large prostates (>100 g), an open prostatectomy may be required, which may be performed through a retropubic, transvesical, or perineal approach. With the advent of laser, holmium laser enucleation of the prostate (HoLEP) can be effectively used in these patients, although this procedure does have a steeper learning curve. A recent systematic review and meta-analysis assessed the safety and effectiveness of HoLEP compared to TURP (Tan et al., 2007). Meta-analysis showed no statistically significant difference between HoLEP and TURP in terms of symptomatic improvement or urinary flow rates at 6 and 12 months follow-up. While TURP was associated with reduced operating time, HoLEP was associated with significant reductions in blood loss, catheterization time, and length of hospital stay. However, the short follow-up of

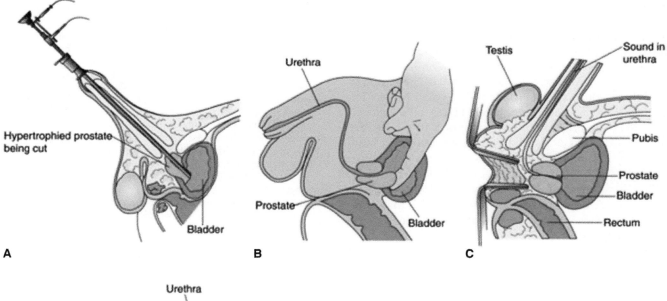

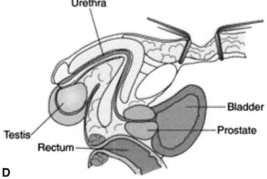

FIGURE 6-12. Types of prostatectomy. **A.** In a transurethral resection of the prostate (TURP), the surgeon connects a wire to a loop of current that is rotated in a cystoscope to remove shavings of the prostate. **B.** In suprapubic prostatectomy, the surgeon enters through the client's abdomen and uses his or her fingers to shell out the prostate. **C.** In perineal prostatectomy, the surgeon uses retractors to view the prostate. **D.** In retropubic prostatectomy, the surgeon makes a low abdominal incision and, working behind the pubic bone, removes the prostate.

patients in these studies limited conclusions on the durability of HoLEP.

In elderly men, those with multiple comorbidities, and those on oral anticoagulants, especially those with relatively small prostates, green light laser photovaporization of the prostate (GLL-PVP) may be an option. GLL-PVP represents one of the latest developments in laser prostate surgery. The potassium titanyl phosphate (KTP) or GreenLight laser emits laser energy that is absorbed by hemoglobin in red blood cells. This causes rapid heating and vaporization of the targeted tissue, as well as coagulation of blood vessels. The procedure requires general or spinal anesthesia. Equivalent improvements may be seen in urinary flow rates and symptoms, with reduced length of stay, length of catheterization, and adverse events for the GLL-PVP group (Bouchier-Hayes et al., 2006; Choong & Emberton, 2000). Longer-term outcomes need to be evaluated.

 Prevention of Urinary Retention

Placebo-controlled trials have shown that treatment with 5α-reductase inhibitors (5-ARIs) for periods of >6 months reduces the risk of AUR by >50% (Emberton & Fitzpatrick, 2008; McConnell et al., 1998). Community-based studies and the placebo arms of long-term randomized studies have identified predictive risk factors for AUR (Emberton & Fitzpatrick, 2008), which include age >70 years with LUTS, an IPSS > 7 (i.e., moderate or severe LUTS), a flow rate of <12 mL/s, and/or a prostate volume of >40 g or a PSA > 1.4 ng/mL (Box 6-2). Studies have suggested that hesitancy may also predict a greater risk of subsequent AUR.

The MTOPS Study was a large-scale, long-term study with a recruitment of 3,047 men with BPH and a mean follow-up period of 4.5 years. The study found that combination therapy with a selective type II 5-ARI (finasteride) and an α1-blocker (doxazosin) provided benefits over either drug as monotherapy in terms of reduction in the risk of clinical progression (McConnell et al., 2003).

The more recent combAT study confirmed the effectiveness of combination therapy using the α1c-blocker, tamsulosin, in combination with a type I and II 5-ARI (dutasteride) in reducing the risk of progression of BPH (Roehrborn et al., 2010). Thus, identifying patients who are high risk for retention of urine and treating them with α1-blockers ±5-ARIs may help prevent urinary retention. It is also essential to ensure follow-up, avoid medications that could precipitate AUR, and prevent constipation.

Conclusion

Urinary retention remains a significant burden for both the patient and health care services. The management of this condition should include modification of risk factors for developing AUR, possible use of a 5-ARI, and potential surgical intervention. Once retention occurs, timing of surgery must be based on the risk of perioperative morbidity and mortality as well as allowing the bladder to recover its contractility. α1-Blockers and TWOC may be useful. Finally, the evidence base for use of SPC for retention patients may support this as a first-line approach.

REFERENCES

Abrams, P. H., Dunn, M., & George, N. (1978). Urodynamic findings in chronic retention of urine and their relevance to results of surgery. *British Medical Journal, 2*(6147), 1258–1260.

Abrams, P., Cardozo, L., Fall, M., et al. (2003). Standardisation Sub-Committee of the International Continence Society. The standardisation of terminology in lower urinary tract function: Report from the standardisation sub-committee of the International Continence Society. *Urology, 61*(1), 37–49.

Abrams, P. H., Shah, P. J., Gaches, C. G., et al. (1980). Role of suprapubic catheterization in retention of urine. *Journal of the Royal Society of Medicine, 73*(12), 845–848.

Ahluwalia, R. S., Johal, N., Kouriefs, C., et al. (2006). The surgical risk of suprapubic catheter insertion and long-term sequelae. *Annals of the Royal College of Surgeons of England, 88*(2), 210–213. doi: 10.1308/003588406X95101.

Ahmed, S. J., Mehta, A., & Rimington, P. (2004). Delayed bowel perforation following suprapubic catheter insertion. *BMC Urology, 4*(1), 16.

Anjum, I., Ahmed, M., Azzopardi, A., et al. (1998). Prostatic infarction/infection in acute urinary retention secondary to benign prostatic hyperplasia. *The Journal of Urology, 160*(3 Pt 1), 792–793.

Armitage, J. (2011). *The epidemiology and management of acute urinary retention: A study based on hospital episode statistics and systematic literature review.* (Doctor of Medicine (Research), University College London). Retrieved from http://eprints.ucl.ac.uk/1318057/1/1318057.pdf.

Armitage, J., & Emberton, M. (2005). Is it time to reconsider the role of prostatic inflammation in the pathogenesis of lower urinary tract symptoms? *BJU International, 96*(6), 745–746. doi: 10.1111/j.1464-410X.2005.05761.x.

Armitage, J. N., & Emberton, M. (2006). Dynamic variables: Novel and perhaps better predictors of progression in benign prostatic hyperplasia. *BJU International, 97*(3), 439–441. doi: 10.1111/j.1464-410X.2006.06067.x.

Barry, M. J., Fowler, F. J., Bin, L., et al. (1997). The natural history of patients with benign prostatic hyperplasia as diagnosed by North American urologists. *The Journal of Urology, 157*(1), 10–14; discussion 14–15.

Bates, T. S., Sugiono, M., James, E. D., et al. (2003). Is the conservative management of chronic retention in men ever justified? *BJU International, 92*(6), 581–583.

Berry, S. J., Coffey, D. S., Walsh, P. C., et al. (1984). The development of human benign prostatic hyperplasia with age. *The Journal of Urology, 132*(3), 474–479.

Bouchier-Hayes, D. M., Anderson, P., Van Appledorn, S., et al. (2006). KTP laser versus transurethral resection: Early results of a randomized trial. *Journal of Endourology/Endourological Society, 20*(8), 580–585. doi: 10.1089/end.2006.20.580.

Cathcart, P., van der Meulen, J., Armitage, J., et al. (2006). Incidence of primary and recurrent acute urinary retention between 1998 and 2003 in England. *The Journal of Urology, 176*(1), 200–204; discussion 204. doi: 10.1016/S0022-5347(06)00509-X.

Choong, S., & Emberton, M. (2000). Acute urinary retention. *BJU International, 85*(2), 186–201.

Emberton, M., & Fitzpatrick, J. M. (2008). The Reten-World survey of the management of acute urinary retention: Preliminary results. *BJU International, 101*(Suppl 3), 27–32. doi: 10.1111/j.1464-410X.2008.07491.x; 10.1111/j.1464-410X.2008.07491.x.

Fitzpatrick, J. M., & Kirby, R. S. (2006). Management of acute urinary retention. *BJU International, 97*(Suppl 2), 16–20; discussion 21–22. doi: 10.1111/j.1464-410X.2006.06100.x.

Garbutt R. B., McD Taylor, D., Lee, V., et al. (2008). Delayed versus immediate urethral catheterization following instillation of local anaesthetic gel in men: A randomized, controlled clinical trial. *Emergency Medicine Australia, 20*(4), 328–332.

George, N. J. R. (1999). Interactive obstructive uropathy: Observations and conclusions from studies on humans. In A. R. Mundy, J. M. Fitzpatrick, D. E. Neal, & N. J. R. George (Eds.), *The scientific basis of urology* (pp. 125–141). London, UK: Isis Medical Media Ltd.

George, N. J., O'Reilly, P. H., Barnard, R. J., et al. (1983). High pressure chronic retention. *British Medical Journal (Clinical Research Ed.), 286*(6380), 1780–1783.

George, N. J., O'Reilly, P. H., Barnard, R. J., et al. (1984). Practical management of patients with dilated upper tracts and chronic retention of urine. *British Journal of Urology, 56*(1), 9–12.

George, N. J., Feneley, R. C., & Roberts, J. B. (1986). Identification of the poor risk patient with "prostatism" and detrusor failure. *British Journal of Urology, 58*(3), 290–295.

Ghalayini, I. F., Al-Ghazo, M. A., & Pickard, R. S. (2005). A prospective randomized trial comparing transurethral prostatic resection and clean intermittent self-catheterization in men with chronic urinary retention. *BJU International, 96*(1), 93–97. doi: 10.1111/j.1464-410X.2005.05574.x.

Ghose, R. R. (1990). Prolonged recovery of renal function after prostatectomy for prostatic outflow obstruction. *BMJ (Clinical Research Ed.), 300*(6736), 1376–1377.

Harrison, S. C. W., Lawrence, W. T., Morley, R., et al. (2011). British Association of Urological surgeons' suprapubic catheter practice guidelines. *BJU International, 107*(1), 77–85.

Hedlund, H., Hjelmas, K., Jonsson, O., et al. (2001). Hydrophilic versus non-coated catheters for intermittent catheterization. *Scandinavian Journal of Urology and Nephrology, 35*(1), 49–53.

Holden, D., George, N. J., Rickards, D., et al. (1984). Renal pelvic pressures in human chronic obstructive uropathy. *British Journal of Urology, 56*(6), 565–570.

Horgan, A. F., Prasad, B., Waldron, D. J., et al. (1992). Acute urinary retention. comparison of suprapubic and urethral catheterisation. *British Journal of Urology, 70*(2), 149–151.

Hunter, K. F., Bharmal, A., & Moore, K. N. (2013). Long-term suprapubic versus urethral catheterization: A scoping review. *Neurourology and Urodynamics, 32*(7), 944–951. doi: 10.1002/nau.22356.

Ichsan, J., & Hunt, D. R. (1987). Suprapubic catheters: A comparison of suprapubic versus urethral catheters in the treatment of acute urinary retention. *Australian & New Zealand Journal of Surgery, 57*(1), 33–36.

Jacobsen, S. J., Jacobson, D. J., Girman, C. J., et al. (1997). Natural history of prostatism: Risk factors for acute urinary retention. *The Journal of Urology, 158*(2), 481–487.

Jahn, P., Beutner, K., & Langer, G. (2012). Types of indwelling urinary catheters for long-term bladder drainage in adults. *Cochrane Database of Systematic Reviews*, (10), CD004997. doi: 10.1002/14651858.CD004997.pub3.

Jones, D. A., Atherton, J. C., O'Reilly, P. H., et al. (1989). Assessment of the nephron segments involved in post-obstructive diuresis in man, using lithium clearance. *British Journal of Urology, 64*(6), 559–563.

Kalejaiye, O., & Speakman, M. J. (2009). Management of acute and chronic retention in men. *European Urology Supplements, 8*(6), 523–529.

Kaplan, S. A., Wein, A. J., Staskin, D. R., et al. (2008). Urinary retention and post-void residual urine in men: Separating truth from tradition. *The Journal of Urology, 180*(1), 47–54. doi: http://dx.doi.org.login.ezproxy.library.ualberta.ca/10.1016/j.juro.2008.03.027.

Lederer, J. W., Jarvis, W. R., Thomas, L., et al. (2014). Multicenter cohort study to assess the impact of a silver-alloy and hydrogel-coated urinary catheter on symptomatic catheter-associated urinary tract infections. *Journal of Wound, Ostomy & Continence Nursing, 41*(5), 473–480. doi: 10.1097/WON.0000000000000056.

Manikandan, R., Srirangam, S. J., O'Reilly, P. H., et al. (2004). Management of acute urinary retention secondary to benign prostatic hyperplasia in the UK: A national survey. *BJU International, 93*(1), 84–88.

McConnell, J. D., Bruskewitz, R., Walsh, P., et al. (1998). The effect of finasteride on the risk of acute urinary retention and the need for surgical treatment among men with benign prostatic hyperplasia. *New England Journal of Medicine, 338*(9), 557–563.

McConnell, J. D., Roehrborn, C. G., Bautista, O. M., et al.; the Medical Therapy of Prostatic Symptoms Research Group. (2003). The long-term effect of doxazosin, finasteride, and combination therapy on the clinical progression of benign prostatic hyperplasia.[see comment]. *New England Journal of Medicine, 349*(25), 2387–2398.

McNeill, S. A., Daruwala, P. D., Mitchell, I. D., et al. (1999). Sustained-release alfuzosin and trial without catheter after acute urinary retention: A prospective, placebo-controlled. *BJU International, 84*(6), 622–627.

McNeill, A. S., Rizvi, S., & Byrne, D. J. (2004). Prostate size influences the outcome after presenting with acute urinary retention. *BJU International, 94*(4), 559–562. doi: 10.1111/j.1464-410X.2004.05000.x.

Meigs, J. B., Barry, M. J., Giovannucci, E., et al. (1999). Incidence rates and risk factors for acute urinary retention: The health professionals follow-up study. *Journal of Urology, 162*(2), 376–382.

Meigs, J. B., Mohr, B., Barry, M. J., et al. (2001). Risk factors for clinical benign prostatic hyperplasia in a community-based population of healthy aging men. *Journal of Clinical Epidemiology, 54*(9), 935–944.

Mishra, V., Allen, D., Nicolaou, C., et al. (2007). Does intraprostatic inflammation have a role in the pathogenesis and progression of benign prostatic hyperplasia? *BJU International, 100*(2), 327–331.

Pruthi, R. S. (2000). The dynamics of prostate-specific antigen in benign and malignant diseases of the prostate. *BJU International, 86*(6), 652–658.

Ramos-Fernandez, M. R., Medero-Colon, R., & Mendez-Carreno, L. (2013). Critical urologic skills and procedures in the emergency department. *Emergency Medicine Clinics of North America, 31*(1), 237–260. doi: 10.1016/j.emc.2012.09.007; 10.1016/j.emc.2012.09.007.

Roehrborn, C. G., McConnell, J. D., Lieber, M., et al. (1999). Serum prostate-specific antigen concentration is a powerful predictor of acute urinary retention and need for surgery in men with clinical benign prostatic hyperplasia. PLESS Study Group. *Urology, 53*(3), 473–480.

Roehrborn, C. G., Malice, M., Cook, T. J., et al. (2001). Clinical predictors of spontaneous acute urinary retention in men with LUTS and clinical BPH: A comprehensive analysis of the pooled placebo groups of several large clinical trials. *Urology, 58*(2), 210–216.

Roehrborn, C. G., Siami, P., Barkin, J., et al.; CombAT Study Group. (2010). The effects of combination therapy with dutasteride and tamsulosin on clinical outcomes in men with symptomatic benign prostatic hyperplasia: 4-year results from the CombAT study. *European Urology, 57*(1), 123–131. doi: 10.1016/j.eururo.2009.09.035; 10.1016/j.eururo.2009.09.035.

Shergill, I. S., Shaikh, T., Arya, M., et al. (2008). A training model for suprapubic catheter insertion: The UroEmerge suprapubic catheter model. *Urology, 72*(1), 196–197. doi: 10.1016/j.urology.2008.03.021; 10.1016/j.urology.2008.03.021.

Siderias, J., Guadio, F., & Singer, A. J. (2004). Comparison of topical anesthetics and lubricants prior to urethral catheterization in males: A randomized controlled trial. *Academic Emergency Medicine, 11*(6), 703–706.

Sparks, M. (2010). *Post-obstructive diuresis.* Retrieved from: http://renalfellow.blogspot.ca/2010/09/post-obstructive-diuresis.html

Spiro, L. H., Labay, G., & Orkin, L. A. (1974). Prostatic infarction. Role in acute urinary retention. *Urology, 3*(3), 345–347.

Tan, A., Liao, C., Mo, Z., et al. (2007). Meta-analysis of holmium laser enucleation versus transurethral resection of the prostate for symptomatic prostatic obstruction. *The British Journal of Surgery, 94*(10), 1201–1208. doi: 10.1002/bjs.5916.

Tuncel, A., Uzun, B., Eruyar, T., et al. (2005). Do prostatic infarction, prostatic inflammation and prostate morphology play a role in acute urinary retention? *European Urology, 48*(2), 277–283. doi: 10.1016/j.eururo.2005.05.001.

Vasdev, N., Kachroo, N., Mathur, S., et al. (2014). Suprapubic bladder catheterisation using the Seldinger technique. *The Internet Journal of Urology, 5*(1). https://ispub.com/IJU/5/1/4324

Verhamme, K. M., Dieleman, J. P., van Wijk, M. A., et al. (2005). Low incidence of acute urinary retention in the general male population: The Triumph project. *European Urology, 47*(4), 494–498. doi: 10.1016/j.eururo.2004.11.011.

Wallace, D. M. (1951). The bladder neck in urinary obstruction. *Proceedings of the Royal Society of Medicine, 44*(6), 434–437.

Zeif, H. J., & Subramonian, K. (2009). Alpha blockers prior to removal of a catheter for acute urinary retention in adult men. *The Cochrane Database of Systematic Reviews*, (4). CD006744. doi: 10.1002/14651858.CD006744.pub2; 10.1002/14651858. CD006744.pub2.

QUESTIONS

1. Following an assessment of urinary functioning, which patient would the continence nurse suspect as having chronic urinary retention (CUR)?
   A. A postpartum female who cannot pass urine
   B. A patient who is unable to pass urine and has a painful, palpable bladder
   C. A patient with a nonpainful palpable bladder and 300-mL residual urine
   D. A male patient with CUR who presents with an episode of AUR

2. A 69-year-old male patient is diagnosed with spontaneous acute urinary retention (AUR). What is a common cause of this condition?
   A. Benign prostatic hyperplasia
   B. Urologic intervention
   C. Anesthesia
   D. Urinary tract infection

3. What common factor would be observed in a patient with acute urinary retention?
   A. A decrease in the prostatic intraurethral pressure caused by decreased α-adrenergic stimulation
   B. An increase in the stromal to epithelial ratio within the prostate
   C. Diverticula in the bladder wall
   D. Evidence of prostatic infarction caused by infection, instrumentation, and/or thrombosis

4. Which condition is NOT a potential complication of urinary retention?
   A. Vesical calculi (bladder stones)
   B. Benign prostatic hypertrophy (BPH)
   C. Hydronephrosis
   D. Urinary tract infection

5. What property of the bladder is one of the most important factors to consider as an etiology when assessing a patient for urinary retention?
   A. Reflux
   B. Compliance
   C. Ability to concentrate urine
   D. Spasticity

6. The practitioner orders a bladder scan for a patient who is manifesting signs and symptoms of urinary retention with moderate discomfort. The continence nurse notes that the findings show the volume of urine drained is a little over 1 L. What condition would the nurse suspect?
   A. Acute-on-chronic retention
   B. Acute retention
   C. Chronic urinary retention
   D. Partial urinary retention

7. A patient with urinary retention is diagnosed with postobstructive diuresis. What is a characteristic of this condition?
   A. Increased tubular reabsorption of sodium
   B. Deceased tubular transit flow time
   C. Decreased production of prostaglandins following relief of obstruction
   D. Inability to maximally concentrate urine

8. For what complication would the continence nurse monitor a patient who develops postobstructive diuresis?
   A. Hyperkalemia
   B. Hypercalcemia
   C. Hypokalemia
   D. Hypophosphatemia

9. A practitioner orders urethral catheterization for a patient diagnosed with chronic urinary retention who is retaining blood clots and urine. Which type of catheter would be the best choice for this patient?
   A. Three-way Foley catheter
   B. Intermittent catheter
   C. Coudé catheter
   D. Robinson catheter

10. A practitioner orders suprapubic catheterization (SPC) for a patient for whom urethral catheterization for urinary retention was unsuccessful. A continence nurse is explaining the procedure to the patient. What statement accurately describes a step in this procedure?
  A. SPC is a relatively painless procedure with proper local anesthesia.
  B. The patient is placed in the supine position for the procedure.
  C. The site of insertion is roughly 10 cm above the pubic symphysis.
  D. A 1-cm suprapubic incision is made on either side of the needle.

11. A trial without catheter (TWOC) is considered for most patients with urinary retention. Which patient would the continence nurse consider at highest risk for TWOC being unsuccessful?
  A. A patient with a drained volume >1 L
  B. A patient with UTI with no previous voiding LUTS
  C. A patient with gross constipation as a precipitating cause
  D. A patient with drained volume/postvoid residual (PVR) <1,000 mL

12. Which type of surgical treatment for urinary retention would be an appropriate option for an elderly man with diabetes mellitus who is on an oral anticoagulant for prevention of DVT?
  A. TURP.
  B. HoLEP.
  C. GLL-PVP.
  D. Surgical treatment is contraindicated in this patient.

ANSWERS: 1.**C**, 2.**A**, 3.**D**, 4.**B**, 5.**B**, 6.**A**, 7.**D**, 8.**C**, 9.**A**, 10.**B**, 11.**A**, 12.**C**

CHAPTER 7

Neurogenic Bladder
Assessment and Management

Mikel Gray

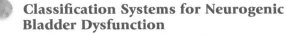

The term "neurogenic" is defined as originating in or caused by the nerves (Oxford English Dictionary, 2014). Neurogenic bladder is defined as lower urinary tract dysfunction arising from a nervous origin, an underlying disease, or disorder of the nervous system. Neurogenic bladder dysfunction is caused by a variety of diseases or disorders directly affecting the central nervous system such as stroke, brain tumors, traumatic brain injury, Parkinsonism, multiple sclerosis, spinal cord injury, vertebral disk disease, transverse myelitis, polio, postpolio syndrome, Guillain-Barré syndrome, and spinal stenosis (Danforth & Ginsberg, 2014). It is also seen in infants, children, and adults with a number of congenital defects affecting central nervous system function and development, including spina bifida (especially myelomeningocele with or without hydrocephalus), anorectal malformations such as imperforate anus, and cerebral palsy. Finally, neurogenic bladder dysfunction can be caused by metabolic or infectious diseases that indirectly influence central nervous system function such as diabetes mellitus or herpetic infections affecting the lumbosacral dermatomes.

CLINICAL PEARL

Neurogenic bladder dysfunction is defined as lower urinary tract dysfunction caused by a disease or disorder of the nervous system, such as spinal cord injury, multiple sclerosis, or myelomeningocele.

Interest in the neurologic function of the bladder and the clinical challenges associated with neurogenic bladder dysfunction can be traced back to the 16th century, when Vicary described the urinary bladder as influenced by nerves that store and let go of urine (Hald & Bradley, 1982). Around the time of the American Civil War, Budge was the first to identify the bladder muscle (detrusor) as innervated by the parasympathetic nervous system (Budge, 1864). Despite these early pioneering works, care of persons with neurogenic bladders remained rudimentary. During World War I, for example, management of neurogenic bladder dysfunction in patients with traumatic spinal cord injuries was primarily limited to indwelling catheterization or containment of urinary incontinence (Silver, 2011), although at least one surgeon described management of neurogenic bladder in five men with spinal cord injuries using intermittent catheterization as early as 1889 (Thorburn, 1889).

Despite these early efforts, 60% of individuals suffering from spinal cord trauma died of complications within 3 years of his or her injury; urinary tract infection (UTI) in the era before antibiotic medications was a leading cause of these deaths (Bodner, 2009). Advances in health care, along with a sharp increase in the number of men who suffered from traumatic spinal cord injury, occurred during World War II and the Korean War. As a result, a number of hospital-based units were created across the globe dedicated to caring for persons with spinal cord injuries, including the Veteran's Administration Hospital in Long Beach, CA (Donovan, 2007). The unit in California was headed by a urologist and a neurologist (E. Bors and A. Comarr, respectively), who focused on management of neurogenic bladder in particular. Their research, combined with advances in antimicrobial therapy to manage UTI (Bors & Comarr, 1971), the introduction of intermittent catheterization in 1966 by Guttman (Guttman & Frankel, 1966), and the popularization of clean intermittent catheterization by Lapides (Lapides et al., 1972) in the early 1970s, provides the cornerstones of the neurogenic bladder management that we continue to use in the 21st century.

CLINICAL PEARL

The introduction of clean intermittent catheterization and development of antibiotics significantly reduced mortality among patients with neurogenic bladder; those developments are key aspects of neurogenic bladder management today.

Classification Systems for Neurogenic Bladder Dysfunction

Various classification systems for neurogenic bladder have been proposed for a variety of dysfunctions associated with this complex clinical challenge (Bors & Comarr, 1971; Lapides et al., 1972). While all of these systems provide clinically relevant insights, none enjoys widespread use owing to their inability to incorporate all of the factors that influence persons with neurogenic bladder dysfunction, including the variable effects of the underlying disease, the effects of bladder outlet obstruction or lower urinary tract dysfunction, and changes occurring over time, especially when neurogenic bladder occurs in an infant or child. Despite their lack of widespread use, two systems have led to the incorporation of concepts still used for neurogenic bladder management today.

Upper versus Lower Motor Neuron Dysfunction

Bors and Comarr (1971) pioneered the concept of upper versus lower motor neuron neurogenic bladder dysfunction based on their clinical experiences with patients with spinal cord injuries. An upper motor neuron neurogenic bladder is characterized by an overactive detrusor (which contracts without voluntary control), while the lower motor neuron neurogenic bladder is characterized by a noncontracting (acontractile or areflexic) detrusor. They further described neurogenic bladders as balanced or imbalanced. A balanced bladder can be roughly defined as one that empties completely and is not associated with recurring UTI or upper urinary tract distress, while an imbalanced bladder does not empty completely and is associated with recurring UTI and/or upper urinary tract distress. Although continence clinicians do not tend to employ these concepts, they are sometimes used by neurosurgeons or rehabilitation clinicians for diagnosis and management of neurogenic bladder dysfunction.

CLINICAL PEARL

An upper motor neuron bladder (lesion above the sacral cord) is characterized by bladder overactivity, while a lower motor neuron bladder (sacral cord lesion) is characterized by bladder underactivity or acontractility.

Lapides Classification System

Lapides (1970) also developed a taxonomy for classifying neurogenic bladder dysfunction. He included a description for reflex neurogenic bladder, which was characterized by detrusor overactivity and incoordination between the detrusor muscle and the striated sphincter mechanism, also referred to as detrusor sphincter dyssynergia. The term reflex incontinence remains widely used in many medical specialties, and it is a nursing diagnosis recognized by the North American Nursing Diagnosis Association and incorporated into the NIC and NOC nursing care schema (Gray, 2008).

● Urinary Continence: A Neurologic Perspective

Normal bladder function can be divided into two stages: filling and storage (Gray, 2007). During bladder filling, the detrusor muscle remains in a relaxed state, allowing the upper urinary tracts to fill the bladder with urine, while the urethral sphincter mechanism remains in a tonic (closed) state, preventing urinary leakage with physical activity. During micurition, the second phase of normal lower urinary tract function, the detrusor muscle contracts and the urethral sphincter mechanism relaxes under neurological control, allowing urine to be expelled from the bladder via the urethra without excessive resistance. Urinary continence is based on three factors: anatomic integrity of the urinary system, neurological control of the detrusor muscles, and an intact urethral sphincter mechanism. For the purposes of this chapter on neurogenic bladder dysfunction, a brief discussion of the physiology of the continent person will be limited to neurological control of the detrusor muscle and urethral sphincter mechanism.

Detrusor Function

The detrusor is a smooth muscle, but it has several properties that distinguish it from other smooth muscle found in the gastrointestinal tract or ureters. Specifically, the detrusor is characterized as single unit rather than multiunit smooth muscle (Yoshimura & Chancellor, 2012). Multiunit smooth muscle cells, such as those found in the ureter or intestinal tract, are linked electrically so that contraction in one smooth muscle cell (in response to stretch) leads to a peristaltic contraction that propels urine from the renal pelvis through the entire ureteral course and into the bladder (Weiss, 2012). Smooth muscle cells in the ureter and gastrointestinal tract share tight junctions, cytoplasmic bridges that create mechanical communication that is independent of nervous system input. This coupling is so efficient that a ureter transplanted along with a donor kidney will continue to transport urine from the renal pelvis through the ureter and into the bladder despite being housed in a new host body. Such an arrangement would be disastrous to continence; a multiunit detrusor muscle would contract as it is filled with urine, resulting in involuntary voiding. Instead, the detrusor muscle has a single-unit arrangement, with a nearly 1:1 ratio of smooth muscle cells to nerve endings (neuromuscular junctions), which provides the neurological governance necessary for the voluntary control of detrusor muscle contractions essential to urinary continence.

Neurotransmitters

The nervous system regulates relaxation and contraction of the urinary bladder using chemical messengers called neurotransmitters (Gray, 2007; Yoshimura & Chancellor, 2012). These neurotransmitters act at specific receptor sites on the smooth muscle; they carry two basic messages: detrusor muscle contract and detrusor muscle relax. The neurotransmitter acetylcholine acts at muscarinic receptor sites on the detrusor muscle cell, signaling the bladder to contract (Andersson, 2011; Frazier et al., 2008; Gray, 2007; Yoshimura & Chancellor, 2012). The neurotransmitter norepinephrine (sometimes called noradrenaline) acts on beta-3 adrenergic receptor sites on the detrusor smooth muscle cell, signaling the bladder to relax (Ursino et al., 2009). Muscarinic and beta-adrenergic receptors are not only essential to neurological control of the detrusor muscle, they are also important pharmacologic targets for management of neurogenic bladder dysfunction.

Urethral Sphincter Mechanism

The urethral sphincter mechanism is best conceptualized as containing two components: elements of compression and muscular elements that promote active urethral closure in response to physical exertion (Gray et al., 1995a). Smooth muscle cells within the bladder base, bladder neck, and proximal urethra are present in women and men. They are particularly abundant in the bladder neck and prostatic urethra in men (Yamata & Ito, 2011). Alpha-1 adrenergic receptors located on these urethral smooth cells cause muscle contraction and urethral closure in response to the neurotransmitter norepinephrine (Kojima et al., 2009). The urethral sphincter mechanism also contains periurethral striated muscle and a rhabdosphincter (formerly called the external sphincter). These muscle cells have nicotinic receptors that react to the neurotransmitter acetylcholine, resulting in contraction of the periurethral and rhabdosphincter muscles and closure of the sphincter mechanism. No drug has been developed that is able to safely change the behavior of the striated muscles of the sphincter mechanism, but the alpha-1 adrenergic blocking drugs are used to reduce urethral resistance to urinary outflow in selected patients with neurogenic bladder.

Bladder–Sphincter Coordination

The central nervous system is ultimately responsible for coordinating lower urinary tract function so that the bladder fills at low pressures with low tone within the detrusor coupled with closure of the urethral sphincter mechanism via contraction of smooth and striated muscles in the bladder neck and urethra (de Groat & Wickens, 2013; Gray, 2007; Griffiths & Fowler, 2013; Yoshimura & Chancellor, 2012). Likewise, the act of voiding relies on input from the central nervous system, resulting in relaxation of smooth and striated muscle within the urethral sphincter mechanism and contraction of the detrusor muscle resulting in evacuation of stored urine from the bladder.

> **CLINICAL PEARL**
> Effective bladder emptying is dependent on both sphincter relaxation and bladder contractility.

Voluntary Control

Prior to toilet training, bladder filling and micturition follow a regular cycle of filling and evacuation without voluntary control. Both bladder filling and micturition are coordinated by neurons in the brain stem; specifically, the pontine micturition center, periaqueductal gray matter, and the M region (de Groat & Wickens, 2013). As the bladder fills and its walls are stretched, afferent signals travel from the bladder to the brain stem via the spinal cord. Approximately once an hour (pending fluid intake and hydration), the bladder will become sufficiently stretched to provoke micturition. Micturition is coordinated by neurons in the periaqueductal gray matter of the brain stem, and the pontine micturition center coordinates detrusor contraction with relaxation of the urethral sphincter mechanism.

Following successful toilet training, the child gains voluntary control over the lower urinary tract that persists throughout adulthood. Advances in functional brain imaging have vastly increased our understanding of how the brain influences both urine filling and storage and micturition in the continent child or adult (Griffiths & Fowler, 2013). While control of bladder filling and the micturition reflex are centered in the brain stem in the infant, neurons in the frontal cortex, cingulate gyrus, and basal ganglia influence bladder filling/storage and voiding. The precise mechanisms underlying the decision to void and the switch from bladder filling/storage to bladder evacuation are unknown; however, a growing body of evidence in humans strongly suggests the brain is not only responsible for deferring micturition until the individual desires to urinate, it also provokes the onset of micturition and ensures the detrusor contraction is of sufficient duration and amplitude to empty the bladder, while maintaining relaxation of muscular elements of the urethral sphincter mechanism.

> **CLINICAL PEARL**
> The ability to voluntarily initiate voiding and to delay voiding until a socially appropriate time and place requires normal central nervous system function and intact pathways between the brain (and brainstem) and the bladder and sphincter.

Etiology and Pathophysiology of Neurogenic Bladder Dysfunction

Trauma or disease affecting the brain, spinal cord, or the rich supply of peripheral nerves required for healthy bladder function cause neurogenic dysfunction of the bladder. The nature of the dysfunction is dictated by the location and nature of the underlying neurological disorder and by lower urinary tract function at the time of the neurological disorder (Fig. 7-1).

While classification schemas for neurogenic bladder dysfunction have failed to gain widespread use, the urodynamic-based system proposed by Wein (1981) will be incorporated in this chapter because of its ability to classify the various pathophysiologic mechanisms that characterize neurogenic bladder dysfunction (Table 7-1). The Wein classification system is based on

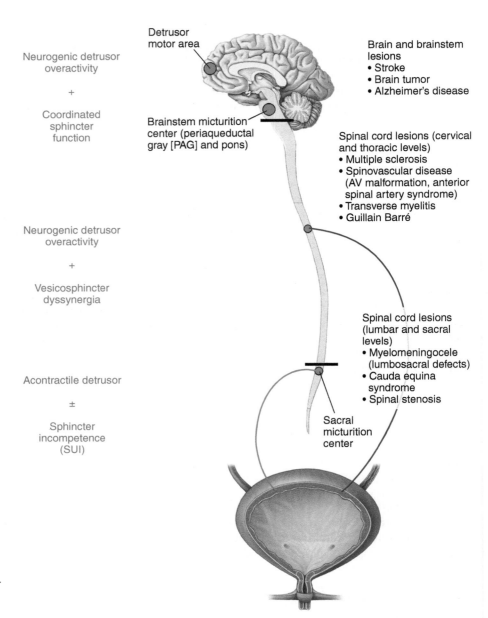

Neurogenic detrusor
overactivity

+

Coordinated
sphincter
function

Neurogenic detrusor
overactivity

+

Vesicosphincter
dyssynergia

Acontractile detrusor

±

Sphincter
incompetence
(SUI)

Detrusor
motor area

Brainstem micturition
center (periaqueductal
gray [PAG] and pons)

Brain and brainstem
lesions
• Stroke
• Brain tumor
• Alzheimer's disease

Spinal cord lesions (cervical
and thoracic levels)
• Multiple sclerosis
• Spinovascular disease
  (AV malformation, anterior
  spinal artery syndrome)
• Transverse myelitis
• Guillain Barré

Spinal cord lesions
(lumbar and sacral
levels)
• Myelomeningocele
  (lumbosacral defects)
• Cauda equina
  syndrome
• Spinal stenosis

Sacral
micturition
center

FIGURE 7-1. Neurological disorders associated with neurogenic detrusor overactivity and urgency and/or urge urinary incontinence.

urodynamic findings, a diagnostic test frequently used to evaluate neurogenic bladder dysfunction; it is particularly useful for characterizing the various dysfunctions that lead to urinary incontinence or retention seen with neurogenic bladder dysfunction. This discussion will be followed by an overview of the link between neurogenic bladder and upper urinary tract distress and its management.

CLINICAL PEARL

The Wein classification system is based on urodynamic findings and classifies lower urinary tract dysfunction as one of the following: failure to store because of the bladder; failure to store because of the sphincter; failure to empty because of the bladder; and failure to empty because of the sphincter.

Failure to Store Urine Because of the Bladder

Failure to store urine because of the bladder is caused by a condition called detrusor overactivity (Abrams et al., 2002; Wein, 1981). Detrusor overactivity is defined as an involuntary detrusor contraction of sufficient magnitude to cause urgency and/or urinary leakage. Neurogenic detrusor overactivity is defined as an overactive detrusor contraction associated with neurogenic bladder. It is one of the most common dysfunctions among patients with neurogenic bladder and is seen in 50.9% of patients with multiple sclerosis, 52.3% of patients with spinal cord injury, 33.1% of persons with Parkinsonism, and 23.6% of all patients who experience a stroke (Ruffion et al., 2013).

Among patients with preserved sensations of the lower urinary tract, detrusor overactivity is typically associated with daytime voiding frequency (more than eight voids in

TABLE 7-1 Wein's Urodynamics-Based Classification System for Neurogenic Voiding Dysfunction

Failure to Store Urine	Failure to Empty Urine
Because of the bladder (Neurogenic detrusor overactivity, low bladder wall compliance) [Urge urinary incontinence, urgency] [Reflex urinary incontinence]	Because of the bladder (Detrusor underactivity*) [Urinary retention†]
Because of the outlet (Urethral sphincter mechanism incompetence) [Stress urinary incontinence]	Because of the outlet (Bladder outlet obstruction) [Urinary retention†]

( ) = urodynamic abnormality.
[ ] = primary lower urinary tract symptom.
*Detrusor underactivity is defined as incomplete bladder emptying due to poor detrusor contraction strength or acontractile or hypocontractile detrusor.
†urinary retention defined as inability to expel any urine from the bladder or chronic residual urine volumes despite the ability to partially evacuate urine from the bladder via micturition.
Data from Wein, A.J. (1981). Classification of neurogenic voiding dysfunction. *Journal of Urology, 125*(5), 605–609.

a 24-hour period or voiding more often than every 2 hours while awake), nocturia (three or more episodes per night), and urgency (a sudden and compelling desire to urinate that cannot be deferred), with or without urge incontinence (urinary leakage associated with urgency). This cluster of lower urinary tract symptoms (LUTS) has been labeled overactive bladder (Abrams et al., 2002). (Refer to Chapter 5 for a more detailed discussion of the assessment and management of this prevalent form of incontinence.) Figure 7-1 lists neurological disorders associated with neurogenic detrusor overactivity and urgency and/or urge urinary incontinence.

CLINICAL PEARL

Neurogenic detrusor overactivity is defined as bladder overactivity associated with neurogenic impairment; it can cause urgency, frequency, nocturia, and urge incontinence in the patient with intact sensation or incontinence without sensory awareness in those with diminished or absent sensation.

Depending on the underlying neurological disorder, persons with neurogenic bladder dysfunction also may experience neurogenic detrusor overactivity with absent or markedly decreased sensations of bladder filling. In contrast to urge incontinence, these individuals experience urinary incontinence without sensory awareness, although clinical experience reveals that some patients with spinal cord injury report atypical sensations associated with detrusor overactivity such as tingling of the jaw or side of the face. Rather than nocturia, these individuals often experience nocturnal enuresis. Neurogenic detrusor overactivity with sensory impairment frequently occurs in patients

with paralyzing spinal disorders such as spinal cord injury or transverse myelitis (Fig. 7-1) (Martens et al., 2010).

Failure to Store Urine Because of the Outlet

Failure to store because of the outlet is caused by incompetence of the urethral sphincter mechanism, which results in stress urinary incontinence (Wein, 1981). Stress urinary incontinence presents as a LUTS or sign on physical assessment or as a urodynamic finding (Abrams et al., 2002). The symptom of stress incontinence is defined as the report of urine loss with coughing, sneezing, or physical activity. The sign of stress urinary incontinence occurs when a clinician observes urinary leakage from the urethra when the patient is asked to raise abdominal pressures by coughing or performing a Valsalva maneuver. Urodynamic stress incontinence is defined as urine loss in response to a rise in abdominal pressure; two urodynamic techniques, the abdominal leak point (Gray, 2011a) and urethral pressure profile (Gray, 2011b), are used to evaluate urodynamic stress urinary incontinence.

Stress urinary incontinence is especially prevalent in adult women (see Chapter 9 for a detailed discussion of the assessment and management of stress UI in women). Among patients with neurogenic bladder dysfunction, urethral sphincter incompetence occurs when disease or trauma damages lumbosacral spinal segments (including Onuf's nucleus), leading to denervation of the striated sphincter muscle (Groen et al., 2012; Kulwin et al., 2013). The resulting stress urinary incontinence varies from mild leakage to nearly continuous urine loss when sphincter function is severely compromised. Neurological conditions associated with denervation of Onuf's nucleus and stress urinary incontinence are shown in Figure 7-1.

CLINICAL PEARL

Stress incontinence (leakage with increased intra-abdominal pressure) is common among individuals with neurogenic bladder, due to loss of voluntary sphincter control.

In addition to denervation of the striated muscle component of the sphincter mechanism, the choice of bladder management program may result in erosion of the urethra and sphincter. Long-term indwelling catheterization has been linked to urethral erosion in both women and men; it often leads to a condition called catheter bypassing, defined as leakage around an indwelling catheter associated with local damage or erosion of the urethral sphincter mechanism (Moore & Rayome, 1995). In severe cases, the entire urethra is involved, leading to a condition called "stove-pipe" urethra where the urethra is unable to exert any closure pressure, resulting in continuous urinary leakage (Chapple et al., 2009).

Failure to Empty Because of the Bladder

Contraction of the detrusor muscle is an essential component of normal micturition. Failure to empty because of the bladder is caused by an underactive detrusor (Wein, 1981).

Detrusor underactivity is defined as a contraction that has inadequate strength and/or duration to empty the bladder of urine in a reasonable period of time (Abrams et al., 2002). Assessment of the strength of a detrusor contraction is difficult; LUTS commonly associated with detrusor underactivity include weak urinary stream, terminal dribble, postvoid dribbling, difficulty urinating, and feelings of incomplete bladder emptying. An elevated urinary residual volume is the most commonly used sign of detrusor underactivity, but the presence of an elevated residual volume is not exclusively caused by an underactive detrusor; incomplete bladder emptying is also caused by bladder outlet obstruction or a combination of detrusor underactivity and obstruction (Gray, 2010, 2012a, 2012b).

Uroflowmetry is often used to evaluate incomplete bladder emptying, but it cannot differentiate an abnormal flow rate caused by detrusor underactivity from one caused by bladder outlet obstruction (Gray, 2010). The voiding pressure flow study provides a more definitive evaluation of detrusor underactivity; this test is used to measure the amplitude (maximal strength) and duration of a detrusor contraction during micturition (Gray, 2012a, 2012b). Unfortunately, normal values for these parameters vary based on age and gender and have not been firmly established. In addition, the performance of the detrusor contraction, similar to all other smooth or striated muscles of the body, varies widely as evidenced by the widely variable residual volumes measured over multiple voiding episodes (Griffiths et al., 1996; Saaby & Lose, 2012).

> **CLINICAL PEARL**
>
> Detrusor underactivity refers to detrusor contractions that lack the strength and duration to effectively empty the bladder in a reasonable period of time.

Detrusor underactivity is prevalent in patients with neurogenic bladder dysfunction; conditions commonly associated with detrusor underactivity include multiple sclerosis, dementia/Alzheimer's disease, Parkinsonism, and disorders affecting lower spinal segments such as spinal stenosis, tethered spinal cord, and cerebrovascular accident (Drake et al., 2014; van Koeveringe et al., 2011). Additional factors leading to detrusor underactivity in patients with neurogenic bladder dysfunction include constipation and antimuscarinic drugs, which are commonly used in the management of neurogenic detrusor overactivity.

Failure to Empty Because of the Outlet

Failure to empty because of the outlet occurs when urethral resistance is great enough to interfere with complete and efficient micturition (Wein, 1981). Similar to detrusor underactivity, there are no specific LUTS or physical signs that can reliably diagnose bladder outlet obstruction. The LUTS most closely associated with bladder outlet obstruction are the same as those linked with detrusor underactivity.

Presence of an elevated residual urine volume is unreliable since it does not differentiate incomplete bladder emptying because of the outlet from incomplete emptying due to detrusor underactivity. Uroflowmetry detects abnormal flow rates, but it does not identify the cause of the abnormal flow (Gray, 2011). Therefore, diagnosis of the presence and magnitude of bladder outlet obstruction relies on the voiding pressure flow study, preferably aided by a more quantitative analysis using a voiding pressure nomogram (Gray, 2012a, 2012b).

A variety of factors can obstruct the bladder outlet, but the condition most closely associated with neurogenic bladder dysfunction is detrusor external sphincter dyssynergia, that is, loss of coordination between the detrusor muscle and external (striated) sphincter. Detrusor sphincter dyssynergia (also called vesicosphincter dyssynergia or detrusor-striated sphincter dyssynergia) occurs when the detrusor and striated sphincter contract simultaneously during micturition. Simultaneous contraction creates a functional obstruction of the bladder outlet that interferes with bladder emptying and increases the risk for UTI (Ahmed et al., 2006; Bacsu et al., 2012). It is caused by trauma or disease affecting spinal segments above S2 (suprasacral lesions) and below spinal segment C2.

In the continent individual, the pontine micturition center coordinates reflex activity of the detrusor and urethral sphincter mechanisms so that the urethral sphincter mechanism is closed (contracted) during bladder filling/storage and open (relaxed) during micturition. During voiding, the detrusor muscle contracts and the urethral sphincter mechanism opens (relaxes), enabling unobstructed outflow of urine. Spinal lesions below the brain stem and above the sacral micturition center (S2–S4) interfere with the pons' ability to coordinate detrusor and sphincter responses, resulting in incoordination (dyssynergia) between these elements of the lower urinary tract. Multiple neurological conditions cause neurogenic bladder dysfunction with detrusor sphincter dyssynergia. Approximately 75% to 87% of patients with spinal cord injuries above spinal segment S2, 35% of patients with multiple sclerosis, and 25% of patients with spina bifida have detrusor sphincter dyssynergia (Ahmed et al., 2006; De Seze et al., 2007; Weld et al., 2000).

> **CLINICAL PEARL**
>
> In the patient with neurogenic bladder dysfunction, failure to empty due to the sphincter is most commonly the result of detrusor external sphincter dyssynergia (persistent contraction of the sphincter during detrusor contraction), resulting from a lesion between the sacral cord and the pons.

Bladder neck dyssynergia (also called detrusor bladder neck dyssynergia) is defined as failure of the smooth muscle of the urethra to relax during a detrusor contraction (Stohrer et al., 1999). Similar to dyssynergia between the detrusor muscle and the striated sphincter, detrusor bladder neck dyssynergia increases resistance within the urethral sphincter mechanism, obstructing the bladder outlet and interfering with bladder emptying. It is uncommon in men without neurogenic bladder dysfunction and extremely rare in neurologically normal women (Coblentz & Gray, 2001; Yamanishi et al., 1997). Detrusor bladder neck dyssynergia is seen in patients with spinal cord injury; it is associated with complete spinal injuries occurring above spinal segment S2 and incomplete spinal injuries (usually T9 or lower) (Al-Ali & Haddad, 1996; Schurch et al., 1994).

Benign prostate hypertrophy (BPH) is defined as enlargement of the prostate and increased tone in the prostatic urethra, which may result in obstruction of the bladder outlet and a variety of LUTS. This condition is discussed in detail in Chapters 6 and 8. Nevertheless, it is emphasized in this discussion because of its prevalence in aging men with Parkinsonism, stroke, and dementia resulting in neurogenic bladder dysfunction. In addition, there is a growing body of evidence suggesting that BPH causes changes in the detrusor muscle that alter not only the local response of smooth muscle cells to the various neurotransmitters but also the spinal reflexes that regulate bladder filling/storage and micturition (Chai et al., 1998; Mirone et al., 2007).

Neurogenic Bladder Dysfunction as a Cause of Upper Urinary Tract Distress

Upper urinary tract distress is defined as impaired function of the upper urinary tracts (the paired kidneys, renal pelves, and ureters), associated with neurogenic bladder dysfunction (Gray, 2011; Killorin et al., 1992). Clinical manifestations include febrile UTI (recurring or chronic pyelonephritis), vesicoureteral reflux, ureterohydronephrosis, and impaired renal function. Two components of neurogenic bladder dysfunction, low bladder wall compliance and increased urethral resistance (bladder outlet obstruction), increase the likelihood of upper urinary tract distress in patients with neurogenic bladder dysfunction (Ghoniem et al., 1989; McGuire et al., 1981; Perez et al., 1993).

Bladder wall compliance is defined as the relationship between bladder volume and intravesical pressure during bladder filling/storage (Gray, 2011; Hosker et al., 2009); in the clinical setting, it is measured during urodynamic testing (Chapter 4). In the healthy bladder, intravesical pressures remain low despite filling to as much as 600 mL or more. Low bladder wall compliance occurs when intravesical pressures rise in proportion with bladder filling; whole bladder compliance ≤ 10 mL/cm H_2O or a detrusor pressure >40 cm H_2O is associated with increased risk for upper urinary tract distress (Gray, 2011). Two characteristics of the bladder wall affect bladder compliance: detrusor smooth muscle tone and the viscoelastic properties of the vesical wall. In a person

with normal bladder wall compliance, the detrusor muscle remains in a relaxed state until its owner makes a voluntary decision to urinate, and the viscoelastic components of the bladder wall (primarily collagen and elastin proteins) promote passive filling at low intravesical pressures.

CLINICAL PEARL

Neurogenic bladder dysfunction is a risk factor for upper tract distress, defined as impaired function of the kidneys and renal pelves.

Urethral resistance is defined as the detrusor pressure required to overcome the urethral sphincter mechanism and create urinary flow (Gray, 2011; Hosker et al., 2009; Schafer, 1995). In the person with normal lower urinary tract function, urethral resistance is defined as the magnitude of detrusor pressure required to open the urethra and initiate urine flow (voiding); it is measured during urodynamic testing as the urethral opening pressure (Gray, 2011, 2012a, 2012b). Bladder outlet obstruction is defined as increased resistance to urethral opening and urinary outflow (failure to empty because of the outlet). As noted previously, common causes of bladder outlet obstruction in the patient with neurogenic bladder dysfunction include detrusor sphincter dyssynergia and prostatic hyperplasia in aging men. However, the magnitude of urethral resistance is also clinically relevant in patients with neurogenic bladder and underactive detrusor function (failure to empty because of the bladder), along with low bladder wall compliance. Among these patients, urethral resistance is measured via the detrusor leak point pressure, defined as the sustained detrusor pressure required to open the urethra and create overflow incontinence (Gray, 2011; McGuire et al., 1981; Ghoniem et al., 1989).

Bladder outlet obstruction with an elevated urethral opening pressure or low bladder wall compliance with an elevated detrusor leak point pressure is sometimes described as an indicator of *hostile bladder function*, indicating a bladder that is likely to produce upper urinary tract distress unless a bladder management program is implemented to reduce urethral opening and/or detrusor leak point pressures while enhancing bladder wall compliance in order to prevent or alleviate upper urinary tract distress (Morrisroe et al., 2005; Perez et al., 1993).

CLINICAL PEARL

Bladder outlet obstruction resulting in elevated detrusor pressures and/or low bladder wall compliance are examples of *hostile bladder conditions* that are common among individuals with neurogenic bladder dysfunction. (Hostile bladder conditions are those that increase the risk of upper tract distress.)

Assessment of the Patient with Neurogenic Bladder: General Principles

Chapter 3 provides a detailed discussion of the assessment of the patient with urinary incontinence, and the principles and approaches described in that chapter apply to all patients with neurogenic bladder dysfunction. The brief discussion in this chapter will focus on components of the overall assessment unique to patients with neurogenic bladder dysfunction.

Focused History: Bladder Management Program

The focused history for patients with urinary incontinence must include assessment of LUTS (Abrams et al., 2002). Pertinent LUTS are subdivided into storage symptoms (daytime voiding frequency, nocturia, urgency, along with stress, urge, or mixed incontinence and incontinence without sensory awareness), voiding LUTS (weak or intermittent urinary stream, hesitancy, and terminal dribbling), and postvoid LUTS (feelings of incomplete bladder emptying and postvoid dribbling). However, many patients with neurogenic bladder dysfunction do not experience the typical cycle of bladder function: filling/storage, followed by micturition, followed by another cycle beginning with bladder filling/storage. Instead, they rely on a specific program to manage their bladder such as intermittent catheterization, involuntary voiding into an external collection device or absorptive brief, indwelling catheterization, or some combination of these management strategies.

Therefore, it is important to first determine if the patient with neurogenic bladder dysfunction manages her or his bladder via spontaneous voiding. If this is not the case, questions about LUTS should be tailored to account for presence of a bladder management program. For example, patients who perform clean intermittent catheterization (CIC) should be queried about the frequency of catheterization, the size and type of catheter used, and whether they use a new catheter each time they catheterize or clean and reuse catheters. Persons who rely on CIC should also be asked if they void between catheterizations or whether they rely on CIC exclusively for bladder emptying. The person who empties his or her bladder using CIC should be asked about nighttime urinary drainage. While most are able to sleep through the night without catheterizing, some will report the need to catheterize once or more per night, and others (especially children with spina bifida) may be drained with

---

CLINICAL PEARL

When conducting the interview for an individual with neurogenic bladder dysfunction, the nurse should ask about the patient's bladder management program (spontaneous voiding, clean intermittent catheterization, involuntary voiding into a collection device, etc.) as well as any problems or concerns associated with the current management program.

---

an indwelling catheter that remains in place overnight, followed by resumption of CIC during waking hours.

Patients who void into an external collection device or absorptive brief should be asked about the type of external collective device that they use (condom catheter or hydrocolloid-based device) (ReliaFit, Eloquest, Ferndale, MI), how often they change their external collection device, and whether they experience leakage due to an incomplete seal between device and penis. Those who involuntarily void into an absorptive brief should be asked about the type of brief they use. The patient and care provider should be asked about skin problems associated with use of an external collection device or absorptive brief. They should also be asked if they perform CIC in addition to voiding into an external collection device.

Persons with neurogenic bladder dysfunction who use a long-term indwelling catheter should be asked about his or her catheterization site (urethral or suprapubic), the cumulative length of time that they have worn an indwelling catheter, the reason they use this bladder management strategy, and problems associated with catheter use. The average frequency of catheter changes should be explored, as well as experiences with catheter blockage resulting in the need to change the catheter urgently. They should be asked about possible problems associated with long-term catheterization including bypassing (leaking around the catheter), bladder spasms with leakage or pain, and episodes of hematuria. Patients using long-term indwelling catheters should be asked about his or her usual drainage system, including use of leg bags, overnight drainage bags, or belly bags. Problems associated with the urinary drainage system should be discussed, including leaks because of problems with their drainage system and skin problems related to leg bag straps (Fowler et al., 2014; Ostaszkiewicz & Paterson, 2012). Nighttime urinary drainage habits should be queried, along with strategies for repeated use of urinary drainage bags and how they are cleaned and prepared for reuse. Patients should be asked about catheter care (how the individual and/or care provider cleanses the perineal skin and exposed portion of the catheter) and how they manage the catheter during general bathing.

Physical Assessment: Cognition, Dexterity, and Mobility, and Natural History of Underlying Disease

Functional and cognitive assessments are routine components of the physical assessment for all patients with urinary incontinence, and they are especially important for the patient with neurogenic bladder dysfunction. Because many patients with neurogenic bladder dysfunction experience incontinence without sensory awareness, a combination of urinary incontinence and incomplete bladder emptying, or hostile neurogenic bladder dysfunction with an increased risk of upper urinary tract distress, CIC is more widely used for bladder management in this population than in able-bodied, community-dwelling persons.

Therefore, physical assessment of the person with neurogenic bladder dysfunction often includes evaluation of suitability for CIC or the need for long-term indwelling catheter use. This assessment should include consideration of body habitus, the physical ability of the patient to perform CIC, motivation to perform CIC, and the availability of a caregiver (partner, family member, paid care provider) to perform CIC if the patient is transiently unable to perform catheterization or able to perform the procedure only with some level of assistance.

The natural history of the underlying neurologic disorder should also be evaluated when considering CIC versus indwelling catheter use in selected patients with neurogenic bladder. For example, the person with a stable neurologic lesion such as a spinal cord injury resulting in paraplegia or relapsing–remitting multiple sclerosis may be expected to retain the ability to perform CIC over an extended period of time (Castel-Lacanal et al., 2013; Gray et al., 1995b). In contrast, the person with rapid physical deterioration due to progressive multiple sclerosis or recently diagnosed Guillain-Barré disease may only be able to perform CIC for a comparatively brief period of time before upper extremity function becomes so compromised that CIC is no longer possible. In this case, indwelling catheter use may be considered, provided all other options for bladder management have been explored and found not feasible.

CLINICAL PEARL

When conducting the physical assessment of an individual with neurogenic bladder, it is particularly important to assess functional status (mobility and dexterity), specifically the ability to access the urethra and perform intermittent catheterization.

Urinalysis Screening

Queries regarding recurrent UTI and screening urinalysis are routine components of evaluation in the community-dwelling adult with urinary incontinence (Gormley et al., 2014; Lucas et al., 2013). UTI is a frequent complication of neurogenic bladder dysfunction, and it is the most prevalent urologic complication among patients who use indwelling catheters (Gormley, 2010; Vasudeva & Madersbacher, 2014). Nevertheless, the purpose of the urinalysis and the use of data obtained from the urinalysis differ in patients with neurogenic bladder dysfunction who manage their bladder with CIC or indwelling urinary catheters. For example, while presence of leukocytes and nitrites on urinalysis indicates the need for additional evaluation in the patient with nonneurogenic stress, urge, or mixed urinary incontinence, these findings are highly prevalent in patients using CIC or an indwelling catheter and should not prompt further investigation unless a symptomatic UTI is suspected.

Urodynamic Testing

According to the American Urological Association/Society for Urodynamics, urodynamic testing is not indicated for the routine evaluation of persons with nonneurogenic urge,

stress, or mixed urinary incontinence; rather, it is indicated in selected cases when surgical intervention that may permanently alter lower urinary tract function is anticipated (Institute of Medicine, Food and Science Board, 2004). However, the guidelines do support consideration of urodynamic testing and the measurement of postvoid residual volume for evaluation of persons with neurogenic bladder dysfunction. The guidelines also support consideration of voiding pressure flow studies, pelvic floor muscle electromyography, and videourodynamic testing in patients with neurogenic bladder dysfunction and incomplete bladder emptying or other urologic symptoms, including suspicion of upper urinary tract distress.

CLINICAL PEARL

Urodynamic testing is commonly indicated for patients with neurogenic bladder dysfunction, to determine detrusor contractility, bladder wall compliance, and the presence and severity of any detrusor external sphincter dyssynergia.

Management of the Patient with Neurogenic Bladder Dysfunction: General Principles

Multiple chapters in this book discuss management of patients with various types of nonneurogenic urinary incontinence and retention. The brief discussion in this chapter will focus on management options especially appropriate for patients with neurogenic bladder dysfunction. Management options will be divided into several categories: behavioral interventions, catheterization techniques, pharmacologic interventions, and surgical options.

CLINICAL PEARL

Management of the patient with neurogenic bladder must be individualized based on patient assessment and specific problems and issues; strategies include behavioral strategies, pharmacologic therapy, and surgical interventions.

Behavioral Interventions

Behavioral interventions such as fluid and dietary modifications or changes in toileting behaviors (scheduled toileting, prompted voiding) have been shown to alleviate LUTS in patients with overactive bladder dysfunction and stress, urge, and mixed incontinence (Gormley et al., 2014; Lucas et al., 2013). They may also be considered in the management of patients with neurogenic bladders, but the precise nature of these interventions varies according to the nature of the lower urinary tract dysfunction and the bladder management program. Patients with neurogenic detrusor overactivity and urge incontinence should be counseled similarly to those with nonneurogenic overactive bladder syndrome. Counseling focuses on maintenance of adequate fluid intake based on recommended daily allowances from the Institute of Medicine (Institute of Medicine, Food and Science Board, 2004) and avoidance or reduction of caffeine intake because of its role as a bladder irritant (Wells et al., 2014). However, there is insufficient evidence to conclude that these behavioral interventions are clinically beneficial for patients with neurogenic detrusor overactivity with decreased or absent sensations of bladder filling, especially when combined with detrusor sphincter dyssynergia. Similarly, advice about fluid and caffeine intake must be individualized for the patient managed by CIC or indwelling catheterization. Prevention of constipation is recommended for maintenance of healthy bladder habits (Lukacz et al., 2011), but this advice must be individualized for those with neurogenic bladder dysfunction who may also utilize a structured bowel program for neurogenic bowel management.

Catheterization

Two forms of catheterization are used in the management of neurogenic bladder dysfunction: clean intermittent catheterization (CIC) and long-term indwelling catheterization.

Clean Intermittent Catheterization

CIC is indicated for patients with urinary retention, with or without urinary incontinence. Self-catheterization is taught whenever possible, and a care provider in the person's home is taught to catheterize as well. Teaching begins with an assessment of the patient's physical ability to manipulate and insert the catheter. This is particularly important for patients whose underlying neurological disorder may compromise upper arm movement, such as multiple sclerosis or cervical spinal cord injuries. This challenge was illustrated in a study of 44 community-dwelling persons practicing CIC for a variety of reasons; 21% of those with neurogenic bladder and multiple sclerosis cited poor dexterity as a problem when engaging in CIC (Bolinger & Engberg, 2013).

The continence nurse should be intimately involved in teaching principles of CIC and counseling patients about self-management of potential complications including symptomatic UTI, difficulty inserting a catheter, and urethral trauma or bleeding (Newman & Willson, 2011; Wyndaele, 2002). For patients with urinary retention with or without urinary incontinence, patients are taught to catheterize every 4 to 6 hours or four times daily while awake. The nurse teaches CIC technique, including hand hygiene prior to catheterization, location of the urethral meatus (especially in women), gentle insertion of the catheter until urine returns, and maneuvers to encourage complete evacuation of the urine from the bladder. Teaching for those living at home should include the patient and at least one care provider.

> **CLINICAL PEARL**
>
> Clean intermittent catheterization is indicated for patients with urinary retention with or without incontinence; a common challenge is the physical mobility and dexterity required to perform the procedure.

Catheter selection is an important component of CIC teaching; adults are typically instructed to use a 14- to 16-French catheter, and families of infants and children are taught to use catheters ranging in size from 6 to 10 French. Patients should be educated about the various types of intermittent catheters, including red rubber, polyvinyl chloride (clear) catheters, prelubricated hydrophilic intermittent catheters, and enclosed catheter systems. Women and girls should be introduced to intermittent catheters of shorter length, and men may be taught to use a coudé-tipped catheter if catheterization with a straight-tipped tube proves difficult. Children are taught to self-catheterize as soon as feasible based on physical ability, cognitive function, maturation, and motivation.

Traditionally, patients managing their bladders with CIC were taught to clean and reuse catheters, but the U.S. Centers for Medicare and Medicaid Services has altered its policies and now covers 200 single catheters per month (WOCN White Paper, 2009). A 2014 Cochrane Review (Prieto et al., 2014) reviewed the evidence regarding single use versus reused catheters for prevention of UTIs and concluded that the evidence is too weak to draw firm conclusions about its impact; regardless, the change in coverage does allow users a new, sterile catheter for every catheterization, eliminating the significant burden associated with catheter cleaning and reuse.

Prevention of complications associated with CIC must be taught, including UTI prevention. Strategies to reduce the risk for recurring UTI include consistent hand hygiene prior to catheter insertion, adherence to prescribed regimens for catheterization, and strategies to enhance complete evacuation of urine, such as catheterizing in an upright position whenever possible and slow removal of the catheter to enhance drainage. Prelubricated hydrophilic catheters and closed intermittent catheterization systems may reduce the potential for bacteriuria and/or UTI, and their use should be considered for patients who experience recurrent symptomatic UTI (Chartier Kastler & Denys, 2011; Day et al., 2002). Overwhelming clinical experience and limited clinical evidence suggests that selected use of coudé-tipped catheters and prelubricated hydrophilic catheters also reduces the risk of urethral trauma (Parker et al., 2009). Whenever any change is made to the bowel or bladder management program (such as a change to a closed system or prelubricated catheter), the continence nurse should track symptom improvement and antibiotic use.

Strategies to reduce the risk of UTI among individuals managing with CIC include consistent hand hygiene, adherence to the prescribed schedule for catheterization, and measures to assure complete emptying.

Indwelling Catheterization

Short-term indwelling catheterization (see also Chapter 6) is often used to manage urinary drainage after an acute neurologic event such as a spinal cord injury or a stroke. These catheters typically remain in place for 30 days or less and should be managed using accepted principles for short-term catheters, including measures for prevention of catheter-associated UTI (Parker et al., 2009). Cyclical clamping and unclamping prior to removal of a short-term indwelling urinary catheter has been attempted in an effort to improve lower urinary tract function following removal of the catheter, but limited evidence demonstrates that this practice provides no benefit when compared to removal without clamping (Moon et al., 2012).

Long-term indwelling catheterization is sometimes used for patients with neurogenic bladder dysfunction and urinary retention (with or without urinary incontinence) that is not amenable to CIC or other bladder management techniques (Wisconsin Department of Health Services, 2001). It is also used in highly selected patients with neurogenic bladder and urinary incontinence who cannot manage with CIC because of specific social or economic circumstances. For example, use of a long-term indwelling catheter may be used for a quadriplegic female who cannot be managed with CIC because of lack of a full-time care provider in her home setting.

Long-term use of indwelling catheters is considered a last resort and should be used only in select situations when other management approaches are not feasible.

The continence nurse plays a primary role in management of the patient with a neurogenic bladder and long-term indwelling catheter. The decision to insert a long-term urinary catheter is typically made by an interdisciplinary team (including a nurse), with the order written by a physician. The team should counsel the patient and family regarding placement of a urethral versus suprapubic catheter. Evidence regarding the benefits and disadvantages of suprapubic versus urethral catheters remains sparse; several studies of patients with neurogenic bladder (due to spinal cord injuries, stroke, multiple sclerosis, and Parkinsonism) found no difference in catheter-associated UTI occurrences, catheter bypassing (from the urethra or suprapubic site, respectively), or serum creatinine (Ahluwalia et al., 2006; Katsumi et al., 2010). Nevertheless,

evidence suggests that some patients prefer suprapubic catheters, while others prefer urethral catheters (Ahluwalia et al., 2006; Fowler et al., 2014). Therefore, the selection between suprapubic versus urethral catheter should be based on a discussion of the advantages and disadvantages of urethral and suprapubic catheters from the perspective of the patient and family.

There is very limited data regarding advantages of urethral versus suprapubic catheters; thus, the decision should be made based on a discussion with the patient and family to determine their preference.

Selection of catheter size, substrate (material of construction), and urinary drainage system is typically a nursing decision. A 14- to 16-French catheter is preferred for a long-term indwelling urethral catheter. Several substrates are available, including latex with a polytetrafluoroethylene coating, latex with a hydrogel coating, latex with a silicone coating, and all-silicone catheters (Curtis & Klykken, 2008). While all catheter substrates are susceptible to biofilm formation and encrustation, hydrogel-coated, silicone-coated, and all-silicone catheters are preferred to polytetrafluoroethylene catheters because they appear to produce less urethral inflammation and discomfort when left in place for a prolonged period of time (Parker et al., 2009). Evidence suggests that catheters impregnated with a silver alloy or antibiotic-coated catheters provide short-term protection against bacteriuria or catheter-associated urinary tract infection (CAUTI); they are not recommended for patients requiring long-term catheterization.

Hydrogel-coated, silicone-coated, and all-silicone catheters are preferred for long-term use because they produce less urethral inflammation when left in place for prolonged periods of time.

Selection of a urinary drainage system is individualized based on patient preference, typical physical activity, and dexterity/ability to drain the system (Gray et al., 2008). While maintenance of a closed drainage system is feasible and desirable for the patient with a short-term indwelling catheter, it is not feasible for persons with long-term indwelling catheters. Daytime urinary drainage may be accomplished using a leg bag or a drainage bag attached to the lower abdominal area.

The optimal drainage bag should be comfortably attached to the patient, remain discreet under clothing, and create minimal noise when partially filled with urine during activity (Curtis & Klykken, 2008; Fowler et al., 2014). Leg straps should remain in place without irritating the underlying skin; in one study of nonneurogenic patients using leg bags, cloth leg straps with secure snaps were preferred over latex straps (Pinar et al., 2009). Patients who experience trouble with leg straps may be counseled regarding use of a cloth pouch device. Consideration should also be given to the backing of the leg bag (cloth is preferred to latex) and the connecting tubing; adjustable length and flexibility underneath clothing have been identified as important features by leg bag users (Fowler et al., 2014; Pinar et al., 2009). Evaluation of an optimal daytime drainage system should also take into account the dexterity required to open the spout, drain the leg bag, return the spout to a closed position, and distinguish between these positions. Overnight drainage usually relies on a bedside urinary drainage bag with sufficient volume to allow drainage without the need for emptying. Patients may be advised to place the bag in a bucket as added protection in the event of leakage (Fowler et al., 2014).

Pharmacotherapy

A number of drugs are used in the management of neurogenic bladder. Drugs may be used to diminish or enhance urethral sphincter resistance, alleviate neurogenic detrusor overactivity, or improve bladder compliance by reducing detrusor muscle tone during bladder filling/storage (Cameron, 2010). Table 7-2 summarizes pharmacologic options for management of neurogenic bladder dysfunction.

TABLE 7-2 Pharmacologic Options for Management of Neurogenic Bladder Dysfunction

Neurogenic Bladder Dysfunction	Drug Class: Examples	Pharmacologic Action	Adverse Effects
Failure to store urine: because of the bladder (neurogenic detrusor overactivity, low bladder wall compliance)	**Antimuscarinics** (anticholinergics): Oxybutynin IR* Oxybutynin ER Oxybutynin TD patch Oxybutynin TD gel Tolterodine ER Fesoterodine Trospium ER Solifenacin Darifenacin	Binds with muscarinic receptors in bladder wall to block acetylcholine and abolish or reduce neurogenic detrusor overactivity	Dry mouth Blurred vision Constipation Flushing of skin Urinary retention
	Beta-3 adrenergic agonists Mirabegron	Adrenergic agonist, activates β-3 receptors causing detrusor muscle relaxation and promoting bladder filling	Hypertension Stuffy nose Urinary tract infection Headache Constipation
	Injectable neurotoxin OnabotulinumtoxinA	Cleaves SNAP-25 proteins preventing release of the neurotransmitter acetylcholine, abolishing or reducing neurogenic detrusor overactivity	Transient hematuria following injection Urinary tract infection Urinary retention Fatigue Constipation
Failure to store urine: because of the outlet (urethral sphincter incompetence)	**No drugs approved for this indication by U.S. FDA*** Alpha-adrenergic agonist pseudoephedrine and the tricyclic antidepressant imipramine have been used off label in the management of neurogenic bladder; imipramine also exerts anticholinergic effects used to alleviate or abolish neurogenic detrusor overactivity.	Alpha-adrenergic agonists promote urethral sphincter closure by increasing smooth muscle tone in the bladder neck and proximal urethra.	Hypertension Nervousness, restlessness Rapid pulse, palpitations Headache Imipramine also exerts anticholinergic side effects similar to antimuscarinic drugs.
Failure to empty urine: because of the bladder (underactive detrusor function)	**Cholinergic agonists** Bethanechol chloride, no longer used for underactive detrusor function due to lack of effectiveness in clinical practice	Synthetic analog of acetylcholine, acts at muscarinic receptors in the detrusor muscle to stimulate and sustained detrusor muscle contraction	Abdominal cramps Nausea Diarrhea Sweating Bronchial constriction

TABLE 7-2 **Pharmacologic Options for Management of Neurogenic Bladder Dysfunction (*Continued*)**

Neurogenic Bladder Dysfunction	Drug Class: Examples	Pharmacologic Action	Adverse Effects
Failure to empty urine: because of the outlet (bladder outlet obstruction, detrusor-striated sphincter dyssynergia, or detrusor bladder neck dyssynergia)	**Alpha-1 adrenergic blockers** Terazosin Doxazosin Tamsulosin Alfuzosin Silodosin	Binds with alpha-1 adrenergic receptors in smooth muscle of urethral sphincter mechanism to reduce urethral resistance to urinary outflow	Postural hypotension Dizziness Nasal congestion Headache Reflex tachycardia
	Skeletal muscle relaxants Baclofen (intrathecal)	Reduces skeletal muscle tone in the rhabdosphincter and periurethral skeletal muscles by inhibiting monosynaptic and polysynaptic reflexes at the spinal level	Drowsiness Dizziness Weakness Fatigue **Adverse side effects for intrathecal delivery** Sedation Respiratory and cardiovascular suppression Meningitis
	Injectable neurotoxin OnabotulinumtoxinA (not approved for this indication by the U.S. FDA*)	Cleaves SNAP-25 proteins preventing release of the neurotransmitter acetylcholine, abolishing or reducing neurogenic detrusor overactivity	Generalized muscle weakness Transient urethral bleeding Transient autonomic dysreflexia

*U.S. Food and Drug Administration.
Data from Amend et al. (2008); Barrett (1981); Cameron (2010); Cruz (2014); Finkbeiner (1985); Kenelly et al. (2009); Lapeyre et al. (2010); Mahfouz & Corcos (2011); Marberger (2013); McIntyre et al. (2014); Mehta et al. (2012); Mertens et al. (1995); Nadulli et al. (2012); Nitti et al. (2014); Rapidi et al. (2007); Soljanik (2013); Trocio et al. (2010).

CLINICAL PEARL

Medications used for neurogenic bladder management primarily include those designed to reduce or eliminate detrusor contractions (antimuscarinics, beta-3 agonists, and onabotulinumtoxinA) and those designed to reduce urethral resistance (alpha-adrenergic antagonists, skeletal muscle relaxants, and onabotulinum toxin A).

Antimuscarinics

Pharmacotherapy is a cornerstone of therapy for neurogenic detrusor overactivity (failure to store because of the bladder). Antimuscarinics, also referred to as anticholinergics, block the neurotransmitter acetylcholine from binding to muscarinic receptors in the detrusor smooth muscle. Multiple pharmacologic options are available, including immediate- and extended-release oral agents, transdermal patches, and transdermal gels. In patients with preserved sensations of bladder filling, neurogenic detrusor overactivity is usually associated with urinary urgency, frequent urination while awake, nocturia or nocturnal enuresis, and urge incontinence. The typical goal of therapy in these patients is alleviation of urge incontinence and related LUTS (nocturia, daytime voiding frequency, and urgency) while preserving spontaneous voiding. Evidence strongly suggests that the clinical benefits of antimuscarinic drugs are enhanced when pharmacotherapy is combined with the behavioral interventions described earlier (Trocio et al., 2010). Refer to Chapter 5 for a more detailed discussion of the use of antimuscarinic drugs in persons with overactive bladder, including long-term use in older patients.

In contrast, patients with paralyzing spinal disorders such as spinal cord injury, transverse myelitis, and multiple sclerosis typically have significantly reduced or absent sensations of bladder filling; these individuals are usually unable to manage their bladders with spontaneous voiding owing to the combination of neurogenic detrusor overactivity and greatly reduced or absent sensory awareness of impending micturition. In addition, these individuals often experience detrusor sphincter dyssynergia, which results in incomplete emptying as well as leakage (a combination of failure to empty and failure to store). In this case, the goal of therapy is to abolish detrusor overactivity so that the bladder stores urine at low intravesical pressures and the individual remains free of incontinence between catheterizations (Amend et al., 2008; Kenelly et al., 2009; Mahfouz & Corcos, 2011; Nadulli et al., 2012). Because the goal is to eliminate detrusor overactivity, these patients often require CIC and higher dosages of a single antimuscarinic agent, more than one oral antimuscarinic drug, an oral antimuscarinic drug combined with a transdermal formulation, or an antimuscarinic combined with a beta-3 agonist. In patients who are prescribed higher antimuscarinic dosages or multidrug therapy, the continence nurse should be particularly alert to the possibility of adverse side effects.

Beta-3 Agonists

Pharmacotherapy for patients with neurogenic detrusor overactivity has expanded to include a new drug class, the beta-3 agonists. Research is ongoing on several potential molecules, and one drug has been approved for clinical use by the U.S. FDA (Nitti et al., 2014). Beta-3 agonists act differently than the antimuscarinics. Rather than blocking muscarinic receptors, they enhance the activity of the neurotransmitter epinephrine as it binds to beta-3 receptors in the bladder wall. Mirabegron may be administered for first-line management of neurogenic detrusor overactivity, or it may be used in combination with an antimuscarinic agent. Although additional research is needed, bladder management using both classes appears attractive for patients who prove refractory to a single agent because of the different sites of pharmacologic activity and different potential side effects.

Onabotulinum Toxin A

Onabotulinum toxin A is an attractive pharmacologic agent for patients with neurogenic detrusor overactivity because of its efficacy and comparatively long duration of action. This neurotoxin is injected directly into the detrusor wall during a cystoscopic procedure (Soljanik, 2013). It cleaves SNAP-25 proteins in the nerve cell, which blocks the release of acetylcholine and thereby prevents contraction of the detrusor muscle (Cruz, 2014). OnabotulinumtoxinA is injected approximately every 9 months. Many patients are able to reduce or discontinue oral or transdermal drugs for neurogenic detrusor overactivity after injection. OnabotulinumtoxinA requires up to 36 injection sites; transient hematuria following injection occurs frequently, and prolonged hematuria was noted in 4.9% of a pooled sample of 2,301 patients with neurogenic detrusor overactivity. Urinary retention and UTIs are common side effects, affecting 23.7% and 16.7%, respectively. Given the high rate of urinary retention, patients with neurogenic bladder dysfunction who manage with spontaneous voiding must be counseled about the possible need to perform CIC following injection of onabotulinumtoxinA.

OnabotulinumtoxinA may also be injected directly into the striated muscles of the urethral sphincter mechanism in patients with detrusor-striated sphincter dyssynergia. Similar to its actions on the smooth muscle of the detrusor, it blocks contraction of the rhabdosphincter and periurethral striated muscles by cleaving SNAP-25 proteins in the nerve cells of the motor unit (Marberger, 2013). Although onabotulinumtoxinA is not officially indicated or approved for treatment of detrusor-striated sphincter dyssynergia, a systematic review identified 2 randomized clinical trials and 6 nonrandomized trials involving 129 subjects with neurogenic bladder associated with spinal cord injury. Pooled analysis of evidence from these trials found that treatment reduced postvoid residual volumes and the magnitude of obstruction caused by dyssynergia 30 days after injection. Findings from 4 studies showed reduction in CIC and results of three studies indicated a 50% reduction in UTI occurrence.

Baclofen

The pharmacologic management of patients with increased urethral resistance caused by detrusor–sphincter dyssynergia (failure to empty because of the outlet) is challenging. This problem is most commonly encountered in patients with neurogenic bladder and paralyzing spinal disorders such as spinal cord injuries, transverse myelitis, or multiple sclerosis. Baclofen administered by intrathecal pump has proved effective for skeletal muscle spasticity in patients with paralyzing spinal disorders (Lapeyre et al., 2010; McIntyre et al., 2014), and limited evidence suggests it may be effective for management of neurogenic detrusor overactivity with detrusor-striated sphincter dyssynergia (Mertens et al., 1995; Rapidi et al., 2007).

Alpha-Adrenergic Antagonists

The alpha-1 adrenergic antagonists reduce urethral sphincter mechanism resistance by blocking adrenergic receptors on the smooth muscle of the bladder neck and proximal urethra. They may be used to reduce urethral resistance in patients with detrusor-striated sphincter dyssynergia and those with detrusor–bladder neck dyssynergia (Ahmed et al., 2006; Yamanishi et al., 1997). They are also used in older men with neurogenic bladder dysfunction complicated by bladder outlet obstruction associated with benign prostatic enlargement (Mehta et al., 2012).

Cholinergic Agonists

Cholinergic agonists have been used in the past in an attempt to treat underactive detrusor function (failure to empty because of the bladder). A single agent, bethanechol chloride, is currently available. However, cholinergic agonists have been shown to be ineffective for improving bladder emptying in multiple studies, and they are no longer recommended for use in the management of neurogenic bladder dysfunction (Barrett, 1981; Finkbeiner, 1985).

Surgical Management

A comprehensive review of surgical options for treatment of neurogenic bladder dysfunction is beyond the scope of this chapter focusing on nursing management. Table 7-3 provides an overview of surgical options for managing the neurogenic bladder (Graham et al., 2007).

TABLE 7-3 **Surgical Management Options for Neurogenic Bladder Dysfunction**

Neurogenic Bladder Dysfunction	Surgical Procedure	Description
Failure to store urine: because of the bladder (neurogenic detrusor overactivity, low bladder wall compliance)	Augmentation enterocystoplasty Implantation of a sacral neuromodulation device	A segment of the bowel is isolated from the gastrointestinal tract, detubularized, and attached to the urinary bladder. A sacral neuromodulation device is implanted into the pelvis and leads are placed at the sacral roots that communicate with a remote control device. Activation of the device inhibits detrusor muscle contraction.
Failure to store urine: because of the outlet (urethral sphincter incompetence)	Injection of suburethral bulking agents (glutaraldehyde cross-linked collagen, calcium hydroxylapatite, pyrolytic carbon-coated beads, polydimethylsiloxane, ethylene vinyl alcohol copolymer) Suburethral sling procedures Artificial urinary sphincter	Biocompatible bulking agents are injected into the urethral submucosa just distal to the rhabdosphincter (membranous urethra in males, midurethra in females) under endoscopic guidance. Suburethral sling procedures using synthetic mesh or bolsters may be used to increase urethral resistance to urine outflow in both women and men. Artificial urinary sphincters may be implanted in both men and women to increase urethral resistance to urine outflow; the device is maintained in a closed position; activation of the sphincter shunts fluid from a urethral cuff to an abdominal reservoir, which transiently opens the cuff to enable spontaneous voiding or intermittent catheterization.
Failure to empty urine: because of the outlet (bladder outlet obstruction, detrusor-striated muscle dyssynergia, or detrusor bladder neck dyssynergia)	Transurethral sphincterotomy Multiple procedures may be used to relieve bladder outlet obstruction; common examples include transurethral or minimally invasive prostatectomy	Uses an endoscopic approach to incise the striated urethral sphincter in men in order to reduce urethral sphincter resistance to urine outflow. Uses an endoscopic approach to visualize the prostatic urethra; excess prostatic tissue is resected using a variety of instruments. Minimally invasive prostatectomy procedures use one of several forms of energy to destroy prostatic tissue such as microwave energy, direct contact laser energy, or high intensity ultrasound.

Data from Atala (2014); Atala et al. (2006); Beirs et al. (2011); Boone (2009); Graham et al. (2007); Joseph et al. (2014); Kari et al. (2013); Liard et al. (2001); Lopez et al. (2006); Nerli et al. (2013); Perkash (1996); Perkash (2009); Peters et al. (2013); Revicky & Tincello (2014); Zuckerman et al. (2014).

Augmentation Enterocystoplasty

Augmentation enterocystoplasty is a reconstructive surgical procedure that enlarges bladder capacity, improves bladder wall compliance, and alleviates or abolishes neurogenic detrusor overactivity (Beirs et al., 2011). A bowel segment (usually the ileum) is isolated from the fecal stream and detubularized to interrupt peristaltic contractions. This segment is attached to the bladder, which is bivalved to create a spherical vesicle for maximum capacity. Patients who have undergone augmentation enterocystoplasty almost always use CIC to manage their bladder postoperatively, and they should be taught techniques to manage mucus production from the bowel segment, including adequate fluid intake and routine irrigation if mucus is significant. Patients must also be counseled about the long-term risk for carcinoma of the augmented bladder, and the importance of routine follow-up with his or her physician.

Autologous Bladder Replacement

Tissue-engineered autologous bladders have been developed and successfully implanted into human hosts (Atala et al., 2006). These bladders are created from autologous cell cultures that are expanded using techniques originally developed and tested in animal models. A neobladder is formed using a scaffold constructed from homologous decellularized bladder submucosa, collagen, and/or a synthetic material used for hernia repair; the construction process requires approximately 7 to 8 weeks prior to surgical implantation. At the time of surgery, the engineered neobladder is attached onto the base of the native bladder and omentum is used to increase the vascularity of the reconstructed neobladder.

The engineered neobladder differs from augmentation enterocystoplasty in several important ways: (1) it replaces rather than augments the existing bladder body, (2) it is constructed from homologous bladder tissue rather than intestinal tissue, (3) surgery does not require loss of bowel from the gastrointestinal tract, and (4) it does not create mucus or reabsorb urinary constituents as does reconstructed bowel. Nevertheless, it must be remembered that CIC is needed for these bladders just as it is for bladders augmented by detubularized bowel. Short-term results in children with neurogenic bladder dysfunction associated with myelomeningocele were promising, but longer-term results have been disappointing (Atala, 2014; Joseph et al., 2014). Additional research and refinement of these techniques are needed, but the promise of this procedure clearly justifies this effort.

Sacral Neuromodulation

Sacral neuromodulation devices may be implanted into the pelvis with the leads placed at the sacral roots (Graham et al., 2007). Activation of this device inhibits neurogenic detrusor overactivity and the resulting urge incontinence or incontinence without sensory awareness. Implanted sacral neuromodulation has been used for a variety of nonneurogenic voiding conditions including detrusor overactivity refractory to more conservative treatments. A study comparing 340 patients with and without neurogenic bladder dysfunction (including persons with stroke, multiple sclerosis, incomplete spinal cord injuries, and Parkinsonism) demonstrated similar outcomes (Peters et al. 2013). Persons contemplating implantation of a neuromodulation device should be counseled about the need for ongoing monitoring of his or her device including adjustment of the electrical signals used to stimulate the lower urinary tract and the potential need for additional surgery to ensure maximum function.

> **CLINICAL PEARL**
>
> Sacral neuromodulation has been used for a variety of non-neurogenic voiding disorders; recent studies indicate this therapy may also be of benefit to individuals with neurogenic bladder dysfunction.

Continent Catheterizable Stoma Construction

Several reconstructive procedures have been designed for persons who experience difficulty with CIC owing to urethral obstruction or prior urethral surgery, discomfort associated with catheterization, or the lack of mobility and dexterity required for urethral catheterization. Two procedures, creation of an appendovesicostomy (attributed to Mitrofanoff) or an ileovesicostomy (attributed to Yang-Monti), allow children and adults with neurogenic bladder dysfunction to perform CIC who might not otherwise be able to perform these procedures (Liard et al., 2001; Nerli et al., 2013). The appendicovesicostomy involves attaching the appendix to the bladder and bringing the appendix to the umbilicus or abdominal wall to create a catheterizable stoma. The ileovesicostomy uses a small segment of reconstructed bowel to create a continent, catheterizable stoma. Research is limited but current evidence suggests that catheterizable abdominal or umbilical stomas remain continent over a 10-year period or longer, enhance adherence to CIC regimens, and reduce the psychosocial burden associated with urethral catheterization in selected children (Kari et al., 2013; Liard et al., 2001; Nerli et al., 2013).

Suburethral Slings

Multiple surgical procedures have been developed for the treatment of urethral sphincter incompetence in women; the most common procedure involves placement of a synthetic mesh creating a suburethral sling (Revicky & Tincello, 2014). Refer to Chapter 9 for a more detailed description of the management of stress incontinence. Suburethral sling procedures have also been adapted for male patients; short-term continence rates are impressive, but longer-term results (>1 year) show less robust dry rates (40%) (Zuckerman et al., 2014).

Artificial Urinary Sphincter

Artificial urinary sphincters (AUS) remain an attractive surgical option for some patients with neurogenic bladder and urethral sphincter incompetence. The sling comprises three components: an abdominal reservoir, a baffling system with a pump implanted in the scrotum in men or underneath the labia majora in women, and a cuff that encircles the urethra distal to the rhabdosphincter (Graham et al., 2007). Similar to other surgical options, implantation of an AUS requires ongoing monitoring and repeated evaluation of its impact on neurogenic bladder dysfunction (Lopez et al., 2006).

Transurethral Sphincterotomy

Multiple surgical procedures have been developed to manage bladder outlet obstruction associated with benign prostatic enlargement or urethral stricture disease. Refer to Chapters 6 and 8 for a more detailed discussion of these procedures. In contrast, transurethral sphincterotomy and associated procedures such as implantation of a urethral stent are used specifically for treatment of male patients with neurogenic bladder dysfunction and detrusor-striated sphincter dyssynergia (Perkash, 1996, 2009). Once considered a mainstay of the management of detrusor sphincter dyssynergia in men with neurogenic bladder and detrusor-striated sphincter dyssynergia caused by spinal cord injury, performance of this procedure has declined dramatically due to less than optimal long-term outcomes.

● Neurogenic Bladder Management: Specific Examples

As noted earlier in this chapter, taxonomies for classifying and managing neurogenic bladder dysfunction have not gained widespread use owing to limitations in their application to clinical practice. These limitations include failure to account for the natural history of the underlying neurologic condition and its impact on options for a bladder management program, the long-term impact of obstruction on lower urinary tract function, the risk for hostile neurogenic bladder dysfunction and upper urinary tract distress, and patient/family preference. The following examples of neurogenic bladder dysfunction associated with prevalent neurologic conditions illustrate the need to consider all of these factors when providing nursing care for these individuals.

Spinal Cord Injury

Spinal cord injury (SCI) is defined as trauma or damage to the spinal cord resulting in loss of motor and/or sensory function (Kirshblum et al., 2014). Approximately 270,000

Americans have an SCI, and 12,000 to 20,000 experience an SCI each year (Ma et al., 2014).

Classification

Spinal cord injuries are classified according to the International Standards for Neurological Classification of Spinal Cord Injury (Kirshblum et al., 2014). This classification schema requires identification of sensory and motor impairments and matching of these deficits with the appropriate dermatome. The result is a spinal injury level that aids clinicians in determining physical rehabilitation needs and options for managing neurogenic bladder and bowel.

The American Spinal Injury Association (ASIA) has developed a complementary system to classify the severity of the impairment associated with SCI. An ASIA A SCI is defined as a "complete injury" with no sensory or motor function below the level of the SCI, and an ASIA B SCI is defined as "sensory incomplete" with preservation of sensory but no motor function below the level of the injury (van Middendorp et al., 2009). An ASIA C SCI is described as "motor complete" with preservation of less than half of the key muscle functions below the level of injury, while an ASIA D SCI indicates a "motor incomplete injury," with preservation of function of 50% or more of the key muscle groups below the level of injury. An ASIA E injury, sometimes referred to as an injury with no neurological deficit, is defined as absence of sensory or motor deficits despite a documented spinal trauma. Neurogenic bladder dysfunction is anticipated in all patients with ASIA A and B SCI and a high proportion of those with ASIA C and D injuries.

Management of neurogenic bladder dysfunction is based on two main goals: preservation of upper urinary tract health and restoration of the greatest degree of continence possible.

Spinal Shock

Following SCI, the individual experiences a period of spinal shock characterized by four phases: (1) absent motor reflexes with flaccid paralysis of skeletal muscles, which lasts approximately 1 day post injury; (2) denervation supersensitivity, which occurs approximately 1 to 3 days post injury and involves initial return of affected skeletal muscle reflexes; (3) onset of hyperreflexia of the affected muscles, which occurs about 1 to 4 weeks after injury; and (4) onset of a chronic state of striated muscle hyperreflexia, which begins as soon as 1 month post injury but can be delayed for as long as 12 months post injury (Ditunno et al., 2004). The bulbocavernosus reflex is a contraction of the bulbospongiosus muscle (one of the pelvic floor muscles) that occurs in response to tapping of the dorsum of the penis, gentle compression of the glans penis, or tapping of the clitoris during physical assessment. This polysynaptic response is mediated by sacral spinal segments 2 to 4, and it is a common component of a physical examination in the person with urinary incontinence. It was historically used to determine the end of spinal shock, but it typically recovers during the first 24 hours following SCI, long before

other signs of recovery from spinal shock in most patients. Despite flaccid paralysis of muscles below the level of injury, the urethral sphincter remains closed and the detrusor remains acontractile during spinal shock, resulting in urinary retention (failure to empty urine: because of the bladder) (Awad et al., 1977; Rossier & Ott, 1976).

An indwelling catheter is inserted immediately following SCI that is likely to remain in place during the early phases of spinal shock. This catheter is managed as a short-term indwelling catheter, and emphasis is placed on prevention of catheter-associated UTI. It serves two purposes, ongoing drainage of urine from the bladder and measurement of urine output. An acute SCI alters urine production, antidiuretic hormone production, and urinary output, predisposing the person to brisk urine production during the night and reduced production during waking hours when sitting upright (Kilinc et al., 1999; Szollar et al., 1995). Intermittent catheterization is begun as soon as nighttime urine volumes diminish to a point that an intermittent catheterization schedule is reasonable; this usually occurs within a period of days to weeks after an acute SCI. Nevertheless, changes in urine production associated with SCI may create the need for an around the clock catheterization schedule until urine nighttime urine production subsides (Kilinc et al., 1999; Szollar et al., 1995).

> **CLINICAL PEARL**
>
> An indwelling catheter is typically required initially post spinal cord injury due to spinal shock; once spinal shock resolves and nighttime urine production normalizes, the catheter can be removed and intermittent catheterization can be initiated.

Selection of Bladder Management Program

Selection of an ongoing bladder management program is an important process based on careful consideration of multiple factors including characteristics of the specific individual's bladder dysfunction, level and severity of the SCI and its impact on mobility and dexterity, resources within the patient's home, patient preference, and long-term impact of the management program selected (Engkasan et al., 2014). Patients with an SCI that damages the sacral micturition center (sacral segments 2 to 4) are likely to experience chronic paralysis of the detrusor (underactive detrusor function), requiring ongoing CIC or continuous drainage using an indwelling urinary catheter. From a clinical perspective, these patients typically present as having ASIA A, B, or C SCI affecting vertebral levels T10–L2 (van Middendorp et al., 2009; Wyndaele, 1997).

Depending on the level of injury and whether spinal trauma has affected Onuf's nucleus, these patients also may experience urethral sphincter incompetence (failure to store because of the outlet), with stress urinary incontinence noted during transfers in and out of the wheelchair or during coughing, sneezing, or straining. Depending on its severity, urethral sphincter incompetence may be

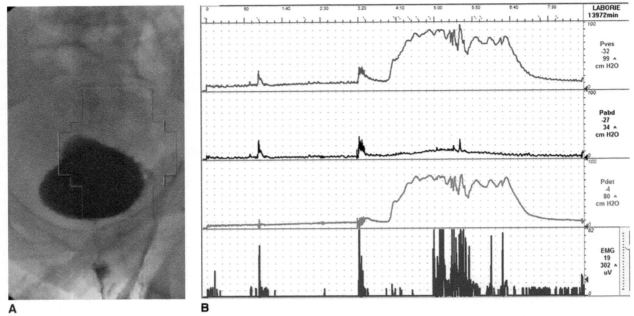

FIGURE 7-2. Management of a female patient with an ASIA A SCI and neurogenic bladder with detrusor neurogenic overactivity and detrusor-striated sphincter dyssynergia. Refer to Case 1.

managed by suburethral injection of a bulking agent, suburethral sling surgery, or implantation of an AUS (Bennett et al., 1995; Chartier Kastler et al., 2011; Davis et al., 2013; Groen et al., 2012).

The majority of patients with ASIA A, B, or C spinal injuries will have suprasacral level lesions, corresponding with injuries of vertebral levels of T10 to as high as C2 (van Middendorp et al., 2009; Wyndaele, 1997). As spinal shock subsides, the bladder exhibits neurogenic detrusor overactivity (failure to store because of the bladder), usually associated with detrusor-striated sphincter dyssynergia (failure to empty because of the outlet). A minority of patients with less severe SCI (ASIA C or D lesions), preserved sensations of bladder filling, and the ability to move to the toilet and prepare his or her clothing for urination may be able to maintain spontaneous voiding. These individuals may be managed by scheduled toileting, maintenance of a recommended daily intake of fluids, and avoidance of caffeine or other bladder irritants. Those with adequate detrusor contraction strength may benefit from an antimuscarinic or beta-3 agonist to reduce detrusor overactivity, possibly in combination with an alpha-1 adrenergic blocker to reduce sphincter resistance during micturition. These persons are at low risk for upper urinary tract distress, but they are at increased risk for UTI and should be monitored regularly (at least annually) to ensure optimal urinary tract function and maintenance of maximal social continence (Anson & Gray, 1993; Killorin et al., 1992).

Persons with neurogenic detrusor overactivity, reduced or absent sensations of bladder filling, and detrusor-striated sphincter dyssynergia are not able to void voluntarily and are typically managed by CIC, involuntary voiding into an

external collection device, or long-term indwelling urinary catheterization (Anson & Gray, 1993; Killorin et al., 1992). Clean intermittent catheterization is preferred in these individuals, because of its ability to prevent upper urinary tract distress, in combination with its ability to maintain continence between catheterizations in most individuals (Gray et al., 1995b; Weld et al., 2000). Intermittent catheterization is typically combined with an antimuscarinic agent, beta-3 agonist, or onabotulinumtoxinA injections. In this case, the goal of therapy is to ablate all overactive detrusor contractions between catheterizations, ensuring continence and preventing upper urinary tract distress. Figure 7-2 and Case 1 describe management of a woman with an ASIA A SCI and neurogenic bladder with detrusor neurogenic overactivity and detrusor-striated sphincter dyssynergia.

Quadriplegic males who are unable to perform CIC owing to motor deficits of their upper extremities or paraplegic males unwilling or unable to perform CIC may be managed by involuntary voiding into an external collection device (this program is sometimes referred to as a reflex, kickoff, or trigger voiding program) (Anson & Gray, 1993; Killorin et al., 1992). Involuntary voiding into an external collection device is dependent on the ability of the detrusor muscle to overcome any bladder outlet obstruction created by detrusor-striated sphincter dyssynergia. If there is sufficient outlet resistance to impede emptying, these men are at risk for recurring UTI and upper urinary tract distress. The risk for recurring UTI or upper urinary tract distress may be reduced by administration of alpha-1 adrenergic blockers to reduce urethral sphincter resistance, injection of onabotulinumtoxinA into the rhabdosphincter, or a surgical sphincterotomy. The effectiveness of the

CASE STUDIES

CASE 1 NEUROGENIC BLADDER IN A 34-YEAR-OLD FEMALE FOLLOWING T6 SPINAL CORD INJURY

Figure 7-2 illustrates the case of TA, a 34-year-old female who suffered a T6 (ASIA A, complete) spinal cord injury following a motor vehicle accident 3 years prior to attending our continence promotion center. She attended her initial evaluation with her partner; they have been together for 7 years. TA reported managing her bladder using adult containment briefs because of urinary incontinence without awareness. She states she performs CIC twice daily. She stated that she originally catheterized every 4 hours and regularly took oxybutynin 5 mg twice daily but stopped the medication and CIC due to frequent episodes of urinary incontinence and occasional UTIs that she attributed to CIC. She began containing urinary leakage with adult absorptive briefs only. However, she restarted catheterizations twice daily when she began experiencing episodes of autonomic dysreflexia and a febrile UTI that required hospitalization and management with parenteral antibiotics. She initially approached her primary care WOC nurse requesting placement of an indwelling catheter. Her primary care provider declined and referred her for further evaluation of her neurogenic bladder. Initial evaluation revealed a thin, alert, motivated Caucasian female with paraplegia and significant spasticity of her lower extremities. Her upper extremity strength was excellent and she reported no difficulty performing CIC. Her medications included nitrofurantoin 50 mg once daily for UTI suppression and baclofen 20 mg three times daily. Inspection of the perineal area revealed inflamed skin with some erosion of the skin surrounding the labia and inner thighs consistent with incontinence-associated dermatitis. Urinalysis revealed positive nitrites and small leukocytes with no red blood cells, glucose, or protein in her urine. Her serum creatinine was 0.6 mg/dL.

Urodynamic testing revealed small cystometric capacity (220 mL) with neurogenic detrusor overactivity causing urinary incontinence without awareness; detrusor-striated sphincter dyssynergia was noted on EMG causing functional obstruction of urinary outflow. Her postvoid residual volume was 150 mL. Testing did not provoke autonomic dysreflexia.

Based on these findings, TA was asked about her willingness to restart a regular CIC program. She expressed her willingness to restart pharmacotherapy and CIC but states she was concerned about the adverse side effects of dry mouth and significant flushing and fatigue when outdoors on warm, humid days. She was initially started on CIC every 4 hours while awake and solifenacin 10 mg daily. On 6-week follow-up, she stated that she was encouraged that her new medication appeared to be more effective than her previous regimen but reported that she still experienced leakage episodes almost daily. After lengthy discussion, she underwent intradetrusor injection of onabotulinumtoxinA. Following injection, she enjoyed complete dryness on her CIC program without any additional pharmacotherapy. She began experiencing UI episodes after a period of 8 months but regained continence after a second injection. She is currently scheduled to receive a third injection after 8 months.

This case illustrates the need for ongoing management in a young adult woman with paraplegia and neurogenic bladder dysfunction following T6 SCI. Her original bladder management program, CIC with an antimuscarinic therapy, was appropriate for her bladder dysfunction, but her initial drug dosage proved insufficient to prevent neurogenic detrusor overactivity and incontinence between catheterizations. As a result, she abandoned her initial bladder management program but returned to care after experiencing autonomic dysreflexia and a febrile UTI. While a second antimuscarinic agent improved continence between catheterizations, it did not completely ablate leakage episodes. Second-line treatment, injection of onabotulinumtoxinA, proved effective in preventing incontinence between catheterizations for a period of just over 8 months. The proposal of indwelling catheterization was not pursued because of its association with an increased risk for urologic complications with long-term use.

program in preventing incontinence is determined by the ability of the external collection device and urinary drainage system to retain urine and prevent urine loss onto the clothing or skin.

Because of challenges associated with normal female anatomy, no reliable external collection device has been developed for women. Therefore, quadriplegic women, or paraplegic women unwilling or unable to perform CIC, may require long-term use of an indwelling urinary catheter for bladder management. There are multiple potential complications associated with long-term use of indwelling catheters; therefore, meticulous management and routine follow-up is essential (see Chapter 13).

Ongoing Monitoring

Regardless of the bladder management program selected, ongoing monitoring and care are important for all patients with SCI. While the neurological impact of a traumatic SCI remains unchanged after spinal shock has subsided, the potential impact on lower urinary tract function is progressive and is affected by the presence and severity of bladder outlet obstruction, the variable impact of the bladder management program, and possibly the cumulative effects of recurring UTI or upper urinary tract distress. Monitoring of patients with SCI and neurogenic bladder is recommended on an annual basis or more frequently when indicated. In a study of 96 patients with SCI and neurogenic bladder who were followed with annual visits for at least 2 years, 47.9% required adjustments in their bladder management programs either to enhance continence or to manage recurring UTI or upper urinary tract distress (Linsenmeyer & Linsenmeyer, 2013).

The risk for upper urinary tract distress among persons with SCI and neurogenic bladder dysfunction is significant (Anson & Gray, 1993; Killorin et al., 1992; Weld et al., 2000), due in part to the underlying bladder dysfunction and in part to the selected bladder management program. Spontaneous voiding and CIC are associated with lower complication rates than involuntary voiding into an external collecting device; thus, these approaches are encouraged and implemented whenever feasible (Anson & Gray, 1993; Killorin et al., 1992). In contrast, the greatest risk for upper urinary tract distress is associated with long-term indwelling catheterization (Anson & Gray, 1993; Killorin et al., 1992; Weld et al., 2000). Therefore, this program is reserved for patients who cannot manage neurogenic bladder dysfunction using an alternative program.

CLINICAL PEARL

Among individuals with neurogenic bladder dysfunction due to SCI, the lowest incidence of upper tract distress is associated with spontaneous voiding and CIC, and the highest incidence of upper tract distress is associated with long-term use of indwelling catheters.

Surgical management is required in some persons with SCI and upper urinary tract distress. Augmentation enterocystoplasty may be indicated for patients with neurogenic detrusor overactivity or low bladder wall compliance who are able to perform CIC. An incontinent urinary diversion (ileal conduit) is performed in highly selected patients with SCI and neurogenic bladder dysfunction that cannot be managed by any other means; individuals managed with diversion tend to be older with more physical limitations than those undergoing augmentation enterocystoplasty (Peterson et al., 2012).

Multiple Sclerosis

Multiple sclerosis (MS) is a chronic, immune-mediated inflammatory disease that affects multiple sites within the central nervous system (Milo & Miller, 2014). Several types of MS have been identified, including relapsing–remitting and primary progressive. Relapsing–remitting is the most common type of MS, accounting for 80% to 85% of all cases, followed by primary progressive, which comprises 10% to 15% of all cases. Additional categories based on the highly variable disease progression of MS have also been identified. Clinically isolated syndrome is defined as the first occurrence of clinical symptoms suggestive of MS. Secondary progressive MS is defined as an initial pattern of relapsing–remitting disease followed by slower progression with occasional remissions or plateaus; about half of patients who initially present with relapsing–remitting MS develop this pattern within 5 years, and 90% develop this pattern within 25 years.

Clinical Presentation

Approximately 400,000 persons living in the United States have some form of MS; the incidence is approximately 3.6 cases per 100,000 person-years in women and 2.0 per 100,000 person-years in men (Ma et al., 2014). The average time from disease onset to difficulty with ambulation is 8 years, and the mean time to complete reliance on assistive walking devices or a wheelchair is 15 to 30 years. Neurogenic bladder dysfunction is prevalent in patients with MS; it is estimated to occur in 80% to 100% over the course of the disease (de Seze et al., 2007; Tubaro et al., 2012). Approximately 60% to 80% of persons with MS will have neurogenic detrusor overactivity with urgency, frequency, nocturia, nocturnal enuresis, and/or urge incontinence. Detrusor-striated sphincter dyssynergia occurs in as many as 25% of persons with MS, and underactive detrusor function is seen in about 20%.

CLINICAL PEARL

Neurogenic bladder dysfunction occurs in 80% to 100% of patients with MS, and sphincter dyssynergia occurs in 25% of these individuals.

Because of the variability in progression of neurological deficits caused by MS, and its ability to impair more than one area of the CNS, it is difficult to identify a predominant or typical type of neurogenic bladder (de Seze et al., 2007; Tubaro et al., 2012). Instead, individualized assessment is required based on LUTS or signs of urological dysfunction present at the time of assessment. Most individuals with MS report urinary incontinence as the most bothersome urinary symptom, though others present because of recurring UTI or weak urinary stream with elevated residual volumes. Evaluation and selection of a bladder management program is based on a careful examination of lower urinary tract function, including routine measurement of residual urine volume and possibly urodynamic testing.

Management Options

Similar to the patient with an SCI, spontaneous voiding is maintained whenever feasible. Many persons with MS will present with LUTS consistent with neurogenic detrusor overactivity (urgency, daytime voiding frequency, nocturia greater than three episodes per night with or without urge incontinence). These LUTS may be managed using behavioral interventions for detrusor overactivity as described earlier, often combined with pharmacologic therapy. This approach also may be employed for persons with neurogenic detrusor overactivity and detrusor-striated sphincter dyssynergia provided their residual volumes are comparatively low (usually ≤200 mL) and they are not experiencing upper urinary tract distress. Alpha-1 adrenergic blocking agents may be considered in selected patients to further reduce residual urine volumes.

Clean intermittent catheterization with pharmacologic therapy designed to prevent all detrusor contractions may be used for patients with MS and markedly reduced or absent sensations of bladder filling. This program is also preferred in patients with neurogenic detrusor overactivity, detrusor-striated sphincter dyssynergia, and higher residual volumes. Although CIC plus pharmacotherapy for neurogenic detrusor overactivity is attractive from a urological perspective, it should be prescribed only after careful evaluation of the patient, who may experience impaired dexterity and difficulty with CIC (Bolinger & Engberg, 2013). Nevertheless, a study of 9,702 persons with MS revealed that 81% reported use of CIC at some point during the course of their disease (Mahajan et al., 2013).

Persons with MS and underactive detrusor function are also managed with CIC whenever possible (de Seze et al., 2007). However, indwelling urinary catheterization is occasionally necessary. Persons with MS who are managed with an indwelling catheter tend to have had the disease for a longer period of time resulting in greater impairment of both dexterity and mobility. Males are also more likely to be managed with an indwelling catheter. Despite the limited situations in which indwelling catheter use is

recommended, 43% of a cohort of 9,702 persons with MS reported using an indwelling catheter at some point during the course of his or her disease (Mahajan et al., 2013).

> **CLINICAL PEARL**
>
> Studies indicate that 81% of individuals with MS use CIC at some point during their illness, and 43% report use of an indwelling catheter at some point.

Ongoing Monitoring

Because of the variable progression of neurologic impairment caused by MS, ongoing urologic monitoring and care is essential (de Seze et al., 2007). It is difficult to determine a routine time frame for follow-up assessments; timing should be based on the success of current bladder management strategies, changes in LUTS, occurrence of urologic complications such as UTI, or progression of MS resulting in a change in dexterity or mobility that affects the person's ability to continue a particular bladder management program.

Multiple sclerosis is associated with an increased likelihood of upper urinary tract distress, but the magnitude of this risk is less than that associated with SCI. In one study, upper urinary tract distress was identified in 12.4% of 89 subjects with MS followed over a period of approximately 12 months (Fletcher et al., 2013). Risk factors associated with upper urinary tract distress include age ≥50 years, low bladder wall compliance, and duration of disease (Fletcher et al., 2013; de Seze et al., 2007). Figure 7-3 and Case 2 describe a 34-year-old male with multiple sclerosis, urinary retention, and underactive detrusor function.

Parkinson's Disease

Parkinson's disease (PD) is a neurodegenerative disease characterized by a combination of motor deficits including

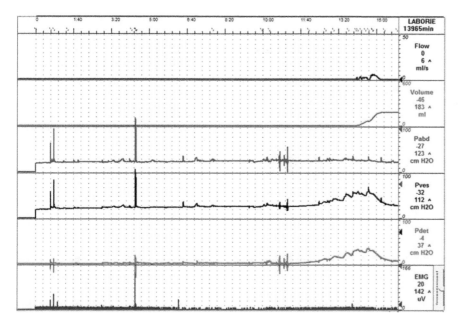

FIGURE 7-3. Neurogenic bladder in a 34-year-old male with multiple sclerosis, urinary retention, and underactive detrusor function. Refer to Case 2.

CASE STUDIES

CASE 2 NEUROGENIC BLADDER IN A 34-YEAR-OLD MALE WITH MULTIPLE SCLEROSIS, URINARY RETENTION, AND UNDERACTIVE DETRUSOR FUNCTION

Figure 7-3 illustrates the case of a 34-year-old male with multiple sclerosis, urinary retention, and underactive detrusor function. AD is a 34-year-old male who was diagnosed with relapsing–remitting multiple sclerosis 8 years prior to evaluation at our continence service. He presented to our service based on self-referral, complaining of weak urinary stream and increasing difficulty urinating. Questioning about lower urinary tract symptoms revealed daytime voiding frequency, urgency with occasional episodes of urge incontinence, two to three episodes of nocturia per night, weak urinary stream, and postvoid dribbling. He reported difficulty initiating urination at times and feelings of incomplete bladder emptying. He denied any prior UTI, dysuria, or hematuria. A review of systems identified increasing weakness of his lower extremities with preservation of upper extremity strength and dexterity. He also reported frequent constipation and erectile dysfunction. Medications included fingolimod 5 mg daily (to prevent exacerbations of MS), baclofen 20 mg twice daily, and vitamin D 5,000 IU daily. He also reported taking the alpha-1 adrenergic blocker tamsulosin 0.4 mg daily but reported it has not improved his urgency as anticipated. Urinalysis was negative; his serum creatinine was 0.9 mg/dL. A 3-day bladder diary revealed voiding every 2 to 3 hours, three episodes of nocturia nightly, and two episodes of urge incontinence.

Urodynamic testing was performed to further evaluate his neurogenic bladder dysfunction. Testing revealed a large cystometric capacity (800 mL), normal bladder wall compliance, and increased sensations of bladder filling. He experienced neurogenic detrusor overactivity with urgency and dribbling UI at 773 mL of filling. Voiding pressure flow study revealed underactive detrusor function (poor detrusor contraction strength); no detrusor sphincter dyssynergia was noted. His voided volume was 373 mL and his residual volume was 400 mL.

Initially, he was informed of the purpose of tamsulosin (reduction of urethral sphincter resistance in an attempt to improve bladder emptying with micturition) rather than suppression of urgency or urge incontinence episodes. Because of the magnitude of his residual volumes in combination with underactive detrusor function, AD was counseled about the need to add CIC to his bladder management strategy. Two options were discussed in detail, CIC with maintenance of spontaneous voiding or CIC with pharmacotherapy to ablate all detrusor contractions and prevent leakage between catheterizations. He reported reluctance to perform CIC or stop spontaneous voiding. He initially agreed to perform CIC once daily before sleep to reduce frequency of nocturia and improve sleep, and he was encourage to add a morning catheterization if he desired. On follow-up 4 weeks later, he reported adding a second catheterization in the morning and expressed an interest in adding a drug to prevent all leakage with catheterization every 4 to 6 hours. Fesoterodine 4 mg was added to his regimen, with dosage titrated to 8 mg after a 2-week trial. On 6-week follow-up appointment, he reported catheterizing four to five times daily with no incontinence episodes over the past month.

This case illustrates a technique for introducing CIC to patient who was initially reluctant to give up spontaneous voiding. In these cases, teaching the patient to catheterize once daily is recommended because it greatly reduces or (as in AD's case) ablates nocturia entirely. Given the success of that strategy, the patient added a second catheterization episode and he ultimately elected a regular CIC program.

bradykinesia and one or more of the following signs: tremor while at rest, rigidity, and/or postural instability (Bhidayasiri & Reichmann, 2013; Mahlknecht & Poewe, 2013). Various classification schemas have been proposed, but none has gained prominence and the diagnosis of Parkinsonism is based on physical assessment and clinical evaluation rather than findings from a definitive diagnostic marker. Approximately 630,000 Americans suffer from PD; its incidence is approximately 13.4 per 100,000 persons making it the second leading form of neurodegenerative disease behind Alzheimer's dementia (Kowal et al., 2013; van den Eeden et al., 2003). While dementia is not a characteristic feature of PD, slightly more than 10% also develop Lewy bodies (abnormal protein aggregates found in nerve cells) resulting in dementia, which further increases the likelihood of developing neurogenic bladder dysfunction (Ransmayr et al., 2008; Savica et al., 2013).

Neurogenic bladder in Parkinson's Disease

The mechanisms that produce neurogenic bladder dysfunction in PD are not entirely understood. Some researchers suggest that the dopaminergic degeneration characteristic of PD causes neurogenic bladder dysfunction, while others state bladder dysfunction is an incidental finding more related to aging or comorbid conditions (Winge & Fowler, 2006). Clinical experience suggests that PD does cause identifiable neurogenic bladder dysfunction that is far more prevalent than can be explained by age or comorbid conditions alone. The reported prevalence of LUTS in persons with PD varies significantly; in a meta-analysis of 28 studies, prevalence rates ranged from as low as 7.7% to as high as 97% (Ruffion et al., 2013).

In a study of 271 males with PD in which the prevalence of LUTS was determined based on a validated instrument, slightly more than 40% of respondents reported at least one bothersome LUTS. The most prevalent was urge incontinence, followed by nocturia and voiding frequency (Robinson et al., 2013). Another study of 74 female and male patients found that nocturia was most prevalent, followed by voiding frequency and incontinence (Campos-Sousa et al., 2003). Clinical experience indicates that a minority of patients with PD experience urinary retention, though the cause of the retention is not well understood. A study of 23 men with PD who underwent transurethral resection of the prostate for benign prostatic enlargement found that 36% had persistent urinary retention postoperatively, indicating that retention in these men was at least partially attributable to underactive detrusor function (failure to empty because of the bladder) (Roth et al., 2009). Another study of 41 women and men correlated urodynamic findings and outcomes of PET scanning. Findings in this study suggest that urinary retention in these individuals was due to detrusor underactivity rather than outlet obstruction (Terayama et al., 2012).

> **CLINICAL PEARL**
>
> While the pathology is not clear, LUTS are common among individuals with PD, ranging from 7.7% to 97%; the most common and problematic symptoms are urge incontinence, nocturia, and frequency. A minority of patients experience retention.

Management Options

Similar to care for patients with other neurological diseases, bladder management is based on the specific lower urinary tract dysfunctions, the physical and cognitive deficits produced by PD, resources in the home, and the patient and family's preferences. Most patients with PD have detrusor overactivity resulting in urge incontinence, frequent urination, and nocturia, as noted above. Because these patients have intact sensations and they do not experience striated sphincter dyssynergia, they are able to void spontaneously. Behavioral interventions comprise first-line interventions, including fluid and dietary counseling along with scheduled toileting. These interventions are usually combined with pharmacotherapy for detrusor overactivity, as described earlier.

Particular attention should be paid to the symptoms of nocturia and nighttime urgency. Persons with PD have been shown to have a higher incidence of falls and hip fractures than age-matched controls, and nocturia and nighttime urgency have been shown to act as independent risk factors for these events (Asplund 2006; Brown et al., 2000; Temml et al., 2009). In the case of patients with PD, nocturia is primarily attributable to two factors: nighttime urine production and detrusor overactivity. Options for managing nocturia include fluid restriction for 2 hours prior to sleep and elevation of the lower extremities prior to sleep for persons with dependent edema. Patients taking a diuretic may be advised to move the dose from morning to late afternoon or evening to reduce urine production at night.

> **CLINICAL PEARL**
>
> Falls and hip fractures are more common among individuals with PD than age-matched controls, and nocturia and nighttime urgency are major risk factors for these events.

Patients with urinary retention and PD are managed with CIC whenever feasible or indwelling catheterization when CIC is not possible. Indwelling catheterization is more often necessary when retention occurs in a patient whose PD is associated with significant deficits in dexterity and mobility or complicated by Lewy bodies and dementia. Men with PD and evidence of prostatic enlargement and obstruction may be managed pharmacologically or with transurethral or minimally invasive prostatectomy procedures to alleviate obstruction. However, they should be counseled first about possible adverse outcomes of these procedures, including persistent urinary retention or urge incontinence due to detrusor overactivity (Roth et al., 2009).

Comorbid Conditions

Because persons with PD tend to be older when the disease is first diagnosed, they are also more likely to have comorbid conditions impacting lower urinary tract function. For example, a study of 271 male patients found that major depression, constipation, and dementia were present in more than half of men with PD and LUTS (Robinson et al., 2013). BPH, a known cause of LUTS, is also prevalent in older men. The impact of these comorbid conditions has not been extensively studied, but the likelihood that these conditions will influence lower urinary tract function is significant and should be accounted for when managing these challenging patients. Figure 7-4 and Case 3 describe a 78-year-old male with PD and neurogenic bladder dysfunction complicated by benign prostatic enlargement.

Stroke

The term *stroke* (sometimes referred to as cerebrovascular accident or brain attack) is defined as an acute, focal injury of the central nervous system owing to a vascular cause such as cerebral infarction, intracerebral hemorrhage, or subarachnoid hemorrhage (Sacco et al., 2013). Strokes associated with cerebral infarction may be classified as ischemic or hemorrhagic. Approximately 6.8 million Americans have experienced a stroke in their lifetime, accounting for nearly 3% of the population (Ma et al., 2014). The physical consequences of a stroke vary

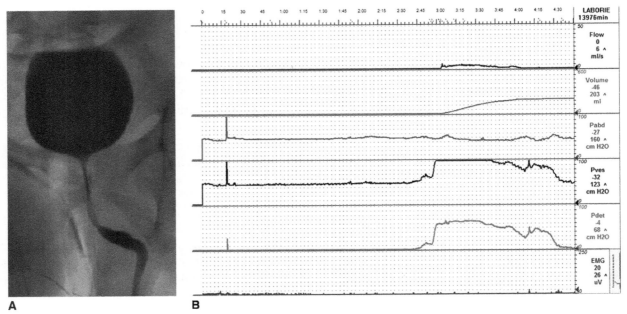

FIGURE 7-4. An elderly man with neurogenic bladder dysfunction complicated by benign prostatic enlargement. Refer to Case 3.

CASE STUDIES

CASE 3 NEUROGENIC BLADDER IN A 78-YEAR-OLD MALE WITH BENIGN PROSTATIC ENLARGEMENT

Figure 7-4 illustrates the case of PA, a 78-year-old male diagnosed with PD 2 years prior to evaluation for neurogenic bladder dysfunction. He is accompanied by his wife, who suffered a stroke approximately 1 year ago. He is able to walk for short distances with the aid of a walker; he requires a wheelchair for longer distances. His speech appears somewhat slowed, but he is alert and able to answer questions without assistance. Lower urinary tract symptoms include nocturia up to six episodes per night, daytime voiding frequency, urgency, and urge incontinence episodes. PA stated that he found paradoxical urgency to urinate, but difficulty initiating micturition when reaching the toilet, to be the most bothersome of all his lower urinary tract symptoms. He also described using an absorptive brief to manage urinary incontinence whenever traveling away from home. Approximately 2 years prior to being diagnosed with PD, PA was evaluated for LUTS associated with benign prostatic enlargement. Notes from that examination revealed nocturia three episodes per night, weak urinary stream, and urgency but no urinary incontinence. Several postvoid residual volumes were measured, which varied from 60 to 90 mL. A minimally invasive prostatectomy was advised but PA declined surgery. He was advised about watchful waiting versus pharmacotherapy for LUTS but elected to pursue no further

therapy at the time. Current medications include amantadine 100 mg twice daily, carbidopa–levodopa 25 to 100 mg three times daily, olmesartan–amlodipine 5/20, and furosemide 40 mg daily. Urinalysis was normal; his serum creatinine was 1.3 mg/dL.

Videourodynamic testing revealed small cystometric capacity (275 mL) with neurogenic detrusor overactivity resulting in urgency and involuntary urination. No detrusor sphincter dyssynergia was noted, but voiding urethrography revealed narrowing and elongation of his proximal (prostatic) urethra; the voiding pressure flow study indicated moderately severe bladder outlet obstruction; his residual volume was 70 mL.

PA was counseled that his bladder dysfunction was attributable to his prostatic enlargement and his PD. He was counseled about fluid and dietary interventions for management of neurogenic detrusor overactivity. He was started on tamsulosin 0.4 mg daily and finasteride 5 mg daily for treatment of his prostatic enlargement. He was also counseled about management of his nocturia. He was provided a urinal to avoid the need to move from bed to his regular toilet, and he was advised about restriction of fluids within two hours of bedtime. He was also advised to move his furosemide dosage from breakfast to dinner in order to reduce nighttime urine production. Follow-up appointment 4 weeks later revealed that his nocturia had declined from six episodes per night to three. He reported that he was able to urinate with less hesitancy, but he also noted that he now had less warning before the onset of urge incontinence. Bladder ultrasound revealed a postvoid residual volume of 90 mL. In order to better manage his neurogenic detrusor overactivity, he began taking darifenacin 7.5 mg daily. After 4 weeks, PA reported that his nocturia had been reduced to two episodes per night, and he was experiencing less than one urge incontinent episode per day. Bladder ultrasound revealed a postvoid residual volume of 75 mL.

This case illustrates the multiple factors that may contribute to LUTS in an older man with neurogenic bladder associated with PD. Initial treatment focused on addressing benign prostatic enlargement. Despite moderately severe bladder outlet obstruction, pharmacotherapy was favored over transurethral resection of the prostate because of concerns that surgery might worsen his underlying neurogenic detrusor overactivity

and urge incontinence if urethral resistance were markedly reduced using a surgical approach. Rather, a pharmacological approach was adopted using one drug (finasteride) that acted to reduce prostate size and a second drug (tamsulosin) that acted to reduce smooth muscle tone within the urethra (Table 7-2).

Nocturia was addressed by altering the patient's environment (providing a urinal) and by reducing nighttime urine production. Two strategies were used to reduce nighttime urine production, restriction of fluids two hours prior to sleep and moving administration of his diuretic medication from the morning to dinner time. A final mediation, darifenacin, was added to reduce the LUTS urgency and urge incontinence. While this addition did not completely eradicate his urge incontinence episodes, it reduced these symptoms to an acceptable level without elevating his postvoid residual volumes.

significantly, but they tend to be more severe among older persons. Approximately 26% of older individuals who suffered a stroke remain dependent for one or more activities of daily living 6 months after the event, and 30% remain unable to walk without assistance. A systematic review and meta-analysis of 61 studies involving stroke patients reported that 64.7% of persons experiencing a stroke also experience neurogenic bladder dysfunction (Ruffion et al., 2013).

Stroke and Urologic Symptoms

Stroke produces a more homogenous group of LUTS than SCI or MS. A neurologic lesion that affects the brain alone tends to produce neurogenic detrusor overactivity with intact sensory function; thus, urgency, frequency, nocturia, and urge incontinence are the most commonly reported LUTS (McKenzie & Badlani, 2012). Several urodynamic studies have found evidence of underactive detrusor function in 33% to 40% of patients following cerebrovascular accident, but the magnitude of detrusor underactivity and its clinical relevance have not yet been established. While MS and PD are characterized by progression of neurologic deficits over time, functional impairments associated with a stroke may improve following the original insult (Hayward et al., 2014). For example, a longitudinal study of 340 patients with LUTS and a stroke found that 35% of the patients who reported new onset of urge urinary incontinence immediately following a stroke experienced resolution of urinary leakage at 12 months (Williams et al., 2012). Risk factors for persistent incontinence in this group included urinary leakage prior to the stroke and female gender.

CLINICAL PEARL

64.7% of individuals who sustain a stroke experience neurogenic bladder dysfunction (overactive bladder), but 35% of these individuals experience spontaneous resolution within 12 months.

Management Options

Similar to the prior specific examples of neurogenic bladder dysfunction, assessment and care of the patient who has experienced a stroke must take into consideration the physical and cognitive disabilities created by the stroke, characteristics of the associated bladder dysfunction, resources in the home, and patient and family preference. Because most patients have intact sensation and do not experience striated sphincter dyssynergia, the vast majority are able to manage their bladder with spontaneous voiding.

Behavioral interventions, including fluid and dietary advice and scheduled toileting, are usual first-line interventions. Ultimately, many individuals will also require pharmacologic management for neurogenic detrusor overactivity. The efficacy of pharmacotherapy is enhanced when combined with behavioral interventions. In addition, because many persons with a stroke recover physical function over time, it is reasonable to consider pharmacotherapy over a 6- to 12-month period, followed by a drug holiday, and to discontinue drug therapy whenever possible. Because of the risk of detrusor underactivity, patients managed pharmacologically should be counseled about the risk of urinary retention and should be monitored with postvoid residual urine measurements as indicated.

The prevalence of stroke is highest among older adults, and management of the male patient should incorporate consideration of the potential for BPH and its impact on neurogenic dysfunction (McKenzie & Badlani, 2012). Because of the risk of obstruction and urinary retention associated with BPH, older men with bladder dysfunction following a stroke should undergo postvoid residual measurement as part of a continence evaluation, and many will benefit from multichannel urodynamic testing.

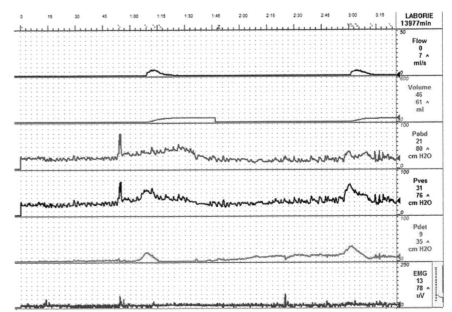

FIGURE 7-5. A 75-year-old female with neurogenic bladder and new onset urge urinary incontinence following a stroke affecting the middle cerebral artery. Refer to Case 4.

Neurogenic bladder dysfunction in patients with stroke is not associated with low bladder compliance or outlet obstruction caused by detrusor-striated sphincter dyssynergia; thus, the risk of hostile bladder dysfunction and upper urinary tract distress is low (McKenzie & Badlani, 2012). Patients who experience febrile UTI, vesicoureteral reflux, or deterioration of renal function should undergo evaluation for other potential causes of upper urinary tract distress. Figure 7-5 and Case 4 describe a 75-year-old female with neurogenic bladder and new onset urge urinary incontinence following a stroke affecting the middle cerebral artery.

CASE STUDIES

CASE 4 NEUROGENIC BLADDER IN A 75-YEAR-OLD FEMALE FOLLOWING A STROKE

Figure 7-5 illustrates the case of MK, a 75-year-old female who experienced an ischemic stroke involving the middle cerebral artery 16 weeks prior to evaluation. Prior to her stroke, she reported mild stress urinary incontinence that did not require regular use of pads. Upon presentation to our clinic, she reported voiding frequency of every hour and frequent incontinence episodes with complete loss of the ability to postpone urination. She tearfully reported the need for absorptive briefs at all times to prevent urinary leakage. She also reported four to five episodes of nocturia per night that usually resulted in incontinence before she was able to reach the toilet. Physical assessment revealed mild left hemiparesis; her speech was clear and she was alert and oriented throughout her evaluation. She was able to ambulate without assistance although she reported her gait as somewhat slowed. Current medications included lisinopril 5 mg daily and clopidogrel 75 mg daily. Urinalysis was normal and her serum creatinine was 0.9 mg/dL.

Urodynamic testing revealed small cystometric capacity (60 to 90 mL) with neurogenic detrusor overactivity and urge incontinence. Voiding pressure flow study demonstrated good detrusor contraction strength and no detrusor-striated sphincter dyssynergia. Residual volumes were 0 mL on sequential examinations.

Because of the severity of her voiding frequency and incontinence episodes, she was initially provided education about behavioral management of neurogenic detrusor overactivity (including dietary and fluid advice along with urge suppression techniques) and begun on a medication to alleviate her neurogenic detrusor overactivity (trospium extended release 60 mg daily). She was also advised that LUTS improve in some patients just as their physical function can improve over time. On follow-up, 3 weeks later, she reported significant improvement in her voiding frequency to every 1.5 hours and reduction of her nocturia to two episodes per night. Bladder ultrasound revealed a residual urine volume of 20 mL. Alternative medications were discussed, but she elected to continue with her current bladder management strategy. Telephone follow-up at 3 months revealed further reductions in daytime frequency to every 2 hours or more and reduction of nocturia to two episodes per night. During a scheduled follow-up visit at 6 months, the possibility of a medication holiday was discussed (stopping her daily antimuscarinic drug). MK expressed some anxiety but agreed to stop her medication. Telephone follow-up revealed that she remained off her medication and had not experienced the return of frequent urination and incontinence she had feared.

This case illustrates management of a sudden onset of urge incontinence caused by neurogenic detrusor overactivity following a stroke. It also emphasizes the importance of considering the natural history of the underlying neurological disorder when managing neurogenic bladder dysfunction. In this case, research has shown that many patients will experience a sudden onset of urge incontinence that may subside over the first 12 months following a stroke as the brain recovers and adapts. By providing a drug holiday, MK was able to determine that she was able to retain continence without ongoing drug therapy.

Conclusions

Neurogenic bladder dysfunction is associated with a variety of underlying disorders resulting in a wide variety of negative consequences to lower urinary tract function. Assessment and treatment of the neurogenic bladder relies on evaluation of bladder dysfunction, combined with knowledge of the patient's physical and cognitive status, social situation, and knowledge of the natural history of the underlying neurological disorder.

REFERENCES

Abrams, P., Cardozo, L., Fall, M., et al. (2002). The standardization of nomenclature for lower urinary tract function. *Neurourology and Urodynamics, 21,* 167–178.

Ahluwalia, R. S., Johal, N., Kouriefs, C., et al. (2006). The surgical risk of suprapubic catheter insertion and long-term sequelae. *Annals of the Royal College of Surgeons England, 88,* 201–203.

Ahmed, H. U., Sherfill, I. S., Arya, M., et al. (2006). Management of detrusor-external sphincter dyssynergia. *Nature Clinical Practice Urology, 3*(7), 368–380.

Al-Ali, M., & Haddad, L. (1996). A 10 year review of the endoscopic treatment of 125 spinal cord injured patients with vesical outlet obstruction: Does bladder neck dyssynergia exist? *Paraplegia, 34,* 34–8.

Amend, B., Hennenlotter, J., Schafer, T., et al. (2008). Effective treatment of neurogenic detrusor dysfunction by combined high dose antimuscarinics without increased side effects. *European Urology, 53*(5), 1021–1028.

Andersson, K. E. (2011). Muscarinic acetylcholine receptors in the urinary tract. *Handbook of Experimental Pharmacology, 202,* 319–344.

Anson, C., & Gray, M. (1993). Secondary complications after spinal cord injury. *Urologic Nursing, 13*(4), 107–112.

Asplund, R. (2006). Hip fractures, nocturia and nocturnal polyuria in the elderly. *Archives of Gerontology & Geriatrics, 43*(3), 319–326.

Atala, A. (2014). Regenerative bladder augmentation using autologous tissue—when will we get there? *Journal of Urology, 191,* 1204–1205.

Atala, A., Bauer, S. B., Soker, S., et al. (2006). Tissue-engineered autologous bladders for patients needing cystoplasty. *Lancet, 367,* 1241–1246.

Awad, S. A., Bryniak, S. R., Downie, J. W., et al. (1977). Urethral pressure profile during the spinal shock stage in man: A preliminary report. *Journal of Urology, 117*(1), 91–93.

Bacsu, C., Chan, L., & Tse, V. (2012). Diagnosing detrusor sphincter dyssynergia in the neurological patient. *BJU International, 109*(Suppl 3), 31–34.

Barrett, D. M. (1981). The effect of bethanechol chloride on voiding in female patients with excessive residual urine: A randomized double-blind study. *Journal of Urology, 126,* 640.

Beirs, S. M., Venn, S. N., & Greenwell, T. J. (2011). The past, present and future of augmentation cystoplasty. *BJU International, 109,* 1280–1293.

Bennett, J. K., Green, B. G., Foote, J. E., et al. (1995). Collagen injections for intrinsic sphincter deficiency in the neuropathic urethra. *Paraplegia, 33*(12), 697–700.

Bhidayasiri, R., & Reichmann, H. (2013). Different diagnostic criteria for Parkinson disease: What are the pitfalls? *Journal of Neural Transmission, 120,* 619–625.

Bodner, D. R. (2009). Comarr memorial reward for distinguished clinical service: The legacy of A. Estin Comarr, MD. *Journal of Spinal Cord Medicine, 32*(3), 213–214.

Bolinger, R., & Engberg, S. (2013). Barriers, complications, adherence and self-reported quality of life for people using clean intermittent catheterization. *Journal of Wound, Ostomy and Continence Nursing, 40*(1), 83–89.

Boone, T. B. (2009). External urethral sphincter stent for dyssynergia. *Journal of Urology, 181,* 1538–1539.

Bors, E., & Comarr, A. E. (1971). *Neurological urology.* Baltimore, MD: University Park Press.

Brown, J. S., Vitinghoff, E., Wyman, J. F., et al. (2000). Urinary incontinence: Does it increase risk for falls and fractures? *Journal of the American Geriatrics Society, 48*(7), 721–725.

Budge, J. (1864). Uber den Einfluss des Nervebsystems auf die Bewegung der Blasé. *Zietschr. F. rationelle Medizin, 21,* 1.

Cameron, A. (2010). Pharmacologic therapy for the neurogenic bladder. *Urologic Clinics of North America, 37,* 495–506.

Campos-Sousa, R. N., Quagliato, E., de Silva, B. B., et al. (2003). Urinary symptoms in Parkinson's disease: Prevalence and associated factors. *Arquivos de Neuro-Psiquiatria, 61*(2B), 359–363.

Castel-Lacanal, E., Game, X., De Boissezon, X., et al. (2013). Impact of intermittent catheterization on the quality of life in patients with multiple sclerosis. *World Journal of Urology, 31*(6), 1445–1450.

Chai, T. C., Gray, M. L., & Steers, W. D. (1998). The incidence of a positive ice water test on bladder outlet obstructed patients: Evidence for altered innervation. *Journal of Urology, 160,* 34–38.

Chapple, C. R., MacDiarmid, S. A., & Patel, A. (2009). *Urodynamics made easy* (3rd ed., pp. 117). Oxford, UK: Elsevier.

Chartier Kastler, E., & Denys, P. (2011). Intermittent catheterization with hydrophilic catheters as a treatment of chronic neurogenic urinary retention. *Neurourology and Urodynamics, 30,* 21–31.

Chartier Kastler, E., Genevois, S., Game, X., et al. (2011). Treatment of neurogenic male urinary incontinence related to intrinsic sphincter insufficiency with an artificial urinary sphincter: A French retrospective multicentre study. *BJU International, 107*(3), 426–432.

Coblentz, T., & Gray, M. (2001). Bladder neck obstruction in the female: A case study. *Urologic Nursing, 21,* 265–272.

Cruz, F. (2014). Targets for botulinum toxin the lower urinary tract. *Neurourology and Urodynamics, 33*, 31–38.

Curtis, J., & Klykken, P. (2008). A comparative assessment of three common catheter materials. Retrieved from http://www.dowcorning.com/content/publishedlit/52-1116.pdf

Danforth, T. L., & Ginsberg, D. A. (2014). Neurogenic lower urinary tract dysfunction: How when and with which patients do we use urodynamics. *Urologic Clinics of North America, 41*, 445–452.

Davis, N. F., Kheradmand, F., & Creagh, T. (2013). Injectable biomaterials for the treatment of stress urinary incontinence: Their potential and pitfalls as urethral bulking agents. *International Urogynecology Journal, 24*(6), 913–919.

Day, R. A., Moore, K. N., & Albers, M. K. (2002). A study comparing 2 methods of intermittent catheterization: Limitations and challenges. *Urologic Nursing, 23*(2), 143–147.

de Groat, W. C., & Wickens, C. (2013). Organization of the neural switching circuitry underlying reflex micturition. *Acta Physiologica (Oxford), 207*, 66–84.

De Seze, M., Ruffion, A., Denys, P., et al. (2007). GENULF study group. The neurogenic bladder in multiple sclerosis: Review of the literature and proposal of management guidelines. *Multiple Sclerosis, 13*, 915–928.

Ditunno, J. F., Little, J. W., Tessler, A., et al. (2004). Spinal shock revisited: A four-phase model. *Spinal Cord, 42*, 383–395.

Donovan, W. H. (2007). Donald munro lecture: Spinal Cord Injury—past, present and future. *Journal of Spinal Cord Medicine, 30*, 85–100.

Drake, M. J., Williams, J., & Bijos, D. A. (2014). Voiding dysfunction due to detrusor underactivity: An overview. *Nature Reviews in Urology, 11*, 454–464.

Engkasan, J. P., Ng, C. J., & Low, W. Y. (2014). Factors influencing bladder management in male patients with spinal cord injury: A qualitative study. *Spinal Cord, 52*(2), 157–162.

Finkbeiner, A. E. (1985). Is bethanechol chloride clinically effective in promoting bladder emptying? A literature review. *Journal of Urology, 134*, 443–449.

Fletcher, S. G., Dillon, B. E., Gilchrist, A. S., et al. (2013). Renal deterioration in multiple sclerosis patients with neurovesical dysfunction. *Multiple Sclerosis, 19*, 1169–1174.

Fowler, S., Godfrey, H., Fader, M., et al. (2014). Living with a long-term indwelling urinary catheter: Catheter user's experiences. *Journal of Wound, Ostomy and Continence Nursing PAP.* Retrieved from http://journals.lww.com/jwocnonline/toc/publishahead

Frazier, E. P., Peters, S. L., Braverman, A. S., et al. (2008). Signal conduction underlying the control of urinary bladder smooth muscle tone by muscarinic receptors and beta-adrenoreceptors. *Naunyn-Schmiedebergs Archives of Pharmacology, 377*(4–6), 449–462.

Ghoniem, G. M., Bloom, D. A., McGuire, E. J., et al. (1989). Bladder compliance in myelomeningocele children. *The Journal of Urology, 141*(6), 1404–1406.

Gormley, E. A. (2010). Urologic complications of the neurogenic bladder. *Urologic Clinics of North America, 37*(4), 601–607.

Gormley, E. A., Lightner, D. J., Burgio, K. L., et al. (2014). Diagnosis and treatment of overactive bladder (non-neurogenic) in adults: AUA/SUFU Guideline. Retrieved from http://www.auanet.org/common/pdf/education/clinical-guidance/Overactive-Bladder.pdf

Graham, S. D., Keane, T. E., & Glenn, J. F. (Eds.), (2007). *Glenn's urologic surgery* (7th ed). Philadelphia, PA: Wolters Kluwer Health.

Gray, M. (2007). An update on the physiology of urinary continence. *Continence UK, 1*(2), 28–36.

Gray, M. (2008). Reflex urinary incontinence. In B. K. Ackely & G. B. Ladwig (Eds.), *Nursing diagnosis handbook* (8th ed., pp. 458–461). Philadelphia, PA: Elsevier.

Gray, M. (2010). Traces: Making sense of urodynamics testing—Part 2: Uroflowmetry. *Urologic Nursing, 30*(6), 321–326.

Gray, M. (2011a). Traces: Making sense of urodynamic testing—Part 6: Evaluation of bladder filling/storage: Bladder wall compliance and the detrusor leak point pressure. *Urologic Nursing, 31*(4), 215–221.

Gray, M. (2011b). Traces: Making sense of urodynamics testing-Part 7: Evaluation of bladder filling/storage: Evaluation of urethral sphincter incompetence and stress urinary incontinence. *Urologic Nursing, 31*(5), 267–277, 289.

Gray, M. (2012a). Traces: Making sense of urodynamics testing—Part 10: Evaluation of micturition via the voiding pressure-flow study. *Urologic Nursing, 32*(2), 71–78.

Gray, M. (2012b). Traces: Making sense of urodynamics testing—Part 11: Quantitative analysis of micturition via the voiding pressure-flow study. *Urologic Nursing, 32*(3), 159–165.

Gray, M., Joseph, A. C., Mercer, D. M., et al. (2008). Consensus and controversies in urinary drainage systems: Indications for improving patient's safety. *Safe Practice in Patient Care, 4*(1), 1–7.

Gray, M., Rayome, R., & Moore, K. N. (1995a). The urethral sphincter: An update. *Urologic Nursing, 15*(2), 40–55.

Gray, M., Rayome, R., & Anson, C. (1995b). Incontinence and clean intermittent catheterization following spinal cord injury. *Clinical Nursing Research, 4*(1), 6–21.

Griffiths, D. J., & Fowler, C. J. (2013). The micturition reflex and its forebrain influences. *Acta Physiologica (Oxford), 207*, 93–109.

Griffiths, D. H., Harrison, G., Moore, K., et al. (1996). Variability of post-void residual urine volume in the elderly. *Urological Research, 24*(1), 23–26.

Groen, L. A., Spinoit, A. F., Hoebeke, P., et al. (2012). The advance male sling as a minimally invasive treatment for intrinsic sphincter deficiency in men with neurogenic bladder sphincter dysfunction: A pilot study. *Neurourology and Urodynamics, 31*(8), 1284–1287.

Guttman, L., & Frankel, H. (1966). The value of intermittent catheterization in the management of traumatic paraplegia and tetraplegia. *Paraplegia, 4*, 63–84.

Hald, T., & Bradley, W. E. (1982) *The urinary bladder: Neurology and dynamics* (pp. 1–4). Baltimore, MD: Williams & Wilkins.

Hayward, K. S., Barker, R. N., Carson, R. G., et al. (2014). The effect of altering a single component of a rehabilitation programme on the functional recovery of stroke patients: A systematic review and meta-analysis. *Clinical Rehabilitation, 28*(2), 107–117.

Hosker, G., Rosier, P., Gajewski, J., et al. (2009). Dynamic testing. In P. Abrams, L. Cardozo, S. Khoury, et al. (Eds.), *Incontinence* (4th ed., pp. 413–522). London, UK: Health Publication Ltd.

Institute of Medicine, Food and Science Board. (2004). Retrieved from http://www.iom.edu/Global/News%20Announcements/~/media/442A08B899F44DF9AAD083D86164C75B.ashx

Joseph, D. B., Borer, J. G., DeFillipo, R. E., et al. (2014). Autologous seeded biodegradable scaffold for augmentation cystoplasty: Phase II study in children and adolescents with spina bifida. *Journal of Urology, 191*, 1389–1395.

Kari, J., Al-Deek, B., Elkhatib, L., et al. (2013). Is Mitrofanoff a more socially acceptable CIC route for children and their families? *European Journal of Surgery, 23*, 405–410.

Katsumi, H. K., Kalisvaart, J. F., Ronningen, L. D., et al. (2010). Urethral versus suprapubic catheter: Choosing the best bladder management for male spinal cord injury patients with indwelling catheters. *Spinal Cord, 48*, 325–329.

Kenelly, M. J., Lemack, G. E., Foote, J. E., et al. (2009). Efficacy and safety of transdermal oxybutynin system in spinal cord injury patients with neurogenic detrusor overactivity and incontinence: An open label, dose titration study. *Urology, 74*(4), 741–745.

Kilinc, S., Akman, M. N., Levendoglu, F., et al. (1999). Diurnal variation of antidiuretic hormone and urinary output in spinal cord injury. *Spinal Cord, 37*(5), 332–335.

Killorin, W., Gray, M., Bennett, J. K., et al. (1992). The value of urodynamics and bladder management in predicting upper urinary tract distress in male spinal cord injury patients. *Paraplegia, 30*, 437–441.

Kirshblum, S. C., Biering-Sorenson, F., Betz, R., et al. (2014). International standards for neurological classification of spinal cord injury: Cases with classification challenges. *Journal of Spinal Cord Medicine, 37*(2), 120–128.

Kojima, Y., Kubota, Y., Sasaki, S., et al. (2009). Translational pharmacology in aging men with benign prostatic hyperplasia: Molecular and clinical approaches to alpha-1 adrenoreceptors. *Current Aging Science, 2*(3), 223–229.

Kowal, S. L., Dall, T. M., Chakrabarti, R., et al. (2013). Current and projected economic burden of Parkinson's disease in the United States. *Movement Disorders, 28*(3), 311–318.

Kulwin, C. G., Patel, N. B., Ackerman, L. L., et al. (2013). Radiographic and clinical outcome of syringomyelia in patients treated for tethered spinal cord without other significant imaging abnormalities. *Journal of Neurosurgery Pediatrics, 11*(3), 307–312.

Lapeyre, E., Kuks, J. B., & Meijler, W. J. (2010). Revisiting the role and the individual value of several pharmacological treatments. *Neurorehabilitation, 27*(2), 193–200.

Lapides, J. (1970). Neuromuscular, vesicle and ureteral dysfunction. In M. F. Campbell & J. H. Harrison (Eds.), *Campbell's urology* (3rd ed., pp. 1343–1379). Philadelphia, PA: Saunders.

Lapides, J., Diokno, A. C., & Silber, S. J. (1972). Clean intermittent catheterization in the treatment of urinary tract disease. *Journal of Urology, 107*(3), 458–461.

Liard, A., Seguier-Lipszyc, E., Mathiot, A., et al. (2001). The Mitrofanoff procedure: 20 years later. *Journal of Urology, 165*(6 Pt 2), 2394–2398.

Linsenmeyer, T. A., & Linsenmeyer, M. A. (2013). Impact of annual urodynamic evaluations on guiding bladder management in individuals with spinal cord injuries. *Journal of Spinal Cord Medicine, 36*(5), 420–426.

Lopez, P. P., Somoza, A. I., Martinez, U. M., et al. (2006). Artificial urinary sphincter: 11 year follow-up in adolescents with congenital neuropathic bladder. *European Urology, 50*(5), 1096–1101.

Lucas, M. G., Bedretdinova, D., Bosch, J. L., et al. (2013). Guidelines on urinary incontinence. European Association of Urology. Retrieved from http://www.uroweb.org/gls/pdf/19_Urinary_Incontinence_LR.pdf

Lukacz, E. S., Sampselle, C., Gray, M., et al. (2011). A healthy bladder: A consensus statement. *International Journal of Clinical Practice, 65*(10), 1026–1036.

Ma, V. Y., Chan, L., & Carruthers, K. J. (2014). Incidence, prevalence, costs, and impact on disability of common conditions requiring rehabilitation in the United States: Stroke, spinal cord injury, traumatic brain injury, multiple sclerosis, osteoarthritis, rheumatoid arthritis, limb loss, and back pain. *Archives of Physical Medicine and Rehabilitation, 95*, 986–995.

Mahajan, S. T., Frasure, H. E., & Marrie, R. A. (2013). The prevalence of urinary catheterization in women and men with multiple sclerosis. *Journal of Spinal Cord Medicine, 36*(6), 632–637.

Mahfouz, W., & Corcos, J. (2011). Management of detrusor external sphincter dyssynergia in neurogenic bladder. *European Journal of Physical & Rehabilitation Medicine, 47*(4), 639–650.

Mahlknecht, P., & Poewe, W. (2013). Is there a need to redefine Parkinson's disease? *Journal of Neural Transmission, 120*(Suppl 1), S9–S17.

Marberger, M. (2013). Medical management of lower urinary tract symptoms in men with benign prostatic enlargement. *Advances in Therapy, 30*(4), 309–319.

Martens, F. M., van Kuppevelt, H. J., Beekman, J. A., et al. (2010). Limited value of bladder sensation as a trigger for conditional neurostimulation in spinal cord injury patients. *Neurourology and Urodynamics, 29*(3), 395–400.

McGuire, E. J., Woodside, J. R., Borden, T. A., et al. (1981). Prognostic value of urodynamic testing in myelodysplastic children. *Journal of Urology, 126*(2), 205–209.

McIntyre, A., Mary, R., Mehta, S., et al. (2014). Examining the effectiveness of intrathecal baclofen on spasticity in individuals with chronic spinal cord injury: A systematic review. *Journal of Spinal Cord Medicine, 37*(1), 11–18.

McKenzie, P., & Badlani, G. H. (2012). The incidence and etiology of overactive bladder in patients after cerebrovascular accident. *Current Urological Reports, 13*, 402–406.

Mehta, A., Hill, D., Foley, N., et al. (2012). A meta-analysis of botulinum toxin sphincteric injections in the treatment of incomplete voiding after spinal cord injury. *Archives in Physical Medicine & Rehabilitation, 93*, 597–603.

Mertens, P., Parise, M., Garcia-Larrea, L., et al. (1995). Long-term clinical electrophysiological and urodynamic effects of chronic intrathecal baclofen infusion for treatment of spinal spasticity. *Acat Neurochiurgica, 64*(Suppl), 17–25.

Milo, R., & Miller, A. (2014). Revised diagnostic criteria of multiple sclerosis. *Autoimmunity Reviews, 13*, 518–524.

Mirone, V., Imbimbo, C., Longo, N., et al. (2007). The detrusor muscle: An innocent victim of bladder outlet obstruction. *European Urology, 51*(1), 57–66.

Moon, H. J., Chun, M. H., Lee, S. J., et al. (2012). The usefulness of bladder reconditioning before indwelling urethral catheter removal from stroke patients. *American Journal of Physical Medicine & Rehabilitation, 91*, 681–688.

Moore, K. N., & Rayome, R. G. (1995). Problem solving and troubleshooting: The indwelling urinary catheter. *Journal of Wound, Ostomy and Continence Nursing, 22*(5), 242–247.

Morrisroe, S. N., O'Connor, R. C., Nanigian, D. K., et al. (2005). Vesicostomy revisited: The best treatment for the hostile bladder is myelodysplastic child? *BJU International, 96*(3), 397–400.

Nadulli, R., Lasavio, E., Ranieri, M., et al. (2012). Combined antimuscarinics for treatment of neurogenic overactive bladder. *International Journal of Immunopathology & Pharmacology, 25*(1 Suppl), 35S–41S.

Nerli, R. B., Patil, S. M., Hiremath, M. B., et al. (2013). Yang-Monti's catheterizable stoma in children. *Nephrourology Monthly, 5*(3), 801–805.

Newman, D. K., & Willson, M. M. (2011). Review of intermittent catheterization and current best practices. *Urologic Nursing, 31*(1), 12–28.

Nitti, V. W., Chapple, C. R., Walters, C., et al. (2014). Safety and tolerability of the beta3- receptor agonist mirabegron for the treatment of overactive bladder: Results of a prospective analysis of three 12 week randomized Phase III trials and of a 1 year Phase III randomized trial. *International Journal of Clinical Practice, 68*(8), 972–985.

Ostaszkiewicz, J., & Paterson, J. (2012). Nurses advice concerning clean or sterile urinary drainage bags for persons with long-term indwelling catheters. *Journal of Wound, Ostomy and Continence Nursing, 39*(1), 77–83.

Oxford English Dictionary. 2014. Retrieved October 1, 2014, from http://www.oed.com/view/Entry/126392?redirectedFrom=neuro genic#eid. Accessed October 1, 2014.

Parker, D., Callan, L., Harwood, J., et al. (2009). Nursing interventions to reduce risk of catheter-associated urinary tract infection. Part 1: Catheter selection. *Journal of Wound, Ostomy and Continence Nursing, 36*(1), 23–34.

Perez, L. M., Barnes, N., MacDiramid, S. A., et al. (1993). Urological dysfunction in patients with diastematomyelia. *Journal of Urology, 149*(6), 1503–1505.

Perkash, I. (1996). Contact laser sphincterotomy: Further experience and longer follow-up. *Spinal Cord, 34*, 227–233.

Perkash, I. (2009). Transurethral sphincterotomy. *Journal of Urology, 181*, 1539–1540.

Peters, K. M., Kandagatla, P., Killinger, K. A., et al. (2013). Clinical outcomes of sacral neuromodulation in patients with neurologic conditions. *Urology, 81*, 738–744.

Peterson, A. C., Curtis, L. H., Shea, A. M., et al. (2012). Urinary diversions in patients with spinal cord injury in the United States. *Urology, 80*, 1247–1251.

Pinar, K., Moore, K. N., Smits, E., et al. (2009). Leg bag comparison. *Journal of Wound, Ostomy and Continence Nursing, 36*(3), 319–326.

Prieto, J. A., Murphy, C., Moore, K. N., et al. (2014). Intermittent catheterization for long-term bladder management (Cochrane Review). *The Cochrane Database of Systematic Reviews, 9*:CD006008. doi: 10.1002/14651858.CD006008.pub3.

Ransmayr, G. N., Hilliger, S., Scheletterer, K., et al. (2008). Lower urinary tract symptoms in Lewy bodies, Parkinson disease, and Alzheimer disease. *Neurology, 70*(4), 299–303.

Rapidi, C. A., Panourias, I. G., Petropoulou, K., et al. (2007). Management and rehabilitation of neuropathic bladder in patients with spinal cord lesions. *Acta Neurochirurgia Supplement, 97*(Pt 1), 307–314.

Revicky, V., & Tincello, D. G. (2014). New surgical approaches for urinary incontinence in women. *Maturitas, 77*(3), 238–242.

Robinson, J. P., Bradway, C. W., Bunting-Perry, L., et al. (2013). Lower urinary tract symptoms in men with Parkinson's disease. *Journal of Neuroscience Nursing, 45*(6), 381–392.

Rossier, A. B., & Ott, R. (1976). Bladder and urethral recordings in acute and chronic spinal cord injury patients. *Urologia Internationalis, 31*(1–2), 49–59.

Roth, B., Studer, U. E., Fowler, C. J., et al. (2009). Benign prostatic obstruction and Parkinson's disease—should transurethral resection be avoided? *Journal of Urology, 181*, 2209–2213.

Ruffion, A., Castro-Diaz, D., Patel, H., et al. (2013). Systematic review of urinary incontinence and detrusor overactivity among patients with neurogenic overactive bladder. *Neuroepidemiology, 41*, 146–155.

Saaby, M. L., & Lose, G. (2012). Repeatability of post void urinary residual >100 ml in urogynecology patients. *International Urogynecology Journal, 23*(2), 207–209.

Sacco, R., Kasner, S. E., Broderick, J. P., et al. (2013). An updated definition of stroke for the 21st century: A statement for healthcare professionals from the American Heart Association/American Stroke Association. *Stroke, 44*, 2064–2089.

Savica, R., Grossardt, B. R., Bower, J. H., et al. (2013). Incidence of dementia with Lewy bodies and Parkinson disease dementia. *JAMA Neurology, 70*(11), 1396–1402.

Schafer, W. (1995). Analysis of bladder outlet function with the linearized passive urethral resistance relation, linPURR, a disease specific approach for grading obstruction: From complex to simple. *World Journal of Urology, 13*(1), 47–58.

Schurch, B., Yasuda, K., & Rossier, A. B. (1994). Detrusor bladder neck dyssynergia revisited. *Journal of Urology, 152*(6, Pt 1), 2066–2070.

Silver, J. R. (2011). Management of the bladder in traumatic injuries of the spinal cord during the First World War and its implications for current practice of urology. *BJU International, 108*, 493–500.

Soljanik, I. (2013). Efficacy and safety of botulinum toxin A intradetrusor injections in adults with neurogenic detrusor overactivity/ neurogenic overactive bladder: A systematic review. *Drugs, 73*, 1055–1066.

Stohrer, M., Goepel, M., Kondo, A., et al. (1999). The standardization of terminology in neurogenic lower urinary tract dysfunction. *Neurourology and Urodynamics, 18*, 139–158.

Szollar, S., North, J., & Chung, J. (1995). Antidiuretic levels and polyuria in spinal cord injury. *Paraplegia, 33*(2), 94–97.

Temml, C., Ponholzer, A., Gutjahr, G., et al. (2009). Nocturia is an age-independent risk factor for hip fracture in men. *Neurourology and Urodynamics, 28*(8), 949–952.

Terayama, K., Sakakibara, R., Ogawa, A., et al. (2012). Weak detrusor contractility correlates with motor disorders in Parkinson's disease. *Movement Disorders, 27*(14), 1775–1780.

Thorburn, W. (1889). *A contribution to the surgery of the spinal cord.* London, UK: Griffin.

Trocio, J. N., Brubaker, L., Schavert, V. F., et al. (2010). Effects of combined behavioral and tolterodine on patient-reported outcomes. *Canadian Journal of Urology, 17*(4), 5283–5290.

Tubaro, A., Puccini, F., De Nunzio, C., et al. (2012). The treatment or lower urinary tract symptoms in patients with multiple sclerosis: A systematic review. *Current Urologic Reports, 13*, 335–342.

Ursino, M. G., Vasina, V., Raschi, E., et al. (2009). The beta-3 adrenoceptor as a therapeutic target: Current perspectives. *Pharmacological Research, 59*(4), 221–234.

Van den Eeden, S. K., Tanner, C. M., Bernstein, A. L., et al. (2003). Incidence of Parkinson's disease: Variation by age, gender and race/ethnicity. *American Journal of Epidemiology, 157*(11), 1015–1022.

Van Koeveringe, G. A., Vahabi, B., Andersson, K. E., et al. (2011). Detrusor underactivity: A plea for new approaches to a common bladder dysfunction. *Neurourology and Urodynamics, 30*, 723–728.

Van Middendorp, J. J., Hosman, A. J., Pouw, M. H., et al.; Em-SCI Study Group. (2009). ASIA impairment scale conversions in traumatic SCI: It is related with the ability to walk? *Spinal Cord, 47*, 555–560.

Vasudeva, P., & Madersbacher, H. (2014). Factors implicated in pathogenesis of urinary tract infections in neurogenic bladders: Some revered, few forgotten, others ignored. *Neurourology and Urodynamics, 33*, 95–100.

Wein, A. J. (1981). Classification of neurogenic voiding dysfunction. *Journal of Urology, 125*(5), 605–609.

Weiss, R. M. (2012). Physiology and pharmacology of the renal pelvic and ureter. In A. J. Wein, et al. (Eds.), *Campbell-Walsh urology* (10th ed., pp.1755–1785). St. Louis, MO: Elsevier.

Weld, K. J., Graney, M. J., & Dmochowski, R. R. (2000). Clinical significance of detrusor dyssynergia type in patients with post-traumatic spinal cord injury. *Urology, 56*(4), 565–568.

Wells, M. J., Jamieson, K., Markham, T. C., et al. (2014). The effects of caffeinated versus decaffeinated drinks on overactive bladder: A double-blind, randomized cross-over study. *Journal of Wound, Ostomy and Continence Nursing, 41*(4), 371–378.

Williams, M. P., Srikanth, V., Bird, M., et al. (2012). Urinary symptoms and natural history of urinary continence after first-ever stroke—a longitudinal population-based study. *Age and Ageing, 41*, 371–376.

Winge, K., & Fowler, C. J. (2006). Bladder dysfunction in Parkinsonism: Mechanisms, prevalence, symptoms and management. *Movement Disorders, 21*(6), 737–745.

Wisconsin Department of Health Services. (2001). Use of a catheter (F315) standard or practice resource. http://www.dhs.wisconsin.gov/publications/p0/p00285.pdf

WOCN White Paper. (2009). Clinical issues in clean intermittent catheterization. Available at: http://c.ymcdn.com/sites/www.wocn.org/resource/resmgr/Publications/Clinical_Issues_in_Clean_Int.pdf

Wyndaele, J. J. (1997). Correlation between clinical neurological data and urodynamic function in spinal cord injured patients. *Spinal Cord, 35*, 213–216.

Wyndaele, J. J. (2002). Intermittent catheterization: Which is the optimal technique? *Spinal Cord, 40*, 432–437.

Yamanishi, T., Yasuda, K., Sakakibara, R., et al. (1997). The nature of detrusor bladder neck dyssynergia in non-neurogenic bladder dysfunction. *Neurourology and Urodynamics, 66*(3), 163–168.

Yamata, S., & Ito, Y. (2011). Alpha-1 adrenoreceptors in the urinary tract. *Handbook of Experimental Pharmacology, 202*, 283–306.

Yoshimura, N., & Chancellor, M. B. (2012). Physiology and pharmacology of the urinary bladder and urethra. In A. J. Wein, et al. (Eds.), *Campbell-Walsh urology* (10th ed., pp. 1786–1853). St. Louis, MO: Elsevier.

Zuckerman, J. M., Edwards, B., Henderson, K., et al. (2014). Extended outcomes in the treatment of male stress urinary incontinence with a transobturator sling. *Urology, 83*(4), 939–945.

QUESTIONS

1. According to Wein's Urodynamics-Based Classification System for Neurogenic Voiding Dysfunction, which of the following is a urodynamic abnormality related to failure to store urine because of the outlet?
   A. Neurogenic detrusor overactivity
   B. Urethral sphincter mechanism incompetence
   C. Bladder outlet obstruction
   D. Detrusor underactivity

2. A continence nurse documents the condition "stove-pipe" urethra. What is the common cause of this alteration?
   A. Short-term indwelling catheterization
   B. Intermittent catheterization
   C. Long-term indwelling catheterization
   D. Surgical intervention

3. A patient is diagnosed with failure to empty urine due to the sphincter. What is the most common cause of this disorder among individuals with a neurogenic condition?
   A. Bladder outlet obstruction
   B. Detrusor external sphincter dyssynergia
   C. Weak pelvic floor
   D. Detrusor underactivity

4. Which of the following is an example of a "hostile bladder condition?"
   A. Low bladder wall compliance
   B. Decreased detrusor pressures
   C. Urgency
   D. Reflex urinary incontinence

5. The continence nurse is assessing a patient with urinary retention who empties his bladder using clean inter-mittent catheterization (CIC). What pertinent assessment question should be part of the focused history?
   A. "Are you experiencing nighttime urinary leakage?"
   B. "Are you experiencing pain upon catheter-ization?"
   C. "What type of external collection device do you use?"
   D. "Are you experiencing any leaking around the catheter?"

6. The continence nurse is instructing patients with urinary retention related to neurogenic bladder and how to perform clean intermittent catheterization (CIC). Which teaching point would the nurse include in the plan?
   A. Adult patients should use a 6- to 10-French catheter for the procedure.
   B. Patients should remove the catheter quickly to prevent drainage.
   C. Patients should clean and reuse catheters.
   D. Catheterization should be performed in an upright position if possible.

7. The continence nurse recommends a silicone-coated catheter for long-term catheterization. What is the advantage of this type of catheter?
   A. Protection against bacteriuria
   B. Reduced urethral inflammation
   C. Ease of insertion
   D. Reduced risk of urinary leakage

8. A patient is diagnosed with detrusor-striated sphincter dyssynergia related to neurogenic bladder. What category of drugs is recommended for this condition?
   A. Alpha-adrenergic antagonists
   B. Beta-3 adrenergic agonists
   C. Cholinergic agonists
   D. Injectable neurotoxin

9. A female patient is diagnosed with urethral sphincter incompetence. What surgical intervention might be recommended for this patient?
   A. Suburethral sling procedure
   B. Augmentation enterocystoplasty
   C. Implantation of a sacral neuromodulation device
   D. Transurethral sphincterotomy

10. A patient with neurogenic bladder undergoes sacral neuromodulation surgery to implant a device into the pelvis with leads placed at the sacral roots. What disorder does this surgery attempt to correct?
    A. Urethral sphincter incompetence
    B. Bladder outlet obstruction
    C. Detrusor-striated muscle dyssynergia
    D. Neurogenic detrusor overactivity

11. Which intervention is typically initiated immediately following spinal cord injury (SCI) for management of neurogenic bladder?
    A. Intermittent catheterization
    B. Insertion of an indwelling catheter
    C. Prophylactic antibiotic therapy
    D. Surgical intervention to create a urinary diversion

12. Which of the following is the typical first-line management strategy for patients experiencing neurogenic bladder related to stroke?
    A. Surgical interventions
    B. Pharmacotherapy
    C. Behavioral interventions
    D. Use of indwelling catheterization to prevent urinary retention

ANSWERS: 1.**C**, 2.**C**, 3.**B**, 4.**A**, 5.**A**, 6.**D**, 7.**B**, 8.**A**, 9.**A**, 10.**D**, 11.**B**, 12.**C**

CHAPTER 8

Voiding Dysfunction and Urinary Incontinence in Men

Michael Clark and Joanne P. Robinson

OBJECTIVES

1. Explain the etiology, pathology, and management of lower urinary tract symptoms in older men.
2. Describe types of voiding dysfunction and urinary incontinence unique to the male patient to include pathology, presentation, and management.
3. Explain the presentation, diagnosis, and treatment modalities for prostate cancer.
4. Explain the pathology and management of urinary incontinence and erectile dysfunction following radical prostatectomy.
5. Discuss the psychosocial impact of prostate cancer on the male and his partner.

Topic Outline

C linicians who provide care for men with lower urinary tract symptoms (LUTS) must have background knowledge that is sufficiently broad to support the development of a trusting, high-quality collaborative relationship and therapeutic plan. This chapter provides an overview of common LUTS in men and interrelated issues of sexuality and intimacy. A running case study is used to model a patient-centered approach to working with men who experience LUTS and erectile dysfunction (ED) due to benign prostatic hyperplasia (BPH) and prostate cancer. Fundamental aspects of epidemiology, pathophysiology, evaluation, treatment, and management of these conditions, including educational and emotional support, are emphasized.

CLINICAL PEARL

LUTS (lower urinary tract symptoms) is a general term that refers to subjective indicators of conditions and diseases that affect the bladder and urethra.

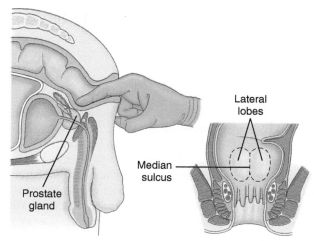

FIGURE 8-1. Digital rectal examination (DRE) and assessment of the prostate gland.

CASE STUDY: PART 1

Mr. Jones is a 58-year-old African American man who presents to his primary care provider for an initial visit. He has just obtained health insurance and he wants to "have everything checked out." On review of systems, he reports that he is getting up approximately three times at night to urinate. He reports urinating small to moderate amounts each time. He also reports that he has a weak urinary stream and doesn't feel that he is always able to empty his bladder completely. On occasion, he admits to a sudden urge to void with one or two episodes of urinary incontinence per week. He also reports mild to moderate discomfort in his midpelvic area just prior to urinating, without radiation to his flanks or back. He denies flank pain, dysuria, penile discharge, fever/chills, and other constitutional symptoms.

Mr. Jones has one cup of coffee per day and does not drink diet sodas. His medical history includes a history of hypertension and hyperlipidemia. He does not have a history of diabetes or cardiovascular disease. His medications include amlodipine and hydrochlorothiazide. On physical exam, Mr. Jones has an enlarged symmetrical prostate with normal texture and no

nodules. The prostate is not boggy or tender. A urine dipstick is negative for leukocytes and blood. He has no suprapubic tenderness.

When Mr. Jones is asked what he thinks of his urinary symptoms, he reports, "I have been bothered by them but felt that they were just normal for my age; however, if you can do something to help, it would be great."

DISCUSSION

Mr. Jones has a number of lower urinary tract symptoms (LUTS), including nocturia, weak urinary stream, sensations of incomplete bladder emptying, urgency, incontinence, and pelvic pain. LUTS is a general term that refers to subjective indicators of conditions and diseases that affect the bladder and urethra (Abrams et al., 2009). LUTS are highly prevalent in men and prevalence increases with age (Rosen et al., 2003). One large international study found that 62.5% of men reported having LUTS (Irwin et al., 2006). In older men, the prevalence of LUTS was estimated at 30% in men aged 65 years or older (Jones et al., 2010) and 70% in men older than 80 years (Parsons et al., 2008).

An initial workup should consider certain modifiable factors that may improve symptoms. Signs and symptoms of a urinary tract infection (UTI), urethritis, or prostate infection should be considered and treated if present. Mr. Jones should be asked about estimated voiding volumes. Symptoms attributed to LUTS may be due to polyuria from such causes as renal disease, poorly controlled diabetes mellitus, and other endocrine conditions such as diabetes insipidus. Mr. Jones lacks signs of infection and polyuria.

His prostate is nontender and firm, which indicates that a prostate infection is not present.

Mr. Jones had a normal prostate exam, with the exception of symmetrical enlargement. If the prostate was boggy or tender on exam, the clinical suspicion for prostate infection (prostatitis) would be increased. Also, if there was any asymmetry or nodules appreciated on exam, Mr. Jones would be worked up for prostate cancer. Figure 8-1 depicts the rectal exam and assessment of the prostate.

Lower Urinary Tract Symptoms

LUTS are generally classified into three groups: storage symptoms, voiding symptoms, and postvoiding symptoms (Lee & Lee, 2014).

Characteristics of LUTS

Storage symptoms include urgency, defined as a sudden urge to void that is difficult to delay; daytime frequency, a perception of excessive frequency of voiding during the day; nocturia, the need to awaken at night to void; urge incontinence, involuntary leakage immediately preceded by urgency; stress incontinence, involuntary leakage resulting from sudden pressure on the bladder; and pain. Voiding symptoms include slow and/or interrupted stream, the perception of reduced flow; hesitancy, difficulty in initiating voiding; straining, the need to use Valsalva or abdominal muscles to void; terminal dribble, prolongation of the last phase of voiding; hematuria, blood in the urine; and dysuria, a burning sensation or general discomfort during voiding. Postvoiding symptoms include sensation of incomplete emptying and postmicturition dribble, the involuntary loss of urine shortly after voiding. Mr. Jones has LUTS in each of the above categories, which is fairly common in men with an enlarged prostate gland.

CLINICAL PEARL

LUTS are classified as storage symptoms (e.g., frequency, urgency, UI, and nocturia), voiding symptoms (e.g., hesitancy, slow stream, terminal dribbling, straining to empty), and postvoiding symptoms (e.g., feelings of incomplete emptying and postvoid dribbling).

Pathophysiology

The prostate is a walnut-sized gland that surrounds the proximal urethra. It sits just below the base of the bladder and just distal to the internal urinary sphincter. Seminal ducts pass through the prostate gland and empty into the urethra proximal to the external urethral sphincter, or rhabdosphincter. The bulbourethral glands or Cowper's glands (not shown) are located on either side of the urethra just distal to the prostate (Fig. 8-2).

The prostate gland along with the seminal vesicles and the bulbourethral glands serve primarily to enhance male sexual functioning and fertility. A normal prostate is important in the production of semen and plays a crucial role in orgasm and ejaculation. The prostate produces a slightly alkaline fluid that comprises the majority of the volume of semen. The alkalinity of this fluid neutralizes the acidity of the vaginal tract and prolongs the life span of sperm. The seminal vesicles store semen, and the bulbourethral glands secrete an alkaline fluid prior to ejaculation that neutralizes the acidity of urine to protect sperm. During orgasm, the nerve plexus surrounding the prostate stimulates rhythmic contractions of the prostate, urethral walls, seminal vesicles, and the bulbourethral glands. The normal anatomy of the prostate and surrounding structures is depicted in Figure 8-2.

CLINICAL PEARL

The primary function of the prostate is to enhance male sexual function and fertility.

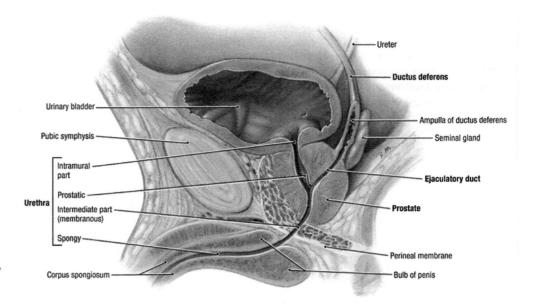

FIGURE 8-2. Normal anatomy of the prostate and surrounding structures.

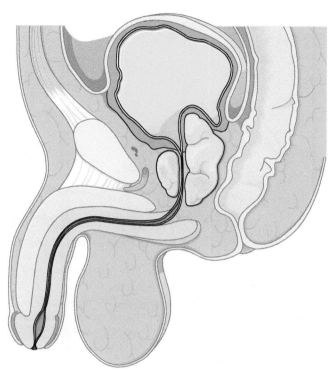

FIGURE 8-3. Anatomic abnormalities of BPH and bladder dysfunction.

Application to Case Study

Mr. Jones has an enlarged prostate without other suspicious findings that would suggest the presence of prostate cancer (nodularity, asymmetries in size or texture). As shown in Figure 8-3, an enlarged prostate causes structural problems with urinary outflow due to a mass effect that constricts the proximal urethra and diminishes urinary flow.

Etiologic Factors

Bladder outlet obstruction is an important but not sole contributing factor to LUTS. The act of voiding requires the coordination of several structures, including the bladder wall or detrusor muscle and the internal urethral sphincter. LUTS in men are commonly due to a complex interaction of structural problems caused by BPH and alterations in neurologic signaling and feedback.

Benign Prostatic Hyperplasia

BPH is the most common benign neoplasm in American men. Its prevalence increases with age, affecting almost three of four men in the seventh decade of life (Wei et al., 2005). The relationship between BPH and LUTS involves the anatomic and physiological effects of hypertrophy but also involves other pathology, including inflammation.

Hypertrophy

BPH is associated with an increase in the size of the prostate due to unregulated proliferation of connective tissue, smooth muscle, and glandular epithelium. This mass effect is static

and causes direct bladder outlet obstruction. BPH is also associated with an increase in the smooth muscle tone of the internal urethral sphincter, a dynamic effect. Both processes lead to the voiding symptoms of LUTS (McVary et al., 2010). In addition, if the enlarged prostate begins to push up on the bladder as noted in Figure 8-3, changes in the mechanics and sensation of bladder filling can occur. The bladder wall (detrusor muscle) may become overactive, resulting in problems with the storage of urine and symptoms of urgency and frequency. ED also frequently coexists with BPH and LUTS, although a causal link has not been clearly identified (Fwu et al., 2014). Estimates of the rate of ED in men with BPH range from 30% to 70% (Roupret et al., 2012). Age and comorbid conditions associated with aging, such as arterial disease and diabetes, confound the relationship between ED and BPH, as does the tendency of men to underreport both conditions to clinicians (Foster et al., 2013).

> **CLINICAL PEARL**
>
> BPH involves enlargement of the prostate and increased smooth muscle tone in the proximal urethra, both of which can contribute to bladder outlet obstruction.

Inflammation

Recent research findings suggest that the pathophysiology of BPH, LUTS, and ED may be related to chronic subclinical inflammation and associated endothelial dysfunction. BPH involves remodeling of prostate tissue and an alteration in prostatic secretions. These changes are associated with an increase in the production and release of inflammatory cytokines, which drive prostatic hyperplasia. Inflammatory cytokines also cause changes in autonomic innervation, which disrupts the normal balance between sympathetic and parasympathetic tone (Agnihotri et al., 2014; Cellek et al., 2014; Yan et al., 2014). This balance is necessary for proper functioning of the detrusor muscle and internal urethral sphincter as well as for achievement of erection and orgasm. Overactivity of the detrusor muscle and failure to appropriately relax the internal urethral sphincter are key features of LUTS.

Alterations in Nerve Signaling

There is increasing awareness of the importance of afferent sensitivity in patients who present with LUTS. In the past, it was thought that LUTS were due to a motor (efferent) problem (detrusor overactivity) and bladder neck dysfunction (outflow obstruction). Recently, attention is being paid to sensory (afferent) components of LUTS (Chapple, 2014). Increased afferent sensitivity may play a significant role in the LUTS experience for some patients, and the efficacy of newer second- and third-line interventions, such as nerve stimulation techniques (Kacker et al., 2013) and tricyclic antidepressants (Athanasopoulos, 2011), in these patients is promising.

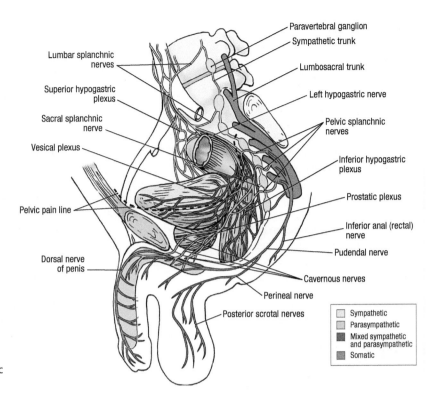

FIGURE 8-4. Innervation of the prostate, pelvic organs, and penis.

The nerves and blood vessels that supply the prostate, seminal vesicles, and bulbourethral glands also supply the penis. Parasympathetic nerve stimulation promotes erection and sympathetic stimulation promotes ejaculation. As shown in Figure 8-4, the neurologic transmission to and among these structures is complex and consists of afferent, efferent, and reflex arc pathways.

CLINICAL PEARL

Increased sensitivity and abnormal function of sensory nerves may be one factor contributing to LUTS; this explains the positive effects of nerve stimulation and tricyclic antidepressants in some men.

Inflammation-associated alterations in these pathways can have a significant impact on sexual function. BPH-associated inflammatory cytokines may contribute to endothelial dysfunction, which leads to a decrease in blood flow to the penis. Endothelial dysfunction impedes the vasodilation needed in order to achieve an erection. This may be particularly problematic for men with underlying vascular problems due to comorbidities such as diabetes and arterial disease.

Initial Evaluation and Workup

Mr. Jones has a mixture of LUTS. He is experiencing obstructive symptoms, including a weak urine stream and sensations of incomplete bladder emptying, most likely due to an enlarged prostate and/or BPH. The size of the prostate and the prevalence of BPH increase steadily with age; in fact, prostate size loosely correlates with the severity of LUTS (Parsons et al., 2008). Technically, enlargement of the prostate alone is not synonymous with BPH. BPH involves histologic changes that preferentially affect different areas of the prostate. In particular, BPH tends to affect the "transitional zone" surrounding the urethra, which may produce obstructive symptoms in excess of those attributable to prostate size alone. It is important to remember that while obstruction is *suggested* by symptoms, the diagnosis should be confirmed by flow studies (McVary et al., 2010).

Mr. Jones is also experiencing irritative symptoms, including nocturia, urgency, and incontinence, most likely due to an overactive bladder. Normally, the detrusor muscle relaxes during bladder filling and contracts during bladder emptying. An overactive detrusor muscle inappropriately contracts during bladder filling, leading to classic signs and symptoms of overactive bladder: nocturia, frequency, and urgency, with or without urge incontinence (McVary et al., 2010).

History and Physical Examination

Initial assessment of the patient with LUTS begins with a careful history and physical. This includes a cognitive and functional assessment since, unlike Mr. Jones, many patients have cognitive and functional limitations that impact the management of symptoms. Serious conditions such as infection, prostate cancer, bladder cancer, and chronic kidney disease should be ruled out. The history should include the nature and frequency of symptoms, symptom progression, family history, and the presence of comorbidities, particularly diabetes or other chronic conditions that cause peripheral or central nervous system (CNS) dysfunction. Perineal sensation and rectal tone should be tested to determine whether voiding dysfunction has neurologic components. A urinalysis should be performed with a follow-up urine culture only if the urine dipstick suggests infection. Any patient with gross or occult hematuria should be referred to a urologist. Finally, clinicians should also assess for daytime sleepiness and fatigue since nocturia can significantly interfere with the quality of sleep. That said, it is important to distinguish the nature of the primary problem. For example, men who have insomnia and early awakening due to depression may void simply because they are awake rather than because of an overactive bladder (Jones et al., 2010).

CLINICAL PEARL

It is important to rule out serious pathology in the man with LUTS (e.g., infection, prostate or bladder cancer, chronic kidney disease). Any patient with gross or occult hematuria should be referred to a urologist.

In performing the initial workup for Mr. Jones, the clinician should decide whether LUTS are likely due to an obstruction that restricts outflow, an overactive bladder, or a combination of both. Typically, obstructive symptoms lead to overflow incontinence while an overactive bladder leads to urge incontinence. The dynamics of overflow and urge incontinence are depicted in Figure 8-5. Treatment should be targeted to the presenting problem(s).

Obstructive problems are initially treated with medications that relax the urethral sphincter as well as medications that decrease the size of the prostate. Treatment of an overactive bladder is approached in a stepwise manner that begins with behavioral interventions.

Types of Incontinence

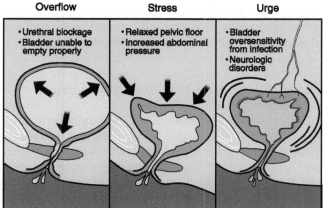

Overflow	Stress	Urge
• Urethral blockage • Bladder unable to empty properly	• Relaxed pelvic floor • Increased abdominal pressure	• Bladder oversensitivity from infection • Neurologic disorders

FIGURE 8-5. Overflow and urge incontinence in BPH/LUTS.

CLINICAL PEARL

In analyzing the data from a male with LUTS, the clinician must determine whether the LUTS are due to obstruction, overactive bladder, or a combination.

Standardized Assessment Tools

The care of patients with LUTS primarily involves symptom management (Jones et al., 2010). Therefore, the use of standardized tools that measure the severity of symptoms and their degree of "bother" to the patient is important. Data from appropriately administered standardized tools are robust and should be used to guide initial treatment decisions and to evaluate changes in symptoms over time and the efficacy of treatment.

The International Prostate Symptom Score (IPSS), also known as the American Urologic Association (AUA) score (AUA, 2003; Barry, 1992), is one of the most common tools employed to assess LUTS in men (Fig. 8-6). The tool assesses frequency of symptoms in seven domains, including sensation of incomplete emptying, urinary frequency, intermittency (starting and stopping of flow), weak stream, need to strain during urination, and need to get up at night to urinate. Each domain is scored on a scale that ranges from 0 to 5 ("not at all" to "almost always"). In addition, the patient is asked, "If you were to spend the rest of your life with your urinary symptoms just the way they are now, how would you feel about that?" This "degree of bother" item is rated on a scale that ranges from 0 to 6 ("delighted" to "terrible").

Treatment decisions are based on the total IPSS (sum of all domain scores) as well as the "degree of bother" item. Categories of symptom burden include mild (0 to 7), moderate (8 to 19), and severe (20 to 35). A cutoff score of 8 or greater is commonly used as an indicator of the need to start or advance treatment, as long as the patient is bothered by the symptoms. No treatment may be indicated when the total IPSS is 7 or less or if the patient is not significantly bothered by the symptoms.

CLINICAL PEARL

The management of LUTS is primarily symptomatic (once serious conditions have been ruled out); thus, determining the degree to which the symptoms "bother" the patient is important.

Treatment of LUTS

Although LUTS in men are known to increase with age, they are not a uniformly progressive problem. Many men experience patterns of worsening and improving LUTS in the absence of treatment (Poyhonen et al., 2014). LUTS are not associated with increased mortality. Treatment should be targeted at relieving symptoms as well as eliminating or mitigating their underlying mechanism(s). The degree to which the patient is bothered by LUTS is a major factor

	Not at all	Less than 1 time in 5	Less than half the time	About half the time	More than half the time	Almost always
	0	1	2	3	4	5
1. INCOMPLETE EMPTYING Over the last month or so, how often have you had a sensation of not emptying your bladder completely after you finished urinating?	O 0	O 1	O 2	O 3	O 4	O 5
2. FREQUENCY During the last month or so, how often have you had to urinate again <2 hours after you finished urinating?	O 0	O 1	O 2	O 3	O 4	O 5
3. INTERMITTENCY During the last month or so, how often have you stopped and started again several times when you urinated?	O 0	O 1	O 2	O 3	O 4	O 5
4. URGENCY During the last month or so, how often have you found it difficult to postpone urination?	O 0	O 1	O 2	O 3	O 4	O 5
5. WEAK STREAM During the last month or so, how often have you had a weak urinary stream?	O 0	O 1	O 2	O 3	O 4	O 5
6. STRAINING During the last month or so, how often have you had to push or strain to begin urination?	O 0	O 1	O 2	O 3	O 4	O 5
7. SLEEPING During the last month, how many times did you most typically get up to urinate from the time you went to bed at night until the time you got up in the morning?	O 0	O 1	O 2	O 3	O 4	O 5

(times at night)

_____ SCORE: (0-35)_____

The <u>International Prostate Symptom Score (IPSS)</u> uses the same 7 questions as the AUA Symptom Index, but adds a "Disease Specific Quality of Life Question" (sometimes referred to as the "bother score") that is scored from 0 to 6 points ("delighted" to "terrible").

If you were to spend the rest of your life with your urinary condition just the way it is now, how would you feel about that?

Delighted	Pleased	Mostly satisfied	Mixed	Mostly disappointed	Unhappy	Terrible
0	1	2	3	4	5	6
O	O	O	O	O	O	O

FIGURE 8-6. International Prostate Symptom Score (IPSS), also known as the American Urologic Association score.

in determining both the initiation and advancement of treatment.

Watchful Waiting

A "watchful waiting" approach is a sound option for the initial treatment of LUTS. In a review of the literature on LUTS and modifiable risk factors (Raheem & Parsons, 2014), progression of untreated LUTS was associated with obesity, problems with mobility, mental health issues, hypertension, and back pain; conversely, a reduced risk of LUTS (and BPH) was related to a healthy diet low in fat and high in vegetables and exercise. Of note is that moderate intake of alcohol was associated with lower risk of BPH but a higher risk for LUTS. Men with LUTS were also more likely to be on medication such as antidepressants that modulated serotonin and GABA. It is postulated that these agents may promote relaxation of the detrusor muscle. Although randomized controlled trials on modifiable lifestyle issues have yet to be conducted, Raheem and Parsons (2014) remind us that it is reasonable to recommend healthy living habits to all men who present with urologic symptoms.

The AUA and International Consultation on Incontinence (ICI) (2013) recommend a stepped approach to the treatment of LUTS, including first-, second-, and third-line therapies for storage, voiding, and postvoiding symptoms (Gormley et al., 2012). Decision making about treatment progression requires collaboration between the patient and his provider to balance the patient's expectations with the risk–benefit ratio of each treatment option. Abrams et al. (2013) provide an evidence-based algorithm that can guide initial and expert evaluation of the male with incontinence.

General Health and Lifestyle Considerations

Developing a treatment plan for LUTS begins by considering the patient's general health and lifestyle. For example, patients with diminished cognitive capacity may not be able to engage in behavioral interventions. Functional limitations that impede access to toileting will also limit the effectiveness of behavioral interventions. An overall lack of physical conditioning not only is associated with higher symptom scores in men with LUTS (Raheem & Parsons, 2014) but also restricts options for behavioral interventions.

There is a positive correlation between LUTS and body mass index. Weight loss is a very important modifiable risk factor (Raheem & Parsons, 2014). Obesity is associated with an increase in the incidence of BPH, LUTS, and prostate cancer (Lee et al., 2012). In one study that tested a weight loss intervention for urinary incontinence (UI) in women, an 8% reduction in body mass index was associated with a 42% reduction in UI, compared to 26% in the control group (Subak et al., 2009).

Medications, fluid intake, and ingestion of substances that irritate the bladder may also contribute to LUTS and should be modified if possible. In general, the use of decongestants and other adrenergic agonists should be avoided. Other options to improve symptoms that have limited research evidence include evening fluid limitation (Hashim & Abrams, 2008), minimizing alcohol intake, avoiding spicy or highly seasoned food (Abrams et al., 2009), and decreasing or eliminating caffeine intake (Bryant et al., 2002).

> **CLINICAL PEARL**
>
> The AUA and ICI recommend a "stepped" approach to the management of voiding LUTS in men; step 1 involves lifestyle modifications such as weight loss (if indicated), avoidance of alpha-adrenergic agonists, and avoidance of potential bladder irritants.

Treatment of Voiding and Postvoiding Symptoms

Mr. Jones has a number of voiding and postvoiding symptoms related to his enlarged prostate. First-line therapy should include behavioral approaches to enhance bladder emptying. Bladder emptying results from an interactive effect between increased intra-abdominal pressure (Valsalva) and decreased outflow restriction (relaxation and distraction). Evidence from studying Iranian men with BPH suggests that voiding in a traditional crouched/squat position may improve emptying because of increased bladder pressure and abdominal pressure transmission with concomitant pelvic floor relaxation (Amjadi et al., 2006). To date, no studies were found that evaluated effective emptying in men sitting on a Western toilet compared to the standing position. Since incomplete bladder emptying is often accompanied by nocturia, sleep habits should

be explored and, if needed, interventions to promote sleep should be offered (Carlson & Palmer, 2014).

Pharmacologic Agents

Medications are considered second-line therapy to enhance bladder emptying. They are introduced in combination with first-line interventions or initially depending on symptom severity of the individual patient's goals. Current medications that enhance bladder emptying in men with BPH work in two ways. One class of agents, alpha-adrenergic antagonists, decreases the tone of the internal urethral sphincter and the other, 5-alpha reductase inhibitors, decreases the size of the prostate. Each may be used alone or in combination. An algorithmic approach to the pharmacologic management of obstructive symptoms is depicted in Figure 8-7 and Figure 8-12 shows an algorithm for PSA and decision-making.

> **CLINICAL PEARL**
>
> For men with bothersome voiding LUTS unresponsive to lifestyle modifications, medications are recommended as the second step (alpha-adrenergic antagonists and 5-alpha reductase inhibitors).

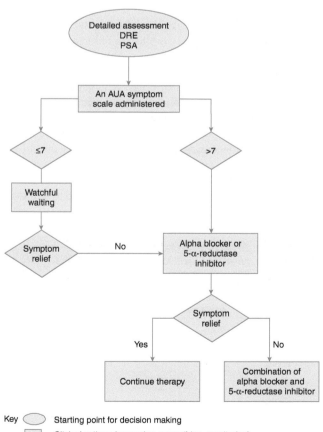

FIGURE 8-7. Treatment approach to the management of obstructive symptoms of LUTS.

Alpha-Adrenergic Antagonists

Five alpha-adrenergic antagonists are currently approved by the Federal Drug Administration. These agents act by altering neural signaling to promote relaxation of the internal urinary sphincter. Among the alpha-adrenergic antagonists, two agents (terazosin and doxazosin) are nonselective and must be used with caution, especially in the elderly, because they interfere with the normal vasoconstrictive response to postural changes. Patients who use these agents should especially be cautioned about getting out of bed abruptly to prevent orthostatic hypotension. Patient teaching should emphasize sitting on the side of the bed for a minute or so to be sure that they are not light-headed or dizzy before standing. They should then stand for a minute or so by the bed before proceeding to the bathroom. Recently, two new alpha-adrenergic antagonists (tamsulosin and silodosin) that are selective for the bladder neck and prostate have become available. These drugs have fewer cardiovascular side effects, although older patients should still use the same precautions when arising from bed.

5-Alpha Reductase Inhibitors

Medications that reduce the size of the prostate are 5-alpha reductase inhibitors. The growth of the prostate is promoted by testosterone and dihydrotestosterone (DHT). Compared to testosterone, DHT is a much more potent stimulant of prostate growth. The conversion of testosterone to DHT is catalyzed by the enzyme 5-alpha reductase, which is inhibited by this class of drugs. Two 5-alpha reductase inhibitors (finasteride and dutasteride) are commonly used to treat BPH. Side effects include reduced libido, erectile dysfunction, breast tenderness, and/or breast enlargement. Patients should be informed of these side effects prior to treatment and encouraged to discuss them with their sexual partners. In addition, these agents affect prostate-specific antigen (PSA) levels. Some suggest that actual PSA levels should be doubled in order to estimate prostate cancer risk for a man using these agents (Gacci et al., 2012). Table 8-1 lists therapeutic effects and side effects of medications used to enhance bladder emptying in men with BPH.

TABLE 8-1 **Effects and Adverse Effects of Medications Used for Symptom Management of BPH**

	Alpha₁-Adrenergic Antagonists	5-Alpha Reductase Inhibitors
Decrease in prostate size	No	Yes
Peak onset	2–4 wk	6–12 mo
Sexual dysfunction	+	++
Hypotensive effects	++	—
Commonly used drugs	Tamsulosin, alfuzosin	Finasteride, dutasteride

Surgical Intervention

Men who continue to have significant difficulty with bladder emptying despite the use of medications may be offered a variety of third-line invasive therapies to remove or ablate prostate tissue in the interest of improved urine flow. The selection of an intervention is influenced by age, prostate size, degree of symptom burden, and potential complications. These third-line therapies are listed and described in Table 8-2.

Transurethral Resection of Prostate

Transurethral resection of the prostate (TURP) is the gold standard third-line intervention with an 80% to 90% efficacy rate as measured by symptom improvement. A number of complications are associated with its use; however, complication rates have decreased with newer techniques such as microprocessor controlled electrocautery units. The most significant complications are clot and urinary retention. Early urge incontinence is experienced by approximately 30% to 40% of patients, but late stress incontinence is rare (<0.5%). The major late complications are urethral stricture (2.2% to 9.8%) and bladder neck contractures (0.3% to 9.2%) (Rassweiler et al., 2006). Newer protocols allow for a 1-day hospital stay and discharge without a catheter (Shum et al., 2014). Figure 8-8 illustrates the most common approach to a TURP.

Total Prostatectomy

Total prostatectomy is indicated only in cases in which the prostate is unusually large or prostate cancer is suspected. The literature on complications associated with total prostatectomy is confusing due to wide variability in reporting types of complications and estimating complication rates (Hakimi et al., 2012). The greatest concerns are rates of postoperative UI and sexual dysfunction. These complications are more of an issue for younger men and men with higher baseline functioning (Brajtbord et al., 2014).

Minimally Invasive Techniques

In recent years, newer minimally invasive techniques have been introduced in the interest of achieving desired outcomes with fewer complications. Ablative techniques involve the use of lasers to vaporize prostatic tissue. Limited data suggest that they have fewer short- and long-term complications (Kumar, 2007). One study suggested that photoselective vaporization of the prostate (PVP) resulted in sustained symptom relief at 5 years and a 43% reduction in prostate size (Otsuki et al., 2014). The prostatic urethral lift is a procedure for men with less pronounced symptoms and involves the placement of implants to reposition the prostate so that urethral patency is optimized. Limited data suggest promising results (Chin et al., 2012; Roehrborn et al., 2013).

CLINICAL PEARL

Surgical reduction of the prostate (and less invasive alternatives) for treatment of voiding LUTS is recommended only for bothersome symptoms not responsive to lifestyle modifications and pharmacologic therapy.

TABLE 8-2 Current Procedures to Reduce Symptoms of BPH/LUTS

Invasive Therapies

Technique	Brief Description	Efficacy	Side Effects Profile
Total prostatectomy	Surgical removal of the prostate through an abdominal or perineal approach Major surgery generally performed only if very large prostate or suspicion of coexisting prostate cancer	Significant improvement in IPSS and quality of life scores	Significant blood loss with transfusion rates about 10% in some studies Long hospital stays (average 5 d) Long duration of indwelling catheter (average 5 d) Long-term complications include incontinence, bladder neck contracture.

Transurethral resection of the prostate (TURP)	Typically an endoscopic introduction of an electrocautery device into the prostatic urethra with layered removal of perurethral prostate tissue	High degree of long-term efficacy	Requires spinal or general anesthesia
			Significant risks:
			    Blood loss
			    Hematuria
			    TUR syndrome
			    Long-term possible complications from urethral stricture or bladder neck abnormality
			    Retrograde ejaculation

Transurethral incision of the prostate (TUIP)	Selective small incisions limited to the bladder neck using endoscopic guidance through the urethra	Indicated for men with smaller prostates and moderate symptoms who are at higher risk for more invasive procedures	Fewer complications compared with TURP

Laser Therapy*

Technique	Brief Description	Efficacy	Side Effects Profile
Holmium laser enucleation	The laser is used to cut and remove the excess tissue that is blocking the urethra. Another instrument, called a morcellator, is then used to chop the prostate tissue into small pieces that are easily removed.	Limited data that suggest acceptable efficacy	Minimal complications and short procedure
Holmium laser ablation of the prostate (HoLAP)	Holmium laser is used to melt away (vaporize) the excess prostate tissue.	Limited data suggest acceptable efficacy.	Minimal short- and long-term complications
Photoselective vaporization of the prostate (PVP)	A laser is used to melt away (vaporize) excess prostate tissue to enlarge the urinary channel.	One study with sustained improvement in symptoms and significant reduction in prostate size	Minimal short- and long-term complications

Minimally Invasive Therapies

Technique	Brief Description	Efficacy	Side Effects Profile
Transurethral radiofrequency needle ablation (TUNA)	Endoscopic transurethral placement of needles across lumen into surrounding prostate with radiofrequency energy used to cause prostate tissue necrosis and subsequent reduction in prostate volume	Short-term outcomes similar to TURP. Long-term outcomes may not be quite as good.	Does not require surgery Less sexual dysfunction including retrograde ejaculation
Transurethral microwave therapy	Transurethral approach that uses devices to heat the prostate tissue while cooling the urethra allowing for maximal prostate tissue ablation while minimizing urethral damage	Probably similar to TUNA but data are limited due to evolving nature of the technology as well as lack of uniformity in study design to measure efficacy and adverse effects. Concerns about long-term efficacy	Does not require surgery Less sexual dysfunction
Prostatic urethral lift	Transurethral placement of small implants to reposition the prostate lobes to optimize urethral patency	Limited data suggest adequate efficacy.	Performed under local anesthesia Minimal to no ejaculatory or sexual dysfunction

*Ablation, the laser melts away excess tissue; enucleation, the laser cuts away excess prostate tissue. In all laser procedures, the laser is introduced into the urethra through a scope.

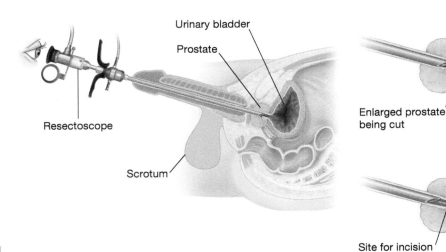

FIGURE 8-8. Transurethral resection of the prostate.

Treatment of Storage Symptoms

Mr. Jones has a number of storage symptoms that are likely due to an overactive bladder. Table 8-3 lists first-, second-, and third-line approaches to the management of overactive bladder and the benefit risk profile associated with each.

Pelvic Floor Muscle Training and Bladder Retraining

First-line treatment for overactive bladder symptoms includes pelvic floor muscle training (Burgio, 2013) and other techniques to enhance bladder control and decrease symptoms of urgency. Bladder training is a strategy to reduce urgency symptoms by purposeful relaxation, distraction, and self-assertions, such as assuring themselves that they can prevent urinary leakage during an episode of urgency, while tightening pelvic floor muscles. Men may also be taught to gradually prolong the intervals between voiding so that bladder capacity increases (Natalin et al., 2013). Lifestyle modifications such as fluid management, reduction in caffeine and alcohol (depending on intake as per bladder diary), and weight loss are typically recommended along with bladder training.

Bladder function is regulated by local and CNS neural signaling. The detrusor muscle is under parasympathetic control, which is associated with the neurotransmitter acetylcholine. Acetylcholine activates the detrusor muscle and increases its tension. In the overactive bladder, anticholinergic agents and newer agents such as beta-3 agonists work to reduce detrusor activity and tension.

The CNS has an indirect effect on bladder functioning through both somatic and autonomic mechanisms. Behavior modification, such as relaxation and voluntary contraction of the pelvic floor muscles and external urethral sphincter (rhabdosphincter), is an important intervention that modifies CNS signaling to reduce bladder activity and tension.

TABLE 8-3 Stepped Approach to the Management of Overactive Bladder

Treatment Category	Types of Interventions	Benefit: Risk Profile
First line	Behavioral, lifestyle, intake modifications	Combination of these approaches has equal efficacy compared with second-line treatments without side effects or risks.
Second line	Antimuscarinic agents	Anticholinergic effects of antimuscarinic agents include dry mouth, constipation, possible worsening of cognitive functioning.
	Beta₃ agonist agents	Beta₃ agonists do not have the side effects associated with anticholinergic agents and they do not provoke excess sympathetic side effects at the doses given (hypertension).
Third line	Intradetrusor onabotulinumtoxin A	Patients must be willing to perform intermittent self-catheterization if they develop urinary retention.
	Peripheral tibial nerve stimulation	12 weekly treatments for 30 min each, possibility of infection and problems with technology
	Sacral neuromodulator	Lead migration in 5%–10% of patients requiring invasive repositioning of implanted electrodes

The bladder diary is a first-line treatment that is especially important for patients with storage symptoms. Use of the bladder diary improves awareness of symptoms and engages the man in the treatment plan. The diary should include the time interval between voids, the number of voids per day, and the volume voided. Recording the volume voided may particularly help to distinguish LUTS from other comorbid conditions associated with polyuria. Diaries also provide a baseline for evaluating the efficacy of interventions (McVary et al., 2011).

Finally, first-line treatment includes providing information about basic anatomy and physiology of the bladder. The patient should also be informed about the complexity of the neural and vascular supply that is shared by the bladder, prostate, and penis. The interaction between bladder functioning and erectile dysfunction, both at baseline and as a result of possible interventions, should be reviewed. Figure 8-9 illustrates the important neural signaling pathways that are associated with bladder function.

> **CLINICAL PEARL**
>
> First-line management of bothersome storage symptoms (urgency, frequency, nocturia) involves pelvic floor muscle training and bladder retraining.

Pharmacologic Agents

Second-line treatments for overactive bladder consist of pharmacologic agents that relax the detrusor muscle. Detrusor contraction is triggered by acetylcholine. Anticholinergic agents that target cholinergic receptors, as well as sympathetic agonists that target beta-3 adrenergic receptors, counteract stimulation of the detrusor muscle by acetylcholine, thereby mitigating the symptoms of overactive bladder. Anticholinergics are the most commonly used agents. Although they are somewhat selective for detrusor receptors, all agents have some possible systemic anticholinergic effects including dry mouth, constipation, dry or itchy eyes, blurred vision, dyspepsia, UTI, urinary retention, and impaired cognition. Beta-3 agonists are newer agents that specifically target and relax the detrusor muscle.

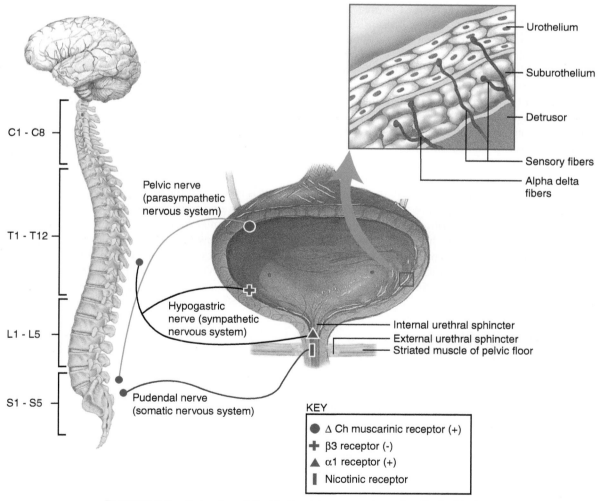

FIGURE 8-9. Innervation of the bladder detrusor muscles and urethral sphincters.

These drugs are recommended in patients who have bothersome symptoms related to the use of anticholinergic agents.

In general, men receiving second-line pharmacologic treatment for overactive bladder should be monitored for symptoms of urinary retention, and postvoid residual volume should be regularly measured in those who are symptomatic (Gormley et al., 2012). In addition, anticholinergic agents should be used with caution in men with postvoid residual volumes in excess of 250 to 300 mL (McVary et al., 2011).

Tibial and Sacral Nerve Stimulation

Third-line treatments for overactive bladder should be considered for patients with symptoms that are refractory to first- and second-line therapies. Tibial and sacral nerve stimulation may be considered in selected patients, although both receive a grade C recommendation from AUA (Gormley et al., 2012). These interventions are thought to diminish abnormal reflex arcs associated with overactive bladder by modulating afferent signals from the bladder to the spinal cord.

Tibial nerve stimulation involves placement of a fine needle electrode near the tibial nerve in the area of the medial malleolus of the ankle, with a grounding pad placed near the heel. An electrical impulse is generated that travels up the tibial nerve to the sacral region. The procedure requires weekly 30-minute treatments for 12 weeks. In individuals sufficiently motivated to complete treatment, favorable short- and long-term improvement comparable or slightly better than with medications have been reported (Peters et al., 2013). Side effects are relatively minor and include local bleeding, mild pain, and skin irritation (Govier et al., 2001).

Sacral neuromodulation involves stimulation of the sacral nerves involved in the spinal reflex arc that controls bladder function. Patients initially have a temporary surface electrode placed to gauge response. If successful, they may elect to have a pulse generator implanted, usually in the upper outer buttock or abdomen. The most common complication is lead migration, which requires readjustment in 5% to 10% of patients. Although much of the research on sacral neuromodulation has been conducted in women with urinary and fecal incontinence, newer studies suggest that the procedure is effective in men with symptoms of overactive bladder (Johnsen et al., 2014).

CLINICAL PEARL

Second- and third-line therapies for bothersome storage LUTS include pharmacologic agents (antimuscarinics) and neuromodulation.

Complementary and Alternative Treatments

Several plant extracts (phytotherapeutic agents) are commonly used by men with LUTS related to BPH. Many use these over-the-counter preparations as dietary supplements and may fail to disclose their use to health care providers (Kennedy et al., 2008) as they do not consider them "medications." History taking should include all medications, over-the-counter preparations, alcohol intake, and smoking.

Serenoa repens is an abstract of the berry of the saw palmetto. It is the most commonly used agent and some evidence supports its use. Therapeutic effects of saw palmetto are most likely due to the same mechanisms as 5-alpha reductase inhibitors; anti-inflammatory and antiproliferative properties are also theorized (Avins & Bent, 2006). Other commonly used agents include the stinging nettle (*Urtica dioica*), extracts of the African plum tree (*Pygeum africanum*), pumpkin seed (*Cucurbita pepo*), South African star grass (*Hypoxis rooperi*), and rye pollen (*Secale cereale*) (Wilt et al., 2002). Most products contain a combination of agents of variable composition and strength. As with other agents that are not regulated by the FDA, there is little information about the quality of any given product and little unbiased evidence to support their benefit.

Empirical evidence on the efficacy of phytotherapeutic agents is mixed and the quality of studies is limited. Agents used singly or in combinations lack evidence based on robust randomized controlled trials with sufficiently long periods of follow-up. In addition, findings are often contradictory. For example, an early Cochrane Review on Serenoa repens (Wilt et al., 2002) suggested its positive effect on symptoms, while a later Cochrane Review indicated no beneficial effects (Tacklind et al., 2012).

CASE STUDY: PART 2

Mr. Jones has never had a workup for prostate health issues, but he is bothered by the nocturia and difficulty with his urinary stream. He does not initially offer specific concerns; however, further questioning reveals that he is worried about prostate cancer. His father died of prostate cancer at age 55. Further discussion results in Mr. Jones stating, "I want everything tested."

DISCUSSION

The decision to undergo PSA testing to screen for prostate cancer is controversial. The decision should be based on the age and race of the patient as well as individual risk factors such as a history of prostate cancer in the family. Mr. Jones' father died of prostate cancer at a young age, which suggests that Mr. Jones may be at high risk of developing prostate cancer.

PSA Testing

The primary purpose of PSA testing is to decrease mortality and morbidity associated with prostate cancer in asymptomatic men. The routine use of PSA testing in the United States began in the late 1980s and early 1990s. Prostate cancer death rates in the United States have decreased more than 40% in the period between the introduction of testing up until 2009 (Hayat et al., 2007); the degree to which this decrease should be directly attributed to PSA testing is highly controversial. Approximately 80% of the prostate cancers that are identified today are confined to the prostate gland. Although localized prostate cancer has a very high cure rate, important "if" and "when" questions about the progression of localized prostate cancers to clinically significant disease remain unanswered (Carroll et al., 2014). Newer recommendations suggest that routine screening may be extended to every 2 years (Cooperberg, 2014).

CLINICAL PEARL

PSA testing for prostate cancer is controversial; the decision to test should be based on age, race, and individual risk factors (such as family history).

Harms of PSA Testing

It is estimated that 1,400 men need to be screened with a PSA test in order to identify one case of prostate cancer. In cases that are detected, it is difficult to determine with any degree of certainty which cases will progress to clinically significant disease. Figure 8-10 illustrates the benefits and risks of PSA screening at the population level.

PSA results may lead to an overdiagnosis of prostate cancer, either due to false-positive results or due to the identification of indolent cancer that would never result in mortality or significant morbidity. The rate of overdiagnosis ranges from 23.5% to 42% (Draisma et al., 2003; Telesca et al., 2008).

Most men in the United States with elevated PSA levels elect to undergo a biopsy of the prostate. Complication rates associated with prostate biopsies are not insignificant. The 30-day risk of hospitalization is 4%, and three quarters of these hospitalizations are due to infection (Loeb et al., 2012; Nam et al., 2013). Infection risk due to antibiotic resistance is also an important consideration given that some men will experience multiple biopsies as part of a treatment plan for active surveillance to track disease progression or recurrence (Cohen et al., 2014).

Although consensus has not been reached, BPH is generally not thought to be associated with an increased risk of prostate cancer (Schenk et al., 2011). LUTS are weak predictors of prostate cancer. PSA values in men with LUTS and/or BPH are thought to be elevated in part due to chronic inflammation. No specific reference range for PSA values in men with LUTS has been established (Agnihotri et al., 2014).

Almost all of the research on the efficacy of screening has involved men in the age range of 50 to 69 years. Within this group, approximately 1,000 men need to be screened in order to prevent one cancer death with 10 years of testing (Schroder et al., 2009). The number needed to be screened may be less if prevention of death is evaluated over a longer period of time (Schroder et al., 2014).

It is of note that the U.S. Preventive Services Task Force recommends against PSA screening and gives the service a grade D recommendation. A grade D recommendation suggests that there is "moderate or high certainty that the service has no net benefit or that the harms outweigh the benefits" (Screening for Prostate Cancer, Topic Page. U.S. Preventive Services Task Force, 2012). Guidelines developed by the AUA recommend selective PSA screening (Carter et al., 2012), including biennial screening of men in the age range of 55 to 69 years if shared decision making is employed. Additional recommendations call for no screening of men age 70 and greater who have a life expectancy of <10 to 15 years (Wein et al., 2011).

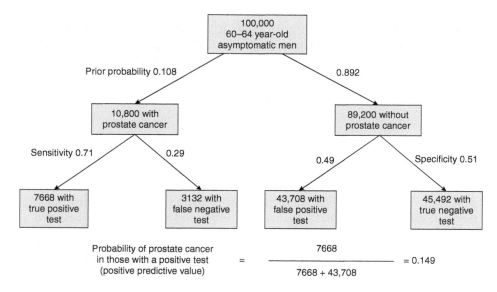

FIGURE 8-10. Benefits and risks of PSA testing in 1,000 men.

Screening should not be routinely recommended to men under the age of 54 without additional risk factors, such as a history of early prostate cancer in first-degree male relatives. For those at risk, counseling should be provided on an individual basis (Cooperberg, 2014). Special consideration may be given to men with a history of prostate cancer in first-degree relatives, especially if there was prostate cancer in multiple generations or a family history of early-onset prostate cancer. Although there is insufficient evidence, African American men may be at higher risk for prostate cancer at an earlier age (Carter et al., 2012). Population studies indicate that in black men, the relative risk of developing prostate cancer is 1.6 times greater than the relative risk for white men (Crawford, 2009). Black men are also at greater risk of being undertreated for prostate cancer (Pettaway et al., 2011).

Shared Decision Making about PSA Testing

Mr. Jones is concerned about the possibility of prostate cancer and elects to undergo PSA testing. Men who undergo PSA testing may be unwittingly committing themselves to a potentially unnecessary sequential series of tests if the PSA value falls within a suspicious range. Patients should be informed that they may be required to make a series of decisions based on the results of subsequent testing, which may include a transrectal ultrasound biopsy of the prostate and possibly prostatectomy. During this process, the man will have to live with the anxiety and stigma associated with diagnostic uncertainty.

Prostate cancer screening is psychologically burdensome for many men and their families. There is considerable distress associated with the decision-making process related to screening as well as with biopsy and treatment choices should the PSA level be elevated. One study found elevated rates of suicide and cardiovascular events associated with a new diagnosis of prostate cancer (Fang et al., 2010). Guidelines from the AUA recommend the use of shared decision-making strategies with men who are making testing and treatment decisions related to prostate cancer. A systematic review conducted by the AUA found high-quality evidence to support claims that shared decision making increased knowledge, reduced decisional conflict, and promoted greater involvement in decision making (Carter et al., 2012). Moreover, a meta-analysis involving 86 trials and 20,000 patients found that patients who used decision aids were able to better identify risk and make decisions that were consistent with their values (Stacey et al., 2014). Newer tools are being developed for patients such as Mr. Jones, who is at greater risk of developing prostate cancer due to his race and family history (Gwede et al., 2014).

Information discussed in the process of shared decision making should include the fact that although many men are diagnosed with prostate cancer, few will die from the disease. The man should understand the limitations of PSA testing, particularly the potential for overdiagnosis. He should understand that PSA values normally fluctuate and that up to 20% of elevated PSA values will return to normal levels within a year (Eastham et al., 2003). Finally, men should understand the risks associated with biopsies of the prostate. One third of all men will experience some type of mild to severe symptom following biopsy, including pain, fever, bleeding, infection, and problems urinating (Nam et al., 2013).

CLINICAL PEARL

Prostate cancer screening and decision making regarding biopsy and treatment are psychologically burdensome for men and their families; shared decision making is associated with reduced levels of patient distress.

Ideally, sexual partners of men who are considering testing or treatment for prostate cancer should be included in the shared decision-making process. The man should be encouraged to invite the sexual partner into all conversations. However, it should not be assumed that all men are comfortable including their sexual partners in the shared decision-making process (Shaw et al., 2013). Special consideration may need to be given to men who are sexually active but not in partnered relationships (Kazer et al., 2011).

CLINICAL PEARL

There is no absolute cutoff value for PSA that reliably distinguishes between presence and absence of prostate cancer or between low- and high-grade malignancies.

CASE STUDY: PART 3

Mr. Jones undergoes PSA testing and his PSA level is 3.5 ng/mL. He asks, "Does this mean that I have prostate cancer?"

DISCUSSION

The terms "normal" and "high" PSA level are misleading. PSA levels correlate with the probability that prostate cancer is present; however, there is no absolute cutoff value that assures the presence or absence of the disease. In addition, PSA levels alone are not sensitive in discriminating low- versus high-grade cancer.

As is the case with Mr. Jones, African Americans without prostate cancer have higher PSA values than their White counterparts. PSA values also increase with the size of the prostate and age of the male. The PSA value increases approximately 4% for each additional milliliter in prostate volume (Wein et al., 2011). Figure 8-11 illustrates the correlation between PSA levels and prostate cancer risk as confirmed by biopsy of the prostate. A clinical decision is required to differentiate among the various grades of prostate cancer.

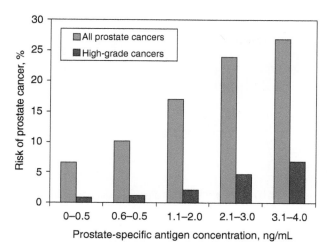

FIGURE 8-11 PSA levels and risk of prostate cancer.

that may be done prior to biopsy. Although a PSA value of >10 ng/mL suggests a clear need for biopsy in most men, the lower limit for performing routine biopsies is more complex. Men who are on 5-alpha reductase inhibitors should have their measured PSA value doubled in order to estimate the "true" value (Wein et al., 2011).

Initially, a PSA value of <4 ng/mL was considered the upper limit of normal; however, many clinicians are now using a threshold of 2.5 to 3.0 ng/mL. While this lower threshold increases the detection rate, it also increases the number of false-positive results and the detection of prostate cancers that are not clinically significant. It is generally recommended that PSA values be repeated in men who have an initial elevated reading as there is considerable variability in PSA values over time in some men (Wein et al., 2011). An algorithm to guide PSA testing and the decision to biopsy is presented in Figure 8-12.

Decision Making about Biopsy

The man and his significant other(s) should be involved in the decision making about proceeding to biopsy. The duty of the clinician is to try to convey an estimate of the risk of clinically significant prostate cancer based on testing

CLINICAL PEARL

A PSA higher than 10 ng/mL generally mandates biopsy; men on 5-alpha reductase inhibitors should have their PSA levels doubled to determine the true value.

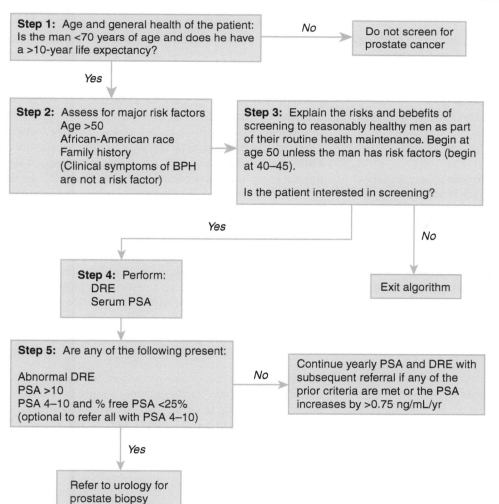

FIGURE 8-12. PSA and biopsy algorithm (note that many clinicians use a PSA cutoff of 2.3 to 3.0 ng/mL and not 4 ng/mL).

It is anticipated that additional clinical decision-making support tools will be developed so that the need for biopsy can be prevented or delayed. Recently, the U.S. Food and Drug Administration approved the Prostate Health Index (PHI), a composite score of tests that are now administered concurrently. The PHI score combines the following values: total PSA; free PSA, which is the fraction that is not protein bound and tends to be lower in men with prostate cancer; and pro-PSA, which is an isoform of PSA. The PHI score is more specific than the score from each individual test. The result is a decrease in false-positive rates in men with PSA values between 2 and 10 ng/mL. Results of randomized controlled trials indicate that use of the PHI may decrease the need for unnecessary biopsies by 7.6% (Catalona et al., 2011). The PHI may be particularly useful in evaluating obese men, who tend to have slightly lower PSA values (Abrate et al., 2014).

CLINICAL PEARL

The FDA has recently approved the use of the Prostate Health Index (PHI), which includes total PSA, free PSA, and pro-PSA; this combination is associated with lower false-positive rates and may reduce unnecessary biopsies.

Men who forgo immediate biopsy should be seen regularly for digital rectal exams and PSA testing. New findings or a significant increase in the PSA value should prompt further discussions with the patient. The rise in PSA value over 1 year is called the PSA velocity; an increase of more than 0.75 ng/mL usually triggers the need for a biopsy (Cooperberg, 2014).

Biopsy Procedure

The most common approach to prostate biopsy is transrectal, although a transperineal approach is occasionally used. Today, the transrectal biopsy of the prostate is performed with an ultrasound-guided needle. The ultrasound probe is introduced into the rectum to ensure that the needle is being inserted correctly into various sites within the prostate gland. Figure 8-13 illustrates this process.

All patients should have a urinalysis and urine culture prior to the biopsy to rule out UTI. If the urinalysis

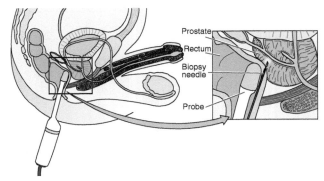

FIGURE 8-13. Transrectal ultrasound-guided biopsy.

suggests an infection and the culture is positive, the procedure should be postponed until the infection clears with an appropriate course of antibiotics.

Preparation for ultrasound-guided biopsy includes prophylactic antibiotics such as a fluoroquinolone. Enemas and other methods of rectal cleansing have not shown increased benefits beyond those provided by antibiotics (Zaytoun et al., 2011). Frequently, an anxiolytic medication is given. In addition to a topical anesthetic, clinicians may also administer ultrasound-guided regional blocks to improve comfort.

There is some evidence that patients on antiplatelet agents, such as low-dose aspirin or warfarin, are not at increased risk for bleeding from the biopsy procedure (Giannarini et al., 2007; Ihezue et al., 2005). Decisions to hold these medications must be individualized based on the risk of interrupting these therapies.

Risks associated with a biopsy of the prostate include infection, urethral and rectal bleeding, and hematospermia. Visible hematuria, which typically does not represent a significant complication, is common and self-limited. The rate of visible hematuria following a biopsy ranges from 10% to 84% (Loeb et al., 2013). Sepsis is a rare but potentially lethal complication of prostate biopsy, and postoperative instruction must include early signs of infection and how to contact the urologist should these develop. Clinicians should consider the possibility of postprocedure obstruction; thus, bladder ultrasound to estimate a postvoid residual should be performed in symptomatic patients.

CASE STUDY: PART 4

Mr. Jones returns a year later and a repeat PSA comes back with a level of 4.1 ng/mL. Mr. Jones elects to have a transrectal ultrasound and biopsy. The biopsy results indicate a Gleason score of 6. Mr. Jones is quite anxious. He states, "Tell me the truth; how much longer do I have to live?"

DISCUSSION

Each step in the workup of prostate cancer causes anxiety—undergoing the test, waiting for results, and wondering "why me?" The potential for subsequent decision making and further anxiety should be considered before engaging in testing. Shared decision making should be employed in each step of the workup. Mr. Jones and his significant other should be invited to share in the decision making about undergoing a biopsy.

Gleason Score

Prostate biopsy samples are analyzed under a microscope in order to assess the cellular architecture of the sample. Samples that closely resemble normal prostate tissue are given a score of 1 on the Gleason scale, and those that are bizarre or highly undifferentiated are given a score of 5. A different number of core samples may be obtained during the prostate biopsy. A higher number of samples increase both the sensitivity and the complication rates for the biopsy. The complication rates are 31.5% for 12 cores, 41.8% for 18 cores, and 57.4 % in 24 or more cores.

The Gleason score, an index of prostate cancer aggressiveness, is assigned by a pathologist, who grades each core sample on the 5-point Gleason scale that represents five histologic patterns of tumor gland formation and infiltration. Gleason grades range from 1 (highly differentiated tissue) to 5 (poorly differentiated tissue), with higher scores indicative of greater prostate cancer aggressiveness (Fig. 8-14).

CLINICAL PEARL

A number of samples are obtained on prostate biopsy, and each is scored according to the Gleason scale, which ranges from 1 (highly differentiated) to 5 (poorly differentiated); the Gleason score is obtained by adding the numbers for the most common and least common histologic patterns (e.g., 2 + 4 = 6). Scores of 6 or less suggest low risk for progression.

The pathologist determines the most prominent and least prominent histologic patterns among the core samples according to the Gleason scale that is illustrated above. The Gleason score is the sum of grades assigned to the most prominent and least prominent patterns. For example, if most of the core samples contain highly differentiated tissue that is close to normal, the pathologist assigns a grade of 1. If the least common pattern among core samples is slightly less differentiated tissue with a grade of 2, the Gleason score would be 1 + 2 = 3. The Gleason score is the first step in the diagnosis and staging of prostate cancer. A score of 6 or less suggests a low risk for cancer progression. A score of 7 suggests an intermediate risk for progression and a score of 8 to 10 a high risk for progression (Carroll et al., 2013).

Patients with low Gleason scores may elect to defer surgery or other treatments and engage in an active surveillance program, which involves a series of follow-up biopsies. Active surveillance may be appropriate for older men with cancers that are thought to be less aggressive. Younger men, particularly those with aggressive cancer (Gleason score of 8 to 10), will be advised to undergo prostatectomy or other first-line therapies when localized disease is suspected (Wein et al., 2011). Other first-line therapies for suspected localized disease include brachytherapy (the implantation of radioactive seeds in the prostate) and external beam radiation (Zerbib et al., 2008). Decision making regarding aggressive treatment for older men depends on the overall health, life expectancy, and man's preferences. Brachytherapy and external beam radiation are options for men with PSA values of <10, which suggests early, localized disease (Carroll et al., 2013).

It is important for Mr. Jones to remember that not all prostate cancers detected on biopsy are destined to become clinically significant disease. Biopsy results are used not only to determine whether prostate cancer is present but also to determine which cancers need immediate attention and which are unlikely to progress.

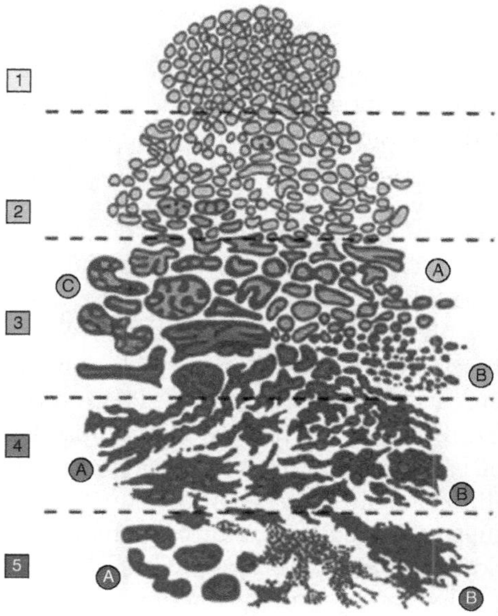

GLANDS

	Differentiation	Distribution
1	'Round,' lined by single layer of cuboidal cells	Close packed in rounded masses; definite edge
2	More variable in size and shape	Separated up to one gland diameter; 'loose' edge
3a	Irregular shape: medium to large size	Irregularly spaced apart; poorly defined 'edge'; surround normal structures
3b	Small to minute glands, not fused or 'chained'	
3c	Masses of cribriform or papillary epithelium with smooth outer surfaces	Very irregular spacing and distribution; no 'edge'; surround normal structures
4a	Ragged masses of fused glandular epithelium; bare tumor cells in stroma	Ragged infiltrating masses that overrun normal structures; No smooth surfaces against stroma
4b	Same as 4a; large clear cells	
5a	Smooth, cribriform to solid masses; often central necrosis 'comedocarcinoma'	Ragged infiltrating masses that infiltrate stroma fibers
5b	Anaplastic carcinoma with vacuoles and glands that suggest adenocarcinoma	

FIGURE 8-14. Gleason score for tissue biopsy cores.

Additional Diagnostic Workup

Although staging of prostate cancer is somewhat complex, the main consideration is whether the cancer is restricted to the prostate gland or whether it has spread by local extension to the surrounding tissue, including the seminal vesicles. More advanced prostate cancer spreads to the bone and lymphatic system with or without distant metastasis. If distant metastasis is present, it is most likely to occur in the lung and less commonly in the bladder, liver, and adrenal glands (Hess et al., 2006). The four stages of prostate cancer are described in Table 8-4 and illustrated in Figure 8-15.

> **CLINICAL PEARL**
>
> Advanced prostate cancer spreads to the bone and lymphatic system; distant metastases usually involve the lung, bladder, liver, and adrenal glands.

Decisions about additional testing to estimate the risk for nodal involvement can be based on both the Gleason score and PSA levels. Computerized tomography (CT) or

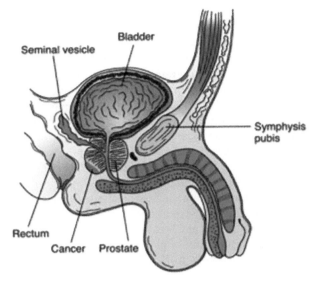

LOCAL CARCINOMA
T1-T2

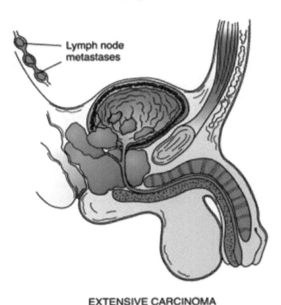

EXTENSIVE CARCINOMA
T3-T4

FIGURE 8-15. Progressive stages of prostate cancer.

magnetic resonance imaging (MRI) may be done in an attempt to identify local lymph node involvement; however, these diagnostic procedures typically have a low yield in patients with a PSA level of <20 ng/mL (Carroll et al., 2013). In fact, studies show that the risk of lymph node involvement is <20% in patients with PSA levels of <20 ng/mL (Scardino, 2005). Similarly, men with a PSA level of 20 ng/mL are at low risk for metastasis to the bone and thus derive little benefit from a bone scan unless clinical symptoms suggest the possibility of bone metastasis. In men who undergo prostatectomy, additional diagnostic and staging information can be obtained from the pathology report.

TABLE 8-4 Characteristics of the Stages of Prostate Cancer

Prostate Cancer Stage	Staging Characteristics	Staging*
1	Cancer is not found on digital rectal exam but may be detected on biopsy or as a result of tissue analysis obtained during other surgeries such as transurethral resection of the prostate (TURP). It is located only in the prostate gland.	T1N0M0 Small confined tumor No nodal involvement No metastasis
2	Can be detected on rectal exam but has not spread outside the prostate	T2N0M0 Somewhat larger confined tumor No nodal involvement No metastasis
3	Cancer has spread outside the prostate, perhaps to the seminal vesicles but no nodal involvement.	T3N0M0 Spread locally beyond the prostate (perhaps to seminal vesicles) No nodal involvement No metastasis
4	Extensive local spread with possible nodal involvement or metastasis	T4 or N1 or M1 Any of the following criteria: Extensive local tumor spread or any nodal involvement or any evidence of metastasis

*T, tumor size/characteristics; N, nodal spread; M, metastasis (0 = no; 1 = yes).

CASE STUDY: PART 5

Mr. Jones states, "I can't live with this thing inside me. I want it taken out." He undergoes a CT scan of the abdomen and pelvis, which is negative for regional lymph node involvement. There does not appear to be evidence of spread beyond the capsule of the prostate.

DISCUSSION

Thus far, test results suggest that Mr. Jones has localized prostate cancer. The computed tomography (CT) scan failed to detect grossly enlarged regional lymph nodes, which is consistent with a clinical picture of disease that is confined to the prostate gland. Although pelvic lymph node dissection (PLND) is the gold standard for confirmation of metastasis to regional nodes, it is generally reserved for men undergoing radical prostatectomy (U.S. Department of Health and Human Services [U.S. DHHS], 2014). A finding of regional lymph node enlargement on CT scan may have triggered a radionucleotide bone scan to detect metastasis to the bone, the most common site of distant tumor spread (U.S. DHHS, 2014). An MRI study, preferably with an endorectal coil, might also have been performed to evaluate the extent of disease beyond the prostate capsule (U.S. DHHS, 2014).

Based on his diagnostic workup, it is very likely that Mr. Jones has Stage 1 prostate cancer as defined by the American Joint Committee on Cancer's TNM classification system: clinically localized Stage T1–T2 disease,

PSA <10 ng/mL, Gleason ≤6, and no evidence of regional lymph node or distant metastasis (Edge et al., 2010). In fact, Stage 1 disease accounts for approximately 90% of all prostate cancers diagnosed annually in the United States (AUA, 2007; Catalona & Han, 2012). Although many Stage 1 prostate cancers remain relatively dormant, younger patients (age 50 to 60 years) with a normal life expectancy are encouraged to consider treatment (U.S. DHHS, 2014). Decision making about the pursuit of treatment should be a shared experience with clinicians and significant others. Physicians can assist with decision making by personalizing the patient's risk for disease progression based on clinical findings, including PSA level, highest/worst Gleason score of biopsy cores, clinical stage of biopsy cores, and disease burden, either the number or percent of biopsy cores with cancer (AUA, 2007). Family history, comorbidities, and values and preferences of the patient and his significant other(s) are also essential considerations in making a decision about treatment.

At age 58, Mr. Jones considers all of the above factors and decides that he wants his prostate "taken out." He is encouraged to learn about all of the standard treatment options for Stage 1 prostate cancer including expectant management, through either watchful waiting or active surveillance; radical prostatectomy; external beam radiation therapy (EBRT); and brachytherapy.

CLINICAL PEARL

Stage 1 prostate cancer (PSA <10 ng/mL, Gleason score ≤6, and localized disease) accounts for 90% of all prostate cancers diagnosed in the United States each year.

 ## Treatment Options for Prostate Cancer

Expectant Management

Watchful waiting and active surveillance are two distinct conservative approaches to prostate cancer treatment. Common to both approaches, however, is the individual's decision to defer immediate curative treatment (Catalona & Han, 2012). Evidence of the slow progression of Stage 1 prostate cancers may prompt men with a life expectancy of <10 to 15 years to defer immediate curative treatment. Younger men with a very small volume of cancer in their biopsies, as well as men whose quality of life is significantly threatened by the potential side effects of curative treatment, may also elect to defer immediate curative treatment (AUA, 2007).

Men with Stage 1 prostate cancer who elect *watchful waiting* make the decision to forego both immediate and future curative treatment. Instead, they are monitored for signs and symptoms of tumor progression and receive palliative care as needed to alleviate symptoms (AUA, 2007; Eastham & Scardino, 2012; U.S. DHHS, 2014).

In contrast, those who elect *active surveillance* make the decision to defer only immediate curative treatment. They are monitored regularly for signs of local tumor progression, at which point, curative treatment is initiated. Essentially, active surveillance is a *just-in-time* approach designed to spare men at low risk for disease progression from unnecessary treatment-related complications while preserving the ability to provide curative treatment if needed (AUA, 2007). At this time, protocols for active surveillance are arbitrary (AUA, 2007; NCI, 2014); however, experts suggest monitoring with a DRE and PSA quarterly or semiannually and biopsy annually or biennially (Catalona & Han, 2012). Research is needed to develop evidence-based selection criteria, monitoring procedures, and intervention trigger points for patients who choose active surveillance (Catalona & Han, 2012; Eastham & Scardino, 2012).

Existing evidence from studies of watchful waiting in those with Stage 1 prostate cancer reports 10-year prostate cancer-specific survival rates that range from 79% to 84% for all ages combined, 81% to 95% for younger patients (age <60 years), and 70% to 95% for older patients (age ≥60 years) (Eastham & Scardino, 2012; U.S. DHHS, 2014). Studies of active surveillance in Stage 1 prostate cancer patients are even more encouraging, with reports of prostate cancer-specific survival rates of 100% and 99% at 5- and 8-year follow-up, respectively, and range from 91% to 100% at 10 years (Eastham & Scardino, 2012; U.S. DHHS, 2014). A metastasis-free survival rate of 99% at 8-year follow-up has also been reported as well as 5- and 10-year progression-free survival rates of 64% and 50%, respectively (Eastham & Scardino, 2012).

Radical Prostatectomy

Radical prostatectomy is considered the gold standard treatment for Stage 1 prostate cancer because it offers the best probability of achieving both cancer control and quality of life (Catalona & Han, 2012; Schaeffer et al., 2012). The procedure can be performed either *openly*, through a single long incision in the lower abdomen or perineum, or *laparoscopically or robotically*, minimally invasive approaches in which the surgeon works with specialized instruments inserted through several small incisions in the abdomen.

Whether it is performed with open or laparoscopic technique, radical prostatectomy involves removal of the prostate gland, seminal vesicles, ampulla of the vas deferens, pelvic lymph nodes as indicated, and affected nerve bundles and surrounding tissue as necessary in order to obtain clean surgical margins (AUA, 2007). The prostatic portion of the proximal urethra, which contains smooth muscle essential to the involuntary continence mechanism, is inevitably removed with the prostate gland. The bladder neck, also comprised of smooth muscle that automatically contracts as the bladder fills, is reconstructed and anastamosed to the membranous portion of the proximal urethra. The membranous urethra is surrounded by the horseshoe-shaped external urethral sphincter or rhabdosphincter, a striated (skeletal) muscle under voluntary

control composed of about two-third Type 1 fatigue-resistant slow-twitch fibers (for "long-distance" contractions), and one-third Type 2 fast-twitch fibers (for short powerful contractions). Care is taken during surgery to incorporate urethral mucosa and submucosa rather than muscle tissue into the anastamosis so that recovery of urinary control is not delayed by traumatized or injured muscle (Dorey, 2006; Schaeffer et al., 2012).

There are two *open* approaches to radical prostatectomy: radical *retropubic* prostatectomy (RRP) and radical *perineal* prostatectomy (RPP). Of the two, the RRP is by far the most commonly performed procedure because it is better suited for the sparing of neurovascular bundles that are important to continence and erectile function (Sohn et al., 2013). The RRP also allows for intraoperative removal of pelvic lymph nodes for either diagnostic or cancer control purposes, which is not possible with the RPP. Compared to the RRP, however, the RPP is associated with shorter operative time, less blood loss, less postoperative pain, and quicker convalescence, although the risks of rectal injury and fecal incontinence are greater. Existing evidence suggests that RRP and RPP offer comparable odds of achieving the "trifecta" of ideal surgical outcomes: cancer control, preservation of urinary continence, and preservation of sexual function (Catalona & Han, 2012; Schaeffer et al., 2012; Sohn et al., 2013).

There are few contraindications to RPP other than conditions of the hip or spine that interfere with tolerance of the exaggerated lithotomy position required during surgery. In fact, RPP is often better suited than RRP for patients with a history of renal transplantation, herniorrhaphy with placement of synthetic mesh, morbid obesity, a large prostate (>100 g), or a narrow pelvis (Schaeffer et al., 2012).

Since the first minimally invasive laparoscopic radical prostatectomy in 1997, a juggernaut of technologic advances has fueled a revolution in the surgical treatment of Stage 1 prostate cancer (Su & Smith, 2012). Today, the vast majority of radical prostatectomies are performed *robotically* using the da Vinci robotic surgical system, with existing evidence that suggests reduced blood loss, less pain, faster recovery, and equivalent long-term outcomes compared to open approaches (Sohn et al., 2013; Su & Smith, 2012). There are just a few contraindications to robotic-assisted laparoscopic prostatectomy (RALP), including bleeding disorders as well as cardiopulmonary conditions and/or morbid obesity to the extent that the deep Trendelenburg position required during surgery would not be tolerated. Although neoadjuvant hormone therapy and prior complex lower abdominal or pelvic surgery are not absolute contraindications to RALP, they are challenging to surgeons because normal anatomy is distorted and adhesions are often present (Su & Smith, 2012).

The major complications of radical prostatectomy are urinary incontinence (UI) and erectile dysfunction (ED). Although most patients experience some degree of UI for several weeks or months following surgery, reports from high-volume centers indicate that more than 90% ultimately achieve "pad-free" control. Recovery of continence appears to be associated with age of the patient and expertise of the surgeon, with younger men (age <60 years) treated at high-volume centers demonstrating the best continence outcomes (Catalona & Han, 2012; Schaeffer et al., 2012; Su & Smith, 2012). In the realm of ED, partial erections begin in most patients during postoperative months 3 to 6 and may continue to improve for as long as 2 to 3 years (Catalona & Han, 2012; Hamilton & Mirza, 2014; Schaeffer et al., 2012). Similar to continence, recovery of erectile function appears to be associated with age of the patient as well as with preoperative erectile function, preservation of both neurovascular bundles, and era of surgery. In fact, a focus of current research is the evaluation of models that predict postprostatectomy ED based on factors such as age, body mass index, diabetes, hypertension, and the use of nerve-sparing procedures (Haskins et al., 2014).

Evidence is mixed with regard to recovery of potency following radical prostatectomy, due in part to imprecise and variable definitions of potency. For example, in one retrospective study based at a large treatment center, only 19.8% of men who underwent nerve-sparing prostatectomy were fully potent 5 years after surgery (Schiavina et al., 2014). Other evidence suggests that up to 85% of younger patients (ages 40 to 60) with normal preoperative erectile function and bilateral nerve-sparing surgery performed at high-volume centers will ultimately recover erections sufficient for penetration and intercourse, while expected recovery rates for older men (age >60) under the same circumstances would likely range from 50% to 75% (Catalona & Han, 2012; Schaeffer et al., 2012).

> **CLINICAL PEARL**
>
> The most common complications following radical prostatectomy are urinary incontinence (approximately 10% long term) and erectile dysfunction (approximately 15% to 50%, depending on age and potency prior to surgery).

Less prevalent complications of radical prostatectomy include urethral stricture, shortening of penile length, lymphedema, inguinal hernia, and fecal incontinence. Urethral stricture, typically at the anastamosed bladder neck, occurs in up to 10% of radical prostatectomy patients and is managed initially with simple dilatation. Strictures that are refractory to dilatation may require internal incision with or without endoscopic injection of glucocorticoids (Catalona & Han, 2012; Schaeffer et al., 2012). Shortening of penile length by an average of 1 to 2 cm has been reported in several studies and is probably related to removal of the prostatic urethra (American Cancer Society [ACS], 2014; U.S. DHHS, 2014). Although the change is noticeable to some men, no effect on penile function has been documented. Removal of lymph nodes carries the risk of lymphedema; however, it is a rare complication and usually responsive to physical therapy (ACS, 2014; Catalona & Han, 2012).

In contrast, observational studies document the occurrence of inguinal hernias in up to 21% of men within 2 years of radical prostatectomy, although this may represent a detection bias given the frequency of follow-up exams and/or diagnostic imaging in this population (ACS, 2014; Catalona & Han, 2012; U.S. DHHS, 2014). Finally, new-onset fecal incontinence is associated mostly with RPP and has been reported in up to 32% of RPP patients (Schaeffer et al., 2012; U.S. DHHS, 2014). Rectal urgency and small amounts of leakage are considered the most common symptoms; however, moderate- and large-volume leakage has been reported. Fecal incontinence is thought to resolve over time; however, gross underreporting to health care providers is suspected.

External Beam Radiation Therapy

External beam radiation therapy (EBRT) is a curative treatment for Stage 1 prostate cancer that is generally recommended to men who are poor surgical candidates for radical prostatectomy (AUA, 2007; U.S. DHHS, 2014). Inflammatory bowel disease and prior radiation therapy to the pelvis are the only contraindications to EBRT (AUA, 2007). Two types of EBRT are in use today: conformal and intensity modulated. Conformal radiation therapy (CRT) was introduced in the 1990s, when the capability of three-dimensional tumor visualization allowed delivery of a radiation beam that conformed to the shape of the treatment target and minimized the dose to surrounding normal tissue (D'Amico et al., 2012). Thus, the goal of CRT for Stage 1 prostate cancer is to maximize the dose of radiation delivered to the prostate while minimizing the dose delivered to unaffected surrounding tissue in the GU and lower GI tracts. Intensity-modulated radiation therapy (IMRT) is an advanced form of CRT that employs a set of radiation beams with changing intensities to deliver very high doses to target tissue and very low doses to surrounding normal tissue compared to conventional CRT (D'Amico et al., 2012). Studies are underway to determine dosage parameters that will maximize cancer control and minimize complications.

In patients with Stage 1 prostate cancer, EBRT is associated with a 5-year PSA failure-free survival rate of >85% as well as only a 5.6% risk of prostate cancer-specific mortality at 10 years following treatment (D'Amico et al., 2012). Complications of EBRT include GI, GU, and sexual dysfunctions that increase gradually as radiation accumulates in the body and generally decline over time as radioactivity dissipates. Compared to radical prostatectomy, rates of UI and early ED are lower with EBRT; however, short-term proctitis and fecal incontinence are common (U.S. DHHS, 2014). Current evidence suggests that IMRT enables the delivery of higher doses of radiation with lower rates of rectal bleeding compared to conventional CRT (D'Amico et al., 2012).

Urinary complications related to EBRT may present years after treatment and are poorly understood. Most rectal complications occur within 2 to 4 years of treatment, and a relationship between rectal complications, radiation dose, and degree of rectal tissue exposure has been demonstrated (D'Amico et al., 2012). ED appears to increase over time after EBRT, with rates of 39% to 53% reported within 5 years of treatment (D'Amico et al., 2012). EBRT is also associated with greater risks of bladder and other types of genitourinary cancer (U.S. DHHS, 2014).

Brachytherapy

Brachytherapy is a definitive treatment for Stage 1 prostate cancer that involves permanent placement of radioactive seeds into or near the tumor (AUA, 2007; D'Amico et al., 2012). Today, brachytherapy is performed as an outpatient procedure, during which radioactive seeds are implanted into interstitial prostate tissue via a closed transperineal approach guided by transrectal ultrasound or CT scanning.

Because image-guided interstitial brachytherapy is a relatively new procedure, long-term survival rates and quality of life outcomes have not yet been determined. However, 5- and 10-year recurrence rates among Stage 1 prostate cancer patients who were treated with modern interstitial brachytherapy range from 5% to 18%, which compare favorably with rates for EBRT and radical prostatectomy (D'Amico et al., 2012). Short-term urinary symptoms, including frequency, urgency, weak stream, and, less often, urinary retention (U.S. DHHS, 2014), occur for an average duration of 19 months and typically resolve by 36 months postimplantation (D'Amico et al., 2012). Rectal bleeding is associated with brachytherapy; however, it is generally minor, self-limiting, and correlated with both radiation dose and volume of highly radiated rectal tissue (D'Amico et al., 2012). Potency rates following brachytherapy are superior to those following EBRT and radical prostatectomy, although evidence suggests that potency declines over time in brachytherapy patients (D'Amico et al., 2012; U.S. DHHS, 2014). Not surprisingly, a direct relationship has been observed between postbrachytherapy ED and radiation dosage to the neurovascular bundles and penile bulb (D'Amico et al., 2012).

Postprostatectomy Stress UI

Pathophysiology

UI following radical prostatectomy likely results from trauma to the external urethral sphincter (rhabdosphincter). With surgical removal of the prostatic urethra and its smooth muscle fibers that contract automatically as the bladder fills, a greater portion of the burden for bladder control falls on the rhabdosphincter and its specialized striated muscle fibers that contract on command to control urination. Radical prostatectomy can traumatize the rhabdosphincter to the extent that it is incompetent to contract with sufficient strength or endurance to prevent urine leakage. Incompetence of the rhabdosphincter is typically temporary and often situational. In the case of stress UI, the rhabdosphincter lacks the capacity to remain sealed in situations when it is stressed by a sudden increase in intra-abdominal pressure.

Fortunately, in most cases, the rhabdosphincter recovers its strength and endurance naturally over time. In addition, limited evidence suggests that systematic exercise and training of pelvic floor musculature can expedite recovery of bladder control following radical prostatectomy (Robinson et al., 2009). The rhabdosphincter is surrounded by the levator ani, a skeletal muscle located deep within the pelvic floor that is comprised of pubococcygeus, ileococcygeus, and puborectalis segments. Together, these three segments of the levator ani form a muscular diaphragm that supports pelvic organs and resists downward thrusts associated with sudden increases in intra-abdominal pressure (Dorey, 2006). The

---

CASE STUDY: PART 6

Mr. Jones undergoes surgery and has an uncomplicated course. One month later, he returns stating that he is experiencing significant urinary incontinence, especially when he coughs or sneezes. The incontinence is a small amount each time. He has started wearing incontinence garments. He states, "I did this surgery so that I could have sex with my wife; now I can't even get close to her in bed due to worrying that I will wet the bed."

DISCUSSION

Postprostatectomy Urinary Incontinence
Mr. Jones has stress UI, a common occurrence following radical prostatectomy. Stress UI involves involuntary urine loss with coughing, sneezing, laughing, or other physical activities that cause pressure within the abdomen to rise.

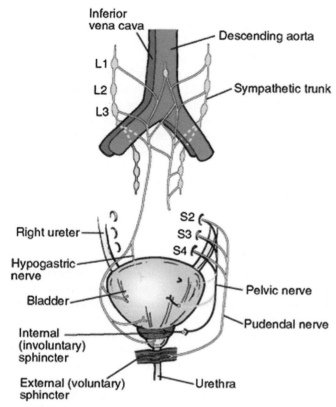

FIGURE 8-16. Innervation for the internal and external urethral sphincters.

pudendal nerve provides most of the innervation to both the levator ani and rhabdosphincter (Fig. 8-16). Thus, activation of the levator ani results in activation of the rhabdosphincter as well (Schaeffer et al., 2012).

> **CLINICAL PEARL**
>
> Incontinence S/P prostatectomy is usually due to damage to the striated sphincter muscle; pelvic floor muscle training may promote earlier resolution.

Pelvic Floor Muscle Rehabilitation

Despite conflicting evidence of overall efficacy (Campbell et al., 2012), systematic exercise of pelvic floor muscles continues to be the mainstay of behavioral interventions for UI following radical prostatectomy (Gray & Moore, 2009a; International Continence Society [ICS], 2013). Pelvic floor muscle rehabilitation essentially involves building awareness, strength, and endurance of the levator ani muscle in the following sequence: (1) mastery of muscle isolation; (2) development of muscle strength sufficient to sustain a contraction of 6 to 12 seconds followed by a relaxation period of equal time; (3) prescription of a daily exercise protocol of 20 to 50 contraction–relaxation repetitions, divided into two or three sets, and performed in sitting, standing, and reclining positions; and (4) neuromuscular re-education to achieve habitual contraction of

pelvic floor muscles prior to activities such as coughing, climbing stairs, or lifting a heavy object in order to prevent stress UI (Gray & Moore, 2009a). Adjuncts to pelvic floor muscle rehabilitation, including biofeedback, electrical stimulation, and passive electromagnetic stimulation, are sometimes employed; however, evidence is equivocal concerning their beneficial effects (Campbell et al., 2012).

Information for men about pelvic floor rehabilitation, including specific instructions for performing pelvic floor muscle exercise, is available online from the National Association for Continence (NAFC) (2013). Of note in this document is that improvement in bladder control is often seen within 6 weeks, but may take as long as 6 months. Similar information is available online from the Simon Foundation for Continence (2014), which additionally emphasizes the importance of ongoing exercise to maintain improvements in muscle function and bladder control.

Absorbent Products

Mr. Jones has started to wear an absorbent product, which is advisable, at least in public, until he is confident about bladder control. Most men benefit from professional guidance regarding product selection. A general rule of thumb for patients is to wear the smallest possible amount of product and to advance gradually to "product-free" living, starting with low-stake circumstances (e.g., around the house), as bladder control begins to return. A variety of absorbent products designed to fit the male pelvic floor are now on the market and all are not alike. An excellent overview of the basic types of absorbent products is available in Chapter 12 and from online sources such as NAFC (2014), which has a comprehensive directory of continence products and services that is updated annually and offered for a nominal fee (NAFC, n.d.). Chapter 12 is dedicated to continence products, and a Web site to assist in decision making on products is found at www.continenceproductadvisor.org.

Men should be encouraged to experiment with different product types and brands to maximize their satisfaction in terms of cost, comfort, absorbency, and availability. Meanwhile, national quality performance standards for adult disposable absorbent products have been developed and their implementation is underway (Muller & McInnis, 2013). Until bladder control is recovered, Mr. Jones should follow evidence-based best practice recommendations for skin care of incontinent patients, which essentially involves gentle cleansing of the perineum twice daily using either a no-rinse skin cleanser or warm water, followed by application of an emollient (Ripley, 2007).

Other Interventions

If Mr. Jones has stress UI that is refractory to pelvic floor muscle rehabilitation alone, pharmacologic, surgical, and alternative/complementary interventions are available. Pharmacologic agents that increase muscle tone in

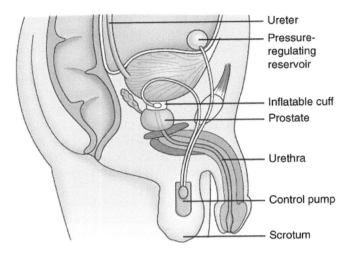

- Ureter
- Pressure-regulating reservoir
- Inflatable cuff
- Prostate
- Urethra
- Control pump
- Scrotum

FIGURE 8-17. Artificial urinary sphincter implant.

the bladder neck and rhabdosphincter include alpha-adrenergic agonists, such as pseudoephedrine; imipramine, a tricyclic antidepressant; and duloxetine, a serotonin and noradrenaline reuptake inhibitor (SNRI). All have demonstrated some beneficial effects on stress UI; however, all also have a side effect profile that restricts their use in many patients (Alhasso et al., 2005; Gray & Moore, 2009b; ICS, 2013; Mariappan et al., 2005).

Injection of a bulking agent, such as collagen, into the submucosa adjacent to the bladder neck is also helpful to many men; however, the need for repeated injections due to migration and/or disintegration of the bulking agent is a drawback (ICS, 2013; Schaeffer et al., 2012). Although required by few radical prostatectomy patients (Catalona & Han, 2012), two surgical interventions are considered definitive therapy for stress UI: implantation of a synthetic sling to restore urethral support and implantation of an artificial urinary sphincter (Fig. 8-17). Synthetic slings are associated with few complications, although success rates in men are lower than in women (ICS, 2013). While effective in eliminating stress UI, implantation of an artificial urinary sphincter is typically the option of last resort and can require surgical revision due to infection, erosion, or atrophy (Gray & Moore, 2009a; Silva et al., 2011).

In the realm of alternative/complementary therapy, the reputation of acupuncture as a credible treatment for stress UI is growing worldwide, as is its availability. The focus of therapy is to reinforce or redirect *qi*, the body's life force, to promote recovery of bladder function. Evidence of the efficacy of acupuncture in alleviating stress UI is, however, currently nil (Wang et al., 2013).

Sexuality and Erectile Dysfunction (ED)

ED is a devastating complication of radical prostatectomy for many men to the extent that some experience profound regret about undergoing prostate cancer treatment (Ratcliff et al., 2013). Mr. Jones' statement about wanting

to have sex with his wife but being unable to "even get close to her in bed" is a signal that he has sexual concerns and is ready to discuss them. Possible confusion related to his expectations of surgery (i.e., "I did this surgery so that I could have sex with my wife"), as well as his preoperative potency, should be explored so that realistic goals for rehabilitation and recovery can be established. The pathophysiology and clinical presentation of stress UI should also be discussed to temper his worry about wetting the bed. Of course, involving Mrs. Jones in all aspects of the evaluation and treatment plan is crucial to building trust; understanding the couple's relationship, concerns, and goals; and providing meaningful and effective guidance (Hamilton & Mirza, 2014; Monturo et al., 2001).

Pathophysiology

If Mr. Jones has new-onset ED, it is likely due to surgical removal or trauma to one or both neurovascular bundles during radical prostatectomy. The neurovascular bundles, located between two layers of fascia at 3 and 9 o'clock positions on the posterior aspect of the prostate, consist of (1) the cavernosal nerve, which is directly responsible for erectile function; (2) branches of the inferior vesical artery; and (3) venous vessels (Sooriakumaran et al., 2013). Trauma to the cavernosal nerve interferes with its ability to both transmit impulses and synthesize nitric oxide, the primary chemical that mediates smooth muscle relaxation and vasodilation of the penis that occurs during erection. When smooth muscle tissue of the penis is deprived of nitric oxide and blood flow, it becomes hypoxic and eventually fibrotic and collagenous, leading to irreversible ED. For this reason, treating ED is a priority following radical prostatectomy, with the goal of insuring adequate blood flow to the penis so that optimal erectile function returns (Albaugh, 2010).

CLINICAL PEARL

Treating ED is a priority following radical prostatectomy, with the goal of ensuring adequate blood flow to the penis so that optimal erectile function returns.

Interventions for ED

Prior to initiating treatment, baseline erectile and sexual function should be determined using a standardized tool such as the International Index of Erectile Function (Rosen et al., 2002). Periodic follow-up measurement with the same instrument as time and treatment progresses will be helpful in trending recovery of function and efficacy of treatment. Potency following radical prostatectomy is considered to be the ability to maintain an erection of sufficient rigidity for penetration and sexual intercourse with or without the aid of a PDE-5 inhibitor (Catalona & Han, 2012). To achieve this outcome, four types of treatment are currently available to men with postprostatectomy ED: oral phosphodiesterase type 5 (PDE-5) inhibitors, venous and vacuum constriction devices, prostaglandin E1 suppositories or injections, and a penile prosthesis.

Of these, oral PDE-5 inhibitors (i.e., sildenafil, vardenafil, tadalafil) are the first-line and most popular treatment. PDE-5 inhibitors contribute to the chemistry of erections by prolonging the bioavailability of guanosine monophosphate (cGMP), an organic molecule released during sexual arousal that induces smooth muscle relaxation and penile engorgement (Albaugh, 2010). Sufficient evidence exists to support the use of PDE-5 inhibitors to treat ED following radical prostatectomy with the expectation of success and few negative effects (Gontero et al., 2005; Hatzimouratidis, 2014; Miles et al., 2007; Pugh et al., 2014). Additional evidence suggests that on-demand rather than nightly dosing of PDE-5 inhibitors is most beneficial to recovery of sexual function (Catalona & Han, 2012; Schaeffer et al., 2012).

CLINICAL PEARL

PDE-5 inhibitors are first-line treatment for ED; if these are ineffective, other options include penile injection therapy, vacuum pump devices, and surgical placement of penile prostheses.

Despite their overall effectiveness, other treatments for ED are no match for the convenience, comfort, cost, and invisibility of PDE-5 inhibitors. Nevertheless, other treatments are often prescribed to supplement a PDE-5 inhibitor when its use alone is ineffective, or as viable alternatives when use of a PDE-5 inhibitor is either contraindicated (i.e., concurrent use of nitrate medications) or cautioned (i.e., concurrent use of alpha blocker medications, renal impairment, or selected heart conditions) (Albaugh, 2010). Noninvasive venous and vacuum constriction devices are used externally on the penis to generate and/or prolong an erection, but are contraindicated in men with a history of priapism, sickle cell anemia, or bleeding disorders (Albaugh, 2010).

Prostaglandin E1, a vasoactive medication either injected or inserted into the penis as a suppository, produces penile engorgement with a high degree of reliability. Injections, in which prostaglandin E1 may be combined with either papaverine or phentolamine, are far superior to suppositories in producing erections sufficient for vaginal intercourse (Montorsi et al., 1997); however, a significant number of men discontinue their use due to reluctance to inject a substance into the penis (Nelson et al., 2013). Intraurethral pain and burning in proportion to dose are common side effects of prostaglandin E1 therapy, albeit rarely serious (Albaugh, 2010; Montorsi et al., 1997; Urciuoli et al., 2004).

The most invasive treatment for ED is the implanted penile prosthesis, the oldest treatment for ED. Currently, penile implants are associated with high patient satisfaction and low rates of mechanical failure and infection, but are the option of last resort since the implant can cause permanent damage to erectile tissue (Albaugh, 2010; Montague & Angermeier, 2000).

Finally, psychosocial interventions have an important role in treating men with ED following radical prostatectomy. Evidence suggests that focused sex group therapy, including psychoeducational and/or psychotherapeutic approaches, can improve ED (Melnik et al., 2007). Evidence also suggests that psychosocial interventions, including one or a combination of cognitive–behavioral, psychoeducational, supportive, and counseling approaches, have a short-term positive impact on knowledge about prostate cancer as well as both physical and cancer-specific dimensions of quality of life (McDonough & Pemberton, 2013). A variety of individual, group, and online psychosocial support programs for prostate cancer patients, their families, and their caregivers are offered by the American Cancer Society (www.cancer.org), UsTOO International (www.ustoo.org), and the Prostate Cancer Foundation (www.pcf.org).

Conclusion

This chapter has addressed male voiding dysfunction. LUTS and BPH are common issues that become more prevalent with age. Symptoms may be modified with first-line strategies such as fluid management and moderation or elimination of caffeine and alcohol intake. In addition, a healthy diet and routine exercise can contribute to symptom reduction. Risk factors for prostate cancer include a direct relative (father, brother) with the disease and African American heritage. Screening for prostate cancer remains controversial as the test can result in false positives and unnecessary biopsies; the decision to screen should be an informed one and should involve both the individual and his physician. Treatment options for early stage prostate cancer include surgery or radiotherapy; treatment of later stages with extension into the prostatic capsule involves radiotherapy. The most common side effects of surgery are erectile dysfunction and urinary incontinence, and behavioral/medical management of these problems should begin early in the recovery period; any surgical intervention is delayed until 6 to 12 months following surgery since spontaneous recovery can continue for several months postoperatively. Adverse effects of radiation therapy include proctitis, urethral strictures, and radiation cystitis; these complications typically develop gradually over the weeks and months following treatment and are treated conservatively. A key element of nursing management for the individual with prostate cancer and his significant other(s) is ongoing education and support.

REFERENCES

Abrams, P., Cardozo, L., Khoury, S., et al. (2013). *Incontinence: 5th International Consultation on Incontinence*. Paris, London: ICUD-EAU. ISBN: 978-9953-493-21-3.

Abrams, P., Chapple, C., Khoury, S., et al. (2009). Evaluation and treatment of lower urinary tract symptoms in older men. *Journal of Urology, 181*(4), 1779–1787.

Abrate, A., Lazzeri, M., Lughezzani, G., et al. (2014). Clinical performance of Prostate Health Index (PHI) for prediction of prostate cancer in obese men: Data from a multicenter European prospective study PROMEtheuS project. *BJU International*. Advance online publication. doi: 10.1111/bju.12907.

Agnihotri, S., Mittal, R. D., Kapoor, R., et al. (2014). Asymptomatic prostatic inflammation in men with clinical BPH and erectile dysfunction affects the positive predictive value of prostate-specific antigen. *Urologic Oncology*. Advance online publication. doi: 10.1016/j.urolonc.2014.03.004.

Albaugh, J. A. (2010). Addressing and managing erectile dysfunction after prostatectomy for prostate cancer. *Urologic Nursing, 30*(3), 167–177.

Alhasso, A., Glazener, C. M. A., Pickard, R., et al. (2005). Adrenergic drugs for urinary incontinence in adults (review). *Cochrane Database of Systematic Reviews, 3*. Article No.: CD001842. doi: 10.1002/14651858.CD001842.pub.2.

American Cancer Society. (2014). *Treating Prostate Cancer Topics: Surgery for Prostate Cancer*. http://www.cancer.org/cancer/prostatecancer/detailedguide/prostate-cancer-treating-surgery

American Urological Association. (2007). *Guideline for the Management of Clinically Localized Prostate Cancer: 2007 Update*. http://www.auanet.org/education/guidelines/prostate-cancer.cfm

Amjadi, M., Madaen, S. K., & Pour-Moazen, H. (2006). Uroflowmetry findings in patients with bladder outlet obstruction symptoms in standing and crouching positions. *Urology Journal, 3*(1), 49–53.

Athanasopoulos, A. (2011). The pharmacotherapy of overactive bladder. *Expert Opinion on Pharmacotherapy, 12*(7), 1003–1005. doi: 10.1517/14656566.2011.554397.

AUA Guideline on Management of Benign Prostatic Hyperplasia. (2003). Chapter 1: Diagnosis and treatment recommendations. *Journal of Urology, 170*(2 Pt 1), 530–547. doi: 10.1097/01.ju.0000078083.38675.79.

Avins, A. L., & Bent, S. (2006). Saw palmetto and lower urinary tract symptoms: What is the latest evidence? *Current Urology Reports, 7*(4), 260–265.

Barry, M. J., Fowler, F. J., O'Leary, M.P., et al. (1992). The American Urological Association symptom index for benign prostatic hyperplasia. The Measurement Committee of the American Urological Association. *Journal of Urology, 148*(5), 1549–1557.

Brajtbord, J. S., Punnen, S., Cowan, J. E., et al. (2014). Age and baseline quality of life at radical prostatectomy—who has the most to lose? *Journal of Urology, 192*(2), 396–401. doi: 10.1016/j.juro.2014.02.045.

Bryant, C. M., Dowell, C. J., & Fairbrother, G. (2002). Caffeine reduction education to improve urinary symptoms. *British Journal of Nursing, 11*(8), 560–565.

Burgio, K. L. (2013). Update on behavioral and physical therapies for incontinence and overactive bladder: The role of pelvic floor muscle training. *Current Urology Reports, 14*(5), 457–464. doi: 10.1007/s11934-013-0358-1.

Campbell, S. E., Glazener, C. M. A., Hunter, K. F., et al. (2012). Conservative management for post-prostatectomy urinary incontinence. *Cochrane Database of Systematic Reviews, 1*. Article No.: CD001843. doi: 10.1002/14651858. CD001843.pub4.

Carlson, B. W., & Palmer, M. H. (2014). Nocturia in older adults: Implications for nursing practice and aging in place. *Nursing Clinics of North America, 49*(2), 233–250. doi: 10.1016/j.cnur.2014.02.009.

Carroll, P. R., Albertsen, P., Greene, K., et al. (2013). *PSA Testing for the Pretreatment Staging and Posttreatment Management of Prostate Cancer: 2013 Revision of 2009 Best Practice Statement*. http://www.auanet.org/education/guidelines/prostate-specific-antigen.cfm

Carroll, P. R., Parsons, J. K., Andriole, G., et al. (2014). Prostate cancer early detection, version 1.2014. *Journal of the National Comprehensive Cancer Network, 12*(9), 1211–1219.

Carter, B. H., Albertsen, C., Barry, M. J., et al. (2012). *Early Detection of Prostate Cancer: AUA Guideline*. http://www.auanet.org/education/guidelines/prostate-cancer-detection.cfm

Catalona, W. J., & Han, M. (2012). Definitive therapy for localized prostate cancer: An overview. In A. J. Wein, L. R. Kavoussi, A. C. Novick, et al. (Eds.), *Campbell-Walsh urology* (10th ed., pp. 2771–2788.e6). Philadelphia, PA: Elsevier.

Catalona, W. J., Partin, A. W., Sanda, M. G., et al. (2011). A multicenter study of [−2]pro-prostate specific antigen combined with prostate specific antigen and free prostate specific antigen for prostate cancer detection in the 2.0 to 10.0 ng/ml prostate specific antigen range. *Journal of Urology, 185*(5), 1650–1655. doi: 10.1016/j.juro.2010.12.032.

Cellek, S., Cameron, N. E., Cotter, M. A., et al. (2014). Microvascular dysfunction and efficacy of PDE5 inhibitors in BPH-LUTS. *Nature Reviews Urology, 11*(4), 231–241. doi: 10.1038/nrurol.2014.53.

Chapple, C. (2014). Chapter 2: Pathophysiology of neurogenic detrusor overactivity and the symptom complex of "overactive bladder". *Neurourology and Urodynamics, 33*(Suppl 3), s6–s13. doi: 10.1002/nau.22635.

Chin, P. T., Bolton, D. M., Jack, G., et al. (2012). Prostatic urethral lift: Two-year results after treatment for lower urinary tract symptoms secondary to benign prostatic hyperplasia. *Urology, 79*(1), 5–11. doi: 10.1016/j.urology.2011.10.021.

Cohen, J. E., Landis, P., Trock, B. J., et al. (2014). Fluoroquinolone resistance in the rectal carriage of men in an active surveillance cohort: Longitudinal analysis. *Journal of Urology*. Advance online publication. doi: 10.1016/j.juro.2014.08.008.

Cooperberg, M. R. (2014). Implications of the new AUA guidelines on prostate cancer detection in the U.S. *Current Urologic Reports, 15*(7), 420. doi: 10.1007/s11934-014-0420-7.

Crawford, E. D. (2009). Understanding the epidemiology, natural history, and key pathways involved in prostate cancer. *Urology, 73*(5 Suppl), S4–S10. doi: 10.1016/j.urology.2009.03.001.

D'Amico, A. V., Crook, J. M., Beard, C. J., et al. (2012). Radiation therapy for prostate cancer. In A. J. Wein, L. R. Kavoussi, A. C. Novick, et al. (Eds.), *Campbell-Walsh urology* (10th ed., pp. 2850–2872.e6). Philadelphia, PA: Elsevier.

Dorey, G. (2006). *Pelvic dysfunction in men: Diagnosis and treatment of male incontinence and erectile dysfunction*. West Sussex, UK: John Wiley & Sons, Ltd.

Draisma, G., Boer, R., Otto, S. J., et al. (2003). Lead times and overdetection due to prostate-specific antigen screening: Estimates from the European Randomized Study of Screening for Prostate Cancer. *Journal of the National Cancer Institute, 95*(12), 868–878.

Eastham, J. A., Kattan, M. W., Riedel, E., et al. (2003). Variations among individual surgeons in the rate of positive surgical margins in radical prostatectomy specimens. *Journal of Urology, 170*(6 Pt 1), 2292–2295. doi: 10.1097/01.ju.0000091100.83725.51.

Eastham, J. A., & Scardino, P. T. (2012). Expectant management of prostate cancer. In A. J. Wein, L. R. Kavoussi, A. C. Novick, et al. (Eds.), *Campbell-Walsh urology* (10th ed., pp. 2789–2800.e2). Philadelphia, PA: Elsevier.

Edge, S. B., Byrd, D. R., Compton, C. C., et al. (Eds.). (2010). *AJCC cancer staging manual* (7th ed.). New York, NY: Springer.

Fang, F., Keating, N. L., Mucci, L. A., et al. (2010). Immediate risk of suicide and cardiovascular death after a prostate cancer diagnosis: Cohort study in the United States. *Journal of the National Cancer Institute, 102*(5), 307–314. doi: 10.1093/jnci/djp537.

Foster, S. A., Annunziata, K., Shortridge, E. F., et al. (2013). Erectile dysfunction with or without coexisting benign prostatic hyperplasia in the general US population: Analysis of US National Health and Wellness Survey. *Current Medical Research and Opinion, 29*(12), 1709–1717. doi: 10.1185/03007995.2013.837385.

Fwu, C. W., Kirkali, Z., McVary, K. T., et al. (2014). Cross-sectional and longitudinal associations of sexual function with lower urinary tract symptoms in men with benign prostatic hyperplasia. *Journal of Urology.* Advance online publication. doi: 10.1016/j.juro.2014.08.086.

Gacci, M., Corona, G., Salvi, M., et al. (2012). A systematic review and meta-analysis on the use of phosphodiesterase 5 inhibitors alone or in combination with alpha-blockers for lower urinary tract symptoms due to benign prostatic hyperplasia. *European Urology, 61*(5), 994–1003. doi: 10.1016/j.eururo.2012.02.033.

Giannarini, G., Mogorovich, A., Valent, F., et al. (2007). Continuing or discontinuing low-dose aspirin before transrectal prostate biopsy: Results of a prospective randomized trial. *Urology, 70*(3), 501–505. doi: 10.1016/j.urology.2007.04.016.

Gontero, P., Fontana, F., Zitella, A., et al. (2005). A prospective evaluation of efficacy and compliance with a multistep treatment approach for erectile dysfunction in patients after non-nerve sparing radical prostatectomy. *BJU International, 95*(3), 359–365. doi: 10.1111/j.1464-410X.2005.05300.x.

Gormley, E. A., Lightner, D. J., Burgio, K. L., et al. (2012). Diagnosis and treatment of overactive bladder (non-neurogenic) in adults: AUA/SUFU guideline amendment. *Journal of Urology, 188*(6 Suppl), 2455–2463. doi: 10.1016/j.juro.2012.09.079.

Govier, F. E., Litwiller, S., Nitti, V., et al. (2001). Percutaneous afferent neuromodulation for the refractory overactive bladder: Results of a multicenter study. *Journal of Urology, 165*(4), 1193–1198.

Gray, M., & Moore, K. N. (2009a). Urinary incontinence. In M. Gray & K. N. Moore (Eds.), *Urologic disorders: Adult and pediatric care* (Chapter 6, pp. 119–159). St. Louis, MO: Elsevier.

Gray, M., & Moore, K. N. (2009b). Surgical procedures. In M. Gray & K. N. Moore (Eds.), *Urologic disorders: Adult and pediatric care* (Chapter 11, pp. 292–340). St. Louis, MO: Elsevier.

Gwede, C. K., Davis, S. N., Wilson, S., et al. (2014). Perceptions of prostate cancer screening controversy and informed decision making: Implications for development of a targeted decision aid for unaffected male first-degree relatives. *American Journal of Health Promotion.* Advance online publication. doi: 10.4278/ajhp.130904-QUAL-463.

Hakimi, A. A., Faleck, D. M., Sobey, S., et al. (2012). Assessment of complication and functional outcome reporting in the minimally invasive prostatectomy literature from 2006 to the present. *BJU International, 109*(1), 26–30; discussion 30. doi: 10.1111/j.1464-410X.2011.10591.x.

Hamilton, Z., & Mirza, M. (2014). Post-prostatectomy erectile dysfunction: Contemporary approaches from a US perspective. *Research and Reports in Urology, 6*, 35–41. doi: 10.2147/rru.s39560.

Hashim, H., & Abrams, P. (2008). How should patients with an overactive bladder manipulate their fluid intake? *BJU International, 102*(1), 62–66. doi: 10.1111/j.1464-410X.2008.07463.x.

Haskins, A. E., Han, P. K., Lucas, F. L., et al. (2014). Development of clinical models for predicting erectile function after localized prostate cancer treatment. *International Journal of Urology.* Advance online publication. doi: 10.1111/iju.12566.

Hatzimouratidis, K. (2014). A review of the use of tadalafil in the treatment of benign prostatic hyperplasia in men with and without erectile dysfunction. *Therapeutic Advances in Urology, 6*(4), 135–147. doi: 10.1177/1756287214531639.

Hayat, M. J., Howlader, N., Reichman, M. E., et al. (2007). Cancer statistics, trends, and multiple primary cancer analyses from the Surveillance, Epidemiology, and End Results (SEER) Program. *The Oncologist, 12*(1), 20–37. doi: 10.1634/theoncologist.12-1-20.

Hess, K. R., Varadhachary, G. R., Taylor, S. H., et al. (2006). Metastatic patterns in adenocarcinoma. *Cancer, 106*(7), 1624–1633. doi: 10.1002/cncr.21778.

Ihezue, C. U., Smart, J., Dewbury, K. C., et al. (2005). Biopsy of the prostate guided by transrectal ultrasound: Relation between warfarin use and incidence of bleeding complications. *Clinical Radiology, 60*(4), 459–463; discussion 457–458. doi: 10.1016/j.crad.2004.10.014.

International Continence Society. (2013). *ICS Factsheets(2013 Edition): Stress Urinary Incontinence.* http://www.ics.org/Documents/Documents.aspx?DocumentID=2172

Irwin, D. E., Milsom, I., Hunskaar, S., et al. (2006). Population-based survey of urinary incontinence, overactive bladder, and other lower urinary tract symptoms in five countries: Results of the EPIC study. *European Urology, 50*(6), 1306–1314; discussion 1314–1305. doi: 10.1016/j.eururo.2006.09.019.

Johnsen, N. V., Osborn, D. J., & Dmochowski, R. R. (2014). The role of electrical stimulation techniques in the management of the male patient with urgency incontinence. *Current Opinion in Urology, 24*(6), 560–565. doi: 10.1097/mou.0000000000000108.

Jones, C., Hill, J., & Chapple, C. (2010). Management of lower urinary tract symptoms in men: Summary of NICE guidance. *British Medical Journal, 340*, c2354. doi: 10.1136/bmj.c2354.

Kacker, R., Lay, A., & Das, A. (2013). Electrical and mechanical office-based neuromodulation. *Urologic Clinics of North America, 40*(4), 581–589. doi: 10.1016/j.ucl.2013.07.002.

Kazer, M. W., Harden, J., Burke, M., et al. (2011). The experiences of unpartnered men with prostate cancer: A qualitative analysis. *Journal of Cancer Survivorship, 5*(2), 132–141. doi: 10.1007/s11764-010-0157-3.

Kennedy, J., Wang, C. C., & Wu, C. H. (2008). Patient disclosure about herb and supplement use among adults in the US. *Evidence-Based Complementary and Alternative Medicine, 5*(4), 451–456. doi: 10.1093/ecam/nem045.

Kumar, S. M. (2007). Rapid communication: Holmium laser ablation of large prostate glands: An endourologic alternative to open prostatectomy. *Journal of Endourology, 21*(6), 659–662. doi: 10.1089/end.2006.0283.

Lee, R. K., Chung, D., Chughtai, B., et al. (2012). Central obesity as measured by waist circumference is predictive of severity of lower urinary tract symptoms. *BJU International, 110*(4), 540–545. doi: 10.1111/j.1464-410X.2011.10819.x.

Lee, S. H., & Lee, J. Y. (2014). Current role of treatment in men with lower urinary tract symptoms combined with overactive bladder. *Prostate International, 2*(2), 43–49. doi: 10.12954/pi.14045.

Loeb, S., van den Heuvel, S., Zhu, X., et al. (2012). Infectious complications and hospital admissions after prostate biopsy in a European randomized trial. *European Urology, 61*(6), 1110–1114. doi: 10.1016/j.eururo.2011.12.058.

Loeb, S., Vellekoop, A., Ahmed, H. U., et al. (2013). Systematic review of complications of prostate biopsy. *European Urology, 64*(6), 876–892. doi: 10.1016/j.eururo.2013.05.049.

Mariappan, P., Alhasso, A. A., Grant, A., et al. (2005). Serotonin and noradrenaline reuptake inhibitors (SNRI) for stress urinary incontinence in adults (Review). *Cochrane Database of Systematic Reviews, 3.* Article No.: CD004742. doi: 10.1002/14651858.CD004742.pub.2.

McDonough, K. S., & Pemberton, M. (2013). Evaluation and development of an ED management model: An effort to optimize patient-centered care. *Journal of Emergency Nursing, 39*(5), 485–490.

McVary, K. T., Roehrborn, C., Avins, A. L., et al. (2010). *American Urological Association guideline: Management of benign prostatic hyperplasia (BPH).* https://www.auanet.org/education/guidelines/benign-prostatic-hyperplasia.cfm

McVary, K. T., Roehrborn, C. G., Avins, A. L., et al. (2011). Update on AUA guideline on the management of benign prostatic hyperplasia. *Journal of Urology, 185*(5), 1793–1803. doi: 10.1016/j.juro.2011.01.074.

Melnik, T., Soares, B., & Nasello, A. G. (2007). Psychosocial interventions for erectile dysfunction. *Cochrane Database of Systematic Reviews, 3.* Article No.: CD004825. doi: 10.1002/14651858.CD004825.pub.2.

Miles, C., Candy, B., Jones, L., et al. (2007). Interventions for sexual dysfunction following treatments for cancer. *Cochrane*

Database of Systematic Reviews, 4. Article No.: CD005540. doi: 10.1002/14651858. CD005540.pub2.

Montague, D. K., & Angermeier, K. W. (2000). Current status of penile prosthesis implantation. *Current Urology Reports, 1*(4), 291–296.

Montorsi, F., Guazzoni, G., Strambi, L. F., et al. (1997). Recovery of spontaneous erectile function after nerve-sparing radical retropubic prostatectomy with and without early intracavernous injections of alprostadil: Results of a prospective, randomized trial. *Journal of Urology, 158*(4), 1408–1410.

Monturo, C. A., Rogers, P. D., Coleman, M., et al. (2001). Beyond sexual assessment: Lessons learned from couples post radical prostatectomy. *Journal of the American Academy of Nurse Practitioners, 13*(11), 511–516.

Muller, N., & McInnis, E. (2013). The development of national quality performance standards for disposable absorbent products for adult incontinence. *Ostomy Wound Management, 59*(9), 40–55.

Nam, R. K., Saskin, R., Lee, Y., et al. (2013). Increasing hospital admission rates for urological complications after transrectal ultrasound guided prostate biopsy. *Journal of Urology, 189*(1 Suppl), S12–S17; discussion S17–S18. doi: 10.1016/j.juro.2012.11.015.

National Association for Continence. (2013). *Pelvic muscle exercises.* http://www.nafc.org/bladder-bowel-health/types-of-incontinence/stress-incontinence/pelvic-muscle-exercises/

National Association for Continence. (2014). *Absorbent products.* http://www.nafc.org/find-a-product/absorbent-products/

National Association for Continence. (n.d.). *Resource guide: Products and services for incontinence.* http://www.nafc.org/online-store/consumer-booklets-and-kits/nafc-educational-booklets/resource-guide-products-and-services-for-incontinence/

Natalin, R., Lorenzetti, F., & Dambros, M. (2013). Management of OAB in those over age 65. *Current Urology Reports, 14*(5), 379–385. doi: 10.1007/s11934-013-0338-5.

Nelson, C. J., Hsiao, W., Balk, E., et al. (2013). Injection anxiety and pain in men using intracavernosal injection therapy after radical pelvic surgery. *The Journal of Sexual Medicine, 10*(10), 2559–2565. doi: 10.1111/jsm.12271.

Otsuki, H., Kuwahara, Y., Kosaka, T., et al. (2014). Sufficient volume ablation with photoselective vaporization of the prostate delivers 5-year durability and improves symptom relief for larger prostates. *Journal of Endourology.* Advance online publication. doi: 10.1089/end.2014.0466.

Parsons, J. K., Bergstrom, J., Silberstein, J., et al. (2008). Prevalence and characteristics of lower urinary tract symptoms in men aged > or = 80 years. *Urology, 72*(2), 318–321. doi: 10.1016/j.urology.2008.03.057.

Peters, K. M., Carrico, D. J., MacDiarmid, S. A., et al. (2013). Sustained therapeutic effects of percutaneous tibial nerve stimulation: 24-month results of the STEP study. *Neurourology and Urodynamics, 32*(1), 24–29. doi: 10.1002/nau.22266.

Pettaway, C. A., Lamerato, L. E., Eaddy, M. T., et al. (2011). Benign prostatic hyperplasia: Racial differences in treatment patterns and prostate cancer prevalence. *BJU International, 108*(8), 1302–1308. doi: 10.1111/j.1464-410X.2010.09991.x.

Poyhonen, A., Hakkinen, J. T., Koskimaki, J., et al. (2014). Natural course of lower urinary tract symptoms in men not requiring treatment—a 5-year longitudinal population-based study. *Urology, 83*(2), 411–415. doi: 10.1016/j.urology.2013.10.003.

Pugh, T. J., Mahmood, U., Swanson, D. A., et al. (2014). Sexual potency preservation and quality of life after prostate brachytherapy and low-dose tadalafil. *Brachytherapy.* Advance online publication. doi: 10.1016/j.brachy.2014.08.045.

Raheem, O. A., & Parsons, J. K. (2014). Associations of obesity, physical activity and diet with benign prostatic hyperplasia and lower urinary tract symptoms. *Current Opinion in Urology, 24*(1), 10–14. doi: 10.1097/mou.0000000000000004.

Rassweiler, J., Teber, D., Kuntz, R., et al. (2006). Complications of transurethral resection of the prostate (TURP)—incidence, management, and prevention. *European Urology, 50*(5), 969–979; discussion 980. doi: 10.1016/j.eururo.2005.12.042.

Ratcliff, C. G., Cohen, L., Pettaway, C. A., et al. (2013). Treatment regret and quality of life following radical prostatectomy. *Supportive Care in Cancer, 21*(12), 3337–3343. doi: 10.1007/s00520-013-1906-4.

Ripley, K. R. (2007). Skin care in patients with urinary and faecal incontinence. *Primary Health Care, 17*(4), 29–34.

Robinson, J. P., Weiss, R., Avi-Itzhak, T., et al. (2009). Pilot-testing of a theory-based pelvic floor training intervention for radical prostatectomy patients [abstract]. *Neurourology and Urodynamics, 28*(7), 682–683.

Roehrborn, C. G., Gange, S. N., Shore, N. D., et al. (2013). The prostatic urethral lift for the treatment of lower urinary tract symptoms associated with prostate enlargement due to benign prostatic hyperplasia: The L.I.F.T. study. *Journal of Urology, 190*(6), 2161–2167.

Rosen, R., Altwein, J., Boyle, P., et al. (2003). Lower urinary tract symptoms and male sexual dysfunction: The multinational survey of the aging male (MSAM-7). *European Urology, 44*(6), 637–649.

Rosen, R. C., Cappelleri, J. C., & Gendrano, N, III. (2002). The International Index of Erectile Function (IIEF): A state-of-the-science review. *International Journal of Impotence Research, 14*(4), 226–244. doi: 10.1038/sj.ijir.3900857.

Roupret, M., Seisen, T., De La Taille, A., et al. (2012). Sexual dysfunctions linked with prostatic diseases. *Progrès en Urologie, 22*(Suppl 1), S14–20. doi: 10.1016/s1166-7087(12)70030-1.

Scardino, P. (2005). Update: NCCN prostate cancer clinical practice guidelines. *Journal of the National Comprehensive Cancer Network, 3*(Suppl 1), S29–S33.

Schaeffer, E. M., Partin, A. W., Lepor, H., et al. (2012). Radical retropubic and perineal prostatectomy. In A. J. Wein, L. R. Kavoussi, A. C. Novick, et al. (Eds.), *Campbell-Walsh urology* (10th ed., pp. 2801–2829.e4). Philadelphia, PA: Elsevier.

Schenk, J. M., Kristal, A. R., Arnold, K. B., et al. (2011). Association of symptomatic benign prostatic hyperplasia and prostate cancer: Results from the prostate cancer prevention trial. *American Journal of Epidemiology, 173*(12), 1419–1428. doi: 10.1093/aje/kwq493.

Schiavina, R., Borghesi, M., Dababneh, H., et al. (2014). Survival, Continence and Potency (SCP) recovery after radical retropubic prostatectomy: A long-term combined evaluation of surgical outcomes. *European Journal of Surgical Oncology.* Advance online publication. doi: 10.1016/j.ejso.2014.06.015.

Schroder, F. H., Hugosson, J., Roobol, M. J., et al. (2009). Screening and prostate-cancer mortality in a randomized European study. *New England Journal of Medicine, 360*(13), 1320–1328. doi: 10.1056/NEJMoa081008.

Schroder, F. H., Hugosson, J., Roobol, M. J., et al., & ERSPC Investigators (2014). Screening and prostate cancer mortality: Results of the European Randomised Study of Screening for Porstate Cancer (ERSPC) at 13 years follow-up. *Lancet, 384*(9959): 2027–2035.

Screening for Prostate Cancer, Topic Page. U.S. Preventive Services Task Force. (2012). http://www.uspreventiveservicestaskforce.org/prostatecancerscreening.htm

Shaw, E. K., Scott, J. G., & Ferrante, J. M. (2013). The influence of family ties on men's prostate cancer screening, biopsy, and treatment decisions. *American Journal of Mens Health, 7*(6), 461–471. doi: 10.1177/1557988313480226.

Shum, C. F., Mukherjee, A., & Teo, C. P. (2014). Catheter-free discharge on first postoperative day after bipolar transurethral resection of prostate: Clinical outcomes of 100 cases. *International Journal of Urology, 21*(3), 313–318. doi: 10.1111/iju.12246.

Silva, L. A., Andriolo, R. B., Atallah, A. N., et al. (2011). Surgery for stress incontinence due to presumed sphincter deficiency after prostate surgery (Review). *Cochrane Database of Systematic Reviews,* (4). Article No.: CD008306. doi: 10.1002/14651858. CD008306.pub2.

Sohn, W., Lee, H. J., & Ahlering, T. E. (2013). Robotic surgery: Review of prostate and bladder cancer. *The Cancer Journal, 19*(2), 133–139.

Sooriakumaran, P., Tan, G. Y., Grover, S., et al. (2013). Anatomical aspects of the neurovascular bundle in prostate surgery. In J. Hubert & P. Wiklund (Eds.), *Robotic Urology* (2nd ed., pp. 199–207). Heidelberg, Germany: Springer-Verlag.

Stacey, D., Legare, F., Col, N. F., et al. (2014). Decision aids for people facing health treatment or screening decisions. *Cochrane Database Systemic Review, 1*, Cd001431. doi: 10.1002/14651858.CD001431. pub4.

Su, L., & Smith, J. A. (2012). Laparoscopic and robotic-assisted laparoscopic radical prostatectomy and pelvic lymphadenectomy. In A. J. Wein, L. R. Kavoussi, A. C. Novick, et al. (Eds.), *Campbell-Walsh urology* (10th ed., pp. 2830–2849.e3). Philadelphia, PA: Elsevier.

Subak, L. L., Wing, R., West, D. S., et al. (2009). Weight loss to treat urinary incontinence in overweight and obese women. *New England Journal of Medicine, 360*(5), 481–490. doi: 10.1056/NEJMoa0806375.

Tacklind, J., MacDonald, R., Rutks, I., et al. (2012). Serenoa repens for benign prostatic hyperplasia. *Cochrane Database of Systematic Reviews, 12*. Article No.: CD001423. doi: 10.1002/14651858. CD001423.pub3.

Telesca, D., Etzioni, R., & Gulati, R. (2008). Estimating lead time and overdiagnosis associated with PSA screening from prostate cancer incidence trends. *Biometrics, 64*(1), 10–19. doi: 10.1111/j.1541-0420.2007.00825.x.

The Simon Foundation for Continence. (2014). *About Incontinence—treatment options—Kegel (Pelvic Floor) exercises for men.* http://www.simonfoundation.org/About_Incontinence_Treatment_Options_Kegels_for_Men.html

Urciuoli, R., Cantisani, T. A., Carlini, M., et al. (2004). Prostaglandin E1 for treatment of erectile dysfunction. *Cochrane Database of Systematic Reviews, (2)*. Article No.: CD001784. doi: 10.1002/14651858. CD001784.pub2.

U.S. Department of Health and Human Services, National Institutes of Health, National Cancer Institute. (2014). *PDQ® Prostate cancer treatment.* http://www.cancer.gov/cancertopics/pdq/treatment/prostate/HealthProfessional

Wang, Y., Zhishun, L., Peng, W., et al. (2013). Acupuncture for stress urinary incontinence in adults. *Cochrane Database of Systematic Reviews, (7)*. Article No.: CD009408. doi: 10.1002/14651858. CD009408.pub2.

Wei, J. T., Calhoun, E., & Jacobsen, S. J. (2005). Urologic diseases in America project: Benign prostatic hyperplasia. *Journal of Urology, 173*(4), 1256–1261. doi: 10.1097/01.ju.0000155709.37840. fe10.1111/j.1541-0420.2007.00825.x.

Wein, A. J., Kavoussi, L. R., Novick, A. C., et al. (2011). Pathology of prostatic neoplasia. In A. J. Wein, L. R. Kavoussi, A. C. Novick, et al. (Eds.), *Campbell-Walsh urology* (10th ed., pp. 2726–2734). Philadelphia, PA: Elsevier Saunders.

Wilt, T., Ishani, A., & MacDonald, R. (2002). Serenoa repens for benign prostatic hyperplasia. *Cochrane Database of Systematic Reviews, (3)*, Cd001423. doi: 10.1002/14651858.cd001423.

Yan, H., Zong, H., Cui, Y., et al. (2014). The efficacy of PDE5 inhibitors alone or in combination with alpha-blockers for the treatment of erectile dysfunction and lower urinary tract symptoms due to benign prostatic hyperplasia: A systematic review and meta-analysis. *Journal of Sexual Medicine, 11*(6), 1539–1545. doi: 10.1111/jsm.12499.

Zaytoun, O. M., Anil, T., Moussa, A. S., et al. (2011). Morbidity of prostate biopsy after simplified versus complex preparation protocols: Assessment of risk factors. *Urology, 77*(4), 910–914. doi: 10.1016/j.urology.2010.12.033.

Zerbib, M., Zelefsky, M. J., Higano, C. S., et al. (2008). Conventional treatments of localized prostate cancer. *Urology, 72*(6 Suppl), S25–S35. doi: 10.1016/j.urology.2008.10.005.

QUESTIONS

1. A 60-year-old male patient tells the continence nurse: "I have to get up to void twice a night and never feel like I'm emptying my bladder completely." The patient also reports urgency and some pelvic pain. A prostate exam indicates a tender, boggy prostate. What condition would the nurse suspect?
   A. Prostate cancer
   B. Prostatitis
   C. Urethritis
   D. Diabetes insipidus

2. A 50-year-old male patient is diagnosed with storage lower urinary tract symptoms (LUTS). What symptom is characteristic of this category of LUTS?
   A. Urgency
   B. Slow interrupted stream
   C. Hesitancy
   D. Involuntary loss of urine shortly after voiding

3. A male patient is diagnosed with hematuria (blood in the urine). This lower urinary tract symptom is grouped as a:
   A. Storage symptom
   B. Voiding symptom
   C. Prevoiding symptom
   D. Postvoiding symptom

4. What is the main function of the prostate gland?
   A. Control the stream of urine
   B. Prevent infection of the urinary tract
   C. Prevent urine from mixing with semen
   D. Production of seminal fluid

5. A 65-year-old male patient is scheduled for a workup for prostate cancer. What symptom is most indicative of this condition?
   A. Firm, nontender prostate
   B. Symmetry in size and texture of the prostate
   C. Enlarged prostate
   D. Boggy prostate

6. The continence nurse is devising a treatment plan for a patient diagnosed with lower urinary tract symptoms (LUTS). What is the recommended first-line treatment for this condition?
   A. Lifestyle modification
   B. Medication therapy
   C. Surgical intervention
   D. Psychological counseling

7. What treatment would be recommended for a patient with an overactive bladder who has symptoms that are refractory to first- and second-line therapies?
   A. Pharmacologic agents that relax the detrusor muscle
   B. Tibial nerve stimulation
   C. Bladder diary
   D. Pelvic floor muscle training

8. A 52-year-old male patient with an elevated PSA value decides to forego immediate biopsy. What future sign would indicate the need for a biopsy?
   A. Urinary retention
   B. Increase in PSA value of more than 0.75 ng/mL
   C. Decrease in PSA value of more than 0.75 ng/mL
   D. Blood in the urine

9. The continence nurse is explaining the procedure for a transrectal biopsy of the prostate to a patient. Which intervention is *not* a common step in this procedure?
   A. Perform a cleansing enema prior to the procedure.
   B. Perform a urinalysis and urine culture prior to the procedure.
   C. Administer prophylactic antibiotics prior to the procedure.
   D. Administer ultrasound-guided regional blocks prior to the procedure.

10. A patient undergoing a prostate biopsy has a Gleason score of 5. What does this finding indicate?
    A. Normal prostate—no risk for cancer
    B. Low risk for cancer progression
    C. Intermediate risk for cancer progression
    D. High risk for cancer progression

11. A continence nurse is counseling a patient with Stage 1 prostate cancer about the treatment options available. Which of the following is currently considered the "treatment of choice" for those wishing to pursue aggressive therapy?
    A. Watchful waiting
    B. Active surveillance
    C. External beam radiation therapy
    D. Radical prostatectomy

12. A patient postsurgery for a radical prostatectomy is diagnosed with erectile dysfunction. What would the practitioner most likely recommend as first-line therapy?
    A. Oral phosphodiesterase type 5 (PDE-5) inhibitors
    B. Venous and vacuum constriction devices
    C. Prostaglandin E1 suppositories or injections
    D. Penile prosthesis

ANSWERS: 1.**B**, 2.**A**, 3.**B**, 4.**D**, 5.**C**, 6.**A**, 7.**B**, 8.**B**, 9.**A**, 10.**B**, 11.**D**, 12.**A**

CHAPTER 9

Urinary Incontinence/Voiding Dysfunction in the Female

Sandra Engberg

Topical Outline

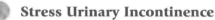

Stress Urinary Incontinence

Stress urinary incontinence (SUI) is the involuntary loss of urine during sudden increases in intra-abdominal pressure. Incontinence occurs when intravesical (bladder) pressure exceeds urethral closure pressure.

Definitions

In their most recent update of the terminology describing female pelvic floor dysfunction, the International Urogynecological Association (IUGA) and the International Continence Society (ICS) defined SUI as a symptom, sign, and urodynamic diagnosis (Haylen et al., 2010). SUI, the symptom, is defined as a "complaint of involuntary loss of urine on effort or physical exertion (e.g., sporting activities), or on sneezing or coughing" (p. 5). The IUGA and ICS also note that calling this "activity-related incontinence" might be advantageous in order to avoid confusion with psychological stress. SUI is also defined as a sign (objective finding): the "observation of involuntary leakage from the urethra synchronous with effort or physical exertion or on sneezing or coughing" (p. 7). Urodynamic SUI is defined as "the involuntary leakage of urine during filling cystometry, associated with increased intra-abdominal pressure, in the absence of a detrusor contraction" (p. 14).

CLINICAL PEARL

Stress incontinence is caused by sphincter dysfunction and involves leakage during activities that cause an increase in intra-abdominal pressure.

Prevalence and Incidence

SUI is primarily a women's health issue. Based on data from 17,850 adults (age 20+ years) participating in the National Health and Nutrition Examination Survey (2001 to 2008), the age-adjusted prevalence of SUI was 51% in women (95% CI 49.4% to 52.4%) as compared to 13.9% in men (95% CI 12.9% to 15.0%). The data also indicated that SUI was the most common subtype of UI among women (24.8% [95% CI 23.4% to 26.3%]) (Markland et al., 2011). While SUI is the most common type of UI in women, the relative prevalence of SUI does vary across the lifespan. A number of studies report the following: SUI is typically first reported during pregnancy or the postpartum period; the prevalence of SUI increases with age, peaking about the fourth or fifth decade; and the prevalence of SUI then decreases, while the prevalence of urge UI (UUI) and mixed SUI and UUI increase (Buckley & Lapitan, 2010; Diokno, 2003; Minassian et al., 2008; Nygaard & Heit, 2004).

Risk Factors

The stress continence mechanism consists of the sphincter mechanism and supporting structures of the pelvic floor (Fig. 9-1) (Delancey, 2010). The sphincteric mechanism includes the bladder neck and the multilayered urethra, which includes the vascular submucosa and several layers of muscle. As it traverses the bladder wall, the urethral lumen is surrounded by the smooth muscle of the trigonal ring. Below this point, the lumen is surrounded by an outer layer of striated muscle (the rhabdosphincter), a middle layer of smooth muscle, and an inner layer of longitudinal (smooth) muscle (Delancey, 2010).

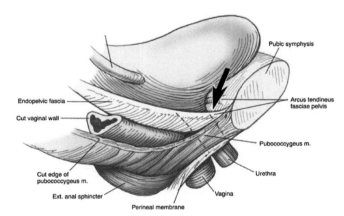

FIGURE 9-1. Stress continence mechanism. The urethra is compressed against the underlying supportive tissues by the downward force (*arrow*) generated by a cough or sneeze.

The urethral support mechanism consists of the anterior vaginal wall, the surrounding muscles (levator ani), and the fascia; specifically, the connections between the vaginal walls and the muscles and fascia influence the position of the urethra, and inadequate urethral support has been thought to play a significant role in SUI. However, in a recent study, Delancey (2010) compared urethral closure pressure, urethral support, levator ani muscle function, and intravesical pressure in 103 women with daily documented SUI and 108 women without SUI; the women were matched in terms of race, age, parity, and hysterectomy status. In this study, urethral closure pressure was a more important factor in SUI than urethral support; maximal urethral closure pressure (MUCP) alone correctly classified 50% of the women with SUI. It should be noted that the level of urethrovaginal support and the cough strength (indicator of force exerted against continence mechanism) also contributed to accurate identification of women with SUI, suggesting that the level of support may be one factor affecting MUCP. Age may be another contributing factor; while there is individual variability in MUCP across all age groups, studies have shown a gradual decline with age. Delancey and colleagues have also found an age-related decrease in both the striated and smooth muscle of the urethra, which may explain the changes seen in MUCP. Although our understanding of the pathophysiology of SUI is increasing, these findings also indicate that our current understanding remains incomplete.

In addition to age, a number of other risk factors for SUI have been identified; these include pregnancy, menopause, hysterectomy, obesity, caffeine, smoking, and genetics. Prevalence of SUI increases during pregnancy with rates varying from 18.6% (*n* = 10,098 in China) (Zhu et al., 2012) to 60% (*n* = 121 in the United States) (Thomason et al., 2007), with most studies reporting prevalence rates between 30% and 50% (Sangsawang & Sangsawang, 2013). In a meta-analysis examining the impact of cesarean section (C-section) on SUI compared to vaginal delivery, the odds of having postpartum SUI were significantly lower (OR = 0.48, 95% CI 0.39, 0.58) in women who had a C-section. There was, however, no significant difference in the odds of developing severe SUI. Findings were similar in the studies that followed women for more than 1 year after delivery (Press et al., 2007). Later studies support findings that women who have vaginal deliveries are at higher risk for developing SUI than those who undergo C-section (Altman et al., 2007a; Gyhagen et al., 2013b; Leijonhufvud et al., 2011).

The EPINCONT study, a large population-based study conducted in Norway, examined the association between other delivery-related characteristics and SUI in a sample of 11,397 women between the ages of 20 and 64 years who had vaginal deliveries. The odds of SUI were significantly greater in women who had a breech delivery (OR = 1.6; 95% CI 1.1, 2.2) and those who had an epidural (OR = 1.4; 95% CI 1.1, 1.8) and significantly lower in those who had a vacuum delivery (OR = 0.7; 95% CI 0.4, 1.0) compared to women without these characteristics. There was no significant association between SUI and gestational age, head circumference, delivery-related injuries, prolonged labor or other functional delivery disorders, or forceps delivery (Rortveit et al., 2003). In a cohort study following women for 10 years following their first vaginal delivery, the prevalence of SUI increased over the 10-year follow-up period. None of the obstetric risk factors examined (age at index delivery, parity, maternal weight or fetal weight at index delivery, perineal lacerations during delivery, or instrumental delivery) were significant risk factors for SUI at 10-year follow-up. However, SUI at 9 months (RR = 12.3, 95% CI 3.9 to 33.1) and 5 years (RR = 14.1, 95% CI 2.5, 18.8) postdelivery were risk factors for SUI at 10 years postdelivery (Altman et al., 2006). In summary, the current evidence indicates that relative to C-section, vaginal delivery increases the risk for developing SUI. It is less clear, however, what obstetric and personal characteristics increase the risk for SUI following vaginal delivery.

Other risk factors examined in relation to SUI include obesity, hysterectomy, caffeine intake, smoking, and genetics. Obesity has been identified as a risk factor for UI in numerous studies, and in most studies, the association was stronger for SUI than for urge urinary incontinence. In most studies, there was also a clear dose–response effect between weight and SUI. The impact of obesity on SUI risk is further supported by studies showing a reduced prevalence of SUI among women who lost weight following surgical or behavioral interventions (Subak et al., 2009). The data regarding the effects of hysterectomy on risk of SUI are mixed; one issue that may contribute to this is the varying definitions used to diagnose SUI. In two studies examining the risk of SUI surgery following hysterectomy, the risk was significantly higher in women who had undergone hysterectomy than those who had not (Altman et al., 2007b; Forsgren et al., 2012). However, in other studies, no significant relationship was demonstrated between

having a hysterectomy and self-reported SUI (De Tayrac et al., 2007; Gustafsson et al., 2006; Miller et al., 2008; van der Vaart et al., 2002). In a systematic review examining the relationship between hysterectomy and UI, Brown et al. (2000) reported that the odds of UI were increased in women age 60 and older (OR = 1.6; 95% CI 1.4, 1.8) but not for women <60 years of age. The association was not examined by subtype of UI.

Another proposed risk factor for UI is caffeine intake; however, the evidence supporting this in relation to SUI is limited, and findings are inconsistent. Two of the studies that examined the relationship between caffeine intake and SUI did not find a significant relationship (Gleason et al., 2013; Jura et al., 2011). In contrast, in the EPINCONT study, coffee had a weak but positive effect on SUI, with an odds ratio of 1.2 (95% CI 1.1, 1.5) for three or more cups per day relative to no coffee intake (Hannestad et al., 2003). Swithinbank et al. (2005) examined the impact of replacing caffeinated beverages with decaffeinated fluids on SUI and found no improvement in SUI symptoms. Smoking is another suggested risk factor for SUI; however, there is limited research examining the association between smoking and SUI and, in the two studies identified, there was no significant association between smoking and SUI (Hannestad et al., 2003; Tahtinen et al., 2011).

Finally, genetics has been suggested as a risk factor, and epidemiological studies do suggest that family history may be a risk factor for SUI; however, the role of genetics is still not clear (McKenzie et al., 2010). In a large twin study designed to examine genetic and environmental influences on SUI, Altman et al. (2008) found that genetic factors accounted for 43% of the variability in SUI after adjusting for age and parity. They also found, however, that nonshared environmental factors accounted for 40% of the variability. Based on these findings, they cautioned that the influence of genetics on SUI should not be overestimated. McKenzie et al. (2010) also reviewed genetic influences on SUI and concluded that, while there is evidence to support the role of genetics, particularly genes encoding extracellular matrix (ECM) proteins, additional research is needed to understand genetic factors in SUI.

CLINICAL PEARL

Some studies suggest that vaginal delivery is a risk factor for stress incontinence; obesity has been clearly demonstrated to be a risk factor.

Pathology and Clinical Presentation

Women with SUI typically present with involuntary urine loss that occurs during activities associated with sudden increases in intra-abdominal pressure such as coughing, sneezing, laughing, lifting, or exercise and that is

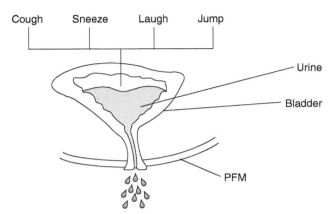

Cough   Sneeze   Laugh   Jump

Urine

Bladder

PFM

FIGURE 9-2. Involuntary urine loss with sudden increases in intra-abdominal pressure, for example, cough.

not associated with a sense of urgency to void (Fig. 9-2). Frail older women with SUI who have difficulty getting up (e.g., from a sitting position) may also report involuntary urine loss when getting up from a chair. Women with SUI typically report leaking small amounts of urine during the activities that precipitate their stress accidents. However, some women with SUI have "low-pressure urethras," which means the urethral sphincter mechanism has limited ability to withstand even minor increases in intra-abdominal pressure (Wilson et al., 2003); as a result, these women report severe SUI and leakage with minimal activity or "always being wet."

Historically, severe SUI has variously been labeled "grade 3 SUI" or "intrinsic sphincter deficiency (ISD)" (McGuire 1981), a classification system based in part on the belief that the pathology of severe SUI was significantly different than the pathology of mild to moderate SUI. However, as knowledge regarding the pathophysiology of SUI evolves, there is increased recognition that the mechanisms underlying ISD and typical SUI (sometimes referred to as bladder neck hypermobility SUI) are not as distinctly different as once believed (Koelb et al., 2013). In addition, while a variety of diagnostic criteria have been proposed for ISD, no precise diagnostic criteria have been identified and agreed upon (Hosker, 2009). These limitations have led some to conclude that the term ISD has limited utility (Smith et al., 2012).

CLINICAL PEARL

As knowledge regarding the pathology of SUI evolves, it is increasingly clear that the mechanisms underlying SUI due to urethral hypermobility and SUI due to intrinsic sphincter deficiency are not as distinctly different as previously thought.

Assessment Guidelines

The Fifth International Consultation on Incontinence (ICI) Committee 5 (Staskin et al., 2013) recommended that the following be components of the initial assessment of all patients presenting with UI, including those with suspected SUI:

History

A complete patient history should be obtained, to include the following:

- Presence, duration, and bother of all urinary, bowel, and pelvic organ prolapse (POP) symptoms. Women should be asked about the situations that are typically associated with involuntary urine loss (e.g., coughing, sneezing, laughing, lifting, and exercise for SUI; urgency, on the way to the toilet, running water, and "key in the door" for UUI; without warning or physical activity; or continuously), the frequency and volume of incontinent episodes, nocturia (including the number of episodes in a typical night), enuresis, urgency, voiding frequency, difficulty emptying their bladder, bladder (lower abdominal) pain, hematuria, dysuria, constipation, fecal incontinence, pelvic discomfort, and dyspareunia. Structured questionnaires such as the International Consultation on Incontinence Modular questionnaires (Bristol Urological Institute, 2014) (http://www.iciq.net/index.html) are useful tools in screening for pelvic floor problems including UI, prolapse, and fecal incontinence.
- The impact of symptoms on sexual function and quality of life (a variety of validated questionnaires are available for this purpose).
- Symptoms suggestive of neurologic disorders and their severity.
- Previous treatments and their effectiveness.
- Comorbid diseases that can affect lower urinary tract/pelvic floor function, for example, chronic obstructive pulmonary disease, asthma, diabetes mellitus, and neurologic diseases.
- Current medications.
- Obstetric and menstrual history.
- Physical impairments, for example, gait or dexterity loss of function.
- Environmental issues: physical, social, and cultural.
- Lifestyle: fluid intake (type and amount), alcohol intake, smoking, and exercise.
- Desire for treatment and acceptable treatment options.
- Goals and expectations for treatment.
- Support systems, including caregiver if relevant.
- Cognitive function.
- Depressive symptoms.

Physical Examination

A complete physical examination for SUI should include:

- Mental status.
- BMI.
- Physical dexterity and mobility.
- Abdominal examination (Fig. 9-3).
- Pelvic examination, including examination of the perineum and external genitalia for tissue quality and sensation, and vaginal examination for atrophic changes and prolapse. Figure 9-4 shows insertion of a vaginal speculum. Step one is the technique used for

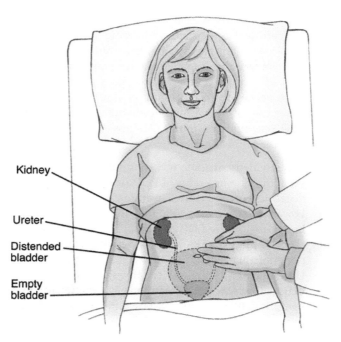

Kidney
Ureter
Distended bladder
Empty bladder

FIGURE 9-3. Abdominal examination.

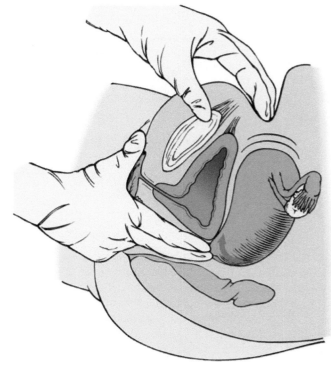

FIGURE 9-5. Palpating the uterus.

the insertion of a speculum into the vagina to view the cervical opening. The blades are held obliquely on entering the vagina. Half of the speculum can be used to retract the anterior and posterior wall to look for prolapse. (POP is discussed in detail later in this chapter.) Bimanual pelvic and anorectal examinations should be conducted to assess for pelvic masses or other abnormalities. Assess pelvic floor muscle (PFM) strength and conduct a stress test for urine loss (have the patient cough deeply while observing the urethral meatus for involuntary urine loss) (Figs. 9-5 and 9-6). During inspection of the vaginal mucosa, the examiner should look for atrophic vaginal changes. When these are present, the vaginal mucosa will generally have a thin, pale shiny appearance with a decrease or loss of vaginal rugae (folds). Alternately, there may be diffuse or patchy erythema and/or petechiae. PFM strength should be assessed as part of the bimanual examination. The modified Oxford scale (Box 9-1)

is a clinically useful method for quantifying PFM strength during vaginal palpation. One or two fingers are inserted into the vagina and the woman is told to squeeze tightly around the examiner's finger(s). The modified Oxford scale has been shown to have moderate interrater reliability (Frawley et al., 2006) and good agreement with perineometic measure of PFM contraction strength (Isherwood & Rane, 2000).

- Neurologic examination.
- PVR if retention is suspected or possible.

CLINICAL PEARL

The physical examination for a woman with stress incontinence should include assessment for atrophic urethritis and assessment of pelvic muscle contractility and endurance.

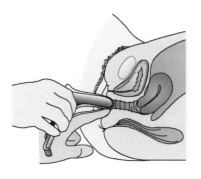
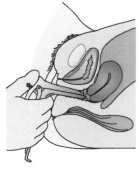
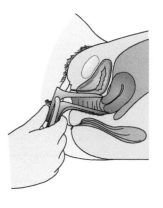

FIGURE 9-4. Pelvic exam with speculum.

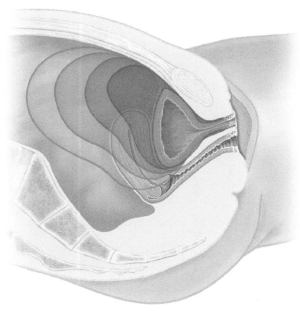

FIGURE 9-6. Contours of the bladder with progressive filling.

Urinalysis

Laboratory evaluation should consist of dipstick test or complete urinalysis. Although the committee recommended routine urinalysis or dipstick as part of the initial evaluation of patients with UI, they reported that the level of evidence supporting this recommendation was based on expert opinion rather than research findings.

Bladder Voiding Diary

Figure 9-7 shows an example of a patient-recorded voiding diary, which is used to assess lower urinary tract symptoms (severity of UI, situations associated with UI, timing and frequency of voiding) and fluid intake.

For most women with SUI, these basic evaluations are sufficient to initiate noninvasive treatment. Additional testing

BOX 9-1.	Oxford Scale for Describing Pelvic Floor Muscle Strength
Score	**Findings When Patient Is Instructed to Squeeze Tightly around the Examiner's Finger**
0	No discernible contraction
1	Barely palpable contraction; flicker
2	Weak but palpable contraction; perceived as slight pressure against the examiner's finger
3	Moderate strength; felt as distinct pressure against the examining finger
4	Good muscle strength with elevation of pelvic floor against light examiner resistance
5	Strong muscle strength; elevation of the examiner's finger against strong resistance

is recommended for women with more complex symptoms such as recurrent or persistent UI despite initial treatment, bladder (lower abdominal) pain, hematuria, recurrent UTI, symptoms suggesting impaired bladder emptying, history of pelvic irradiation or radical pelvic surgery, suspected fistula, or severe pelvic prolapse (Abrams et al., 2010). Depending on the nature of the woman's presentation, the ICI International Scientific Committee (Abrams et al., 2010) recommended the following specialized assessments:

- Uroflowmetry: women with symptoms of voiding dysfunction, physical signs of POP, or evidence of bladder distention on abdominal examination.
- Lower urinary tract/pelvic imaging (e.g., ultrasound): hematuria, severe POP, or pain.
- Lower urinary tract endoscopy: hematuria, pain, or suspected fistula.
- Urodynamic testing: when invasive treatments are planned, when initial treatment was ineffective, or in complicated SUI

Despite recommendations regarding indications for urodynamic studies in women with SUI (Abrams et al., 2010), the role of urodynamic testing and postvoid residual in the assessment and management of uncomplicated SUI is controversial (Dillon & Zimmern, 2012; Nager, 2012). While routine assessment of PVR is standard in many practices, it is questionable if it is always necessary in straightforward cases of UI. Staskin et al. (2009) state that "Female patients who present with storage specific symptoms, with normal sensation and no complaints of decreased bladder emptying, and no anatomical, neurological, organ-specific, or co-morbid risk factors for retention may be assessed for bladder emptying by history and physical examination alone, depending on the potential morbidity of the failure to diagnose and the nature of the intended therapy" (p. 338). The value of routine urodynamic testing is also questionable, even when surgical intervention is planned. In a randomized controlled trial (RCT) examining whether women with SUI who had urodynamic testing prior to stress incontinence procedures had better outcomes than those who did not, there were no differences in outcomes for the two groups of women (Nager et al., 2012). The author concluded that for most women, an office-based stress test can be used instead of urodynamics to confirm the diagnosis of SUI. The test should be performed with a full bladder (instruct women to come to the evaluation with a comfortably full bladder) and in a standing position. The woman should be instructed to place one foot on the examining table step or on a footstool while the examiner positions himself/herself so that the urethral meatus is visible. The woman is then asked to cough deeply. If there is no urine loss during the cough, the Valsalva maneuver can be performed. Urine loss during the cough or Valsalva maneuver is a positive stress test and an objective indicator of SUI (Fig. 9-8).

Column # Directions

    1 Urination in toilet: check, measure, or count # of seconds.

    2 Make a check if a urine leak occurs, note small or large.

    3 Note the reason for the accident (jump, sneeze, lift, water, urge).

    4 Note type and amount of fluid intake.

Fill in the day and date at the top of each column.

Name_____   Acct.#_____

DAY												
	toilet	leak	reason	fluid	toilet	leak	reason	fluid	toilet	leak	reason	fluid
6 am												
7 am												
8 am												
9 am												
10am												
11am												
12am												
1pm												
2pm												
3pm												
4pm												
5pm												
6pm												
7pm												
8pm												
9pm												
10pm												
11pm												
12pm												
1am												
2am												
3am												
4am												
5am												
TOTAL												
# of pads												

Stop Test Results_____   Patient's Signature_____

Type of pad used _____

FIGURE 9-7. Voiding diary.

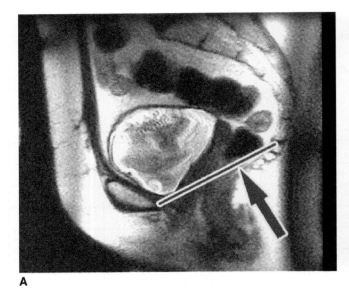
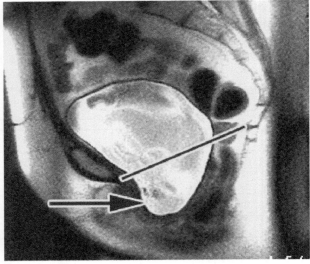

A   **B**

FIGURE 9-8. Dynamic imaging of pelvic floor relaxation shows the position of the bladder base above the sacrococcygeal to inferior pubic line (*arrow*) at rest **(A)**, with subsequent descent during Valsalva maneuver **(B)**.

CLINICAL PEARL

Urodynamic studies are not routinely indicated for women with stress urinary incontinence; urine loss during cough or Valsalva is a positive stress test.

Although bladder diaries are recommended, concerns about their use include patient burden, optimal duration, and optimal content and format. Bright et al. (2011) reviewed English language literature on bladder diaries and concluded that the duration needed to reliably provide information on incontinence and voiding habits is unknown, though most authors recommend that data be collected for at least 3 days. Bright and colleagues also reported that there is no research addressing optimal diary content or format. Given the patient burden associated with keeping a bladder diary, Bradley et al. (2011) examined the agreement between self-report UI questions and a 7-day bladder diary. Using the bladder diary diagnosis of SUI as the gold standard, the self-report questionnaires had a sensitivity of 0.79 to 0.82 and a specificity of 0.76 to 0.77; this means that self-report correctly identified 79% to 82% of the women with SUI based on their bladder diary data and correctly identified 76% to 77% of those without SUI. Agreement between self-report and bladder diary in regard to voiding frequency and frequency of incontinent episodes was good to moderate, respectively ($r = 0.61$ to 0.65; and $r = 0.41$ to 0.56). These findings suggest that the use of self-report is an adequate method for diagnosis of SUI and measurement of UI and voiding frequency when the use of bladder diaries is not feasible.

Shamliyan et al. (2012) conducted an Agency for Healthcare Research and Quality (AHRQ) comparative effectiveness review focusing on the diagnosis and nonsurgical management of urinary incontinence in women. Based on their extensive review of diagnostic studies, the authors concluded that there was a high level of evidence that in clinic settings, women can be accurately diagnosed with UI based on a clinical history and evaluation, a bladder diary to determine the predominate type of incontinence, and a cough stress test. In this review, a high level of evidence was defined as, "High confidence that the evidence reflects the true effect. Further research is very unlikely to change our confidence in the estimated effect" (p. 10).

Management Options

First-line (initial) management options for SUI include lifestyle interventions and PFM training (Bettez et al., 2012; Moore et al., 2013). Additional options include pessaries, vaginal cones, electrical stimulation, urethral inserts, pharmacotherapy, urethral bulking agents, and surgery. Each option will be described along with current evidence regarding its effectiveness in treating SUI. Systematic reviews are generally considered to provide the highest level of evidence to support clinical decision making. Consequently, where such evidence is available, it will be presented.

Lifestyle Interventions

There is strong evidence to support weight loss in obese women (Subak et al., 2009). Women who are overweight or obese should be educated about the impact of obesity on the risk for UI and the evidence that weight loss improves continence. They should be advised to lose weight and provided with specific recommendations or referral to a nutritionist to help them achieve this goal. Given the weak evidence to support the impact of caffeine on SUI, women can be advised to reduce their caffeine intake and monitor its impact on their incontinence. If there is no impact, normal caffeine intake can be resumed. Women with high baseline caffeine intake should be advised to gradually reduce their caffeine intake to reduce the likelihood of caffeine withdrawal symptoms. Women with high baseline fluid intake should be advised to reduce their fluid intake and to monitor its impact on their SUI severity. While it is important to advise women to drink sufficient fluid to prevent dehydration (generally about 1,500 mL/d), results of a small RCT examining the impact of fluid intake on incontinence frequency in women with SUI ($n = 39$) suggest that a reduction in fluid intake may reduce UI episodes in women with high levels of fluid intake at baseline. In this study, restricting caffeine intake had no significant impact on UI episodes (Swithinbank et al., 2005).

Pelvic Floor Muscle Training

There is good evidence to support pelvic floor muscle training (PFMT) as first-line treatment in motivated women with uncomplicated SUI. Physiologically, there are reasons to expect PFMT to be beneficial. First, during a strong PFM contraction, the levator ani muscles are lifted upward and forward, which compresses the urethra and increases urethral closure pressure. Secondly, toned PFMs provide support for the bladder neck and proximal urethra; a well-supported urethra remains essentially in position with limited descent during activities that increase intra-abdominal pressure, which helps to prevent urine leakage. There is research evidence demonstrating that, compared to continent women, women with SUI have lower PFM tone and strength (Dumoulin et al., 2014). In a study of women with SUI, ultrasound imaging was used to compare changes in urethral morphology in women randomly assigned to a PFMT group (12 weekly physiotherapy sessions plus home PFM exercise practice) or a no-intervention control group. In women in the PFMT group, urethral cross-sectional area increased following the 12 treatment sessions while it appeared smaller in the control group. The authors postulated that the PFMT caused hypertrophy of the urethral striated muscle, which, in turn, improved sphincter function (McLean et al., 2013). Indeed, there is strong evidence to support the effectiveness of PFMT in reducing SUI. In a systematic review prepared for the AHRQ, Shamliyan et al. (2012) concluded that there was a high level of evidence to support the benefits of PFMT for women with SUI. The findings of a 2014 Cochrane review comparing PFMT to no treatment or an inactive control treatment also support the effectiveness of PFMT in treating SUI (Dumoulin et al., 2014). Women with SUI in the PFMT groups of the included studies were significantly more likely to report that they were continent (RR = 8.38, 95% CI 3.68 to 19.07) than women in the control groups. They were 17 times more likely to report that their UI was either cured (continent) or improved (RR = 17.33, 95% CI 4.31 to 69.64).

One question about PFMT that remains unanswered is the specific components of an optimal training regimen. PFMT programs can be designed to

1. Increase PFM strength (the maximal force of contraction)
2. Increase PFM endurance (the time that a contraction can be sustained)
3. Improve PFM coordination (contraction prior to or during activities associated with leaking) (Dumoulin et al., 2011).

However, there are no evidence-based guidelines that clinicians can use in developing a PFMT protocol. Available evidence suggests that training can be successfully provided on a one-to-one basis or in a group setting (see Box 9-2 for an example of a consumer-focused PFMT brochure), that the frequency and duration of treatment visits can vary, and that instructions on how to perform the contractions can be verbal, written, taught during the pelvic examination, or taught using biofeedback. The prescribed type of PFM contractions (strength and/or duration focused), the number and frequency of exercises, the positions in which women are taught to perform the exercises, and the addition of resistance to training also vary. In the studies included in systematic reviews, the characteristics of the PFMT intervention varied considerably, and yet, in most of the studies, the majority of women reported continence or reduced SUI (Dumoulin et al., 2014; Shamliyan et al., 2012). One approach is to recommend 40 to 45 PFM exercises per day in three or four sets (either 15 or 10 exercises/set); to suggest that exercises be done in the supine, sitting, and standing positions; to advise patients to avoid use of their abdominal and buttocks muscles during PFM

CLINICAL PEARL

Lifestyle interventions (e.g., weight loss) and pelvic floor muscle training represent first-line treatment for women with stress incontinence.

BOX 9-2. Patient Education: Pelvic Floor Muscle Kegel Exercises

Purpose: To strengthen and maintain the tone of the pubococcygeal muscle, which supports the pelvic organs, reduce or prevent stress incontinence and uterine prolapse, enhance sensation during sexual intercourse, and hasten postpartum healing.

1. Become aware of pelvic floor muscle function by "drawing in" the perivaginal muscles and anal sphincter as if to control urine or defecation, but not contracting the abdominal, buttock, or inner thigh muscles.
2. Sustain contraction of the muscles for up to 10 seconds, followed by at least 10 seconds of relaxation. Another variation is to include several sets of rapid contraction and relaxation each day.
3. Perform these exercises 30 to 80 times daily in supine, sitting, and standing positions.
4. As these exercises can be done inconspicuously, perform them with other daily activities (e.g., brushing teeth, in a car or bus, talking on the telephone, standing in line) as well as before rising from bed and after retiring at night.

Training and exercise should be individualized for each patient.

contractions; and to instruct patients to gradually increase the contraction and relaxation time with an end goal of contracting and relaxing the PFM for 10 seconds with each exercise. (The initial time is based on the baseline assessment of the woman's PFM strength, which is reassessed at each treatment visit.) Some clinicians also ask women to perform repeated unsustained maximal force contractions (quick flicks) as part of the exercise regimen. Most exercise protocols include instruction in a stress strategy also known as the "knack"; that is, the patient is taught to contract her PFM strongly before and during activities associated with involuntary urine loss (Miller et al., 2001).

Other clinicians and researchers have, however, used different PFMT routines with similar outcomes. In a Cochrane systematic review, Hay-Smith et al. (2011) compared approaches to PFMT in relation to improvements in UI. They included RCTs and two-group quasi-experimental trials; the women enrolled in the trials had SUI, UUI, or mixed UI. Each study included at least two groups that received PFMT, with variations in the training protocol between the groups that included one or more of the following: (1) direct versus indirect approach to pelvic muscle contraction; in the direct approach, women were asked to focus specifically on contracting their PFMs, and in the indirect approach, women were instructed to perform PFM contractions along with cocontractions of another related muscle group, for example, the abdominal, hip, or gluteal muscles; (2) differences in exercise parameters (strength of contractions; inclusion of the "knack"; the position during exercises; the number of exercises per set, day, or week; and the duration of contractions); (3) the addition of a resistance factor to contractions (e.g., intravaginal resistance device); (4) approach used for instruction (e.g., verbal, written, individual, or group); (5) differences in the type and amount of health care provider supervision; or (6) the addition of measures (e.g., alarms or text messages) to enhance adherence. Based on the 21 studies included in the review, the authors concluded that there "was insufficient evidence to make strong recommendations about the best approach to PFMT" (p. 2). They did state, however, that based on the limited data available, regular supervision of PFMT (e.g., weekly) was better than little or no supervision. It was not clear, however, whether individual or group supervision was better. The authors also noted a number of limitations in this area: the limited number of studies; the fact that, in a number of the studies, there were multiple differences in the two approaches being compared; the risk of reporting bias due to inability to blind the participants; and the incomplete description of the interventions being compared. Additional research is needed in order to identify the best approach to PFMT.

Biofeedback

The Hay-Smith et al. (2011) review did not examine the impact of biofeedback on outcomes of PFMT. However, a separate Cochrane review (Herderschee et al., 2011) compared PFMT with and without biofeedback to determine if biofeedback improved outcomes in women being treated for SUI and/or UUI. Twenty-four RCTs or quasi-experimental studies were included and nine compared self-reported improvement or cure of UI among women who received PFMT plus biofeedback versus women who received PFMT alone. Those who received PFMT alone were significantly less likely to report that their UI was improved or cured (RR = 0.75, 95% CI 0.66 to 0.86). The authors concluded that, based on the findings of this review, use of biofeedback to teach PFMT may have added benefit in reducing UI; however, they noted that other differences in the treatment regimens (e.g., more contact with the health care provider) could have also accounted for the greater improvement in the biofeedback group (Herderschee et al., 2011). In contrast to the findings in the Cochrane review, the AHRQ comparative effectiveness review compared the impact of PFMT with and without vaginal EMG probe biofeedback on incontinence and found no significant difference in outcomes (Shamliyan et al., 2012). Based on the studies included in their review, Shamliyan and colleagues concluded that there was a high level of evidence to indicate no differences in outcomes in the PFMT groups with and without biofeedback. The differences in findings may have been related to differences in eligibility criteria used in the two reviews; specifically, the Cochrane review included studies that were not included in the AHRQ review. An RCT conducted in Japan and published after these two reviews compared PFMT with and without biofeedback in women with SUI and found no significant differences between the groups in posttreatment reduction in incontinent episodes as measured by bladder diary (Hirakawa et al., 2013).

Alternate Exercises for SUI

Several other exercise regimens have been proposed as treatments for SUI. In a systematic review (Bø & Herbert, 2013), several alternative exercise programs for SUI were identified. One involves deep abdominal muscle training; the theoretical basis for this approach is that deep abdominal muscle contraction will cause the PFMs to cocontract and that combined PFM and deep abdominal muscle contraction is more effective than PFMT alone in promoting continence. Bø and Herbert concluded that the evidence from RCTs is currently mixed and does not provide strong support for this training method. Another alternative is the Paula method (contraction of the muscles of the mouth and eyes), which is based on the theory that all sphincters in the body work simultaneously and that exercising the ring muscles of the mouth, eyes, or nose will cause cocontraction and strengthening of the PFMs (Liebergall-Wischnitzer et al., 2005). Two studies, however, failed to demonstrate cocontraction of the PFMs during contraction of the mouth or eyes, and two trials comparing Paula therapy to PFMT found no evidence to support the efficacy of the Paula method. Theoretically, nonspecific exercises such as Pilates, yoga, breathing exercises, general fitness training, and postural re-education could strengthen or improve PFM function. However, there are no RCTs comparing these alternative exercises to no treatment and no conclusive evidence to support their use in clinical practice.

Electrical Stimulation

Transvaginal electrical stimulation has been theorized to be effective in treating SUI by causing PFM contraction and increasing the number of muscle fibers recruited during rapid contractions (Schreiner et al., 2013). Schreiner et al. (2013) published a systematic review of studies examining the impact of transvaginal electrical stimulation (E-stim) on UI in women. Ten studies on E-stim in the treatment of SUI met eligibility criteria. Both the E-stim intervention protocols and the control conditions varied from study to study. Outcome measures also varied and included pad tests, self-report, bladder diaries, and quality of life. Across these studies, findings were mixed in relation to SUI. In contrast, in the AHRQ review, Shamliyan et al. (2012) concluded that there was a high level of evidence to indicate that E-stim increases continence rates and improves SUI compared to sham stimulation. They also concluded that there was a moderate level of evidence indicating no difference between E-stim and PFMT in relation to continence outcomes among women with SUI. In this review, the strength of evidence was graded as moderate "when RCTs with a medium risk of bias reported consistent treatment effects or large observational studies reported consistent associations" and there was "moderate confidence that the evidence reflects the true effect. Future research may change our confidence in the estimate of effect and may change the estimate" (p. 10). The AHRQ review also examined evidence related to magnetic stimulation in the treatment of UI. Five RCTs compared magnetic stimulation with sham stimulation in women with UI ($n = 1$), SUI ($n = 2$), mixed UI ($n = 1$), and predominant UUI ($n = 1$). Based on the review, Shamliyan et al. (2012) concluded that there was a moderate level of evidence that magnetic stimulation did not improve urinary continence more than sham stimulation.

Vaginal Cones

Weighted vaginal cones have been recommended as a method to assist women to strengthen their PFMs. Women are instructed to insert the heaviest cone that they can retain while in an upright position and to leave it in place for 15 minutes twice a day while up and moving around. Over a period of time (usually 1 month or more), they gradually increase the weight of the cone inserted. Theoretically, holding the cone in place requires PFM contraction, and slippage of the cones may provide a form of biofeedback, which may promote both contraction and coordination of the PFMs (Herbison & Dean, 2013). Herbison and Dean conducted a systematic review of RCTs and quasi-experimental studies comparing cones to a control condition; the control condition did not include active PFMT

($n = 5$ studies). The outcome in relation to continence was based on self-report and involved failure to cure or improve UI. Failure to cure was significantly less likely in the cone group (RR = 0.84, 95% CI 0.76 to 0.94), as was failure to improve UI (RR = 0.72, CI 0.52 to 0.99), compared to the control condition. The authors also included studies comparing cone therapy to active PFMT ($n = 13$ studies) and found no significant difference in the two groups in (1) self-reported cure or improvement in UI (RR = 0.97, 95% CI 0.75 to 1.20 in 6 studies), (2) self-reported cure ($n = 5$ studies; RR = 1.10, 95% CI 0.91 to 1.13), (3) UI episodes/day ($n = 4$ studies; mean difference = 0.00, 95% CI –0.20 to 0.20), (4) pad test results ($n = 6$ studies; RR = 1.00, 95% CI 0.76 to 1.31), or (5) PFM strength (mean difference = 0.61; 95% CI –2.49 to 1.27). Overall, this review found that weighted vaginal cones were better than no active treatment and equivalent to PFMT in treating UI in women.

Continence Pessaries

Continence pessaries are usually round with a knob and may or may not have a supporting diaphragm in the center (e.g., the ring or dish; Fig. 9-9). Since the goal is to stabilize and support the bladder neck and to compress the urethra to prevent urine leakage during increased intra-abdominal pressure, the pessary should be inserted with the knob positioned against the anterior vaginal wall, behind the symphysis pubis, and ideally at the level of the urethrovesical junction (Keyock & Newman, 2011) (Fig. 9-10). There is limited research examining the effectiveness of incontinence pessaries in treating SUI. Richter et al. (2010) compared self-reported improvement as measured by the Patient Global Impression of Improvement scale (much or very much better) and the stress incontinence subscale of the Urogenital Distress Inventory (absence of bothersome SUI symptoms) in women treated with a ring or dish pessary, behavioral therapy (PFMT and stress and urge strategies), or combination therapy at 3 and 12 months posttreatment. Using intention-to-treat when analyzing the outcomes, at 3 months, significantly more women in

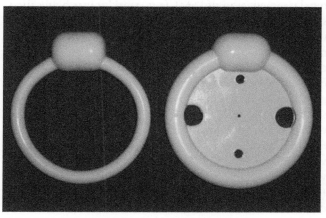

FIGURE 9-9. Ring pessary with knob.

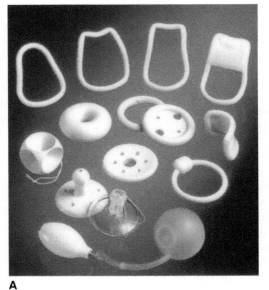
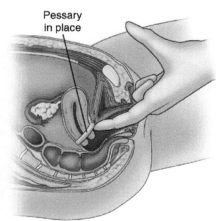

Pessary in place

FIGURE 9-10. Examples of pessaries **(A)** and pessary in position **(B)**. **A** **B**

the combination group (53.3%) reported that they were much or very much better than in the pessary only group (39.6%, $p = 0.02$). There were no significant differences between the pessary and behavioral (49.3%) therapy only groups. Significantly more women in the combined treatment group (44.0%) and in the behavioral therapy only group (48.6%) reported no bothersome SUI symptoms at 3 months than those in the pessary only group (32.9%, $p = 0.05$ and 0.006 respectively). At 12 months, there were no significant group differences for either outcome. When the outcomes were analyzed only for those women who completed the interventions (per protocol analysis), there were no significant group differences at either 3 or 12 months. There is a need for additional research examining the effectiveness of pessaries in the treatment of SUI.

Urethral Inserts

There is currently one urethral insert available in the United States (Keyock & Newman, 2011). It is the FemSoft, a sterile disposable, single use, intraurethral device (http://www.rocm.com/femsoft/). It consists of a narrow, silicone tube encased entirely in a soft, thin, mineral oil-filled sleeve that forms a balloon at the internal tip and comes with a disposable applicator for insertion. It comes in various sizes and is prescribed by a health care provider. It is easily removed for voiding and should be removed at least once every 6 hours (Keyock & Newman, 2011). One single group, quasi-experimental study examining the long-term safety, efficacy, and acceptability of the device in women with SUI was identified (Sirls et al., 2002). One hundred fifty ($n = 150$) women were enrolled in the study. Of these women, 77 (51%) withdrew by the 12-month follow-up visit. The reasons for withdrawal were variable with 33 (43%) doing so for reasons not related to the device. Based on intention-to-treat analysis, 57% of the 112 women had a >50% reduction in total weekly incontinent episodes and

did not withdraw secondary to adverse events or dissatisfaction. The most common adverse events were bacteriuria ($n = 58$ women, 38.7%) and symptomatic UTI (31.3%). Additional research is needed to examine the effectiveness of intraurethral inserts on SUI-related outcomes.

Pharmacotherapy

In the United States, there are currently no FDA-approved drugs to treat SUI. There are, however, recent systematic reviews examining the clinical effectiveness of estrogen therapy and duloxetine in treating SUI. Estrogen receptors have been identified in tissues of the vagina, bladder, urethra, and PFMs. Estrogen deficiency may play a role in the development of UI and estrogen has been used in the treatment of UI including SUI (Cody et al., 2012). The Cochrane review (Cody et al., 2012) included studies examining both systemic and topical estrogen while the AHRQ review (Shamliyan et al., 2012) focused on topical administration. Seventeen of the studies (RCTs or quasi-experimental studies) in the Cochrane review focused on SUI although findings were not reported separately for SUI. The authors concluded that systemic estrogen may actually worsen UI. In contrast, topical estrogen treatment may improve UI. The long-term effects and the impact of discontinuing treatment are currently unknown. In the AHRQ review of pharmacotherapy for SUI, Shamliyan et al. (2012) reported that, "Evidence from individual RCTs indicates greater continence and improvement in UI with vaginal estrogen formulations and worsening UI with transdermal patches" and "Evidence was insufficient to draw conclusions about the clinical efficacy of different topical estrogen treatments for UI" (p. 44). Duloxetine is classified as an SNRI (serotonin and noradrenaline reuptake inhibitor) and has been shown in cat studies to suppress parasympathetic activity and increase sympathetic and somatic neural activity in the lower urinary tract.

These effects are thought to increase rhabdosphincter activity and, consequently, urethral closure pressure (Mariappan et al., 2005). In a Cochrane review published in 2005, Mariappan and colleagues reported that duloxetine reduced UI episodes and improved quality of life in women with SUI. It had little impact on cure rates and side effects, although not serious, were common. In the AHRQ report published in 2012, Shamliyan and colleagues concluded that there was (1) a low level of evidence indicating that it was worse than placebo in resolving UI, (2) a high level of evidence that UI was improved, and (3) a high level of evidence indicating significantly higher adverse event rates relative to placebo, resulting in discontinuation of treatment due to nausea, dizziness, headache, fatigue, diarrhea, and constipation. The authors concluded that, "Duloxetine has an unfavorable balance between improvement in stress UI and treatment discontinuation due to adverse effects" (p. 121).

Urethral Bulking Agents

For women with complicated SUI who do not respond satisfactorily to initial therapy, the ICI committee recommends either surgical intervention or urethral bulking agents (Abrams et al., 2010). Intra- or periurethral injection of bulking agents is used to plump up the urethral mucosa; this creates artificial urethral cushions that can improve urethral coaptation and restore continence (Kirchin et al., 2012). Agents used for urethral bulking in the United States include carbon beads, copolymers, and polyacrylamide hydrogels (Keyock & Newman, 2011). Kirchin et al. (2012) conducted a systematic review of RCTs and quasi-experimental studies where at least one study arm involved urethral injection therapy. The authors concluded that evidence is insufficient to guide clinical practice. In the AHRQ review, Shamliyan et al. (2012) concluded that a low level of evidence suggests that urethral bulking agents do not result in improvement in UI compared to placebo (low level of evidence means low confidence that current evidence reflects the true effect and an acknowledgment that additional research is likely to change the conclusions). Evidence from uncontrolled studies reported high improvement rates, but also adverse events.

Surgical Procedures

There are a number of different surgical procedures used to treat SUI. The two most common are colposuspension (Burch colposuspension) and midurethral sling procedures (Fig. 9-11). Colposuspension, done either as an open lower abdominal procedure or laparoscopically, lifts and stabilizes the bladder neck, which enhances urethral sphincter function during increases in intra-abdominal pressure (Keyock & Newman, 2011). While this was considered the gold standard in the past, the midurethral sling has become much more common and is now considered by many to be the gold standard surgery for SUI (Geller & Wu, 2013). Multiple entry techniques (retropubic, suprapubic, and transobturator) have been utilized

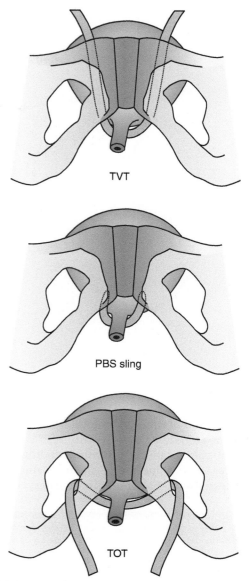

FIGURE 9-11. Mid-urethral slings. TVT, tension-free vaginal tape; PBS, public bone stabilization sling; TOT, transobturator tape.

for insertion of the sling, which is permanently implanted to support the urethra at midpoint between the bladder neck and the urethral meatus. Both retropubic and transobturator slings are widely used today. There are a number of sling materials used, including cadaver fascia lata and various synthetic materials including mesh slings (e.g., tension-free vaginal tape) (Lue & Tanagho, 2014). According to Geller and Wu (2013), the most recent innovation in the midurethral sling is the introduction of the minisling; the newer adjustable minislings can be tightened in the office during postoperative visits. These mesh slings consist of lightweight macroporous polypropylene mesh designed to maximize urethral support while minimizing the risk of erosion. While surgical advances have improved outcomes and allowed surgery to be performed

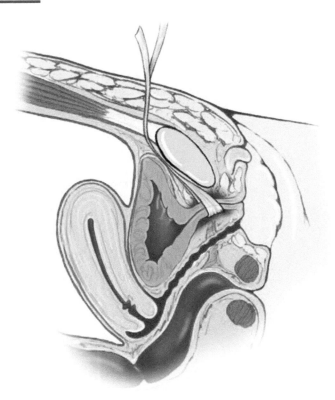

FIGURE 9-12. Traditional suburethral sling.

in a shorter period of time, under local anesthetic, and as an outpatient procedure, there are still treatment failures and surgical complications, including voiding dysfunction, bladder injuries, mesh erosion, and pain. In 2008, the FDA released a Safety Communication describing over

BOX 9-3.	Postoperative Teaching for Women Who Have Had Stress Urinary Incontinence Surgery

Although specific postoperative instructions may vary, they often include:

Resume normal diet.

Administer prescribed pain medications as needed to control pain.

Most women can resume normal physical activity including walking and going up and down steps once home.

Lifting should be restricted to light objects.

Avoid strenuous physical activity and heavy lifting for 4 to 8 weeks.

Avoid sexual intercourse for 4 to 6 weeks.

Depending on the nature of woman's job, work can generally be resumed in 2 to 6 weeks.

Notify health care provider if having

Difficulty voiding or unable to empty bladder

Excessive or recurrent vaginal bleeding

Malodorous vaginal discharge

Pain or burning on urination

Blood in urine

1,000 cases of mesh-related complications; the report was updated in 2011 (Geller & Wu, 2013). A Cochrane review published in 2009 compared procedures involving the traditional suburethral sling (Fig. 9-12) and the minimally invasive sling and concluded that they were equally effective and there were fewer adverse events with the minimally invasive sling (Ogah et al., 2009). Long-term outcome data comparing the minisling and traditional mesh slings are not yet available (Geller & Wu, 2013). Box 9-3 summarizes postoperative teaching for women who have had SUI surgery.

CLINICAL PEARL

The midurethral sling is currently considered by many to be the gold standard for surgical treatment of SUI.

Pelvic Organ Prolapse

POP is the herniation of a pelvic organ toward and through the vaginal introitus (Fig. 9-13). The prolapse can include the anterior vaginal wall, the posterior wall, or the apex (Abed & Rogers, 2008). The most common prolapse is of the anterior vaginal wall, which usually includes descent of the bladder and is thus called a cystocele. Posterior wall prolapses can include small or large bowel, while apical prolapses entail either the uterus or posthysterectomy vaginal cuff and can also include small intestine (enterocele) (Jelovsek et al., 2007). Wu et al. (2014) used the National Health and Nutrition Examination Survey to examine the prevalence of pelvic floor disorders including POP. Self-reported data on a validated questionnaire—"*Do you see or feel a bulge in the vaginal area?*"—were available for 7,071 nonpregnant women. Women with an affirmative response were classified as having a prolapse. Overall, 2.9% of women had POP. Since POP is often asymptomatic, this estimate likely underestimates the prevalence. Using the ICS definition of POP as any prolapse even if asymptomatic, the prevalence rates have been estimated between 27% and 98% (Abed & Rogers, 2008). The Wu-reported prevalence of 2.9% (2014) is consistent with previously reported prevalence rates for bothersome POP, typically a prolapse extending beyond the hymen (Abed & Rogers, 2008).

Pathophysiology and Risk Factors

POP occurs due to weakening of the pelvic floor support structures as a result of direct damage (e.g., tears or breaks) to the supporting structures and/or to neuromuscular dysfunction (Gleason et al., 2012). The levator ani muscles (pubococcygeus, puborectalis, and ileococcygeus) and the connective tissue attachments to the bony pelvis provide anatomical support for the pelvic organs. The levator ani muscles are normally tonically contracted at rest, closing the genital hiatus and acting as a platform to support the pelvic organs. The endopelvic fascia envelops the pelvic organs, holding the vagina and uterus in their

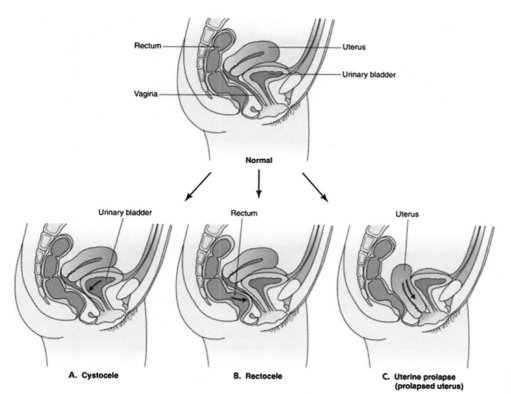

FIGURE 9-13. Pelvic organ prolapse.

normal anatomical position while allowing for sufficient mobility to permit storage of urine and feces, coitus, parturition, and defecation (Jelovsek et al., 2007). Damage or dysfunction of either or both of these components can eventually lead to POP. A variety of pathological changes have been identified as potential causative factors for POP including denervation or direct damage to the levator ani muscles, neuropathic injuries (e.g., related to vaginal delivery or chronic straining), disruption or stretching of the endopelvic fascia attachments, connective tissue abnormalities, smooth muscle abnormalities, and variations in the orientation and shape of the bony pelvis (Jelovsek et al., 2007). Risk factors for POP include age (Awwad et al., 2012; Miedel et al., 2009; Wu et al., 2014), vaginal delivery (Awwad et al., 2012; Elenskaia et al., 2013; Gyhagen et al., 2013a; Rortveit et al., 2007), high BMI (Awwad et al., 2012; Gyhagen et al., 2013a; Miedel et al., 2009), vaginal hysterectomy (Forsgren et al., 2012), parity (Miedel et al., 2009), family history (Miedel et al., 2009; McLennan et al., 2008), an occupation involving heavy lifting (Miedel et al., 2009), and chronic constipation (Miedel et al., 2009; Rortveit et al., 2007). Figure 9-14 shows the tension placed on the pelvic organs with prolapse.

Clinical Presentation

Women with POP can present with a range of symptoms directly related to the prolapse including bulging sensation, feeling or seeing a bulge, pelvic pressure, or heaviness. Some women may also describe symptoms related to coexisting bladder, bowel, or pelvic floor dysfunction:

UI, frequency, urgency, weak or slow urine stream, hesitancy, sensation of incomplete bladder emptying, or the need to shift positions or manually reduce the prolapse in order to void. Bowel symptoms can include fecal incontinence, sensation of incomplete bowel emptying, straining in order to defecate, bowel urgency, and need for digital evacuations or maneuvers to manually reduce the prolapse

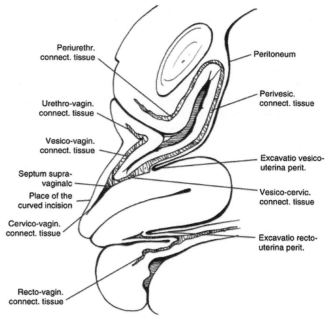

FIGURE 9-14. Traction on pelvic organs from prolapse.

in order to complete defecation. Women may also experience dyspareunia (pain/discomfort during sexual intercourse). The symptomatic presentation of POP varies from relatively minor to having a major effect on quality of life (Jelovsek et al., 2007). Several investigators have examined the prevalence of specific symptoms and the association between the extent of prolapse and the presence of symptoms. Ellerkmann et al. (2001) examined self-reported symptoms (measured by questionnaire) in women who subsequently underwent urogynecologic examination (n = 237) and found a weak to moderate association between the severity of prolapse and specific symptoms related to bowel and bladder function. The correlations were moderate for prolapse-specific symptoms (visualized bulging and pelvic discomfort). In another study examining the relationship between the degree of prolapse and symptoms (n = 296 women), investigators found that prolapse of 0.5 cm distal to the hymen was sensitive and specific for bulging and protrusion symptoms; however, they were unable to identify a prolapse severity threshold for other symptoms (Gutman et al., 2008). Finally, Swift et al. (2003) examined the association between symptoms and the degree of POP in 477 women. As the POP stage increased, the average number of symptoms increased; however, the increase was not statistically significant (p = 0.22 for reported symptoms and p = 0.23 for bothersome symptoms).

CLINICAL PEARL

The clinical impact of pelvic organ prolapse varies from minimal to major impact on quality of life.

Assessment

The pelvic exam is the gold standard for the diagnosis of POP. The basic examination is done with the patient in a supine position and the head of the bed at 45 degrees (Abed & Rogers, 2008). The bladder should be empty; in addition to being uncomfortable for the patient when examined, a full bladder has been shown to restrict the degree of descent and may result in underestimation of the severity of the prolapse (Haylen et al., 2010). While observing the vaginal introitus, the examiner should ask the woman to perform a Valsalva maneuver and observe for bulging. To determine which compartment of the vagina is involved (anterior, posterior, or apical), a split speculum (one blade) is inserted to retract the posterior and then anterior wall and to observe each portion of the vagina sequentially (Fig. 9-4). If the observed prolapse is not consistent with the degree of protrusion the woman reports experiencing, the examiner should have her stand so the maximum descent can be observed.

Figure 9-15 shows progressive stages of prolapse.

Although there are a number of grading systems for POP, the only system that is internationally acceptable with high interexaminer reliability is the Pelvic Organ Prolapse Quantitative Examination (POPQ) (Persu et al., 2011). This

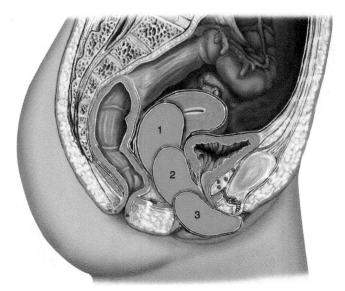

FIGURE 9-15. Progression of prolapse.

system was developed by a multidisciplinary committee of the ICS, the Society of Gynecologic Surgeons, and the American Urogynecologic Society (AUGS). The goal was to establish a standardized system for evaluating and describing POP (Luft, 2006). It describes the topographic positions of six vaginal sites and provides information about perineal descent and changes in the axis of the levator plate based on increases in genital hiatus and perineal body measurements (Auwad et al., 2004) (Fig. 9-16). While the POPQ was developed to provide an objective and reproducible tool for describing and staging POP, it is not widely used in clinical practice. Auwad et al. (2004) conducted a Web-based survey of 667 ICS and AUGS members to determine their use of the POPQ. Of the 380 surveys that were completed, 373 members answered the question about the use of POPQ in clinical practice. Only 150 (40.2%) reported that they routinely used it; 147 (39.2%) did not use it. The second question asked participants if they used POPQ for research; 251 (67.1%) of those who responded (n = 374) reported that

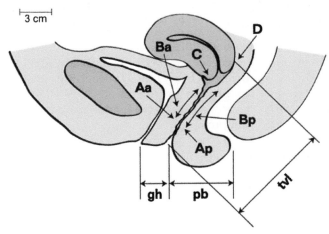

FIGURE 9-16. POPQ assessment guide.

they routinely used it in research. The most common reasons that participants reported not using POPQ were that it was too time consuming (24.2%), colleagues did not use it (20%), and it was too confusing (17.9%).

The most recent International Urogynecological Association (IUGA) and ICS report on terminology for pelvic floor dysfunction in women uses the following method for staging POP (Haylen et al., 2010):

Stage 0: No prolapse is demonstrated.
Stage 1: Most distal portion of the prolapse is more than 1 cm above the level of the hymen.
Stage 2: Most distal portion of the prolapse is 1 cm or less proximal to or distal to the plane of the hymen.
Stage 3: The most distal portion of the prolapse is more than 1 cm below the plane of the hymen.
Stage 4: Complete eversion of the total length of the lower genital tract is demonstrated (p. 8).

Management

Many women have some degree of POP. Current recommended management options for POP include observation, pessary support, PFMT, or surgery.

Observation

Clinical observation is a viable treatment option for many women with POP. Observation is warranted in asymptomatic women with stage 1 or 2 prolapse and, with regular evaluation to monitor for development or worsening of urinary or bowel symptoms, is also an option for those with stage 3 or 4 POP who are asymptomatic (Abed & Rogers, 2008). Handa and colleagues conducted a longitudinal observational study to describe the natural history of POP in postmenopausal women. The study cohort was 412 women with grade 1 (in the vagina), grade 2 (to the introitus), or grade 3 (outside the vagina) prolapses who completed two to eight annual pelvic examinations (mean = 5.7). In this study, regression of the prolapse was common, particularly for grade 1 POP, where the probability of regression was greater than for progression of the prolapse. In contrast, Gilchrist et al. (2013) found minimal changes in POP in a sample of 64 women who selected observation as the primary treatment of the prolapse. Most of the women had stage 2 (48%) or 3 (48%) POP. Over the observation period (medium = 16 months; range, 6 to 91 months), 78% of patients had no change in the leading edge of their prolapse, 3% demonstrated regression (2 cm reduction), and 19% had progression (≥2 cm increase in the leading edge).

Pessaries

Vaginal pessaries are generally considered the cornerstone of nonsurgical treatment of POP (Abed & Rogers, 2008). They have been used to treat women with POP since 400 BC (Jelovsek et al., 2007). Pessaries can be offered as a first-line treatment option for women who prefer nonsurgical treatment, who plan a future pregnancy, who have lower stage or asymptomatic prolapses, or who are not surgical candidates. The limited contraindications associated with pessary use make them a viable option for most women with POP. They should not be used in women with an active pelvic infection or ulcerations in the vagina, who are allergic to silicone or other materials in the pessary, or who are noncompliant and unlikely to attend follow-up visits (Jones & Harmanli, 2010). When pessaries are used in postmenopausal women, clinicians often also prescribe vaginal estrogen therapy to improve health of the vaginal epithelium and help prevent vaginal erosions. Findings from a study examining long-term outcomes associated with pessary use in women with POP (n = 429), however, suggest that topical estrogen cream may not protect women against the occurrence of erosions (Ramsay et al., 2011). Additional research is therefore needed to provide guidance about estrogen use in postmenopausal women fitted for pessaries.

Current pessaries are generally made of silicone plastic, which does not absorb vaginal secretions and prevents odors (Luft, 2006). When selecting and fitting a pessary, considerations need to include the nature and extent of the prolapse and the patient's cognitive status, manual dexterity, and level of sexual activity (Jelovsek et al., 2007). Pessaries are available in many different shapes and sizes, allowing a variety of options depending on the nature and extent of the prolapse as well as the characteristics of the individual patient. Pessaries can be classified as support or space-occupying pessaries. Support pessaries such as the ring sit in the posterior fornix usually resting against the pubic bone anteriorly and/or the pelvic floor. Space-occupying pessaries, such as the cube and donut, occupy a larger space than the introitus and are generally used for larger prolapses. The Gellhorn is a combination of support and space-occupying device (Robert et al., 2013). In general, support pessaries do not need to be removed for intercourse while space-occupying pessaries do (Jones & Harmanli, 2010). While each type has advantages and disadvantages and there is no consensus about which is optimal, the ring and Gellhorn are popular options in the United States (Abed & Rogers, 2008). Ring pessaries are generally the first-line choice for clinicians because they are easy to insert and remove.

Insertion

The ring pessary is folded in half and a small amount of lubricant placed on the tip to aid insertion. It is removed by gently pulling and folding it in half. Many women can be taught to manage their own pessary (Jones & Harmanli, 2010), removing it daily or weekly for cleaning or as infrequently (assuming there are no adverse events) as every 3 months. The Gellhorn is generally the best option for women with more advanced prolapse or in women who are no longer sexually active. It is more difficult to insert and remove so this generally needs to be done by the clinician. According to Jones and Harmanli (2010), "to insert the Gellhorn, the pessary is folded in half with the use of lubricant on the leading edge to ease insertion. Once the pessary is behind the pubic symphysis, it will expand and rest against the leading edge of prolapse, forming suction. To remove the Gellhorn, the knob is grasped, generally with the help of a ring forceps, while the concave end of the pessary is rotated to release the suction and the pessary is pulled downward, folded and removed" (p. 5).

Size of Pessary

In sizing a pessary, the provider estimates the size of the vagina and then selects the largest pessary that she/he thinks will fit comfortably. Following insertion, the clinician should assure that she/he is able to place a finger between the pessary and the walls of the vagina. After fitting, the woman should be asked to perform various activities (e.g., standing, walking, and bearing down) to make sure she can retain the pessary and that there is no discomfort. It is also critical to ensure that she can void before she leaves the clinic/office. Following initial fitting and insertion, the woman should be seen in 2 to 4 weeks to determine if she is satisfied with the pessary or if a different size or style is needed (Robert et al., 2013). If the woman is self-managing her pessary, there is no consensus about the frequency of follow-up visits although every 3 to 6 months is generally recommended. If the woman is unable to self-manage the pessary, it will need to be removed and reinserted by the health care provider, usually every 3 months (Jelovsek et al., 2007; Jones & Harmanli, 2010; Robert et al., 2013). During each follow-up visit, the pessary should be removed and cleansed with soap and water (Robert et al., 2013). The vagina should be inspected for mechanical erosions or other lesions and the pessary should be examined for evidence of damage. Robert et al. recommends removal of the pessary for 2 to 4 weeks and considering the use of topical estrogen if there are erosions. If neglected, these can lead to ulcers or fistula formation. Lesions that persist despite treatment should be biopsied. Serious complications such as fistulas are rare and generally seen in women who do not receive regular follow-up care. Bugge et al. (2013) published a Cochrane review designed to determine the effectiveness of pessaries for POP. Only one RCT was found that assessed pessary use for POP and it compared the ring and Gellhorn pessaries. Both were effective for approximately 60% of the women who completed the study with no significant differences between the two pessaries. The authors concluded that there is currently no consensus on the use of different types of devices, the indications for their use, how often they should be replaced, or how often women require follow-up care. There is a need for well-designed RTCs to address pessary use in comparison to observation, PFMT, and surgery.

CLINICAL PEARL

Many women have some degree of pelvic organ prolapse. Current recommended management options for POP include observation, pessary support, PFMT, or surgery.

Pelvic Floor Muscle Training

The PFMs provide structural support for the pelvic organs. Consequently, it can be theorized that PFMT, by improving muscle function, could improve this structural support (Hagen & Stark, 2011). Research examining the impact of PFMT on POP severity and symptoms is relatively new (Hagen & Stark, 2011). Bø (2012) reviewed five RCTs examining the impact of PFMT on POP severity and/or POP symptoms. Across the five RCTs included in her review, all favored PFMT; two reported statistically significant improvements in symptoms and three in prolapse rates compared to the control subjects. The ICI committee on conservative management of UI in adults (Moore et al., 2013) reviewed six RCTs comparing the impact of PFMT to a control intervention in women with POP. These studies examined the impact of PFMT on POP severity and/or symptoms. This review included one RCT not included in Bø's review. The Committee concluded that there was a high level of evidence to support that PFMT can improve the severity of POP and POP symptoms. In a subsequently published multicenter RCT (Hagen et al., 2014), 447 women (most with a stage 2 or 3 prolapse) were randomly assigned to a PFMT training group ($n = 225$) or control group ($n = 222$). The primary outcome was POP symptoms at 6 and 12 months post intervention and data were analyzed using an intention-to-treat approach. Women in the PFMT group reported a significantly greater reduction in symptoms at 6 and 12 months compared to control subjects and were significantly more likely to report that their prolapse was better. Women in the control group were significantly more likely to report receiving additional treatments at 12 months than those in the PFMT group (50% vs. 24%, respectively). Among women with a follow-up pelvic examination at 6 months, there was not a statistically significant difference in regression or progression of the prolapse in the two groups. Given the low risk of adverse events associated with PFMT, existing evidence supports the use of this intervention for women with POP.

Surgery

The goals of POP surgery are to restore normal vaginal anatomy and normal bladder, bowel, and sexual function. The two main surgical approaches are vaginal and abdominal approaches. Within each of these approaches, there are multiple potential procedures. For example, vaginal approaches include vaginal hysterectomy and anterior or posterior wall repair; abdominal procedures include hysterectomy, sacral colpopexy, and paravaginal repair and can be performed through an open incision, laparoscopically, or robotically (Maher et al., 2013). According to Rogo-Gupta (2013), there has been a significant evolution in the surgical treatment of POP over the past decade. Historically, the most common procedures were inpatient laparotomy, which included hysterectomy. Since the mid-1990s, minimally invasive ambulatory procedures have become popular. Advances in prolapse repair materials have also resulted in changes in surgical practices with surgical mesh gaining popularity. However, recent adverse event reports associated with the use of mesh have caused concerns and there has been some decline in its use since 2008. A 2013 Cochrane review of surgical procedures for POP (Maher et al., 2013) included RCTs and quasi-experimental studies ($n = 56$) comparing the outcomes of various surgical approaches. There were no trials comparing surgery to other treatment options. After reviewing trials comparing surgical options, the authors concluded that:

> Sacral colpopexy has superior outcomes to a variety of vaginal procedures including sacrospinous colpopexy, uterosacral colpopexy and transvaginal mesh. These benefits must be balanced against a longer operating time, longer time to return to activities of daily living, and increased cost of the abdominal approach. The use of mesh or graft inlays at the time of anterior vaginal wall repair reduces the risk of recurrent anterior wall prolapse on examination. Anterior vaginal polypropylene mesh also reduces awareness of prolapse; however, these benefits must be weighed against increased operating time, blood loss, rate of apical or posterior compartment prolapse, de novo stress urinary incontinence, and reoperation rate for mesh exposures associated with the use of polypropylene mesh. Posterior vaginal wall repair may be better than transanal repair in the management of rectocele in terms of recurrence of prolapse. The evidence is not supportive of any grafts at the time of posterior vaginal repair. Adequately powered randomized, controlled clinical trials with blinding of assessors are urgently needed on a wide variety of issues, and they particularly need to include women's perceptions of prolapse symptoms. Following the withdrawal of some commercial transvaginal mesh kits from the market, the generalizability of the findings, especially relating to anterior compartment transvaginal mesh, should be interpreted with caution (p. 2).

Postoperative care following prolapse surgery is generally similar to the care following surgery for SUI. Patients may be advised to avoid strenuous exercise, lifting (more than light objects) and sexual intercourse for a longer period of time (up to 8 weeks following surgery).

Vesicovaginal Fistula

Common sites for fistulas are vesicovaginal (bladder to vagina), urethrovaginal (urethra to vagina), vaginoperineal (vagina to the perineum), ureterovaginal (ureter to vagina), and rectovaginal (rectum to vagina) (Fig. 9-17).

Vesicovaginal fistula (VVF) is an abnormal tract that forms between the bladder and vagina, allowing urine to continuously drain into the vagina. While most fistulas develop between the bladder and vagina, they can occur between the urethra and vagina as well. The woman with a VVF leaks urine continuously, which can have a devastating impact on quality of life (Demirci et al., 2013).

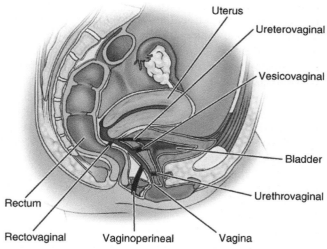

FIGURE 9-17. Common sites for fistulas.

Etiology

In the developing world, the most common cause of VVF is attempted vaginal delivery in the setting of cephalopelvic disproportion. The prolonged pressure of the fetal head causes ischemia and necrosis, which leads to fistula formation. Young, poorly educated primiparas living in rural areas of the developing world are at highest risk for prolonged (obstructed) labor and, thus, fistula formation. The effects on young women in these resource poor areas are devastating (De Ridder, 2009). The estimated incidence of obstetric fistulas is low in developed countries; in North America and Europe, it is about 0.01% (McVary & Marshall, 2002). The primary cause of VVF in developed countries is surgical trauma during gynecologic surgery, especially hysterectomy (Demirci et al., 2013). The incidence rate following hysterectomy is, however, very low at <1% (Forsgren & Altman, 2010). With radical hysterectomy, the incidence increases to an estimated 1% to 4%. Possible mechanisms are direct injury to the bladder or urethra or pressure necrosis secondary to sutures incorporated into the bladder. Data from observational studies have identified a number of characteristics that may increase the risk of hysterectomy-associated VVF. These include older age, laparoscopic or abdominal approaches during the hysterectomy, smoking, and pelvic adhesions (Forsgren & Altman, 2010). Other risk factors include pelvic radiation and, less commonly, destruction of tissue secondary to malignant tumors, ulceration from a foreign body (e.g., pessary), direct trauma, tuberculosis, schistosomiasis, calculi, and endometriosis (McVary & Marshall, 2002).

Clinical Presentation

The diagnosis is obvious in most patients due to the continuous leakage of urine and the observation of urine draining from the vagina. McVary and Marshall (2002) recommend the following diagnostic studies in all patients with VVF: (1) urinalysis, (2) urine culture, (3) intravenous urography, and (4) cystoscopy and vaginoscopy. Successful surgical repair is dependent on determining the exact location of the fistula, its size, and the underlying causes. Other tests should be performed as needed, such as a CT scan, MRI, and/or retrograde ureteropyelogram. A number of systems exist for classifying VVF although there is currently no universally accepted system (De Ridder, 2011). Frajzyngier et al. (2013) examined the diagnostic performance of five current classification systems and concluded that all of the systems were rather complex and none had good prognostic value for successful fistula closure. According to the authors, there is a need for a prognostic classification system that is evidence-based, simple, and easy to use.

Management

Patients with VVF leak urine continuously, which places them at high risk for incontinence-associated dermatitis. Routine cleansing of the perineal area and the application of a moisture barrier product to prevent further damage are an important part of the management. Definitive management options for VVF include conservative management, surgical repair, and urinary diversion (McVary & Marshall, 2002). While small fistulas are sometimes managed conservatively with prolonged catheter drainage to allow healing and closure, the reported success rate in achieving closure has generally been low (McVary & Marshall, 2002; Narayanan et al., 2009). Currently, surgery is considered the preferred treatment for most patients. According to De Ridder (2011), the surgical approach is dependent on the characteristics of the fistula (e.g., size and location) as well as the expertise of the surgeon (Creanga & Genadry, 2007). In the developed world, a variety of approaches are described. These include vaginal, abdominal, laparoscopic, minimally invasive, and robotic-assisted approaches. Depending on the amount of urethral or bladder damage associated with the fistula, some women will experience persistent SUI despite successful closure (Creanga & Genadry, 2007; de Ridder, 2011). When a fistula cannot be repaired or has failed previous closure attempts, urinary diversion may be indicated. Nursing care needs related to the care of patients with VVF will vary with the type of surgery performed. In the early postoperative period, women will have an indwelling catheter and measures need to be taken to minimize the risk of catheter-associated infection. Women need to be monitored for postoperative complications including infections (urinary tract and wound) and hemorrhage. If a woman experiences SUI following surgical closure of the fistula, PFMT is indicated. Nurses need to be aware of the cultural issues related to UI associated with VVF or occurring for other reasons. For instance, Sange et al. (2008) reported that UI has a more devastating impact on the quality of life of Muslim women than for many other women. Muslims have to perform ritual cleansing prior to prayers, which are performed five times a day. If a woman leaks urine, she must perform the cleansing ritual again. This repeated need for cleansing can lead to guilt and perceptions of punishment. As a result of guilt, women may be reluctant to seek treatment for their UI.

CLINICAL PEARL

Surgery is a definitive treatment for most women with a vesicovaginal fistula.

 ## Conclusion

Stress UI and POP are common problems among women. While VVF is relatively rare, it is a devastating problem for women who experience it. SUI generally presents as involuntary loss of small amounts of urine occurring during activities associated with sudden increases in intra-abdominal pressure. Unless the initial evaluation suggests complicated SUI, initial treatment can be initiated following a limited baseline evaluation (history, focused physical examination, cough stress test, and, where feasible, a 3-day bladder diary). PFMT is the best initial treatment option for most women with SUI. While POP is common, most cases are mild and asymptomatic. Observation and PFMT are viable treatment options for women with lower stage POP. Pessaries are the main nonsurgical treatment option for women with POP. The ideal pessary type and size will vary with the severity of the POP as well as other patient characteristics.

VVF is a rare clinical condition with a major impact on the quality of women's lives. In developing countries, it is usually seen in young primigravidas with obstructed labor due to the fetal head being too large to pass through the pelvis. In the United States, it is generally a surgical complication and occurs most often as a result of a hysterectomy. Women present with continuous leakage of urine from the vagina and skin care is an important consideration. Treatment is usually surgical, but depending on the size and location of the fistula and the amount of damage to surrounding tissue, women may continue to experience SUI following surgical correction.

CLINICAL PEARL

- A history, focused physical examination (abdominal, pelvic, and neurological), cough stress test, and 3-day bladder diary provide an adequate basis for treating SUI in most women.
- There is a high level of research to support the effectiveness of PFMT in treating SUI in women. The ideal method of teaching PFMT and the optimal training regimen are, however, yet to be determined. While a variety of training approaches have been shown to be effective, more frequent clinician contact is probably beneficial.
- While some degree (stage) of pelvic prolapse is common among women, most prolapses are mild (stage 1 or 2) and can often be observed and monitored over time. Pessaries are a good option for many women when treatment is indicated. The best type of pessary will depend on the severity of the prolapse as well as other patient characteristics.

CASE STUDY

Mrs. J, a 51-year-old white female, presents with urinary incontinence. Her history reveals that she leaks urine when she coughs and sneezes or if she lifts something heavy. She does not exercise regularly but denies leaking with ordinary physical activities such as walking or changing position. She admits to occasional urgency but this is not associated with involuntary urine loss. Typically, accidents are small, usually "a few drops," and occur one to two times a day. She only wears a pad if she is going out for an extended period of time or if she has a cold and is coughing a lot. She has had occasional incontinent episodes for the past 3 to 4 years, but they have increased in frequency over the past year, which is what prompted her to seek treatment at this time. She does not believe that the incontinence is having a major impact on the quality of her life at present but would like to treat it before it "gets worse." She is sexually active with her husband and denies UI having any negative impact. She has had no previous treatment for UI. She voids six to seven times a day and usually does not get up at night to urinate unless she has coffee or drinks a lot of fluid in the late evening; she has no enuresis. She typically drinks three to four cups of regular coffee per day, one can of diet Coke, and one to two glasses of water or milk; she has an occasional glass of wine or beer when out or has guests. She denies difficulty emptying her bladder, dysuria, lower abdominal or pelvic pain or pressure, hematuria, and dyspareunia. Her bowels usually move daily. She has occasional "dietary-related" constipation and denies fecal incontinence. History includes three uncomplicated vaginal deliveries; the babies weighed 6.1, 7.5, and 8.2 pounds, respectively. She does recall having occasional leaking during her last pregnancy, which subsided by the 8th week postpartum. She is having menopausal symptoms with hot flashes and irregular, but heavy menstrual periods; her last menstrual period was 3 months ago. Her husband uses condoms during sexual intercourse; she denies the possibility of pregnancy.

She describes herself as generally healthy without any physical limitations. Her only medical problem other than "needing to lose some weight" is hypertension. She takes hydrochlorothiazide daily and BP is "usually good." She denies smoking. Her past medical history is negative for urinary tract infections, arthritis, diabetes mellitus, asthma, chronic pulmonary disease, neurologic disorders, or depression.

The physical examination reveals overweight, but healthy-looking, alert, cognitively intact middle-aged woman without any obvious functional limitations. Her vital signs are as follows: BP 138/82, HR 76,

and BMI 30.2. Her abdomen is obese but soft and nontender without masses or organomegaly and no suprapubic dullness on percussion. On neurologic examination, her gait is normal, cranial nerves are intact, and deep tendon reflexes are normal; she has full range of motion and no sensory deficits. On pelvic examination, there is a stage 1 pelvic prolapse of the anterior vaginal wall. The vaginal mucosa is pink and moist, her ovaries are not palpable, and the uterus is midline, mobile, nontender, and normal in size. She is able to voluntarily contract her PFMs with verbal instructions and the strength is moderate with slight retraction of the examiner's fingers; she is able to hold the contraction for 3 to 4 seconds times 3 attempts. The rectal examination is negative for masses and stool. The cough stress test, done in a supine position, is positive for involuntary urine loss.

Diagnosis: SUI by history and mild, asymptomatic cystocele

Following the visit, the patient completed a 3-day bladder diary in which she documented 3 UI episodes associated with coughing or sneezing, an average of 6 voids/d, and no nocturia or enuresis. Average fluid intake was 48 oz/d with 32 of those being caffeinated beverages (coffee or diet coke). At the second visit, the treatment plan was discussed including recommendations for weight loss with review of dietary and physical activity recommendations, reducing caffeine intake and PFMT. During digital vaginal examination, the patient was taught to perform PFM contractions. The patient was instructed to perform three sets of 15 exercises each day, one set supine and two sitting, and instructed to contract her PFMs for 3 seconds followed by 3 seconds of relaxation for each repetition, to breathe normally, and to avoid contracting her abdominal or buttock muscles. She was told that once she could comfortably contract and relax her PFMs for 3 seconds for all 15 exercises per set, the duration of the contraction and relaxation period could be increased to 4 seconds and then 5 seconds with each exercise. Given that her POP was only stage 1 and she was asymptomatic, no additional treatment (other than the PFMT) was deemed necessary. She was instructed to complete a bladder diary for the 3 days prior to her next scheduled visit in 2 weeks. Progress was assessed at that visit. She reported adhering to the exercise regimen and being able to contract and relax her PFMs for 5 seconds; she documented two SUI episodes in the 3-day diary. She had reduced her caffeine intake to 1 cup per day without any noted impact on her incontinence. She was instructed to continue to do three sets of exercises/day but to do one set standing, one sitting, and one supine. She was told to gradually increase her contraction and relaxation time with a goal of 10 seconds each; she was taught the "knack"—to contract her PFM when she coughed or sneezed and prior to and while lifting heavy objects. Caffeine intake was no longer restricted. She completed three additional visits over the next 8 weeks and reported that her incontinence was much improved with rare urinary accidents. Weight loss strategies were reinforced at each visit, but she only lost 2 pounds. She was referred for nutritional counseling. Follow-up visits will be scheduled on an as-needed basis.

REFERENCES

Abed, H., & Rogers, R. G. (2008). Urinary incontinence and pelvic organ prolapse: Diagnosis and treatment for the primary care physician. *Medical Clinics of North America, 92*(5), 1273–1293, xii. doi: 10.1016/j.mcna.2008.04.004.

Abrams, P., Andersson, K. E., Birder, L., et al. (2010). Fourth International Consultation on Incontinence Recommendations of the International Scientific Committee: Evaluation and treatment of urinary incontinence, pelvic organ prolapse, and fecal incontinence. *Neurourology and Urodynamics, 240*, 213–240. doi:10.1002/nau.

Altman, D. J., Ekström, A., Forsgren, C., et al. (2007a). Symptoms of anal and urinary incontinence following cesarean section or spontaneous vaginal delivery. *American Journal of Obstetrics and Gynecology, 197*(5), 512.e1–512.e7. doi:10.1016/j.ajog.2007.03.083.

Altman, D. J., Ekstrom, A., Gustafsson, C., et al. (2006). Risk of urinary incontinence after childbirth. *Obstetrics and Gynecology, 108*(4), 873–878.

Altman, D., Forsman, M., Falconer, C., et al. (2008). Genetic influence on stress urinary incontinence and pelvic organ prolapse. *European Urology, 54*(4), 918–922. doi: 10.1016/j.eururo.2007.12.004.

Altman, D., Granath, F., Cnattingius, S., et al. (2007b). Hysterectomy and risk of stress-urinary-incontinence surgery: Nationwide cohort study. *Lancet, 370*(9597), 1494–1499. doi: 10.1016/S0140-6736(07)61635-3.

Auwad, W., Freeman, R. M., & Swift, S. (2004). Is the pelvic organ prolapse quantification system (POPQ) being used? A survey of members of the International Continence Society (ICS) and the American Urogynecologic Society (AUGS). *International Urogynecology Journal and Pelvic Floor Dysfunction, 15*(5), 324–327. doi: 10.1007/s00192-004-1175-3.

Awwad, J., Sayegh, R., Yeretzian, J., et al. (2012). Prevalence, risk factors, and predictors of pelvic organ prolapse: A community-based study. *Menopause, 19*(11), 1235–1241. doi: 10.1097/gme.0b013e31826d2d94.

Bettez, M., Tu, L. M., Carlson, K., et al. (2012). 2012 update: Guidelines for adult urinary incontinence collaborative consensus document for the Canadian urological association. *Canadian Urologic Association Journal, 6*(5), 354–363.

Bø, K. (2012). Pelvic floor muscle training in treatment of female stress urinary incontinence, pelvic organ prolapse and sexual dysfunction. *World Journal of Urology, 30*(4), 437–443. doi: 10.1007/s00345-011-0779-8.

Bø, K., & Herbert, R. D. (2013). There is not yet strong evidence that exercise regimens other than pelvic floor muscle training can reduce stress urinary incontinence in women: a systematic review. *Journal of Physiotherapy, 59*(3), 159–168. doi: 10.1016/S1836-9553(13)70180-2.

Bradley, C. S., Brown, J. S., Van Den Eeden, S. K., et al. (2011). Urinary incontinence self-report questions: Reproducibility and agreement with bladder diary. *International Urogynecology Journal, 22*(12), 1565–1571. doi: 10.1007/s00192-011-1503-3.

Bright, E., Drake, M. J., & Abrams, P. (2011). Urinary diaries: Evidence for the development and validation of diary content, format, and duration. *Neurourology and Urodynamics, 352*, 348–352. doi: 10.1002/nau.

Bristol Urological Institute. (2014). International Consultation on Incontinence Modular Questionnaire (ICIQ). Retrieved from http://www.iciq.net/index.html

Brown, J. S., Sawaya, G., Thom, D. H., et al. (2000). Hysterectomy and urinary incontinence: A systematic review. *Lancet, 356*(9229), 535–539. doi: 10.1016/S0140-6736(00)02577-0.

Buckley, B. S., & Lapitan, M. C. M. (2010). Prevalence of urinary incontinence in men, women, and children—current evidence: findings of the Fourth International Consultation on Incontinence. *Urology, 76*(2), 265–270. doi: 10.1016/j.urology.2009.11.078.

Bugge, C., Adams, E. J., Gopinath, D., et al. (2013). Pessaries (mechanical devices) for pelvic organ prolapse in women. *Cochrane Database of Systematic Reviews, 2*, CD004010. doi: 10.1002/14651858.CD004010.pub3.

Cody, J. D., Jacobs, M. L., Richardson, K., et al. (2012). Oestrogen Therapy for urinary incontinence in post-menopausal women. *Cochrane Database of Systematic Reviews, 10*, CD001405. doi: 10.1002/14651858.CD001405.pub3.

Creanga, A. A, & Genadry, R. R. (2007). Obstetric fistulas: A clinical review. *International Journal of Gynaecology and Obstetrics, 99*(Suppl 1), S40–S46. doi: 10.1016/j.ijgo.2007.06.021.

Delancey, J. O. (2010). Why do women have stress urinary incontinence? *Neurourology and Urodynamics, 29*, S13–S17. doi: 10.1002/nau.

Demirci, U., Fall, M., Göthe, S., et al. (2013). Urovaginal fistula formation after gynaecological and obstetric surgical procedures: clinical experiences in a Scandinavian series. *Scandinavian Journal of Urology, 47*(2), 140–144. doi: 10.3109/00365599.2012.711772.

De Ridder, D. (2009). Vesicovaginal fistula: a major healthcare problem. *Current Opinion in Urology, 19*(4), 358–361. doi: 10.1097/MOU.0b013e32832ae1b7.

De Ridder, D. (2011). An update on surgery for vesicovaginal and urethrovaginal fistulae. *Current Opinion in Urology, 21*(4), 297–300. doi: 10.1097/MOU.0b013e3283476ec8.

DeTayrac, R., Chevalier, N., Chauveaud-Lambling, A., et al. (2007). Is vaginal hysterectomy a risk factor for urinary incontinence at long-term follow-up? *European Journal of Obstetrics, Gynecology, and Reproductive Biology, 130*(2), 258–261. doi: 10.1016/j.ejogrb.2006.01.032.

Dillon, B. E., & Zimmern, P. E. (2012). When are urodynamics indicated in patients with stress urinary incontinence? *Current Urology Reports, 13*(5), 379–384. doi: 10.1007/s11934-012-0270-0.

Diokno, A. C. (2003). Incidence and prevalence of stress urinary incontinence. *Advanced Studies in Medicine, 3*, 824–828.

Dumoulin, C., Glazener, C., & Jenkinson, D. (2011). Determining the optimal pelvic floor muscle training regimen for women with stress urinary incontinence. *Neurourology and Urodynamics, 30*, 746–753. doi: 10.1002/nau.

Dumoulin, C., Hay-Smith, E. J. C., & Mac Habée-Séguin, G. (2014). Pelvic floor muscle training versus no treatment, or inactive control treatments, for urinary incontinence in women. *Cochrane Database of Systematic Reviews, 5*, CD005654. doi: 10.1002/14651858.CD005654.pub3.

Elenskaia, K., Thakar, R., Sultan, A. H., et al. (2013). Effect of childbirth on pelvic organ support and quality of life: A longitudinal cohort study. *International Urogynecology Journal, 24*(6), 927–937. doi: 10.1007/s00192-012-1932-7.

Ellerkmann, R. M., Cundiff, G. W., Melick, C. F., et al. (2001). Correlation of symptoms with location and severity of pelvic organ prolapse. *American Journal of Obstetrics and Gynecology, 185*(6), 1332–1337; discussion 1337–1338. doi: 10.1067/mob.2001.119078.

Forsgren, C., & Altman, D. (2010). Risk of pelvic organ fistula in patients undergoing hysterectomy. *Current Opinion in Obstetrics and Gynecology, 22*(5), 404–407. doi: 10.1097/GCO.0b013e32833e49b0.

Forsgren, C., Lundholm, C., Johansson, A. L. V., et al. (2012). Vaginal hysterectomy and risk of pelvic organ prolapse and stress urinary incontinence surgery. *International Urogynecology Journal, 23*(1), 43–48. doi: 10.1007/s00192-011-1523-z.

Frawley, H. C., Galea, M. P., Phillips, B. A., et al. (2006). Reliability of pelvic floor muscle strength assessment using different test positions and tools. *Neurourology and Urodynamics, 25*(3), 236–242. doi:10.1002/nau.20201.

Frajzyngier, V., Guohua, L., Larson, E., et al. (2013). Development and comparison of prognostic scoring systems for surgical closure of genitourinary fistula. *American Journal of Obstetrics and Gynecology, 208*(2), 112.e1–11. doi:10.1016/j.ajog.2012.11.040.

Geller, E. J., & Wu, J. M. (2013). Changing trends in surgery for stress urinary incontinence. *Current Opinion in Obstetrics & Gynecology, 25*(5), 404–409. doi: 10.1097/GCO.0b013e3283648cdd.

Gilchrist, A. S., Campbell, W., Steele, H., et al. (2013). Outcomes of observation as therapy for pelvic organ prolapse: A study in the natural history of pelvic organ prolapse. *Neurourology and Urodynamics, 32*, 383–386. doi: 10.1002/nau.

Gleason, J. L., Richter, H. E., Redden, D. T., et al. (2013). Caffeine and urinary incontinence in US women. *International Urogynecology Journal, 24*(2), 295–302. doi: 10.1007/s00192-012-1829-5.

Gleason, J. L., Richter, H. E., & Varner, R. E. (2012). Pelvic organ prolapse. In J. S. Berek (Ed.), *Berek & Novak's gynecology* (15th ed., pp. 1–46). Lippincott Williams & Wilkins.

Gustafsson, C., Ekström, A., Brismar, S., et al. (2006). Urinary incontinence after hysterectomy—three-year observational study. *Urology, 68*(4), 769–774. doi: 10.1016/j.urology.2006.04.001.

Gutman, R. E., Ford, D. E., Quiroz, L. H., et al. (2008). Is there a pelvic organ prolapse threshold that predicts pelvic floor symptoms? *American Journal of Obstetrics and Gynecology, 199*(6), 683.e1–7. doi:10.1016/j.ajog.2008.07.028.

Gyhagen, M., Bullarbo, M., Nielsen, T. F., et al. (2013a). A comparison of the long-term consequences of vaginal delivery versus caesarean section on the prevalence, severity and bothersomeness of urinary incontinence subtypes: a national cohort study in primiparous women. *BJOG: An International Journal of Obstetrics and Gynaecology, 120*(12), 1548–1555. doi: 10.1111/1471-0528.12367.

Gyhagen, M., BullarBo, M., Nielsen, T. F., et al. (2013b). Prevalence and risk factors for pelvic organ prolapse 20 years after childbirth: A national cohort study in singleton primiparae after vaginal or caesarean delivery. *BJOG: An International Journal of Obstetrics and Gynaecology, 120*(2), 152–160. doi: 10.1111/1471-0528.12020.

Hagen, S., & Stark, D. (2011). Conservative prevention and management of pelvic organ prolapse in women. *Cochrane Database of Systematic Reviews, 12*, CD003882. doi: 10.1002/14651858.CD003882.pub4.

Hagen, S., Stark, D., Glazener, C., et al. (2014). Individualised pelvic floor muscle training in women with pelvic organ prolapse (POPPY): a multicentre randomised controlled trial. *Lancet, 383*(9919), 796–806. doi: 10.1016/S0140-6736(13)61977-7.

Hannestad, Y. S., Rortveit, G., Daltveit, A. K., et al. (2003). Are smoking and other lifestyle factors associated with female urinary incontinence? The Norwegian EPINCONT Study. *BJOG: An International Journal of Obstetrics and Gynaecology, 110*, 247–254. doi:10.10161/S1470-0328(02)02927-0.

Hay-Smith, E. J. C., Herderschee, R., Dumoulin, C., et al. (2011). Comparisons of approaches to pelvic floor muscle training for urinary incontinence in women. *Cochrane Database of Systematic Reviews, 12*, CD009508. doi: 10.1002/14651858.CD009508.

Haylen, B. T., Ridder, D. De, Freeman, R. M., et al. (2010). An International Urogynecological Association (IUGA)/International Continence Society (ICS) joint report on the terminology for female pelvic floor dysfunction *International Urogynecology Journal, 20*, 4–20. doi:10.1002/nau.

Herbison, G. P., & Dean, N. (2013). Weighted vaginal cones for urinary incontinence. *Cochrane Database of Systematic Reviews, 7*, CD002114. doi: 10.1002/14651858.CD002114.pub2.

Herderschee, R., Hay-Smith, E. J. C., Herbison, G. P., et al. (2011). Feedback or biofeedback to augment pelvic floor muscle training for urinary incontinence in women. *Cochrane Database of Systematic Reviews, 7*, CD009252. doi: 10.1002/14651858.CD009252.

Hirakawa, T., Suzuki, S., Kato, K., et al. (2013). Randomized controlled trial of pelvic floor muscle training with or without biofeedback for urinary incontinence. *International Urogynecology Journal, 24*(8), 1347–1354. doi: 10.1007/s00192-012-2012-8.

Hosker, G. (2009). Is it possible to diagnose intrinsic sphincter deficiency in women? *Current Opinion in Urology, 19*(4), 342–346. doi: 10.1097/MOU.0b013e32832ae1cb.

Isherwood, P. J., & Rane, A. (2000). Comparative assessment of pelvic floor strength using a perineometer and digital examination. *BJOG: An International Journal of Obstetrics and Gynaecology, 107*(8), 1007–1011.

Jelovsek, J. E., Maher, C., & Barber, M. D. (2007). Pelvic organ prolapse. *Lancet, 369*(9566), 1027–1038. doi: 10.1016/S0140-6736(07)60462-0.

Jones, K. A., & Harmanli, O. (2010). Pessary use in pelvic organ prolapse and urinary incontinence. *Reviews in Obstetrics and Gynecology, 3*(1), 3–9. doi: 10.3909/riog0110.

Jura, Y. H., Townsend, M. K., Curhan, G. C., et al. (2011). Caffeine intake, and the risk of stress, urgency and mixed urinary incontinence. *Journal of Urology, 185*(5), 1775–1780. doi: 10.1016/j.juro.2011.01.003.

Keyock, K. L., & Newman, D. K. (2011). Understanding stress urinary incontinence. *Nurse Practitioner, 36*(10), 24–36; quiz 36–37. doi: 10.1097/01.NPR.0000405281.55881.7a.

Kirchin, V., Page, T., Keegan, P. E., et al. (2012). Urethral injection therapy for urinary incontinence in women. *Cochrane Database of Systematic Reviews, 2*, CD003881. doi: 10.1002/14651858.CD003881.pub3.

Koelb, H., Igawa, T., Salvatore, S., et al. (2013). Pathophysiology of urinary incontinence, faecal incontinence and pelvic organ prolapse. In A. Abrams, L. Cardozo, S. Khoury & A. Wein (Eds.), *Incontinence* (5th ed., pp 263–359). European Association of Urology. ISBN: 978-9953-493-21-3.

Leijonhufvud, A., Lundholm, C., Cnattingius, S., et al. (2011). Risks of stress urinary incontinence and pelvic organ prolapse surgery in relation to mode of childbirth. *American Journal of Obstetrics and Gynecology, 204*(1), 70.e1–7. doi:10.1016/j.ajog.2010.08.034.

Liebergall-Wischnitzer, M., Hochner-Celnikier, D., Lavy, Y., et al. (2005) Paula method of circular muscle exercises for urinary stress incontinence—A clinical trial. *International Urogynecology Journal and Pelvic Floor Dysfunction, 16*, 345–351.

Lue, T. F., & Tanagho, E. A. (2014). Urinary incontinence. In J. W. McAninch & T. F. Lue (Eds.), *Smith & Tanagho's general urology* (18th ed., pp. 1–28). McGraw-Hill Companies, Inc.

Luft, J. (2006). Pelvic organ prolapse: Current state of knowledge about this common condition. *Journal for Nurse Practitioners, 2*(3), 170–177.

Maher, C., Feiner, B., Baessler, K., et al. (2013). Surgical management of pelvic organ prolapse in women. *Cochrane Database of Systematic Reviews, 4*, CD004014. doi: 10.1002/14651858.CD004014.pub5.

Mariappan, P., Alhasso, A. A., Grant, A., N'Dow, J. M. O. (2005). Serotonin and noradrenaline reuptake inhibitors (SNRI) for stress urinary incontinence in adults. *Cochrane Database of Systematic Reviews, 3*, CD004742. doi: 10.1002/14651858.CD004742.pub2.

Markland, A. D., Richter, H. E., Fwu, C.-W., et al. (2011). Prevalence and trends of urinary incontinence in adults in the United States, 2001 to 2008. *Journal of Urology, 186*(2), 589–593. doi: 10.1016/j.juro.2011.03.114.

McGuire, E. J. (1981). Urodynamic findings in patients after failure of stress incontinence operations. *Progress in Clinical and Biological Research, 78*, 351–360.

McKenzie, P., Rohozinski, J., & Badlani, G. (2010). Genetic influences on stress urinary incontinence. *Current Opinion in Urology, 20*(4), 291–295. doi: 10.1097/MOU.0b013e32833a4436.

McLean, L., Varette, K., Gentilcore-Saulnier, E., et al. (2013). Pelvic floor muscle training in women with stress urinary incontinence causes hypertrophy of the urethral sphincters and reduces bladder neck mobility during coughing. *Neurourology and Urodynamics, 32*(8), 1096–1102.

McLennan, M. T., Harris, J. K., Kariuki, B., et al. (2008). Family history as a risk factor for pelvic organ prolapse. *International Urogynecology Journal and Pelvic Floor Dysfunction, 19*(8), 1063–1069. doi: 10.1007/s00192-008-0591-1.

McVary, K. T., & Marshall, F. F. (2002). Vesicovaginal fistula. In J. Y. Gillenwater, J. T. Grayhack, S. S. Howards, M. E. Mitchell (Eds.), *Adult and Pediatric Urology* (4th ed., pp. 1272–1278). Lippincott Williams & Wilkins.

Miedel, A., Tegertedt, G., Moehle-Schmidt, M., et al. (2009). Nonobstetric risk factors for symptomatic pelvic organ prolapse. *Obstetrics and Gynecology, 113*(5), 1089–1097.

Miller, J. M., Perucchini, D., Carchidi, L. T., et al. (2001). Pelvic floor muscle contraction during a cough and decreased vesical neck mobility. *Obstetrics and Gynecology, 97*(2), 255–260. Retrieved from http://www.pubmedcentral.nih.gov/articlerender.fcgi?artid=1226460&tool=pmcentrez&rendertype=abstract.

Miller, J. J. R., Botros, S. M., Beaumont, J. L., et al. (2008). Impact of hysterectomy on stress urinary incontinence: An identical twin study. *American Journal of Obstetrics and Gynecology, 198*(5), 565. e1–4. doi:10.1016/j.ajog.2008.01.046.

Minassian, V. A., Stewart, W. F., & Hirsch, A. G. (2008). Why do stress and urge incontinence co-occur much more often than expected? *International Urogynecology Journal and Pelvic Floor Dysfunction, 19*(10), 1429–1440. doi: 10.1007/s00192-008-0647-2.

Moore, K. N., Dumoulin, C., Bradley, C., et al. (2013). Committee 12: Adult conservative management. In A. Abrams, L. Cardozo, S. Khoury & A. Wein (Eds). *Incontinence* (5th ed., pp. 263–359). European Association of Urology. ISBN: 978-9953-493-21-3.

Nager, C. W. (2012). The urethra is a reliable witness: Simplifying the diagnosis of stress urinary incontinence. *International Urogynecology Journal, 23*(12), 1649–1651. doi: 10.1007/s00192-012-1892-y.

Nager, C. W., Brubaker, L., Litman, H. J., et al.; The Urinary Incontinence Treatment Network. (2012). A randomized trial of urodynamic testing before stress-incontinence surgery. *New England Journal of Medicine, 366*, 1987–1997. doi: 10.1016/j.juro.2012.12.078.

Narayanan, P., Nobbenhuis, M., Reynolds, K. M., et al. (2009). Fistulas in malignant gynecologic disease: Etiology, imaging, and management. *Radiographics, 29*(4), 1073–1083. doi: 10.1148/rg.294085223.

Nygaard, I. E., & Heit, M. (2004). Stress urinary incontinence. *Obstetrics and Gynecology, 104*(3), 607–620. doi: 10.1097/01.AOG.0000137874.84862.94.

Ogah, J., Cody, J. D., Rogerson, L. (2009). Minimally invasive synthetic suburethral sling operations for stress urinary incontinence in women. *Cochrane Database of Systematic Reviews, 4*, CD006375. doi: 10.1002/14651858.CD006375.pub2.

Persu, C., Chapple, C. R., Cauni, V., et al. (2011). Pelvic organ prolapse quantification system (POP-Q)—A new era in pelvic prolapse staging. *Journal of Medicine and Life, 4*(1), 75–81.

Press, J. Z., Klein, M. C., Kaczorowski, J., et al. (2007). Does cesarean section reduce postpartum urinary incontinence? A systematic review. *Birth, 34*(3), 228–237. doi: 10.1111/j.1523-536X.2007.00175.x

Ramsay, S., Bouchard, F., Tu, L. M. (2011). Long term outcomes of pessary use in women with pelvic organ prolapse. *Neurourology and Urodynamics, 30*(6), 1105–1106.

Richter, H. E., Burgio, K. L., Brubaker, L., et al. (2010). Behavioral therapy or combined therapy: A randomized controlled trial. *Obstetrics and Gynecology, 115*(3), 609–617.

Robert, M., Schulz, J. A., Harvey, M.-A., et al. (2013). Technical update on pessary use. *Journal of Obstetrics and Gynaecology Canada, 35*(7), 664–674. Retrieved from http://www.ncbi.nlm.nih.gov/pubmed/23876646.

Rogo-Gupta, L. (2013). Current trends in surgical repair of pelvic organ prolapse. *Current Opinion in Obstetrics and Gynecology, 25*(5), 395–398. doi: 10.1097/GCO.0b013e3283648cfb.

Rortveit, G., Brown, J. S., Thom, D. H., et al. (2007). Symptomatic pelvic organ prolapse: Prevalence and risk factors in a population-based, racially diverse cohort. *Obstetrics and Gynecology, 109*(6), 1396–1403.

Rortveit, G., Daltveit, A. K., Hannestad, Y. S., et al. (2003). Vaginal delivery parameters and urinary incontinence: The Norwegian EPINCONT study. *American Journal of Obstetrics and Gynecology, 189*(5), 1268–1274. doi: 10.1067/S0002-9378(03)00588-X.

Sange, C., Thomas, L., Lyons, C., et al. (2008) Urinary incontinence in Muslim women. *Nursing Times, 104*(25), 49–52.

Sangsawang, B., & Sangsawang, N. (2013). Stress urinary incontinence in pregnant women: A review of prevalence, pathophysiology, and treatment. *International Urogynecology Journal, 24*(6), 901–912. doi: 10.1007/s00192-013-2061-7.

Schreiner, L., Guimarães, T., Borba, A., et al. (2013). Electrical stimulation for urinary incontinence in women: A systematic review. *International Braz J Urol, 39*(4), 454–464. doi: 10.1590/S1677-5538.IBJU.2013.04.02.

Shamliyan, T., Wyman, J., & Kane, R. L. (2012). *Nonsurgical treatments for urinary incontinence in adult women: Diagnosis and comparative effectiveness.* Comparative Effectiveness Review No. 36. (Prepared by the University of Minnesota Evidence-based Practice Center under Contract No. HHSA 290-2007-10064-I.) AHRQ Publication No. 11(12)-EHC074- EF. Rockville, MD. Agency for Healthcare Research and Quality. Available at: www.effectivehealthcare.ahrq.gov/reports/final.cfm.

Sirls, L. T., Foote, J. E., Kaufman, J. M., et al. (2002). Original article long-term results of the FemSoft 1 urethral insert for the management of female stress urinary incontinence. *International Urogynecology Journal, 13*, 88–95.

Smith, P. P., van Leijsen, S. A. L., Heesakkers, J. P. F., et al. (2012). Can we, and do we need to, define bladder neck hypermobility and intrinsic sphincteric deficiency?: ICI-RS 2011. *Neurourology and Urodynamics, 312*, 309–312. doi: 10.1002/nau.

Staskin, D., Kelleher, C., Bosch, R., et al. (2009). Initial assessment of urinary and faecal incontinence in adult male and female patients. In P. Abrams, L. Cardozo, S. Khoury, et al. (Eds.), *4th International Consultation on Incontinence*. Health Publications Ltd.

Staskin, D., Kelleher, C., Bosch, R., et al. (2013). Initial assessment of urinary incontinence in adult male and female patients (5A). In P. Abrams, L. Cardozo, S. Khoury, et al. (Eds.), *5th International Consultation on Incontinence* (pp. 361–388). London, UK: European Association of Urology.

Subak, L. L., Richter, H. E., & Hunskaar, S. (2009). Obesity and urinary incontinence: Epidemiology and clinical research update. *Journal of Urology, 182*(6 Suppl), S2–S7. doi: 10.1016/j.juro.2009.08.071.

Swift, S. E., Tate, S. B., & Nicholas, J. (2003). Correlation of symptoms with degree of pelvic organ support in a general population of women: What is pelvic organ prolapse? *American Journal of Obstetrics and Gynecology, 189*(2), 372–377. doi: 10.1067/S0002-9378(03)00698-7.

Swithinbank, L., Hashim, H., & Abrams, P. (2005). The effect of fluid intake on urinary symptoms in women. *Journal of Urology, 174*(1), 187–189. doi: 10.1097/01.ju.0000162020.10447.31.

Tahtinen, R. M., Auvinen, A., Cartwright, R., et al. (2011). Smoking and bladder symptoms in women. *Obstetrics and Gynecology, 118*(3), 643–648. doi: 10.1097/AOG.0b013e318227b7ac.

Thomason, A. D., Miller, J. M., & Delancey, J. O. (2007). Urinary incontinence symptoms during and after pregnancy in continent and incontinent primiparas. *International Urogynecology Journal and Pelvic Floor Dysfunction, 18*(2), 147–151. doi: 10.1007/s00192-006-0124-8.

Van der Vaart, C., van der Bom, J., de Leeuw, J. R., et al. (2002). The contribution of hysterectomy to the occurrence of urge and stress urinary incontinence symptoms. *BJOG: An International Journal of Obstetrics and Gynaecology, 109*(2), 149–154. Retrieved from http://www.sciencedirect.com/science/article/pii/S1470032802013320.

Wilson, T. S., Lemack, G. E., & Zimmern, P. E. (2003). Management of intrinsic sphincteric deficiency in women. *Journal of Urology, 169*(5), 1662–1669. doi: 10.1097/01.ju.0000058020.37744.aa.

Wu, J. M., Vaughan, C. P., Goode, P. S., et al. (2014). Prevalence and trends of symptomatic pelvic floor disorders in U.S. women. *Obstetrics and Gynecology*, *123*(1), 141–148. doi: 10.1097/AOG.0000000000000057.

Zhu, L., Li, L., Lang, J. H., et al. (2012). Prevalence and risk factors for peri- and postpartum urinary incontinence in primiparous women in China: A prospective longitudinal study. *International Urogynecology Journal*, *23*(5), 563–572.

QUESTIONS

1. A 54-year-old female patient tells the continence nurse: "Every time I take my exercise class, I leak a little urine." What condition would the WOC nurse expect?
    A. Stress urinary incontinence
    B. Reduced bladder capacity
    C. Urinary tract infection
    D. Pelvic organ prolapse

2. Which patient would the continence nurse consider at higher risk for stress urinary incontinence related to her labor and delivery history?
    A. A woman who had a C-section
    B. A woman who experienced prolonged labor
    C. A woman who experienced a forceps delivery
    D. A woman who had a breech delivery

3. A continence nurse is counseling a female patient diagnosed with stress urinary incontinence. What is a recommended first-line management option for this condition?
    A. Vaginal cone
    B. Urethral bulking agents
    C. Pelvic floor muscle training
    D. Pharmacotherapy

4. The continence nurse is explaining treatment options to a female patient diagnosed with stress urinary incontinence. Which statement by the nurse accurately describes current therapy?
    A. There is a great amount of research to support the use of urethral inserts for SUI.
    B. Based on currently available evidence, the Paula method and deep abdominal muscle training should not be utilized in the treatment of SUI.
    C. There are various FDA-approved medications that may be prescribed for the treatment of SUI.
    D. While there are a variety of treatment options for SUI, for most women, the best initial treatment is vaginal cones or incontinence pessaries.

5. The continence nurse is caring for a female patient diagnosed with a cystocele. Which areas of the pelvic organs are involved in this condition?
    A. Anterior vaginal wall
    B. Posterior wall
    C. Apex
    D. Small or large bowel

6. The continence nurse is preparing a patient for a pelvic exam to diagnose suspected pelvic organ prolapse. Which instructions accurately describe a step in the procedure?
    A. The patient should be placed in a prone position.
    B. The patient should be examined with a full bladder.
    C. The patient should be asked to perform a Valsalva maneuver.
    D. The patient should be instructed to sit up to observe the prolapse.

7. The continence nurse is reading the report of a patient diagnosed with stage 3 pelvic organ prolapse. Which findings indicate this level of staging?
    A. The most distal portion of the prolapse is more than 1 cm above the level of the hymen.
    B. The most distal portion of the prolapse is 1 cm or less proximal to or distal to the plane of the hymen.
    C. The most distal portion of the prolapse is more than 1 cm below the plane of the hymen.
    D. Complete eversion of the total length of the lower genital tract is demonstrated.

8. A female patient is diagnosed with stage 2 pelvic organ prolapse and is asymptomatic. What is the first line of treatment for this condition?
    A. Observation
    B. Vaginal pessary
    C. Surgery
    D. Pharmacological treatment

9. A postpartum 32-year-old female is diagnosed with vesicovaginal fistula. What is the most common cause of this condition?
    A. Emergency C-section following prolonged labor
    B. Use of high forceps during delivery
    C. Induced labor
    D. Attempted vaginal delivery in the setting of cephalopelvic disproportion

10. What treatment would the continence nurse expect for a patient who is newly diagnosed with vesicovaginal fistula due to a surgical complication?
    A. PFMT alone
    B. Surgery to close the fistula
    C. Pharmacological treatment
    D. Hysterectomy

ANSWERS: 1.**A**, 2.**D**, 3.**C**, 4.**B**, 5.**A**, 6.**C**, 7.**C**, 8.**A**, 9.**D**, 10.**B**

CHAPTER 10

UI and Lower Urinary Tract Symptoms in the Older Adult

Mary H. Palmer

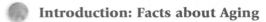
Introduction: Facts about Aging

The portion of the world's population of adults aged 60 years and over is projected to increase from 11% in 2000 to 22% in 2050 and the number of older adults aged 80 years and over is expected to quadruple (World Health Organization, 2012a, 2012b). The United States mirrors this growth in the older adult

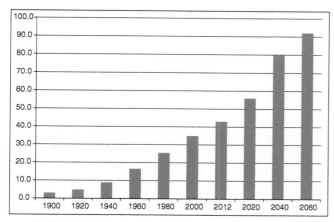

FIGURE 10-1. Number of persons 65+, 1900 to 2060.

population; 21% of the population is projected to be over 65 years of age in 2040 and the 85 years and over group is expected to triple by 2040 (Department of Health and Human Services Administration on Aging, 2013). The World Health Organization notes that in no other time in history have so many middle-aged and older adults had living parents as now (World Health Organization, 2012a). Figure 10-1 depicts changes in the aging population from 1900 to 2060.

This demographic shift has already impacted health care systems by increasing the need for specialized geriatric acute and long-term care services. WOC nurses will continue to play a central role in the care of this aging population due to the prevalence of urinary incontinence and other lower urinary tract symptoms in this population. In one study, 43.8% of older adults living in the community reported urinary leakage, 39% of older adults residing in residential care facilities were reported to have urinary incontinence in the 7 days preceding the study, 45.4% of home care patients reported difficulty with bladder control, and 46.1% of short-term and 75.8% of long-stay nursing home residents experienced incomplete bladder control in the 14 days preceding the study (Gorina et al., 2014).

Collecting, understanding, and using information about aging-related changes in body systems, the impact of comorbid conditions and polypharmacy on function, and the role the environment plays in enhancing and maintaining independence and health will be requisite skills for the WOC nurse in addressing UI and lower urinary tract symptoms in older adults. The lifelong learning process of the WOC nurse must include development and refinement of geriatric competencies that include interdisciplinary collaborations to (1) foster older adults' function, independence, quality of life, and dignity; (2) consider the needs and preferences of older adults and their family and other caregivers in treatment plans; and (3) help older adults and their families with advance planning and with end-of-life decisions about continence care.

Changes in Lower Urinary Tract Associated with Aging

The major role of the lower urinary tract, storing urine and releasing it periodically throughout the day, continues throughout the life span. Although the prevalence of urinary incontinence and overactive bladder (OAB) increases with age, *age alone does not cause urinary incontinence.*

> **CLINICAL PEARL**
>
> Although the prevalence of urinary incontinence and overactive bladder increases with age, age alone does not cause urinary incontinence.

Changes in the bladder related to age include decreased urine flow, reduced bladder capacity due to deposits of collagen and fibrosis, increased sensitivity to neurotransmitters (Siroky, 2004), impaired contractility, and increased postvoid residual volumes, usually 50 mL or less (Dubeau, 2006). In an animal study, aged animals were found to have fewer caveolae in the bladder smooth muscle and alterations in protein expression when compared to young animals (Lowalekar et al., 2012). These authors concluded that contractility of the detrusor muscle may be altered with aging, since caveolae regulate signal transduction. Changes also occur in the urothelium, which produces neurotransmitters and mediators including adenosine triphosphate (ATP). These changes include an increase in ATP-dependent detrusor contractions, fewer cholinergic contractions, and fewer M_3 (muscarinic) receptors (Wagg et al., 2014).

Some age-related changes in bladder and sphincter function are gender based. Because there are estrogen receptors throughout the female genitourinary tract, the decline in estrogen that occurs with menopause is thought to affect lower urinary tract function (Ellsworth et al., 2013). Reduced levels of estrogen are associated with thinning of the urethral urothelium and reduced vascularity of the urethral submucosa (Dubeau, 2006). However, the role of menopause on pelvic floor function is not well-understood and no evidence exists that hormone replacement therapy prevents pelvic organ prolapse or urinary incontinence (Mannella et al., 2013). As men age, they experience prostatic enlargement, which, in some cases, can cause bladder outlet obstruction (BOO) (Ellsworth et al., 2013).

The use of magnetic resonance imaging (MRI) in research has demonstrated the importance of brain white matter hyperintensities (WMH) on urine control. Researchers found that for each 1% increase in percentage of WMH in the brain, there was a corresponding 1.5 to 2.4 times increased risk for diminished function in voiding, mobility, and cognition (Wakefield et al., 2010). These findings reinforce other research and clinical findings that factors outside the lower urinary tract are important contributors to lower urinary tract symptoms in late life. The relationships among factors affecting continence are complex and multifactorial and include age-related changes in central nervous system control and lower urinary tract function, the effects of life events such as childbirth, and the impact of chronic diseases such as diabetes, obesity, and dementia. Chronological age plays a role in the function of the lower urinary tract and in the development of urinary incontinence and other lower urinary tract symptoms, but other influences such as comorbid conditions and non-genitourinary factors cannot be overlooked.

> **CLINICAL PEARL**
>
> Factors outside the urinary tract are important contributors to lower urinary tract symptoms in the elderly.

Nocturia

The International Continence Society (ICS) defined nocturia as "the interruption of sleep one or more times at night to void, with each void being preceded and followed by sleep" (van Kerrebroeck et al., 2002). Nocturia is one of four symptoms (urgency, urgency urinary incontinence, frequency, and nocturia) included in the definition of OAB (Abrams et al., 2002). Urgency is considered the "driver" for nocturia, causing increased nighttime voids at reduced volume (Abrams et al., 2012). Nocturia affects approximately 29% to 59% of men and 28% to 62% women aged 70 years and older (Weiss et al., 2013) and is associated with daytime fatigue and falls (Burgio et al., 2010). Nocturia is often underreported by older adults, with many assuming that waking multiple times at night is a normal part of aging (Bliwise et al., 2009). Many older adults do not differentiate between waking from a primary sleep disorder and waking due to the need to void (Dubeau, 2006). Evidence exists that there is a causative relationship among sleep-disordered breathing, primarily obstructed sleep apnea, and nocturia (Weiss et al., 2013).

> **CLINICAL PEARL**
>
> Nocturia is a common problem among the elderly and is associated with increased daytime fatigue and increased incidence of falls.

Pathology

Several underlying mechanisms for nocturia have been identified, including 24-hour polyuria, nocturnal polyuria, and reduced bladder capacity (Cornu et al., 2012). Twenty-four–hour polyuria in adults is defined as urine volume in 24 hours that is greater than 40 mL/kg (Cornu et al., 2012). It is seen in diabetes mellitus, diabetes insipidus, primary polydipsia, hypercalcemia, excessive fluid intake, and in some cases with the ingestion of certain medications (i.e., phenothiazines and anticholinergics) (Carlson & Palmer, 2014). With the increasing prevalence of obesity and diabetes mellitus in the adult population, including older adults, undiagnosed or poorly controlled diabetes mellitus should be considered during the assessment of nocturia.

Nocturnal polyuria has been traditionally thought of as a condition in which the day/night ratio of urine production is reversed. The International Continence Society proposed use of the nocturnal polyuria index (NPi), which is the ratio between nocturnal urine volume and the 24-hour urine volume. Nocturnal polyuria in older adults was defined as $NPi \geq 0.33$, that is, nocturnal urine output greater than 33% of the 24-hour urine volume (van Kerrebroeck et al., 2002). Some researchers are calling for a revision in the definition of nocturnal polyuria to include nocturnal urine production only (Hofmeester et al., 2015). An important finding in nocturnal polyuria is an abnormally low level of antidiuretic hormone (ADH) (Hirayama et al., 2011). When lower limb edema is present in the evening, ADH production may not occur; as a result, there will be increased production of dilute urine during nighttime hours (Hirayama et al., 2011). Older adults who experience nocturnal polyuria may feel light-headed at night when they stand, as a result of the altered nighttime fluid balance; this may increase their risk of falling (Asplund, 2007).

> **CLINICAL PEARL**
>
> Nocturia may be caused by excessive 24-hour urine production, excessive nighttime urine production, or inadequate bladder capacity.

Reduced nocturnal bladder capacity may be a symptom of several neurogenic conditions, including Parkinson's disease, multiple sclerosis, stroke, or spinal cord injury. Conditions intrinsic to the lower urinary tract that reduce bladder capacity include lower urinary tract cancer and calculi (Cornu et al., 2012). In older men, benign prostatic enlargement (BPE) can lead to reduced nocturnal bladder capacity (van Doorn & Bosch, 2012). Recent research has found that the probability of detrusor overactivity is independently associated with increasing age and BOO (Oelke et al., 2008). Because nocturia has many causes, assessment and identification of the underlying causes are essential to effective treatment.

Assessment

Nocturia is a patient-reported symptom; thus, eliciting information from the older adult is essential to a comprehensive assessment. The International Continence Society provides clinicians and researchers a validated and reliable instrument to screen for and assess the impact of nocturia on quality of life. This instrument, ICIQ-Nocturia (www.iciq.net/ICIQ.Nmodule.html), consists of two items (i.e., frequency and nocturia) and is easy to administer.

A bladder record or voiding diary provides valuable information and helps to differentiate between 24-hour polyuria and nocturnal polyuria. Assessment of nocturia in individuals with cognitive or literacy impairments will rely on surrogate report by family members or caregivers. Therefore, health care providers must stress the importance of accurate information. See Tables 10-1 and 10-2 for Elements of the History and Assessment/Physical Examination for Nocturia and Differential Diagnosis of Nocturia.

Because ingestion of fluids influences urine output, obtaining accurate information about fluid volume ingested and types of fluids (i.e., water, alcohol, and caffeinated) is also necessary. Assessing cardiovascular status, the quality of sleep, and the presence of sleep apnea is important since nocturia is closely associated with cardiovascular disease and sleep disorders.

Management

Management of nocturia is determined by the findings from the assessment. More than one issue (e.g., 24-hour polyuria, nocturnal polyuria, and/or reduced bladder capacity) may be present and each condition should be treated.

TABLE 10-1 Elements of History and Assessment/Physical Examination for Nocturia

Component	Areas of Investigation	
	History	**Assessment/Physical Examination**
Urinary assessment	Lower urinary tract symptoms Voiding patterns Perceived bother Elimination of other urinary tract pathology	Digital rectal examination to rule out constipation Review results of 3-day bladder diary
Comorbidities	Obesity Heart failure Hypertension Diabetes mellitus/insipidus Urologic/gynecologic disorders Renal disease Neurologic disease, including stroke	Calculate BMI Heart failure, peripheral edema BP, vital signs HbA_{1c} serum level Urologic/gynecologic disorders Assess strength

Medication Review	Diuretics
	β-Blockers
	Calcium channel blockers
	Carbonic anhydrase inhibitors
	Xanthines (also found in coffee and chocolate)
	Antihistamines
	Cholinesterase inhibitor
	Polydipsia
	  Phenothiazines
	  Anticholinergics
	Central diabetes insipidus
	  Ethanol
	  Phenytoin (e.g., Dilantin)
	  Low-dose morphine
	  Glucocorticoids
	  Fluphenazine (e.g., Prolixin)
	  Haloperidol (e.g., Haldol)
	  Atypical antipsychotics (e.g., risperidone)
	  Promethazine (e.g., Sominex)
	  Oxilorphan
	  Butorphanol
	  Lithium
	  Demeclocycline (e.g., Declomycin)
	  Cisplatin (e.g., Platin)
	  Tetracycline
	Nephrogenic diabetes insipidus
	  Amphotericin B (e.g., Fungizone)
	  Foscarnet (e.g., Foscavir)
	  Ifosfamide (e.g., Ifex)
	  Clozapine (e.g., Clozaril)
		Neuro exam
		Assess drug–drug interaction
		Adverse drug effects

(Continued)

TABLE 10-1 Elements of History and Assessment/Physical Examination for Nocturia (*Continued*)

Component	Areas of Investigation	
	History	Assessment/Physical Examination
Sleep patterns	Usual bedtimes and wake times, number of times awakened from sleep, total hours spent in bed Daytime drowsiness/naps Reasons for awakening Usual place for nighttime sleeping, quality of mattress, room temperature, television, noise, lights Comfort in bed, pain, discomfort Pet or human bed partners Ability to fall asleep after rising to void Anxiety, troublesome thoughts Snoring, restless sleep Waking with shortness of breath or sweating	Sleep study if indicated
Fall risk assessment	Falls history Room lighting, pathways to bathroom, spectacles	Mobility, gait, balance Toileting ability Check for orthostatic hypotension
Self-management strategies	Past and current strategies for nocturia and their perceived effectiveness Desired outcomes of treatment Preferences for treatment	

From Carlson, B., & Palmer, M. (2014). Nocturia in older adults: Implications for nursing practice and aging in place. *Nursing Clinics of North America*, *49*(2), 233–250, Elsevier Inc.

Treatment of sleep disorders and management of chronic medical conditions such as cardiovascular disease, diabetes mellitus, and prostatic enlargement are necessary, and the impact of such treatment on nocturia should be evaluated.

Lifestyle interventions are considered the first-line treatment option for nocturia (Cornu et al., 2012). When lifestyle interventions, for example, diet and exercise, are used for diabetes control, there is evidence that nocturia also improves (Asplund, 2005). The relationship between insulin resistance and nocturia is unclear, especially for older adults. One study of older adults with chronic kidney disease reported that individual components of metabolic syndrome, including insulin resistance, did not increase the risk of two or more voids at night (Wu et al., 2012). Other lifestyle interventions include "preemptive" voiding (voiding before going to bed) and restricting fluids prior to

TABLE 10-2 Differential Diagnosis of Nocturia

Condition	Diminished or reduced nocturnal bladder capacity	24-hour polyuria	Nocturnal polyuria
Presentation	Urine production is within normal limits; increased frequency, small voided volumes (clear definition lacking), especially at night	24-hour urine production exceeding 40 mL/kg body weight	Nocturnal urine volumes >33% of total 24-hour volume
Possible cause	Overactive bladder Bladder outlet obstruction, including benign prostatic hypertrophy or obstruction Interstitial cystitis, urinary tract infection, bladder hypersensitivity, calculi, cancer, neurogenic detrusor overactivity	Poorly controlled diabetes mellitus (type 1 or type 2) Diabetes insipidus Hypercalcemia Polydipsia	Excessive evening fluid/alcohol/caffeine intake Impaired circadian rhythm of arginine vasopressin secretion Renal insufficiency Heart failure Diuretic use Estrogen deficiency Sleep apnea Venous insufficiency, peripheral edema Hypoalbuminemia

From Carlson, B., & Palmer, M. (2014). Nocturia in older adults: Implications for nursing practice and aging in place. *Nursing Clinics of North America*, *49*(2), 233–250, Elsevier Inc.

bedtime, but there is limited evidence regarding the effectiveness of restricting fluid intake (Weiss et al., 2012) and avoiding caffeine and alcohol prior to bedtime. It is suggested that diuretics be taken during midafternoon hours to minimize sleep disruption at night (Cornu et al., 2012). Older adults who have leg edema are encouraged to wear compression stockings and to elevate their legs in the evening to promote mobilization of fluid, thus reducing episodes of nocturia (Weiss et al., 2012).

The impact of fluid manipulation has been a subject of research, and current data indicate that a 25% reduction in fluid intake can improve nocturia (Hashim & Abrams, 2008). For example, in a study conducted with men experiencing nocturia (ages 53 to 91, mean age 72), subjects were instructed to adjust their food and water intake to produce 24-hour urine volumes less than or equal to 30 mL/kg. The men were encouraged to reduce the volume of fluid ingested during the day rather than the frequency of fluid ingestion. All men were instructed to drink at least one liter daily and to drink whenever they felt thirsty. There was significant improvement in nocturia in men who reduced their daytime fluid volume. The authors suggested that daytime, as well as evening, reduction of fluid intake would improve nocturia (Tani et al., 2014).

Another study indicated that behavioral therapy to control urgency may also reduce nocturia. Women aged 50 years and over who reported nocturia participated in a study comparing the effects of behavioral therapy and drug therapy. Those who received behavioral therapy (i.e., pelvic floor contractions to suppress urgency) had significantly improved nocturia symptoms as compared to women in the drug therapy group (oxybutynin IR) and those in the control group (Johnson et al., 2005).

CLINICAL PEARL

Behavioral therapy (pelvic muscle contractions to suppress urgency) has been shown to reduce nocturia among women. Medications (e.g., desmopressin) must be used with caution in older adults.

Medications are often used to treat nocturnal polyuria, specifically desmopressin, daytime administration of diuretics, and some anticholinergic medications (Committee for Establishment of the Clinical Guidelines for Nocturia of the Neurogenic Bladder Society, 2010). However, pharmacologic treatment should be used with caution in older adults. Over 40% of adverse drug effects in older adults living in nursing homes are considered preventable (Guiding principles for the care of older adults with multimorbidity: an approach for clinicians, 2012), and polypharmacy is a top priority for nursing home research (Morley et al., 2014). There is also heightened awareness about drug–drug interactions and their effects on cognitive and physical functioning (Tannenbaum, 2013). Consultation with geriatric pharmacists and resources

such as the Beers Criteria for Potentially Inappropriate Medications for Older Adults is recommended prior to administering these medications. This document is available from the American Geriatrics Society Web site: www.americangeriatrics.org.

Nocturia can disrupt sleep, an essential component of health. Effective interventions that reduce nocturia, minimize sleep disruption, and improve sleep quality are within the scope of practice for WOC nurses. Collaborating with geriatric specialists is an important role for the WOC nurse to ensure comprehensive assessment of nocturia and implementation of strategies to optimize the quality of sleep for older adults.

Functional Urinary Incontinence

Urinary incontinence can occur as a result of factors outside the genitourinary tract; this is often referred to as functional urinary incontinence. Multiple nongenitourinary tract risk factors for functional urinary incontinence have been identified and are listed in Table 10-3. Over 50% of older adults live with three or more chronic diseases (Guiding principles for the care of older adults with multimorbidity: An approach for clinicians, 2012), which presents challenges that include life-threatening adverse or sentinel events (i.e., adverse drug effects and falls), physical and emotional pain (i.e., osteoarthritis and grief), and accommodation (i.e., adapting lifestyle to be compliant or adherent to treatment and management strategies). In addition to managing chronic diseases and their treatment regimes, older adults often find themselves dealing

TABLE 10-3 Nongenitourinary Factors Related to Urinary Incontinence

Comorbid Disease	Medications
Diabetes	α-Adrenergics (blockers and agonists)
Congestive heart failure	
Degenerative joint disease	Cholinergics (blockers and agonists)
	Angiotensin-converting enzyme inhibitors
Sleep apnea	
Severe constipation	Calcium blockers
	Diuretics
	Opiates
	Anticholinergics (antidepressants, antipsychotics)
Neurologic/ Psychiatric	**Function and Environment**
Stroke	Impaired cognition
Parkinson's disease	Impaired mobility
Normal pressure hydrocephalus	Inaccessible toilets
	Lack of caregivers
Dementia	
Depression	

From Dubeau, C. (2006). The aging lower urinary tract. *Journal of Urology, 175* (3 Pt 2), S11–S15.

with symptoms that arise from treatments or interactions among treatments for different diseases and conditions (e.g., drug side effects like dry mouth). They also continue to seek preventive health care, such as vaccinations. Thus, for many older adults, especially those living in the community, life is filled with an array of medical appointments, medications, special diets, and treatment regimes. Despite disease and treatment burden, older adults are generally satisfied with life (Jivraj et al., 2014). Yet, many times, older adults do not seek care for urinary incontinence and other lower urinary tract symptoms because of the mistaken belief they are an unavoidable part of aging (Ostaszkiewicz et al., 2012).

The older adult population is heterogeneous; people live through different life experiences, have different levels of resources available to them throughout their lives, and respond to life events in multiple ways. Thus, an individualized approach to care for older adults, including those with cognitive impairments, is essential. The aim of geriatric medicine and nursing is to promote function through holistic patient-centered care (Morley, 2012). WOC nurses may need to collaborate with other health care providers with expertise in geriatrics to prevent urinary incontinence from developing or worsening and to provide effective and dignified care to older adults who experience functional urinary incontinence.

In frail older adults, urinary incontinence is viewed as a geriatric syndrome because of the number of nongenitourinary tract risk factors. For example, changes in the central nervous system may contribute to urgency, and the presence of comorbid conditions and their symptoms can affect older adults' ability to toilet, fully empty their bladders, or recognize and appropriately respond to the sensation of bladder fullness. Many older adults require assistance from another person to use the toilet. This care dependency may act as a risk factor for incontinence (Wagg et al., 2013). Severe impairments in the ability to perform activities of daily living were a strong risk factor for urinary incontinence in older women living in residential care facilities (De Gagne et al., 2013).

The environment itself can exert an influence on health and health behaviors in people of all ages. The impact of the environment on older adults' toilet access and voiding behaviors should not be underestimated. When older adults have difficulty carrying out activities of daily living, including toileting, they can begin to experience functional impairments and disabilities. The World Health Organization defined disability as "the result of interactions between health conditions and environmental and personal factors" (World Health Organization, 2012b). The relationship between disability and urinary incontinence is complex and can result in different functional pathways. For example, older adults who are frail or who have physical and cognitive impairments that lead to functional decline may, over time, develop toileting and mobility disabilities

that result in urinary incontinence (Coll-Planas et al., 2008). Yet, other older adults may be incontinent of urine and subsequently experience a fall that results in a hip fracture. Functional decline and ultimate mobility disability may follow, leading to intractability of the incontinence. Understanding the nature of the relationship between urinary incontinence, functional decline, and disability and creating a treatment or management plan that halts or reverses the specific pathway can be challenging and requires interdisciplinary collaboration and consultation.

CLINICAL PEARL

Functional incontinence is caused by factors outside the urinary tract as opposed to a problem with bladder function or sphincter function.

Many older adults who are continent but who have impairments, disabilities, and comorbidities become incontinent during hospitalization. New cases of urinary incontinence during hospitalization have been reported in older women admitted for hip fracture repair. Risk factors included preadmission use of wheelchair or device for walking, presence of confusion, and admission from a nursing home (Palmer et al., 2002). The use of absorbent products for urine containment during hospitalization has been shown to increase the risk that the individual will be incontinent of urine at the time of discharge (Zisberg et al., 2011). Nursing staff must be attentive to their rationale for and the consequences of using absorbent products in the hospital setting.

About 1.2 million (3.5%) older adults in the United States reside in long-term care facilities (Gorina et al., 2014), and approximately 75% of those residents are incontinent of urine (Fig. 10-2) (Gorina et al., 2014). Dependency in activities of daily living is prevalent, with over half of nursing home residents requiring extensive or full assistance with bathing, toileting, and dressing (Jones et al., 2009). Thus, requisites to effective toileting and continence programs are an adequate number of educated and supervised staff to provide physical and emotional assistance to older adults and information to other health care providers about the effectiveness of the care plan related to continence and toileting.

In summary, the prevalence of urinary incontinence is high in institutional settings such as hospitals and nursing homes. The high number of older adults who have complex care needs resulting from functional and cognitive impairments translates into a demand for attentive health care providers who can provide safe and timely access to toilets. Dependency on others can make the difference between being incontinent and being dry. Staff education and supervision are important to ensure that toileting assistance and behavioral interventions are being performed and evaluated.

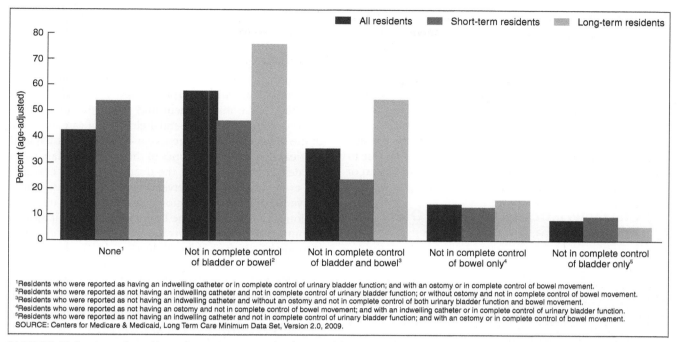

FIGURE 10-2. Age-adjusted incontinence among nursing home residents aged 65 years and over, by type of incontinence and length of stay, 2009.

Comorbid Conditions

There are a number of comorbid conditions that increase the risk of incontinence among older adults. Some of the most common are frailty, cognitive impairment, and mobility impairment.

> **CLINICAL PEARL**
>
> Comorbid conditions commonly associated with functional incontinence include frailty, cognitive impairment, and mobility impairment.

Frailty

Physical frailty is defined as "a medical syndrome with multiple causes and contributors that is characterized by diminished strength, endurance, and reduced physiologic function that increases an individual's vulnerability for developing increased dependency and/or death" (Morley et al., 2013). Frailty is not a disability; some older adults may be frail and disabled, while others may only be frail (Chen et al., 2014). Physical frailty is especially prevalent in older adults with comorbidities and those over 80 years of age. Approximately 11% of community-dwelling older adults are considered frail and 44% are considered prefrail (Collard et al., 2012). Women are more likely than men to be frail (Morley et al.). Screening tools are available, including the FRAIL Questionnaire (Morley et al., 2012), that include items about fatigue and weight loss, ability to walk upstairs and one block, and having concurrent illnesses. Because frailty increases the potential for

progressive dependency, it is also associated with increased risk for incontinence.

Cognitive Impairment

Urinary incontinence is prevalent in older adults who have cognitive impairment. Deterioration in functional, mental, and physical processes is the hallmark of dementia. Urinary incontinence may be due to the older adult not recognizing the need to void or not remembering the location of the toilet or how to prepare for toileting. Many older adults with mild cognitive impairment (MCI) and dementia can remain continent if provided adequate toileting cues and assistance with toileting. However, older adults with advanced dementia can react to toileting assistance with distress; thus, caregivers must be able to "read" the behavioral cues of older adults with cognitive impairments who are unable to express their needs (Ostaszkiewicz et al., 2012). It is critical for caregivers to realize that some forms of dementia, such as normal pressure hydrocephalus (NPH), are potentially reversible. Cardinal signs include gait disturbance (sometimes described as appearing as if the person was walking on a boat), urinary incontinence, and cognitive decline (Rosseau, 2011). If NPH is suspected, appropriate referrals must be made, and any newly occurring or suddenly worsening cognitive impairment requires evaluation.

Mobility Impairment

Impairments in mobility increase the risk for and prevalence of urinary incontinence (Wagg et al., 2014). Urinary incontinence and nocturia in older adults are also associated with increased risk of falls (Rafiq et al., 2014). In the long-term care setting, urinary incontinence has been identified as an independent risk factor for falls (Hasegawa et al., 2010). Because of the relationship between incontinence and falls, assessment of continence status was included in guidelines for fall prevention in the United Kingdom, although adherence to the guideline was found to be low (Edwards et al., 2011). Mobility difficulties often accompany chronic conditions such as arthritis, obesity, and cardiovascular diseases; therefore, a screening test to evaluate gait, balance, and walking speed should be part of continence assessments and patient safety programs.

Characteristics of UI in the Older Adult

Diagnostic Studies/Guidelines for Older Adults

Implementing a toileting trial is an effective method for determining the potential effectiveness of a behavioral intervention. A toileting trial consists of offering toileting assistance to the older adult every 2 hours over a 3-day period (Rahman et al., 2014). Responsiveness to the trial is determined by a reduction in incontinent episodes; previous research has shown that about 25% to 40% of nursing home residents experience a reduction in incontinent episodes from three to four per day to one or less per day. Rahman et al. (2014) found that the toileting trial was a stronger predictor of long-term improvement in continence status than was the cognitive and functional status of the older adult.

CLINICAL PEARL

A toileting trial provides valuable information regarding the probable benefit of a toileting program; results of the toileting trial are a better predictor of positive results than the individual's cognitive and functional status.

In the long-term care setting, the Minimum Data Set (MDS 3.0) is used to gather information on bladder and bowel function (Section H). The purpose is to identify and assess nursing home residents who are incontinent or at risk of becoming incontinent. Facilities must provide individualized treatment to "achieve or maintain as normal elimination function as possible" (Centers for Medicare & Medicaid Services, 2013). The Centers for Medicare and Medicaid Services has provided surveyors with guidance regarding assessment and treatment of urinary incontinence and appropriate utilization and management of indwelling catheters in the tag F315 Urinary Incontinence and Urinary Catheters (http://www.cms.gov/Regulations-and-Guidance/Guidance/Transmittals/downloads/R8SOM.pdf). The Minimum Data Set and guidance to surveyors may undergo revisions; therefore, WOC nurses who work in nursing homes should be aware of updated versions and revisions to these important documents.

Management Options/Guidelines

Management of urinary incontinence is contingent on findings from the assessment. Optimizing overall health through chronic disease management and restorative therapies to improve function is an essential element of care. Inclusion of the older adult's preferences for care and personal goals for treatment are cornerstones of the treatment plan. Creating desired end points for the treatment plan is critical to the evaluation of the interventions' effectiveness. Noninvasive behavioral interventions are the first-line treatment option for older adults. The International Consultation on Incontinence provides a treatment algorithm for urinary incontinence in frail older adults (Fig. 10-3). The National Guideline Clearinghouse located at www.guideline.gov provides a comprehensive list of guidelines for management of urinary incontinence in older adults.

Reversible Factors/Barriers

Urinary incontinence that suddenly occurs or worsens may have been precipitated by a sentinel event or acute health event. Therefore, acute changes in health status, medications, or environment should be assessed. The acronym DIPPERS is often used to help guide assessment (Fig. 10-3).

Delirium

Delirium is an acute worsening of cognitive status, a potentially fatal condition that is often underdetected. It is also called acute brain failure and has multiple risk factors including dementia, functional impairment, visual impairment, history of alcohol misuse, and age over 70 years. Precipitating factors include polypharmacy and the use of psychoactive medications and physical restraints (Inouye et al., 2014). Delirium can present as hyperactive or hypoactive psychomotor disturbances. Key diagnostic factors include acute-onset and fluctuating symptoms, inattention, disorientation, memory impairment, and language changes (Inouye et al., 2014). Treatment is dependent on the underlying cause. The use of a standardized instrument, such as the Confusion Assessment Method (CAM) or Months of the Year Backwards (MOYB), to detect delirium is crucial (O'Regan et al., 2014). Patient safety is a paramount concern until delirium is corrected.

Infection

Infections can lead to new or worsened urinary incontinence via several mechanisms. Fatigue and anergia (i.e., lack of energy) often accompany systemic infection, which in turn can make the act of moving to the toilet an effort that requires a great deal of physical and mental exertion. When the older adult recovers from the acute illness and fatigue and anergia recede, the preillness continence level

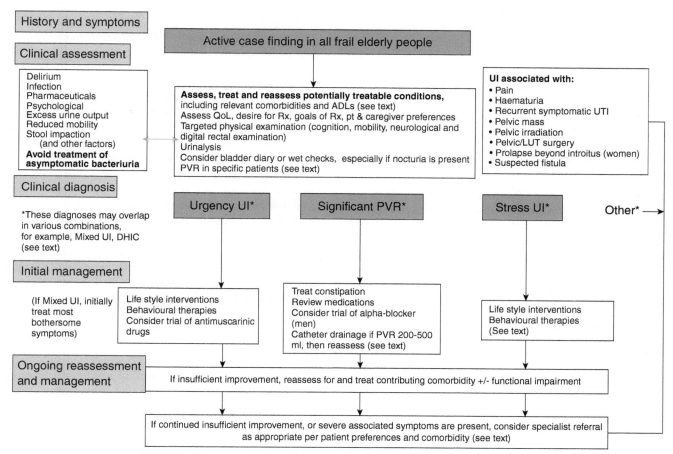

FIGURE 10-3. Management of urinary incontinence in frail older men and women.

should return. In the case of upper respiratory infections, urinary incontinence can develop or worsen when the abdominal pressure transmitted to the pelvic floor during coughing exceeds the intraurethral pressure, resulting in urinary leakage. Urinary incontinence can also occur with symptomatic urinary tract infections, especially in older women (Mody & Juthani-Mehta, 2014). Urgency or frequency may worsen and may be accompanied by one or more of the following symptoms: fever, acute dysuria, suprapubic tenderness, or costovertebral angle pain or tenderness. Older adults with musculoskeletal pain or stiffness that slows walking time or comorbidities that lead to mobility and cognitive impairments are at risk of becoming incontinent in the presence of a symptomatic urinary tract infection.

Pharmaceuticals

New medications, changed doses of existing medication, and drug–drug interactions can lead to urinary incontinence. Older adults, especially those with comorbidities, are often prescribed multiple medications, including medications added to address symptoms caused by other prescribed medications, also known as a prescribing cascade (Tannenbaum & Johnell, 2014). Diuretics can produce urine volumes that overwhelm the bladder and cause

incontinent episodes. Medications that alter consciousness can precipitate incontinent episodes by reducing awareness of the need to void, impairing the ability to communicate the need to void, or impairing the ability to safely navigate to the toilet. Angiotensin-converting enzyme (ACE) inhibitors can cause a cough that precipitates stress urinary incontinence. Consulting with pharmacists, using resources such as the Beers Criteria for Potentially Inappropriate Medications for Older Adults, and conducting a comprehensive medication review are important when assessing acute-onset or transient urinary incontinence.

> **CLINICAL PEARL**
>
> DIPPERS is an acronym for common acute (transient) factors contributing to incontinence: Delirium, Infection, Pharmaceuticals, Psychological Issues, Excess Urine Production, Restricted Mobility, Stool Impaction (constipation).

Psychological

Depression is associated with urinary incontinence. Older adults who experience new-onset urinary incontinence should be screened for depression.

Excess Urine Output

Excess urine output may overwhelm the bladder and lead to incontinent episodes, especially in older adults with mobility impairments. Excess fluid output could be the result of excessive fluid intake, uncontrolled diabetes mellitus, or nocturnal polyuria. Documenting fluid intake and urinary output will help determine the underlying cause of excess urine output.

Reduced Mobility

A sentinel event, such as hip fracture, can abruptly change an older adult's mobility status and, consequently, access to the toilet. Other possible reasons for reduced mobility include exacerbations in arthritis or musculoskeletal pain and stiffness that affect transfer ability. History of a recent fall should be assessed. Consultation or referral to physical therapy to assess gait speed, balance, and transfer ability may be warranted. Pain management to facilitate movement and minimize distress is essential.

Stool Impaction

Constipation is a frequently reported condition among older adults with prevalence estimates of 30% to 40% in people 65 years and older. Of adults admitted to medical wards without constipation, 43% developed it within 3 days of admission (Noiesen et al., 2013). Women report constipation more than men and it is commonly found in the presence of polypharmacy (Dennison et al., 2005). One complication of constipation is stool impaction, which is implicated in the development or worsening of urinary and fecal incontinence (Dennison et al., 2005). Therefore, prevention and treatment of constipation are recommended. Privacy during defecation is considered important. One study showed that adults living in acute and long-term care settings who had dependency needs and fecal incontinence rarely had full privacy (Akpan et al., 2006). Additional preventive measures include adequate intake of dietary fiber, adequate fluid intake, and avoidance of medications with a constipating effect (Dennison et al., 2005).

Interventions for Functional Urinary Incontinence

Scheduled Voiding/Habit Training

Scheduled voiding/habit training is a behavioral intervention that is used with older adults who would not benefit from prompted voiding or other interventions designed to restore continence or voiding patterns (Wagg et al., 2014). The goal of scheduled voiding is to preempt an incontinent episode by toileting the older adult on a schedule based on the older adult's current voiding pattern. To be successful in reducing the number of incontinent voids, there must be staff adherence to the schedule of timely toilet access.

Prompted Voiding

Prompted voiding is a behavioral intervention developed by psychologists for use in nursing homes in the 1980s. The intervention was originally a two-pronged approach. One prong of this intervention was directed toward the nursing staff. Nursing home staff members were given feedback by their supervisor about the number of toiletings they performed and the dryness level of the resident they toileted (Palmer, 2004; Palmer, 2005). The second prong, the prompted voiding protocol, was directed at the nursing home resident. This protocol involved approaching the older adult and asking if he or she was dry or wet. After a response was obtained, the caregiver physically checked the older adult and gave verbal feedback about the accuracy of his or her response. The caregiver then assisted the older adult to the toilet and provided praise when the older adult voided in the toilet. After returning the older adult to the same location before toileting, the caregiver reminded him or her when the next toileting opportunity would occur.

Prompted voiding is a labor and time-intensive intervention intended to increase self-initiated toileting requests and decrease the number of wet episodes. Evidence exists that prompted voiding results in decreased daytime incontinent episodes in the short term (Eustice et al., 2000; Wagg et al., 2014). Prompted voiding is appropriate for older adults who have dementia who can toilet successfully at least 66% of the time or who achieve 20% or more reduction in incontinent episodes during a toileting trial (Wagg et al., 2013). Caregivers must adhere to the protocol to provide toileting assistance for prompted voiding to be effective in reducing the number of incontinent episodes. Prompted voiding is sometimes combined with exercise and food and fluid interventions (Wagg et al., 2013).

Containment/Absorptive Products and Skin Care

Absorbent products are often necessary for older adults who would not benefit from behavioral or pharmacologic intervention for incontinence. The absorbent product should be selected according to the individual's need and skin should be frequently checked to detect incontinence-associated dermatitis and pressure ulcer development (Doughty et al., 2012). Products that can be easily removed and reapplied, if appropriate, should be used for older adults who can self-toilet. There is some evidence that the use of absorbent products by older women who are continent can increase the risk of becoming incontinent, although the mechanism is not clear. Indwelling urinary catheters are to be avoided unless there is a medical justification for their use. If an indwelling catheter is used, the justification for its use should be regularly reassessed and it should be removed as soon as practicable.

● **Conclusion**

Interdisciplinary teamwork is at the core of geriatric care. WOC nurses will need to consult with nurses, physical therapists, physicians, nutritionists, and social workers with expertise in geriatrics in order to provide comprehensive continence care to older adults, especially frail older adults. Integrating geriatric clinical competencies into practice allows the WOC nurse to provide holistic care and draw on the strengths and resources of older adults and their families.

The evidence base for care of older adults who have incontinence and other lower urinary tract symptoms is rapidly increasing. WOC nurses must remain abreast of the latest research, especially in preservation and restoration of cognitive and physical functioning and in end-of-life care. WOC nurses play a pivotal role in providing high-quality continence care to older adults and in contributing to the clinical and research evidence for the appropriate and dignified care for older adults.

CASE STUDY

Mrs. Grant is 87 years old and of Irish–German descent. She is widowed and has one daughter who lives out of state. Mrs. Grant was admitted to the Vista View Healthcare Facility 10 days ago after her discharge from the hospital for surgical repair of her left hip fracture. She was admitted with a stage II pressure ulcer on her sacrum that is healing. Her medical history reveals that she has arthritis in both of her knees and hands, hypertension, diabetes, history of myocardial infarction 2 years ago, and cataract surgery 3 years ago. She requires the help of one person to rise from a chair. She reluctantly uses a walker saying that she is afraid of falling again and she walks slowly, taking frequent rest stops. On some mornings, she forgets the day of the week and where her room is located. Lately she has had a poor appetite and she has been fretful saying, "I want to go home! What will happen to me?"

There is no mention in the medical record about urinary incontinence prior to her hip fracture or during hospitalization. An indwelling catheter had been inserted in the emergency department before her surgery and it was removed 48 hours after surgery.

During the physical examination, Mrs. Grant was not febrile and said she did not have pain when voiding. She did not have suprapubic tenderness or costovertebral angle pain or tenderness. Mrs. Grant winced with pain when she turned onto her operative hip. She noted that the pain was in her knees and hesitantly rated her pain at 7 saying, "it's hard to put a number on it." There was no evidence of incontinence-associated dermatitis. The postvoid residual was 110 mL. A digital rectal exam revealed hard stool in the rectum; there was no documentation of a bowel movement in the past 72 hours. Using validated screening tools, there was no evidence of delirium, depression, or dementia.

Mrs. Grant was distressed by being incontinent, saying that it started in the hospital after surgery and has gotten worse in the past few days. She said that the urine "came without warning." She said she tried to go to the toilet every hour to prevent accidents and because she walked so slowly. She also wore an absorbent brief and used disposable absorbent pads on her bed and chair. She said that she didn't use her call light because "the girls are so busy with people worse off than me." She went on to say that the pain in her knees was "just horrible" and had been worse since the surgery. She also said that at home, she had used a small thin pillow between her knees to sleep, but now, no one would get a pillow for her to use. She also used a topical lotion that helped relieve the pain at home. She was upset that the nurses "give me sleeping pills, because I feel so funny from them in the morning." She also said that she didn't drink much because "that water (indicating her water container) tastes bad." When asked what she drank at home, she said she drank hot water with lemon at breakfast and then drank room temperature tap water with lemon slices at meals and rarely drank fluids between meals.

Medications:

Hypertension: Hydrochlorothiazide 25 mg, every day
Atenolol 25 mg at bedtime
Constipation: Milk of magnesia 30 m/L at bedtime, prn
Pain: Acetaminophen 650 mg every 4 to 6 hours, prn
Sleep: Diphenhydramine 15 mg at bedtime, prn

A 3-day bladder and fluid intake record revealed that Mrs. Grant drank about 800 mL/day and voided 10 times/24-hour period, often in small incontinent amounts. She was usually incontinent in bed upon awakening and within an hour before or after meals. She was also incontinent in the evening before retiring and once during the night hours. Other voids that were recorded on the bladder record had been continent and, upon questioning Mrs. Grant, they had been preemptive voids; that is, she voided before feeling the need in order to prevent urine leakage. In reviewing the medication list, the WOC nurse noted that hydrochlorothiazide was given at 10 AM; diphenhydramine was given every night; three doses of acetaminophen had been administered since Mrs. Grant's admission; and no milk of magnesia had been given since the first night after admission.

Several factors placed Mrs. Grant at risk for developing incontinence:

1. Impaired mobility
2. Medications that affected urine volume and cognition
3. Pain that caused sleep disruption and reluctance to move
4. Low oral fluid intake
5. Constipation
6. Reluctance to ask for help
7. Psychological factors, that is, fear of falling and concern about an uncertain future
8. Use of an indwelling catheter during hospitalization
9. Use of absorbent products that were difficult to remove for self-toileting

Mrs. Grant was asked about her preferences for care. She stated "Of course, I hate leaking urine and I would like to go to the bathroom on my own but..." and her voice drifted off. The WOC nurse asked her if she would like to have a bedside commode in the room for use at night. Mrs. Grant was receptive and the WOC nurse suggested that Mrs. Grant continue to use the toilet according to an individualized schedule, sitting on it until she thought her bladder was empty, and, if she wished, to use a pad insert in her panties to contain the small volumes of leakage. She also encouraged Mrs. Grant to keep her own bladder record and share information on it with the nursing staff.

The WOC nurse talked with the physical therapist assigned to Mrs. Grant and asked about having a commode near the bed at night and also asked the physical therapist to assess Mrs. Grant's musculoskeletal pain, especially in relation to using the toilet. The physical therapist recommended a set of exercises to help relieve pain and increase lower extremity strength. The physical therapist agreed that the bedside commode would be helpful to Mrs. Grant and also provided a pillow to support Mrs. Grant's legs at night. Since Mrs. Grant found relief from the over-the-counter topical lotion she used at home, the physical therapist suggested that Mrs. Grant resume using it and also advised her to take acetaminophen for pain on a regular basis until the pain was under control.

The WOC nurse talked with the nursing staff members who cared for Mrs. Grant and noted Mrs. Grant's reluctance in asking for help. She suggested using a toileting schedule that matched Mrs. Grant's voiding pattern and cueing Mrs. Grant about her exercise regime and about her pain and hydration levels. The WOC nurse talked with the charge nurse and suggested giving the diuretic at 2 PM instead of 10 AM and having Mrs. Grant rest with her feet elevated before her evening meal. She also suggested discontinuing the use of diphenhydramine as a sleep aid because of its potential to affect Mrs. Grant's cognitive status. She asked the staff to be attentive to Mrs. Grant's increased need to use the toilet after administering her diuretic and to use nonpharmacological measures to facilitate Mrs. Grant's sleep. The WOC nurse also suggested giving Mrs. Grant a stool softener and milk of magnesia to relieve constipation and help Mrs. Grant establish a regular time to move her bowels to promote regular elimination.

Based on the WOC nurse recommendation, a dietician visited Mrs. Grant and reviewed her food and fluid likes and dislikes. She talked with Mrs. Grant about the importance of hydration to her overall health and in helping her bowels be regular. She suggested to Mrs. Grant to drink small amounts of fluids throughout the day and with Mrs. Grant's help set up a daily schedule so that Mrs. Grant was drinking about 1,500 mL/day, with about 200 mL coming from high–water-content foods and with most of the oral fluids ingested during daytime hours. The dietician told Mrs. Grant about the availability of single use packets of crystallized lemon, lime, and orange that she could add to water to enhance its taste. The dietician also developed a high-fiber diet including foods with high water content for Mrs. Grant and, because of Mrs. Grant's diabetes, suggested that she use a dietary fiber supplement to prevent constipation.

In summary, several nongenitourinary factors were associated with Mrs. Grant's incontinence. When the staff began addressing them and as Mrs. Grant increased her mobility, her incontinence and overall attitude improved.

REFERENCES

Abrams, P., Cardozo, L., Fall, M., et al.; Standardisation Subcommittee of the International Continence Society. (2002). The standardisation of terminology of lower urinary tract function: Report from the standardisation sub-committee of the International Continence Society. *Neurourology and Urodynamics, 21*(2), 167–178. doi:10.1002/nau.10052 [pii].

Abrams, P., Chapple, C. R., Junemann, K. P., et al. (2012). Urinary urgency: A review of its assessment as the key symptom of the overactive bladder syndrome. *World Journal of Urology, 30*(3), 385–392. doi:10.1007/s00345-011-0742-8.

Akpan, A., Gosney, M. A., & Barrett, J. (2006). Privacy for defecation and fecal incontinence in older adults. *Journal of Wound, Ostomy, and Continence Nursing, 33*(5), 536–540. doi: 00152192-200609000-00012 [pii].

Asplund, R. (2005). Nocturia in relation to sleep, health, and medical treatment in the elderly. *BJU International, 96*(Suppl 1), 15–21. doi: BJU5653 [pii].

Asplund, R. (2007). Pharmacotherapy for nocturia in the elderly patient. *Drugs and Aging, 24*(4), 325–343. doi: 2445 [pii].

Bliwise, D. L., Foley, D. J., Vitiello, M. V., et al. (2009). Nocturia and disturbed sleep in the elderly. *Sleep Medicine, 10*(5), 540–548. doi: 10.1016/j.sleep.2008.04.002.

Burgio, K. L., Johnson, T. M., II, Goode, P. S., et al. (2010). Prevalence and correlates of nocturia in community-dwelling older adults. *Journal of the American Geriatrics Society, 58*(5), 861–866. doi: 10.1111/j.1532-5415.2010.02822.x.

Carlson, B. W., & Palmer, M. H. (2014). Nocturia in older adults: Implications for nursing practice and aging in place. *The Nursing Clinics of North America, 49*(2), 233–250. doi: S0029-6465(14)00014-0 [pii].

Centers for Medicare & Medicaid Services. (2013). MDS 3.0 RAI manual. Retrieved 2014, from http://www.cms.gov/Medicare/Quality-Initiatives-Patient-Assessment-Instruments/NursingHomeQualityInits/MDS30RAIManual.html

Chen, X., Mao, G., & Leng, S. X. (2014). Frailty syndrome: An overview. *Clinical Interventions in Aging, 9*, 433–441. doi:10.2147/CIA.S45300.

Collard, R. M., Boter, H., Schoevers, R. A., et al. (2012). Prevalence of frailty in community-dwelling older persons: A systematic review. *Journal of the American Geriatrics Society, 60*(8), 1487–1492. doi: 10.1111/j.1532-5415.2012.04054.x.

Coll-Planas, L., Denkinger, M. D., & Nikolaus, T. (2008). Relationship of urinary incontinence and late-life disability: Implications for clinical work and research in geriatrics. *Zeitschrift Fur Gerontologie Und Geriatrie, 41*(4), 283–290. doi: 10.1007/s00391-008-0563-6.

Committee for Establishment of the Clinical Guidelines for Nocturia of the Neurogenic Bladder Society. (2010). Clinical guidelines for nocturia. *International Journal of Urology, 17*(5), 397–409. doi: 10.1111/j.1442-2042.2010.02527.x.

Cornu, J. N., Abrams, P., Chapple, C. R., et al. (2012). A contemporary assessment of nocturia: Definition, epidemiology, pathophysiology, and management—a systematic review and meta-analysis. *European Urology, 62*(5), 877–890. doi: 10.1016/j.eururo.2012.07.004.

De Gagne, J. C., So, A., Oh, J., et al. (2013). Sociodemographic and health indicators of older women with urinary incontinence: 2010 national survey of residential care facilities. *Journal of the American Geriatrics Society, 61*(6), 981–986. doi: 10.1111/jgs.12258.

Dennison, C., Prasad, M., Lloyd, A., et al. (2005). The health-related quality of life and economic burden of constipation. *PharmacoEconomics, 23*(5), 461–476. doi: 2356 [pii].

Department of Health and Human Services Administration on Aging. (2013). *A Profile of Older Americans*. Washington, DC: DHHS.

Doughty, D., Junkin, J., Kurz, P., et al. (2012). Incontinence-associated dermatitis: Consensus statements, evidence-based guidelines for prevention and treatment, and current challenges. *Journal of Wound, Ostomy, and Continence Nursing, 39*(3), 303–15; quiz 316–7. doi: 10.1097/WON.0b013e3182549118.

Dubeau, C. E. (2006). The aging lower urinary tract. *Journal of Urology, 175*(3 Pt 2), S11–S15. doi: S0022-5347(05)00311-3 [pii].

Edwards, R., Martin, F. C., Grant, R., et al. (2011). Is urinary continence considered in the assessment of older people after a fall in England and Wales? Cross-sectional clinical audit results. *Maturitas, 69*(2), 179–183. doi: 10.1016/j.maturitas.2011.03.018.

Ellsworth, P., Marschall-Kehrel, D., King, S., et al. (2013). Bladder health across the life course. *International Journal of Clinical Practice, 67*(5), 397–406. doi: 10.1111/ijcp.12127.

Eustice, S., Roe, B., & Paterson, J. (2000). Prompted voiding for the management of urinary incontinence in adults. *Cochrane Database of Systematic Reviews (Online), (2)*, CD002113. doi: 10.1002/14651858.CD002113.

Gorina, Y., Schappert, S., Bercovitz, A., et al. (2014). Prevalence of incontinence among older Americans. *Vital & Health Statistics. Series 3, Analytical and Epidemiological Studies/[U.S. Dept. of Health and Human Services, Public Health Service, National Center for Health Statistics], (36)*, 1–33.

Guiding principles for the care of older adults with multimorbidity: An approach for clinicians. (2012). Guiding principles for the care of older adults with multimorbidity: An approach for clinicians:

American geriatrics society expert panel on the care of older adults with multimorbidity. *Journal of the American Geriatrics Society, 60*(10), E1–E25. doi: 10.1111/j.1532-5415.2012.04188.x.

Hasegawa, J., Kuzuya, M., & Iguchi, A. (2010). Urinary incontinence and behavioral symptoms are independent risk factors for recurrent and injurious falls, respectively, among residents in long-term care facilities. *Archives of Gerontology and Geriatrics, 50*(1), 77–81. doi: 10.1016/j.archger.2009.02.001.

Hashim, H., & Abrams, P. (2008). How should patients with an overactive bladder manipulate their fluid intake? *BJU International, 102*(1), 62–66. doi: 10.1111/j.1464-410X.2008.07463.x.

Hirayama, A., Torimoto, K., Yamada, A., et al. (2011). Relationship between nocturnal urine volume, leg edema, and urinary antidiuretic hormone in older men. *Urology, 77*(6), 1426–1431. doi: 10.1016/j.urology.2010.12.030.

Hofmeester, I., Kollen, B. J., Steffens, M. G., et al. (2015). Impact of the international continence society report on the standardisation of terminology in nocturia on the quality of reports on nocturia and nocturnal polyuria: A systematic review. *BJU International, 115*(4), 520–536. doi: 10.1111/bju.12753.

Inouye, S. K., Kosar, C. M., Tommet, D., et al. (2014). The CAM-S: Development and validation of a new scoring system for delirium severity in 2 cohorts. *Annals of Internal Medicine, 160*(8), 526–533. doi: 10.7326/M13-1927.

Jivraj, S., Nazroo, J., Vanhoutte, B., et al. (2014). Aging and subjective well-being in later life. *Journals of Gerontology. Series B, Psychological Sciences and Social Sciences, 69*(6), 930–941. doi: gbu006 [pii].

Johnson, T. M., II, Burgio, K. L., Redden, D. T., et al. (2005). Effects of behavioral and drug therapy on nocturia in older incontinent women. *Journal of the American Geriatrics Society, 53*(5), 846–850. doi: JGS53260 [pii].

Jones, A. L., Dwyer, L. L., Bercovitz, A. R., et al. (2009). The national nursing home survey: 2004 overview. *Vital and Health Statistics. Series 13, Data from the National Health Survey, (167)*, 1–155.

Lowalekar, S. K., Cristofaro, V., Radisavljevic, Z. M., et al. (2012). Loss of bladder smooth muscle caveolae in the aging bladder. *Neurourology and Urodynamics, 31*(4), 586–592. doi: 10.1002/nau.21217.

Mannella, P., Palla, G., Bellini, M., et al. (2013). The female pelvic floor through midlife and aging. *Maturitas, 76*(3), 230–234. doi: 10.1016/j.maturitas.2013.08.008.

Mody, L., & Juthani-Mehta, M. (2014). Urinary tract infections in older women: A clinical review. *Journal of the American Medical Association, 311*(8), 844–854. doi: 10.1001/jama.2014.303.

Morley, J. E. (2012). Geriatric principles: Evidence-based medicine at its best. *Journal of the American Medical Directors Association, 13*(1), 1–2.e1–e2. doi: 10.1016/j.jamda.2011.10.004.

Morley, J. E., Caplan, G., Cesari, M., et al. (2014). International survey of nursing home research priorities. *Journal of American Medical Directors Association, 15*(5), 309-312.

Morley, J. E., Malmstrom, T. K., & Miller, D. K. (2012). A simple frailty questionnaire (FRAIL) predicts outcomes in middle aged African Americans. *Journal of Nutrition, Health and Aging, 16*(7), 601–608.

Morley, J. E., Vellas, B., van Kan, G. A., et al. (2013). Frailty consensus: A call to action. *Journal of the American Medical Directors Association, 14*(6), 392–397. doi: 10.1016/j.jamda.2013.03.022.

Noiesen, E., Trosborg, I., Bager, L., et al. (2013). Constipation—prevalence and incidence among medical patients acutely admitted to hospital with a medical condition. *Journal of Clinical Nursing, 23*(15–16), 2295–2302. doi: 10.1111/jocn.12511.

Oelke, M., Baard, J., Wijkstra, H., et al. (2008). Age and bladder outlet obstruction are independently associated with detrusor overactivity in patients with benign prostatic hyperplasia. *European Urology, 54*(2), 419–426. doi: 10.1016/j.eururo.2008.02.017.

O'Regan, N. A., Ryan, D. J., Boland, E., et al. (2014). Attention! A good bedside test for delirium? *Journal of Neurology, Neurosurgery, and Psychiatry, 85*(10), 1122–1131. doi: 10.1136/jnnp-2013-307053.

Ostaszkiewicz, J., O'Connell, B., & Dunning, T. (2012). Residents' perspectives on urinary incontinence: A review of literature. *Scandinavian Journal of Caring Sciences, 26*(4), 761–772. doi: 10.1111/j.1471-6712.2011.00959.x.

Palmer, M. H. (2004). Use of health behavior change theories to guide urinary incontinence research. *Nursing Research, 53* (6 Suppl), S49–S55.

Palmer, M. H. (2005). Effectiveness of prompted voiding for incontinent nursing home residents. In B. M. Melnyk, & E. Fineout-Overholt (Eds.), *Evidence-based practice in nursing & healthcare: A guide to the best practice* (pp. 20–30). Philadelphia, PA: Lippincott Williams & Williams.

Palmer, M. H., Baumgarten, M., Langenberg, P., et al. (2002). Risk factors for hospital-acquired incontinence in elderly female hip fracture patients. *Journals of Gerontology. Series A, Biological Sciences and Medical Sciences, 57*(10), M672–M677.

Rafiq, M., McGovern, A., Jones, S., et al. (2014). Falls in the elderly were predicted opportunistically using a decision tree and systematically using a database-driven screening tool. *Journal of Clinical Epidemiology, 67*(8), 877–886. doi: 10.1016/j.jclinepi.2014.03.008.

Rahman, A. N., Schnelle, J. F., & Osterweil, D. (2014). Implementing toileting trials in nursing homes: Evaluation of a dissemination strategy. *Geriatric Nursing (New York, N.Y.), 35*(4), 283–289. doi: S0197-4572(14)00134-7 [pii].

Rosseau, G. (2011). Normal pressure hydrocephalus. *Disease-a-Month: DM, 57*(10), 615–624. doi: 10.1016/j.disamonth.2011.08.023.

Siroky, M. (2004). The aging bladder. *Reviews in Urology, 6*(Suppl 1), S3.

Tani, M., Hirayama, A., Torimoto, K., et al. (2014). Guidance on water intake effectively improves urinary frequency in patients with nocturia. *International Journal of Urology, 21*(6), 595–600. doi: 10.1111/iju.12387.

Tannenbaum, C. (2013). How to treat the frail elderly: The challenge of multimorbidity and polypharmacy. *Canadian Urological Association Journal = Journal De L'Association Des Urologues Du Canada, 7*(9–10 Suppl 4), S183–S185. doi: 10.5489/cuaj.1619.

Tannenbaum, C., & Johnell, K. (2014). Managing therapeutic competition in patients with heart failure, lower urinary tract symptoms and incontinence. *Drugs and Aging, 31*(2), 93–101. doi: 10.1007/s40266-013-0145-1.

van Doorn, B., & Bosch, J. L. (2012). Nocturia in older men. *Maturitas, 71*(1), 8–12. doi: 10.1016/j.maturitas.2011.10.007.

van Kerrebroeck, P., Abrams, P., Chaikin, D., et al.; Standardisation Sub-committee of the International Continence Society. (2002). The standardisation of terminology in nocturia: Report from the standardisation sub-committee of the International Continence Society. *Neurourology and Urodynamics, 21*(2), 179–183. doi: 10.1002/nau.10053 [pii].

Wagg, A., Gibson, W., Johnson, T., III, et al. (2014). Urinary incontinence in frail elderly persons: Report from the 5th international consultation on incontinence. *Neurourology and Urodynamics,* doi: 10.1002/nau.22602.

Wagg, A., Kirschiner-Hermanns, R., Kuchel, G., et al. (2013). Incontinence in the frail elderly. In P. Abrams, L. Cardozo, S. Khoury, et al. (Eds.), *Incontinence* (5th ed., p. 1003). ICUD-EAU. Bristol, UK: International Consultation on Urological Diseases.

Wakefield, D. B., Moscufo, N., Guttmann, C. R., et al. (2010). White matter hyperintensities predict functional decline in voiding, mobility, and cognition in older adults. *Journal of the American Geriatrics Society, 58*(2), 275–281. doi: 10.1111/j.1532-5415.2009.02699.x.

Weiss, J. P., Blaivas, J. G., Blanker, M. H., et al. (2013). The New England Research Institutes, Inc. (NERI) nocturia advisory conference 2012: Focus on outcomes of therapy. *BJU International, 111*(5), 700–716. doi: 10.1111/j.1464-410X.2012.11749.x.

Weiss, J. P., Bosch, J. L., Drake, M., et al. (2012). Nocturia think tank: Focus on nocturnal polyuria: ICI-RS 2011. *Neurourology and Urodynamics, 31*(3), 330–339. doi: 10.1002/nau.22219.

World Health Organization. (2012a). Ageing and life course. interesting facts about ageing. Retrieved 2014, from http://www.who.int/ageing/about/facts/en

World Health Organization. (2012b). *Disability. Report by the secretariat.* Geneva, Switzerland: World Health Organization.

Wu, M. Y., Wu, Y. L., Hsu, Y. H., et al. (2012). Risks of nocturia in patients with chronic kidney disease—do the metabolic syndrome and its components matter? *Journal of Urology, 188*(6), 2269–2273. doi: 10.1016/j.juro.2012.08.008.

Zisberg, A., Gary, S., Gur-Yaish, N., et al. (2011). In-hospital use of continence aids and new-onset urinary incontinence in adults aged 70 and older. *Journal of the American Geriatrics Society, 59*(6), 1099–1104. doi: 10.1111/j.1532-5415.2011.03413.x.

QUESTIONS

1. The continence nurse caring for patients in a long-term care facility should consider what age-related change to the bladder of the older adult when planning care?
   A. Increased urine flow
   B. Reduced bladder capacity
   C. Decreased sensitivity to neurotransmitters
   D. Decreased postvoid residual volumes

2. The continence nurse is caring for an elderly patient who states: "Every night I fall asleep, wake up to pass urine, and fall back to sleep again. This happens two or three times a night." What symptom of overactive bladder would the nurse suspect?
   A. Frequency
   B. Urgency
   C. Urgency urinary incontinence
   D. Nocturia

3. Which patient test result confirms the diagnosis of nocturnal polyuria?
   A. NPi = 35
   B. NPi = 24
   C. NPi = 18
   D. NPi = 10

4. Which patient would the continence nurse place at high risk for reduced nocturnal bladder capacity?
   A. A patient who has Down syndrome
   B. A patient who has rheumatoid arthritis
   C. A patient who has Parkinson's disease
   D. A patient who has SLE

5. An older adult receiving home care services is experiencing urinary incontinence. Upon further assessment by the nurse, which patient finding suggests a diagnosis of functional incontinence?
    A. Impaired mobility
    B. Urinary tract infection
    C. Nocturia
    D. BPH

6. The continence nurse assesses a patient and documents the following: "gait disturbance, urinary incontinence, and cognitive decline." What potentially reversible condition might be causing these findings?
    A. Dementia
    B. Normal pressure hydrocephalus
    C. Alzheimer disease
    D. Spinal cord injury

7. Which assessment would be a first priority for a newly admitted resident of a nursing home who is incontinent of urine?
    A. Depression screening
    B. I and O monitoring
    C. Dietary consultation
    D. Fall risk assessment

8. A continence nurse is planning care for older adults in a long-term care facility who are incontinent of urine. What would be a priority intervention for these patients?
    A. Providing the resident with absorbent pads and underwear
    B. Keeping the resident's room free from urine odors
    C. Arranging for a toileting schedule based on the resident's voiding patterns
    D. Reassuring the resident that incontinence is a normal part of aging

9. When using the DIPPERS acronym to assess for urinary incontinence, the WOC nurse would include an assessment for:
    A. Delirium
    B. Insipidus diabetes
    C. Polyuria
    D. Electrolyte imbalances

10. A continence nurse is initiating a prompted voiding program in a long-term nursing care facility. For which type of resident would this program be most appropriate?
    A. An older adult who does not have dementia and can toilet successfully at least 40% of the time
    B. An older adult who has dementia and can toilet successfully at least 66% of the time
    C. An older adult who does not have cognitive disorders and can toilet 66% of the time
    D. An older adult who can achieve 50% more reduction in incontinent episodes during a toileting trial

ANSWERS: 1.**B**, 2.**D**, 3.**A**, 4.**C**, 5.**A**, 6.**B**, 7.**D**, 8.**C**, 9.**A**, 10.**B**

CHAPTER 11

Voiding Dysfunction and Urinary Incontinence in the Pediatric Population

Darcie Kiddoo

Introduction

The International Children's Continence Society (ICCS) recently published an update to their standardized document on bowel and bladder dysfunction (Austin et al., 2014). In it, they describe 10 conditions for children presenting with bowel and bladder dysfunction (Box 11-1). This chapter will highlight toilet training, enuresis, overactive bladder, and voiding postponement as these are conditions commonly seen within the bladder dysfunction category. Vaginal reflux and giggle incontinence are mentioned due to the uniqueness in the pediatric population. A more exhaustive differential for conditions causing urologic symptoms is presented in Table 11-1.

Overactive bladder

Voiding postponement

Underactive bladder

Dysfunctional voiding

Bladder outlet dysfunction

Stress incontinence

Vaginal reflux

Giggle incontinence

Extraordinary daytime only urinary frequency

Bladder neck dysfunction

 ## Acquisition of Continence/Toilet Training

Babies begin life with a bladder capacity of only 10 mL and a discoordinated voiding pattern (Guerra et al., 2014). The process leading to continence is gradual and complex.

Physiologic and Psychologic Readiness

As the child grows older, bladder volume increases and voiding frequency decreases. There are also physiologic changes that inhibit overnight bladder contractions and reduce nocturnal urine output. To achieve continence, children must possess the ability to store urine for prolonged periods, have the motor skills to use a toilet and empty in a coordinated fashion, and have the understanding to complete this in a socially acceptable manner.

Parents put significant effort into toilet training their children and are always in search of the fastest and most successful method. Toilet training behaviors are extremely variable, with limited data to support one over another. Some parents begin toilet training at a very early age by recognizing cues in their babies that indicate readiness to void (Sun & Rugolotto, 2004). However, most parents follow a child-centered approach to toilet training described by Brazelton (1962). This involves recognizing when a child is interested in toilet training and possesses the motor skills to void on a toilet, which typically occurs between 18 months of age and 28.5 months. In another, now classic, paper, Foxx and Azrin (1973) discussed child readiness, identified specific tasks to determine readiness, and then described a stepwise process to toilet training. Operant conditioning (OC) has also been proposed as a toilet training strategy; OC uses positive and negative reinforcement to achieve dryness (Sun & Rugolotto, 2004).

CLINICAL PEARL

Approaches to toilet training are extremely variable, with limited data to support one over another.

Evidence Regarding Best Approach to Toilet Training

There is no evidence to support any method of toilet training over another (Klassen et al., 2006) nor the ideal age at which to begin or complete toilet training, though there is ongoing research to determine how age affects toilet training. The following studies illustrate the challenge of determining best age to begin toilet training. Based on survey questionnaires of parents and follow-up of 3,249 children in the Netherlands, Bakker et al. (2002) suggest that toilet training after 18 months of age places the child at risk for later problems. Joinson et al. (2009) studied 8,000 UK children ages 4.5 to 9 years and reported that toilet training after 24 months could lead to increased risk of daytime wetting and delayed acquisition of daytime control or relapse; and Barone et al. (2009), in a case control study of 218 US children aged 4 to 12 (n = 58 symptomatic children; N = 157 asymptomatic controls), suggest that toilet training post-32 months places the child at risk for urge symptoms. On the other hand, in another US-based study, 378 children were followed from 17 months until acquisition of continence (Blum et al., 2004), and the authors found no relationship between age and toilet training outcomes. However, they did find that children who completed training post-42 months of age ("later trainers") were more likely "to have stool toileting refusal, to hide when defecating, to be frequently constipated, and to have lower language score at 18 months" (p. 109). Chen et al. (2009) and Yang et al. (2011), however,

TABLE 11-1	**Conditions Causing Urologic Symptoms**
Bowel and bladder dysfunction	Enuresis (nighttime wetting)
	Overactive bladder
	Voiding postponement
	Dysfunctional voiding
	Vaginal reflux
	Giggle incontinence
	Extraordinary daytime frequency
	Underactive bladder
	Obstruction
	Stress incontinence (rare)
CNS malformations	Myelomeningocele, lipomyelomeningocele
	Tethered cord
	Sacral agenesis
Acquired neurologic conditions	Cerebral palsy
	Multiple sclerosis
	Trauma
	Transverse myelitis
Smooth muscle	Muscular dystrophy
Structural conditions	Bladder/cloacal exstrophy; epispadias
	Cloacal anomalies
	Ectopic ureter
	Prune belly
	Posterior urethral valves

found no difference in urinary tract infections (UTI) or reflux based on age at toilet training, and da Fonseca et al. (2011) indicated that toilet training before or after 24 months did not bear a relationship to voiding dysfunction. These studies all illustrate the difficulty in determining both the effect of toilet training and the best age to begin it.

Recommendations

While little evidence exists to support a specific method of toilet training, there is substantial evidence to show that poor toileting behaviors once toilet trained can result in recurrent UTI and daytime incontinence (Maternik et al., 2014; Sillen et al., 2010; Van Batavia et al., 2013). Stressing to parents the importance of appropriate water intake for body weight, avoidance of caffeinated beverages, dietary fiber to maintain regular soft stools, and regular voiding is likely to be more important to long-term bladder health than the specific age or method of toilet training.

CLINICAL PEARL

Stressing to parents the importance of appropriate water intake, avoidance of caffeinated beverages, intake of sufficient fiber to prevent constipation, and regular voiding is probably more important to long-term bladder health than the specific method or age of toilet training.

Frequency, Urgency, and Urinary Incontinence

Urinary frequency, urinary urgency, and incontinence are common reasons for children to see a physician or nurse. Daytime incontinence is found in 6% of girls and 3.8% of boys at age 7 (Schulman, 2004) and can cause a significant impact on the quality of life of children and families (Equit et al., 2014). This can ultimately impact school performance, which can have a longlasting effect. Simple nighttime incontinence (enuresis), while not as medically alarming, can cause significant psychological distress.

Clinical Presentation

In addition to complaints of frequency, urgency, and incontinence, children may also complain of dysuria or genital pain; this could be caused by vaginal or foreskin irritation from the wetness or could be the result of referred pain from constipation. Parents who identify the incontinence and are present during toileting may notice a change in the urinary stream including hesitancy (difficulty initiating the stream), straining, intermittency (stream that is not continuous), or a weak stream. They may also notice holding behaviors; girls may sit on their heels (often called Wilson's curtsey), hold their perineum, or dance around, and boys may hold their penis.

Assessment

While all of these symptoms may result from a functional condition, in rare cases, these findings can portend a serious anatomic condition. As a result, a standard approach should be taken in the evaluation of these children that avoids unnecessary and often traumatic investigations. Most symptoms will be found to relate to bladder or bowel dysfunction, and management strategies can be instituted to address this.

History and Voiding Diary/Stool Diary

As in all areas in nursing and medicine, a complete history and physical may be all that is necessary to diagnose and treat children presenting with urologic symptoms. Having children and families complete a voiding/fluid intake and stool diary prior to their clinic visit can be very helpful during the evaluation process. The history should focus on voiding behaviors including frequency and time taken to void. Holding behaviors should be discussed as well as dietary habits. Children in today's society drink little water, and often, their only fluid intake is from caffeinated beverages. Many parents are not aware of healthy alternatives. Dietary fiber intake should be discussed along with bowel movement frequency and stool consistency; the Bristol stool chart (Lewis & Heaton, 1997) (Fig. 11-1) is a validated tool that can be used to determine whether constipation is present. It is also helpful to discuss daytime routines as the school environment can be stressful for children, and often, there is little access to the bathroom. Finally, it is important to ask about psychological conditions including anxiety and attention deficit/hyperactivity disorder (ADHD) or major depressive disorder (MDD) as well as

Bristol Stool Chart

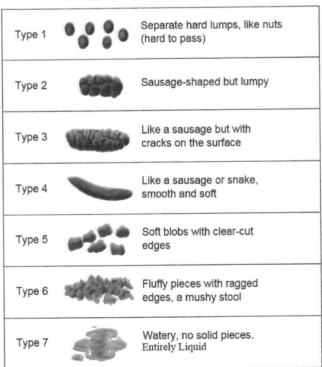

Type 1	Separate hard lumps, like nuts (hard to pass)
Type 2	Sausage-shaped but lumpy
Type 3	Like a sausage but with cracks on the surface
Type 4	Like a sausage or snake, smooth and soft
Type 5	Soft blobs with clear-cut edges
Type 6	Fluffy pieces with ragged edges, a mushy stool
Type 7	Watery, no solid pieces. Entirely Liquid

FIGURE 11-1. Bristol stool chart.

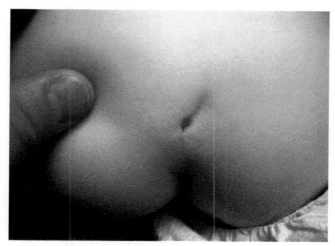

FIGURE 11-2. Sacral dimple within the gluteal fold.

learning delays, which have been identified as risk factors for bladder dysfunction (von Gontard & Equit, 2014).

To be successful, management for children with voiding dysfunction must include attention to any psychological or cognitive issues. Finally, questionnaires can be administered to assess the impact the symptoms have on the child's quality of life and to track progress. The two questionnaires commonly used are the Dysfunctional Voiding Symptoms Score (Farhat et al., 2000) and the Pediatric Urinary Incontinence Quality of Life Score (PIN-Q) (Bower et al., 2006).

Physical Examination

Physical assessment includes an abdominal exam to palpate for retained stool and for a distended bladder. The back should be examined to rule out sacral dimples (Fig. 11-2) or hairy patches, which may suggest a spinal cord pathology. Genital findings to watch for include vaginal redness in girls, continuous leaking, and meatal or foreskin abnormalities in boys such as balanoposthitis—cellulitis (Fig. 11-3).

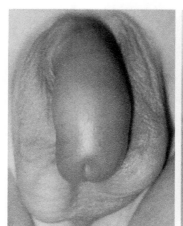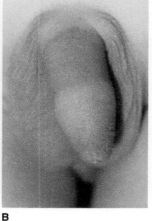

A   B

FIGURE 11-3. **A.** Balanoposthitis—cellulitis of normal foreskin with erythema, edema, and tenderness. **B.** Normal foreskin after treatment of balanoposthitis with antibiotics and warm soaks.

Bladder scanning for pre- and postvoid volumes can be very helpful in the clinic; however, the cost of the machine may prohibit this in smaller centers.

> **CLINICAL PEARL**
>
> Initial workup for the child with frequency, urgency, and incontinence should focus on voiding and defecation patterns, ruling out constipation, and screening for indicators of neurologic dysfunction.

Uroflow

Uroflow is a noninvasive evaluation tool whereby children sit on a commode to void and a scale underneath records various measurements. These include voided volume, maximum flow, and voiding pattern. The addition of an EMG tracing during voiding may be helpful in determining whether the sphincter is active during voiding (dyssynergia), which would prevent effective emptying. Uroflow can aid in the diagnosis of bladder dysfunction; however, it is not available in many centers. The ability of uroflow diagnosis to improve outcomes has not been proven (Nelson et al., 2004), and the initial care for children does not depend on this tool.

Imaging Tests

Imaging with ultrasound and abdominal x-ray may be necessary. Ultrasound may be of particular benefit in children who also present with UTI. Anatomic conditions leading to infections may be found; however, it is important to recognize that ultrasound is not sensitive and may miss anatomic conditions such as vesicoureteral reflux (VUR) (Fig. 11-4) and ectopic ureters (Fig. 11-5). Ultrasound imaging should be performed pre- and postvoid to assess for changes with bladder emptying. X-ray may demonstrate a spinal malformation or ureteric calculus. X-ray can also be used to confirm the presence of fecal loading for parents who need evidence of a problem before they are willing to begin bowel management. Figures 11-6 and 11-7 outline the guidelines for the assessment and treatment of constipation in the pediatric population (Constipation Guideline Committee of the North American Society for Pediatric Gastroenterology, Hepatology and Nutrition, 2006).

Video Urodynamics (see also Chapter 4)

Children who fail initial management may require further investigation. This typically involves video urodynamics; a urethral catheter, rectal catheter, and EMG pads are placed, the bladder is filled under fluoroscopic imaging, and filling pressures are recorded. If the child is able to voluntarily initiate voiding, he/she is asked to void and emptying pressures are recorded. In older children, the urine during leaks and voids is collected and measured; however, in babies, this may be difficult. Urodynamics may demonstrate abnormal bladder contractions in the child with an overactive or neurogenic bladder. In severe cases, the pressure may increase significantly during filling, which is indicative of poor compliance and portends

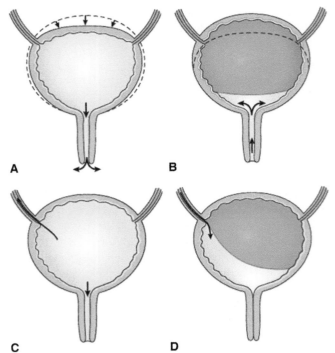

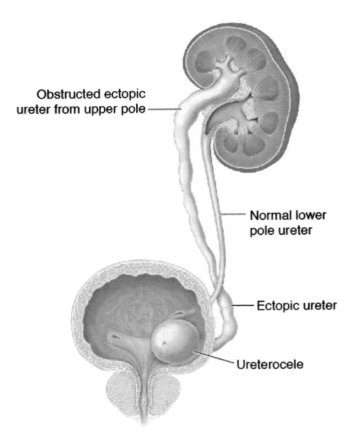

FIGURE 11-4. Urethrovesical and vesicoureteric reflux. With coughing and straining, bladder pressure rises, which may force urine from the bladder into the urethra **(A)**. When bladder pressure returns to normal, the urine flows back to the bladder **(B)**, which introduces bacteria from the urethra to the bladder. Vesicoureteric reflux: With failure of the ureterovesical valve, urine moves up the ureters during voiding **(C)** and flows into the bladder when voiding stops **(D)**. This prevents complete emptying of the bladder. It also leads to urinary stasis and contamination of the ureters with bacterium-laden urine.

FIGURE 11-5. Duplicated collecting system and ectopic ureter.

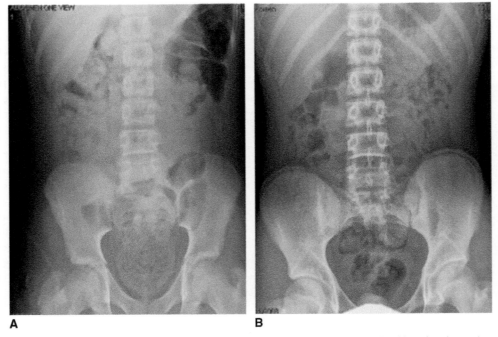

FIGURE 11-6. Abdominal radiographs showing fecal loading. **A.** The rectum is widened and contains a large fecal impaction. **B.** Rectum is less widened and the stool is less compacted.

CONSTIPATION, TREATMENT (PEDIATRIC)

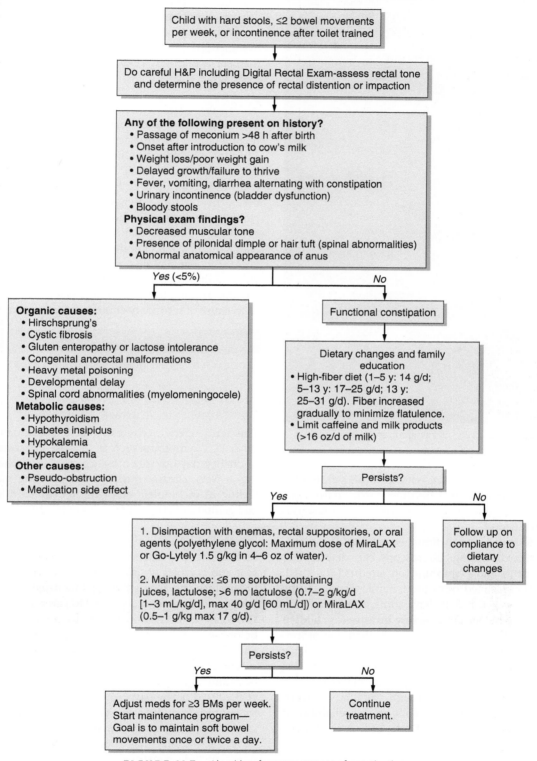

FIGURE 11-7. Algorithm for management of constipation.

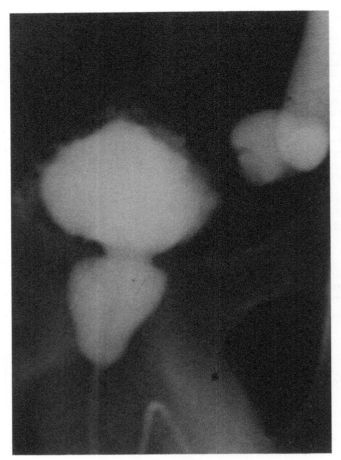

FIGURE 11-8. Spinning-top urethra.

a worse prognosis. In children who hold off voiding for long periods, the bladder may become atonic; in this case, the bladder can be filled to large volumes with no sensation or contractions.

In the child with a dysfunctional external sphincter producing obstructed voiding, fluoroscopy can detect VUR, bladder diverticuli, and a "spinning top" urethra (Fig. 11-8). The information gleaned from urodynamic testing can be very helpful; however, it does have some drawbacks. First of all, the test can be perceived as very invasive for children and a negative experience may worsen their symptoms. Urodynamic findings have also been shown to have a large interobserver variability (Bael et al., 2009) and may not reflect what is happening during natural bladder filling. This issue may be partly resolved with ambulatory urodynamics; however, there are little data on the reliability of this test, particularly in children (Deshpande et al., 2012).

⬤ Enuresis

Enuresis is a common condition affecting 8% of 9.5-year-olds (Kiddoo, 2012). Standardized terminology to describe enuresis and lower urinary tract function or dysfunction has been developed by the International Children's Continence Society (ICCS) (Franco et al., 2013; Nijman et al., 2013). Enuresis has been categorized as monosymptomatic (no urinary symptoms and normal urinalysis) or nonmonosymptomatic (coexisting symptoms of lower urinary tract dysfunction) (Fig. 11-9) such as diabetes melitus (DM), detrusor overactivity (DO), chronic renal failure (CRF) or sleep apnea (OSA).

Monosymptomatic Enuresis

This term is used to denote enuresis in children who have no other lower urinary tract symptoms and who do not have a history of bladder dysfunction; it may be either primary or secondary (Nevéus et al., 2006). *Primary enuresis* refers to enuresis in children who have never achieved a satisfactory period of nighttime dryness and includes the majority of children presenting with nighttime wetting. *Secondary enuresis* refers to enuresis that develops after a dry period of at least 6 months; it is typically related to an unusually stressful event (e.g., parental divorce, birth of a sibling) at a time of vulnerability in a child's life. Stool retention and suboptimal daytime voiding habits also may play a role. However, the exact cause of secondary enuresis remains unknown.

CLINICAL PEARL

Enuresis is a very common condition, affecting 8% of children aged 9.5 years.

Nonmonosymptomatic Enuresis

This term refers to enuresis that is accompanied by any other LUT symptoms such as increased/decreased voiding frequency, daytime incontinence, urgency, hesitancy, straining, a weak stream, intermittency, holding maneuvers, a feeling of incomplete emptying, postmicturition dribble, and genital or LUT pain (Nevéus et al., 2006, p. 319).

Natural History and Pathology

Enuresis has a spontaneous resolution rate of over 15% per year and is typically only diagnosed in children 5 years or older since the acquisition of nighttime continence may take up to 5 years to achieve. However, the need for sensitive care of both the child and parent may be required before age 5 if parents are unrealistic in expecting dry nights and if the enuresis is contributing to child and family stress.

The condition is common, with over 8% of 8-year-old boys and slightly fewer girls still wetting the bed (Nijman et al., 2013). There have been many proposed mechanisms for enuresis including excessive urine output at night, small bladder capacity, and deep sleep and an abnormal sleep cycle. Factors that may predispose to nighttime incontinence include constipation (Halachmi & Farhat, 2008), poor daytime voiding habits, and obstructive sleep apnea. Investigations to determine the cause of the nighttime wetting include urodynamics, nocturnal urine collection to determine volume, sleep studies, and stool and voiding diaries. Recent studies propose that children with enuresis

ENURESIS

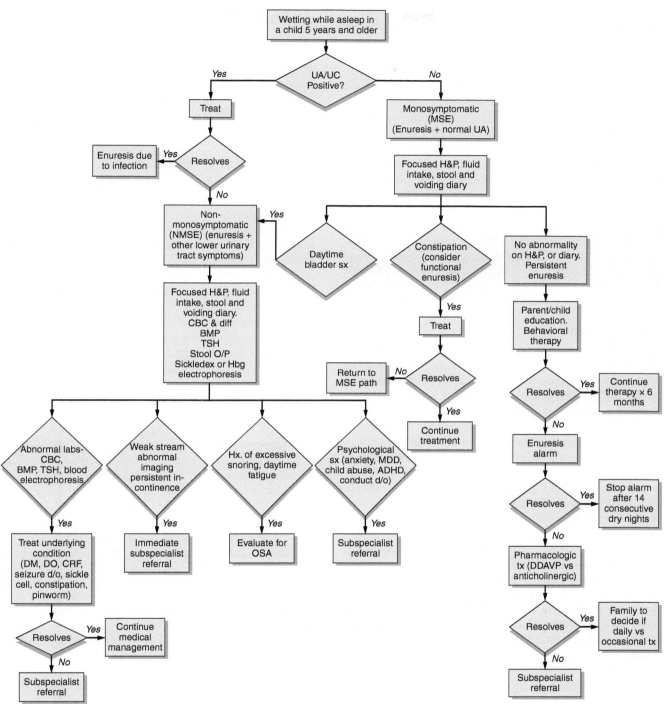

FIGURE 11-9. Algorithm for management of enuresis.

may have increased sleep fragmentation as compared to children without enuresis, suggesting a central nervous system role in the condition (Dhondt et al., 2014). Sleep apnea may cause the same disruption in sleep patterns, and in some studies, enuresis improved after tonsillectomy and adenoidectomy (Jeyakumar et al., 2012).

CLINICAL PEARL

Proposed pathologic mechanisms for enuresis include excessive nighttime production of urine, reduced bladder capacity, and abnormally deep sleep or an abnormal sleep cycle that prevents waking to the sensation of a full bladder.

Evaluation

Children who present with pure nighttime incontinence do not need extensive testing. A standard history and physical should typically suffice. Urinalysis is suggested, but there is no evidence that even a urinalysis affects management. In the absence of daytime incontinence, urinary frequency, or UTI, treatment can be implemented immediately. If parents want further investigation prior to beginning treatment, overnight urine collection is suggested. Excessive urine output is defined as greater than $20 \times (age + 9)$ mL. Urine collection can be challenging in the presence of enuresis and would involve pre– and post–pad weighing as well as measurement of any voided volumes (if the child is taken to the toilet at night).

CLINICAL PEARL

For children with enuresis but no daytime incontinence and no issues with frequency or UTI, treatment can begin immediately without further testing.

Management

Various management strategies have been employed, based on the proposed pathologic mechanisms. All begin with counseling parents on the age ranges for achieving nighttime dryness, emphasizing that it is not the fault of the child and that punishment will not assist but hinder resolution of the issue. It is also important to determine the child's feelings about being wet and whether they are ready to work with the parents to improve the situation; effective management requires "buy-in" and adherence to management recommendations by both the child and family. Recommendations usually include lifestyle management strategies such as regular voiding during the day, management of constipation, and fluid restriction before going to bed. The most successful and well-studied medical interventions include the bed alarm system and DDAVP (desmopressin).

Bed Alarm System

The bed alarm may alter neurologic signaling and has a documented success rate of 66% (Glazener et al., 2005). Parent involvement is critical to success as they must wake the child when the alarm sounds if the child does not wake on his/her own. The parent then takes the child to the bathroom to void; this should be done even if the child has already emptied completely in bed. The goal is to teach the child to wake to the sensation of a full bladder. It should be noted that this treatment approach is different from waking the child at set times, which has not proven successful in treating bed-wetting (though it may decrease the volume voided). Various factors may make it difficult for the parents and child to adhere to alarm therapy. For example, during school, the sleep disruption may be harmful to the child's academic performance, and this may stress an already difficult relationship. Siblings may also share a room and parents may not want the sibling disturbed. Nevertheless, when employed diligently, most children can attain nighttime dryness with this intervention.

CLINICAL PEARL

Alarm therapy and pharmacologic therapy with DDAVP are the strategies with the greatest documented success in treatment of enuresis.

DDAVP

The mainstay in pharmacologic treatment of enuresis is DDAVP (desmopressin), a synthetic analogue of the natural pituitary hormone 8-arginine vasopressin (ADH), an antidiuretic hormone that affects renal water conservation. DDAVP acts on the collecting tubule to reabsorb rather than excrete water, thus concentrating the urine and reducing urine volume. It is available in a tablet, melt form, and nasal spray. In one study, the melt was found to be more effective than tablet in treating nighttime wetting (Juul et al., 2013). Unfortunately, once the medication is discontinued, the child will return to wetting the bed, and therefore, this is not an actual cure. Tricyclic antidepressant medications have also been used to treat bed-wetting although very few parents or physicians feel comfortable prescribing this in a healthy, happy child. Alternative therapies that have been tried for bed-wetting include hypnotherapy, acupuncture, chiropractic, and psychotherapy. To date, there is very weak evidence to support any of these for the successful treatment of bed-wetting.

Enuresis is a common condition that does not require extensive investigation. Children and families should be reassured that there is a high likelihood of cure without intervention and that the condition is not behavioral. Reward systems are not helpful given that the children do not have control over the wetting. The anxiety caused by the condition, however, should not be minimized, and treatment is reasonable if the child and parents are willing. Figure 11-9 provides an algorithm of systematic steps for the management of enuresis.

● Overactive Bladder

Overactive bladder is defined as urinary urgency, frequency, and often nocturia that is not due to a neurologic cause. It is reported as one of the most frequent urologic conditions in children. These children may also have incontinence depending on whether they can reach the toilet on time. The urgency associated with overactive bladder should be differentiated from the normal urgency that occurs when a child postpones voiding while busy and has to rush to the bathroom because the bladder is very full. The best way to confirm abnormal frequency and urgency is with a voiding diary; in the absence of a diary, the clinician can ask specific questions about voiding frequency, such as the child's ability to tolerate long car rides or to sit through a movie. Teachers' comments can also help confirm abnormal voiding frequency. Parents may need to advocate for their child if school policy does not allow children to leave the class without permission to use the bathroom.

Etiologic Factors

Lifestyle factors can play a significant contributing role in overactive bladder. Consumption of caffeinated beverages may cause increased bladder irritability in addition to its diuretic effect; the combined effects can cause increased frequency and urgency. Many parents do not recognize the impact of caffeine on the bladder and may not realize the need to limit intake of these fluids.

Constipation can also cause urinary frequency and is one of the biggest causes of bladder symptoms in the pediatric population (Veiga et al., 2013); the negative impact of fecal loading on bladder function has been confirmed through urodynamic studies (Panayi et al., 2011). Fecal loading can also cause problems with infrequent voiding, insufficient emptying, and VUR. Anxiety disorders can also play a role in bladder overactivity; in children with OAB and anxiety, stressful situations may amplify the symptoms. An overactive bladder in childhood may predict bladder problems as an adult; however, at this time, there is no evidence that specific interventions can prevent later problems (Fitzgerald et al., 2006; Minassian et al., 2006).

Evaluation

Initial investigation should focus on the voiding and bowel history as well as a psychological assessment. If the condition is severe and associated with incontinence, the patient may require urodynamics to determine whether a neurologic assessment is necessary. Frequent bladder contractions on urodynamics do support the diagnosis of overactive bladder (Fig. 11-10); however, an MRI may

be necessary to rule out a spinal cord malformation, especially if initial management is unsuccessful.

Management

Once a diagnosis of overactive bladder is made, management is initiated and should be multimodal. The first step is to ensure that irritating beverages are avoided and that the bowel is under control. An x-ray demonstrating improvement in fecal loading can be helpful though this is not a validated instrument. Bowel management is critically important for children with OAB, because the medications used to treat this condition can cause significant constipation. Psychological referral may also be necessary if there is a large component of anxiety, and special consideration should be given to providing support for the child at school.

Many new medications have been introduced to treat adult overactive bladder; these are discussed in detail in Chapter 5. Anticholinergic medications are beneficial in improving overactive bladder symptoms in children as well and fortunately can be used on a long-term basis (Nijman et al., 2007). While short-acting oxybutynin is the only medication with pediatric approval, in reality, pediatric urologists or nurse practitioners will try all adult medications (at pediatric doses), particularly when side effects and practicality become a problem. Pediatric-friendly formulations include oxybutynin gel and patch and long-acting antimuscarinic medications that retain pharmacokinetics when crushed, such as solifenacin (Nadeau et al., 2014). Practitioners must remember that most children struggle to swallow pills and short-acting medications are difficult to administer when children are at school.

> **CLINICAL PEARL**
>
> Management of OAB in children mirrors OAB management in adults and involves behavioral strategies (e.g., bowel management, elimination caffeinated fluids), antimuscarinic medications if needed, and neuromodulation for refractory cases.

Newer treatment strategies, which have been used less frequently in children, include transcutaneous nerve stimulation (TENS), posterior tibial nerve stimulation (PTNS), sacral neuromodulation via implant (SNM), and Botox injections (De Gennaro et al., 2011).

In a few small studies, TENS has been shown to improve symptoms in up to 73% of patients (Malm-Buatsi et al., 2007; Hagstroem et al., 2009). It has also been shown to improve slow transit constipation, which may help to improve bladder symptoms (Ismail et al., 2009). PTNS has shown some success in children with a mean age of 11.7 years and is well tolerated (Hoebeke et al., 2002). SNM has also been shown to improve voiding symptoms; however, there can be up to a 50% risk of reoperation (Dwyer et al., 2014). Botox is an acceptable treatment for children who already perform intermittent catheterization

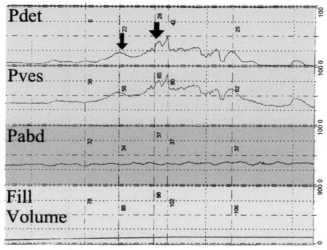

FIGURE 11-10. Detrusor overactivity on filling cystometrography. The patient begins to sense urgency, accompanied by an unstable bladder contraction, when 88 mL of water is instilled into the bladder. The detrusor pressure rises, and when 96 mL of water is instilled, she leaks. (Pabd, abdominal pressure; Pves, vesical pressure; Pdet, detrusor pressure.)

as a result of a neurogenic bladder but is of limited use in children with overactive bladder, because very few children and families will accept the risk of requiring catheterization. However, one study in children did show a significant improvement in symptoms with only 1 of 21 children requiring intermittent catheterization and only for a short period (Hoebeke et al., 2006).

Overactive bladder can disrupt a child's life as well as the family dynamics. Investigation should ensure that there is not a neurologic reason for the symptoms. Lifestyle measures should be optimized initially as avoidance of medications is preferable in children. In the absence of improvement, anticholinergic medication has been found beneficial in children and should be prescribed. Neuromodulation and Botox can be considered in refractory cases.

Voiding Postponement and Dysfunctional Voiding

Children often prefer to play rather than use the toilet on a regular basis. As a result, they may present with urinary incontinence and/or UTI as a result of urine holding. These children may also delay defecation, causing bowel dysfunction as well. Parents may notice little girls sitting on their heels or holding their perineum or boys holding their penis, but may not realize there is a problem until the child has an accident while urgently running to the bathroom. If these behaviors are allowed to continue long term, the child may develop dysfunctional voiding, which is defined as voluntary contraction of the urinary sphincter and pelvic floor during voiding (detrusor sphincter dyssynergia). Children with dysfunctional voiding ultimately develop large postvoid residuals and may present with significant incontinence and UTI. Figure 11-11A shows discoordination (dyssynergia) between bladder contraction and pelvic floor relaxation that results in incomplete emptying; Figure 11-11B shows a chronically distended bladder resulting from chronic voiding postponement.

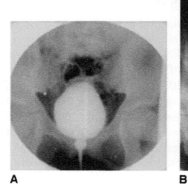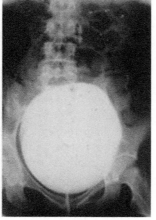

A   **B**

FIGURE 11-11. Video urodynamics. **A.** Detrusor–sphincter dyssynergia in a child. **B.** Atonic bladder due to chronic urinary holding.

CLINICAL PEARL

If voiding postponement behaviors are not identified and corrected, they can result in dysfunctional voiding, chronic bladder distention, and frequent UTIs.

Evaluation

A properly performed voiding diary will quickly point to voiding postponement as a cause for the child's urologic symptoms. If available, a uroflow with EMG tracing and a postvoid residual can also help to diagnose dysfunctional voiding; the EMG tracing will demonstrate abnormal sphincter activity during voiding, and the uroflow will reveal an intermittent "staccato" voiding pattern. If the child also presents with UTI, she/he may need a renal bladder ultrasound with particular attention to the postvoid residual.

Management

Treatment for voiding postponement focuses on timed voiding, increasing water intake, and treating constipation. This becomes critically important with school-aged children, because the child may feel embarrassed to ask to use the bathroom or may only be allowed to go to the bathroom at specific intervals. Vibrating watches can help remind children to void, and the clinician can send letters to the school to ensure teacher cooperation with voiding routines and access to water bottles. PEG 3350 can be used as a stool softener for the child with persistent constipation, and timed bowel elimination attempts are suggested following a meal. It is also critical to treatment success to try to elucidate the child's reasons for postponement, as helping the child with the root cause will greatly improve likelihood of treatment success.

CLINICAL PEARL

Management of voiding postponement involves management of constipation, adequate water intake, and timed voiding. Biofeedback may be of benefit in management of dysfunctional voiding.

Children with voiding postponement may be extremely strong willed and may test the child/parent relationship. If this is the case, a psychologist may be necessary to address the behavioral aspect of care. For the child with dysfunctional voiding, two additional treatments include biofeedback and alpha blockers such as doxazosin.

Biofeedback is an intensive but successful treatment for children as it helps them learn to coordinate pelvic muscle relaxation in order to improve bladder emptying. Improved emptying can also reduce or eliminate incontinence, which improves the child's quality of life (Berry et al., 2014). Patch electrodes are placed on the abdomen and perineal area and connected to a computer software program that looks like a video game. Children learn to properly isolate and relax the pelvic floor muscles and are also educated about healthy bladder and bowel habits. Biofeedback is typically performed weekly for 6 weeks though there is not enough evidence to give definitive advice about length of treatment. Various nonrandomized studies have shown an improvement in UTI (83%) and incontinence (80%) with biofeedback. One randomized trial did not show a statistical difference but did demonstrate an improvement (Desantis et al., 2011).

Biofeedback tends to be favored by parents who prefer a nonmedical approach. Unfortunately, the treatment is not available in all centers, requires time out of school, and may stress a family who must travel a substantial distance. Treatment may not be covered by health insurance, placing a financial strain on the family. In this setting, alpha-blockers can be used to relax the smooth muscle and improve emptying. While there is little evidence that alpha-blockers cure dysfunctional voiding, there is a randomized trial that demonstrated subjective improvement as reported by patients and families (Kramer et al., 2005). Another study demonstrated changes in uroflow parameters with use of the medication (Van Batavia et al., 2010). Alpha-blockers can also be used as adjunctive therapy for the child being managed with biofeedback.

Voiding postponement is common in school-aged children and can lead to significant morbidity and voiding dysfunction. Obtaining a reliable voiding history is critical to management. Children and families must be instructed on regular emptying of the bladder and bowel. In more severe situations, biofeedback can be a powerful tool in treating the condition. Finally, psychological support may be necessary to address behavioral issues and family stress.

Vaginal Reflux

Vaginal voiding or vaginal reflux is a benign condition that can cause troublesome symptoms. It is caused by the passage of urine into the vagina during voiding. With a careful history, the child will describe dribbling after she gets up from the toilet. This can be seen on an ultrasound or a voiding cystourethrogram when urine enters the vagina during voiding. Girls should be instructed to sit forward on the toilet with their legs spread to ensure that the vagina empties. They should also allow some time before standing up after a void. These simple measures typically cure the condition.

Giggle Incontinence

Giggle incontinence is a unique condition seen in girls where laughter triggers complete incontinence of urine (Glahn, 1979). This can understandably cause a significant amount of anxiety for girls who experience this phenomenon. The pathophysiology is not well understood; girls with this condition are completely dry outside of the giggle episodes and have normal anatomy. If the history and physical do not clearly rule out significant pathology, urodynamics should be considered.

> **CLINICAL PEARL**
>
> Giggle incontinence is a poorly understood and highly distressing condition; management involves lifestyle modification (bowel management, avoidance of caffeinated fluids, and scheduled voiding) and sympathomimetic agents to enhance sphincter tone.

Despite the lack of clarity regarding etiology and pathology, treatment to date has focused primarily on improving sphincter tone and enhancing sympathetic stimulation. Currently recognized treatments include stimulants such as methylphenidate (Chang et al., 2011; Berry et al., 2009) and pseudoephedrine and biofeedback (Richardson & Palmer, 2009). Lifestyle measures such as bowel management, regular voiding, and avoiding caffeine should be encouraged to ensure optimum treatment.

Conclusion

Bladder control is a basic function that many people take for granted. The steps to become toilet trained should occur "naturally," although many parents struggle with this process. Once a child is toilet trained, many things may impact continence. While health care professionals may first think of anatomic factors, in reality, psychological and behavioral factors are responsible for the majority of problems. In this fast-paced world, healthy toileting and dietary habits seem to be forgotten. As such, the investigation and management of children presenting with incontinence should focus on a thorough history and bowel and bladder management. If this fails, children may require more invasive investigation and referral to a pediatric urologist.

REFERENCES

Austin, P. F., Bauer, S. B., Bower W., et al. (2014). The standardization of terminology of lower urinary tract function in children and adolescents: Update report from the Standardization Committee of the International Children's Continence Society. *The Journal of Urology, 191*(6), 1863–1865.

Bael, A., Verhulst, J., Lax, H., et al.; European Bladder Dysfunction Study EBC. (2009). Investigator bias in urodynamic studies for functional urinary incontinence. *The Journal of Urology, 182*(4 Suppl), 1949–1952.

Bakker, E., Van Gool, J. D., Van Sprundel, M., et al. (2002). Results of a questionnaire evaluating the effects of different methods of toilet training on achieving bladder control. *BJU International, 90*(4), 456–461.

Barone, J. G., Jasutkar, N., & Schneider, D. (2009). Later toilet training is associated with urge incontinence in children. *Journal of Pediatric Urology, 5*(6), 458–461.

Berry, A. K., Zderic, S., & Carr, M. (2009). Methylphenidate for giggle incontinence. *The Journal of Urology, 182*(4 Suppl), 2028–2032.

Berry, A., Rudick, K., Richter, M., et al. (2014). Objective versus subjective outcome measures of biofeedback: What really matters? *Journal of Pediatric Urology.* Advance online publication. doi: 10.1016/j.jpurol.2014.06.003.

Blum, N. J., Taubman, B., & Nemeth, N. (2004). Why is toilet training occurring at older ages? A study of factors associated with later training. *The Journal of Pediatrics, 145*(1), 107–111.

Bower, W. F., Wong, E. M., & Yeung, C. K. (2006). Development of a validated quality of life tool specific to children with bladder dysfunction. *Neurourology and Urodynamics, 25*(3), 221–227.

Brazelton, T. B. (1962). A child-oriented approach to toilet training. *Pediatrics, 29,* 121–128.

Chang, J. H., Lee, K. Y., Kim, T. B., et al. (2011). Clinical and urodynamic effect of methylphenidate for the treatment of giggle incontinence (enuresis risoria). *Neurourology and Urodynamics, 30*(7), 1338–1342.

Chen, J. J., Ahn, H. J., & Steinhardt, G. F. (2009). Is age at toilet training associated with the presence of vesicoureteral reflux or the occurrence of urinary tract infection? *The Journal of Urology, 182*(1), 268–271.

Constipation Guideline Committee of the North American Society for Pediatric Gastroenterology, Hepatology and Nutrition. (2006). Evaluation and treatment of constipation in infants and children: Recommendations of the North American Society for Pediatric Gastroenterology, Hepatology and Nutrition. *Journal of Pediatric Gastroenterology and Nutrition, 43*(3), e1–e13.

da Fonseca, E. M., Santana, P. G., Gomes, F. A., et al. (2011). Dysfunction elimination syndrome: Is age at toilet training a determinant? *Journal of Pediatric Urology, 7*(3), 332–335.

De Gennaro, M., Capitanucci, M. L., Mosiello, G., et al. (2011). Current state of nerve stimulation technique for lower urinary tract dysfunction in children. *The Journal of Urology, 185*(5), 1571–1577.

Desantis, D. J., Leonard, M. P., Preston, M. A., et al. (2011). Effectiveness of biofeedback for dysfunctional elimination syndrome in pediatrics: A systematic review. *Journal of Pediatric Urology, 7*(3), 342–348.

Deshpande, A. V., Craig, J. C., Caldwell, P. H., et al. (2012). Ambulatory urodynamic studies (UDS) in children using a Bluetooth-enabled device. *BJU International, 110*(Suppl 4), 38–45.

Dhondt, K., Baert, E., Van Herzeele, C., et al. (2014). Sleep fragmentation and increased periodic limb movements are more common in children with nocturnal enuresis. *Acta Paediatrica, 103*(6), e268–e272.

Dwyer, M. E., Vandersteen, D. R., Hollatz, P., et al. (2014). Sacral neuromodulation for the dysfunctional elimination syndrome: A 10-year single-center experience with 105 consecutive children. *Urology, 84*(4), 911–918.

Equit, M., Hill, J., Hubner, A., et al. (2014). Health-related quality of life and treatment effects on children with functional incontinence, and their parents. *Journal of Pediatric Urology.* Advance online publication. doi: 10.1016/j.jpurol.2014.03.002.

Farhat, W., Bagli, D. J., Capolicchio, G., et al. (2000). The dysfunctional voiding scoring system: Quantitative standardization of dysfunctional voiding symptoms in children. *The Journal of Urology, 164*(3 Pt 2), 1011–1015.

Fitzgerald, M. P., Thom, D. H., Wassel-Fyr, C., et al. (2006). Childhood urinary symptoms predict adult overactive bladder symptoms. *The Journal of Urology, 175*(3 Pt 1), 989–993.

Foxx, R. M., & Azrin, N. H. (1973). Dry pants: A rapid method of toilet training children. *Behaviour Research and Therapy, 11*(4), 435–442.

Franco, I., von Gontard, A., De Gennaro, M., et al. (2013). Evaluation and treatment of non monosymptomatic nocturnal enuresis: A standardization document from the International Children's Continence Society. *Journal of Pediatric Urology, 9,* 234–243.

Glahn, B. E. (1979). Giggle incontinence (enuresis risoria). A study and an aetiological hypothesis. *British Journal of Urology, 51*(5), 363–366.

Glazener, C. M., Evans, J. H., & Peto, R. E. (2005). Alarm interventions for nocturnal enuresis in children. *The Cochrane Database of Systematic Reviews,* (2), CD002911.

Guerra, L., Leonard, M., & Castagnetti, M. (2014). Best practice in the assessment of bladder function in infants. *Therapeutic Advances in Urology, 6*(4), 148–164.

Hagstroem, S., Mahler, B., Madsen, B., et al. (2009). Transcutaneous electrical nerve stimulation for refractory daytime urinary urge incontinence. *The Journal of Urology, 182*(4 Suppl), 2072–2078.

Halachmi, S., & Farhat, W. A. (2008). The impact of constipation on the urinary tract system. *International Journal of Adolescent Medicine and Health, 20*(1), 17–22.

Hoebeke, P., De Caestecker, K., Vande Walle, J., et al. (2006). The effect of botulinum-A toxin in incontinent children with therapy resistant overactive detrusor. *The Journal of Urology, 176*(1), 328–330; discussion 330–321.

Hoebeke, P., Renson, C., Petillon, L., et al. (2002). Percutaneous electrical nerve stimulation in children with therapy resistant nonneuropathic bladder sphincter dysfunction: a pilot study. *The Journal of Urology, 168*(6), 2605–2607; discussion 2607–2608.

Ismail, K. A., Chase, J., Gibb, S., et al. (2009). Daily transabdominal electrical stimulation at home increased defecation in children with slow-transit constipation: A pilot study. *Journal of Pediatric Surgery, 44*(12), 2388–2392.

Jeyakumar, A., Rahman, S. I., Armbrecht, E. S., et al. (2012). The association between sleep-disordered breathing and enuresis in children. *The Laryngoscope, 122*(8), 1873–1877.

Joinson, C., Heron, J., Von Gontard, A., et al. (2009). A prospective study of age at initiation of toilet training and subsequent daytime bladder control in school-age children. *Journal of Developmental and Behavioral Pediatrics, 30*(5), 385–393.

Juul, K. V., Van Herzeele, C., De Bruyne, P., et al. (2013). Desmopressin melt improves response and compliance compared with tablet in treatment of primary monosymptomatic nocturnal enuresis. *European Journal of Pediatrics, 172*(9), 1235–1242.

Kiddoo, D. A. (2012). Nocturnal enuresis. *Canadian Medical Association Journal, 184*(8), 908–911.

Klassen, T. P., Kiddoo, D., Lang, M. E., et al. (2006). The effectiveness of different methods of toilet training for bowel and bladder control. *Evidence Report/Technology Assessment, 147,* 1–57.

Kramer, S. A., Rathbun, S. R., Elkins, D., et al. (2005). Double-blind placebo controlled study of alpha-adrenergic receptor antagonists (doxazosin) for treatment of voiding dysfunction in the pediatric population. *The Journal of Urology, 173*(6), 2121–2124; discussion 2124.

Lewis, S. J., & Heaton, K. W. (1997). Stool form scale as a useful guide to intestinal transit time. *Scandinavian Journal of Gastroenterology, 32*(9), 920–924.

Malm-Buatsi, E., Nepple, K. G., Boyt, M. A., et al. (2007). Efficacy of transcutaneous electrical nerve stimulation in children with overactive bladder refractory to pharmacotherapy. *Urology, 70*(5), 980–983.

Maternik, M., Krzeminska, K., & Zurowska, A. (2014). The management of childhood urinary incontinence. *Pediatric Nephrology.* Advance online publication. doi: 10.1007/s00467-014-2791-x.

Minassian, V. A., Lovatsis, D., Pascali, D., et al. (2006). Effect of childhood dysfunctional voiding on urinary incontinence in adult women. *Obstetrics and Gynecology, 107*(6), 1247–1251.

Nadeau, G., Schroder, A., Moore, K., et al. (2014). Long-term use of solifenacin in pediatric patients with overactive bladder: Extension of a prospective open-label study. *Canadian Urological Association Journal, 8*(3–4), 118–123.

Nelson, J. D., Cooper, C. S., Boyt, M. A., et al. (2004). Improved uroflow parameters and post-void residual following biofeedback therapy in pediatric patients with dysfunctional voiding does not correspond to outcome. *The Journal of Urology, 172*(4 Pt 2), 1653–1656; discussion 1656.

Nevéus, T., von Gontard, A., Hoebeke, P., et al. (2006). The standardization of terminology of lower urinary tract function in children and adolescents: Report from the Standardisation Committee of the International Children's Continence Society. *Journal of Urology, 176*(1), 314–324.

Nijman, R. J., Borgstein, N. G., Ellsworth, P., et al. (2007). Long-term tolerability of tolterodine extended release in children 5–11 years of age: Results from a 12-month, open-label study. *European Urology, 52*(5), 1511–1516.

Nijman, R., Tekgul, S., Chase, J., et al. (2013). Diagnosis and management of urinary incontinence in childhood. In P. Abrams, L. Cardozo, S. Khoury, et al., (Eds.), *5th International Consultation on Incontinence* (pp. 729–825). London, UK: European Association of Urology.

Panayi, D. C., Khullar, V., Digesu, G. A., et al. (2011). Rectal distension: The effect on bladder function. *Neurourology and Urodynamics, 30*(3), 344–347.

Richardson, I., & Palmer, L. S. (2009). Successful treatment for giggle incontinence with biofeedback. *The Journal of Urology, 182*(4 Suppl), 2062–2066.

Schulman, S. L. (2004). Voiding dysfunction in children. *The Urologic Clinics of North America, 31*(3), 481–490.

Sillen, U., Brandstrom, P., Jodal, U., et al. (2010). The Swedish reflux trial in children: v. Bladder dysfunction. *The Journal of Urology, 184*(1), 298–304.

Sun, M., & Rugolotto, S. (2004). Assisted infant toilet training in a Western family setting. *Journal of Developmental and Behavioral Pediatrics, 25*(2), 99–101.

Van Batavia, J. P., Ahn, J. J., Fast, A. M., et al. (2013). Prevalence of urinary tract infection and vesicoureteral reflux in children with lower urinary tract dysfunction. *The Journal of Urology, 190*(4 Suppl), 1495–1499.

Van Batavia, J. P., Combs, A. J., Horowitz, M., et al. (2010). Primary bladder neck dysfunction in children and adolescents III: Results of long-term alpha-blocker therapy. *The Journal of Urology, 183*(2) 724–730.

Veiga, M. L., Lordelo, P., Farias, T., et al. (2013). Constipation in children with isolated overactive bladders. *Journal of Pediatric Urology, 9*(6 Pt A), 945–949.

von Gontard, A., & Equit, M. (2014). Comorbidity of ADHD and incontinence in children. *European Child & Adolescent Psychiatry.* Advance online publication. doi: 10.1007/s00787-014-0577-0.

Yang, S. S., Zhao, L. L., & Chang, S. J. (2011). Early initiation of toilet training for urine was associated with early urinary continence and does not appear to be associated with bladder dysfunction. *Neurourology and Urodynamics, 30*(7), 1253–1257.

QUESTIONS

1. The continence nurse examines the back of a child experiencing urinary incontinence to check for sacral dimples or hairy patches. What condition would these findings suggest?
   A. Renal tumors
   B. Juvenile diabetes
   C. Addison's disease
   D. Spinal cord pathology

2. A continence nurse is counseling parents of toddlers who are toilet training their children. Which statement accurately describes a teaching point?
   A. Ideally, children should be potty trained by the age of 2.5 years.
   B. Children who complete training post-24 months of age are more likely to have stool toileting refusal.
   C. Fluid restriction, high-fiber consumption, and timed voiding are more important to long-term bladder health than early toilet training.
   D. There is no evidence that timing of toilet training (before or after 24 months) is a causative or contributing factor for voiding dysfunction.

3. A parent of a child with constipation is using the Bristol stool chart to classify the child's stool. The stool is mushy with fluffy pieces and ragged edges. What type stool is the child experiencing?
   A. Type 4
   B. Type 5
   C. Type 6
   D. Type 7

4. The continence nurse notes that, during urodynamics, the bladder pressure of a child increases significantly during filling. What condition is this indicative of?
   A. Poor compliance
   B. Abnormal bladder contractions
   C. Urinary retention
   D. Ectopic ureters

5. A 5-year-old child is diagnosed with nonmonosymptomatic enuresis. Which of the following describes this condition?
   A. Enuresis that is accompanied by any other LUT symptom
   B. Enuresis that develops after a dry period of at least 6 months
   C. Enuresis that is not associated with a history of bladder dysfunction
   D. Enuresis that has a high spontaneous resolution rate

6. Parents of a child who is experiencing enuresis without daytime incontinence, urinary frequency, or UTI insist on further investigation prior to beginning treatment. What testing is recommended?
   A. Video urodynamics
   B. Urine collection
   C. Imaging tests
   D. Uroflow

7. What is the ultimate goal of treatment when using the bed alarm system to treat childhood enuresis?
   A. Help the parents wake their child prior to an accident
   B. Teach the child to wake to the sensation of a full bladder
   C. Enable the child to experience the negative effect of being wet
   D. Praise the child for staying dry during the night

8. Which of the following is a mainstay in the treatment of enuresis with proven success rates?
   A. Acupuncture
   B. Hypnotherapy
   C. Psychotherapy
   D. Pharmacologic treatment with DDAVP

9. A continence nurse is devising a treatment plan for a child diagnosed with overactive bladder. What should be the first step in this plan?
   A. Fluid restriction
   B. Pharmacologic management
   C. Bowel management
   D. Surgical intervention

10. Which of the following test results point to voiding postponement as a cause for a child's urologic symptoms?
    A. An EMG tracing demonstrating abnormal sphincter activity during voiding
    B. Uroflow revealing a bell-shaped voiding pattern
    C. Postvoiding dribbling seen on a voiding cystourethrogram
    D. Frequent bladder contractions detected with urodynamics

ANSWERS: 1.**D**, 2.**D**, 3.**C**, 4.**A**, 5.**A**, 6.**B**, 7.**B**, 8.**D**, 9.**C**, 10.**A**

CHAPTER 12

Appropriate Use of Containment Devices and Absorbent Products

Mary H. Wilde and Mandy Fader

OBJECTIVES

1. Identify situations in which containment devices or absorbent products are appropriate for management of urinary and/or fecal incontinence.
2. Describe appropriate use of currently available containment devices, to include indications, contraindications, and guidelines for use.
3. Discuss decision-making guidelines related to use of absorbent products.
4. Outline current recommendations for prevention and management of incontinence-associated dermatitis.

Topic Outline

    Wear Position
    Attachment/Suspension System
    Connecting Tube
    Drainage Tap
    Sampling Port
    Comfort Backing
    Discretion
    Antikinking/Twisting Feature
    Infection Reduction Features
Night Drainage Bags

Incontinence-Associated Dermatitis (IAD)
Pathology of IAD
Assessment of IAD
Prevention and Management of IAD
    Superabsorbent Polymers
    Frequent Checks and Prompt Change for
      Wet or Soiled Products
    Preventive Skin Care
Management of IAD

Conclusion

Correct use of continence products can ensure appropriate containment, healthy skin, and user satisfaction. This chapter is aimed primarily at health care professionals seeking to make informed decisions as they choose—or help their patients to choose—between continence product categories and then to select a specific product within the chosen category. The chapter includes a section for each of the major product categories, each section reviewing published data and recommendations for product selection and use. Prevention of incontinence-associated dermatitis (IAD) is also addressed.

Not all incontinence can be cured completely and even individuals who are ultimately successfully treated may have to live with incontinence for a time (e.g., while waiting for surgery or for pelvic floor muscle training to yield its benefits). Still others, depending on their frailty, severity of incontinence, and/or personal priorities, may not be candidates for treatment or may choose management over attempted cure. For all such people, the challenge is to discover how to address incontinence and minimize its impact on quality of life. This usually involves using some type of continence product(s). Managing incontinence successfully with products is often referred to as *contained incontinence, managed incontinence, or social continence*, in recognition of the substantial benefits it can bring to quality of life even if cure has not been achieved (Fonda & Abrams, 2006).

CLINICAL PEARL

Incontinence managed successfully with products is often referred to as contained incontinence, managed incontinence, or social continence.

Guidelines for Selecting Continence Products

Selecting suitable products is critical for the well-being and quality of life of users and caregivers. The ability to contain and conceal incontinence enables individuals to maintain their public identity as a "continent person" and to avoid the stigma associated with incontinence (Paterson, 2000). Failure to do so can result in limited social and professional opportunities, place relationships in jeopardy, and detrimentally affect emotional and mental well-being (Mitteness & Barker, 1995). The ability to contain and conceal incontinence enables caregivers to feel confident that the person(s) they care for will not be embarrassed publicly and reduces challenges related to hygiene and skin integrity as well as costs and burdens associated with laundry of linens (Paterson et al., 2003).

CLINICAL PEARL

The ability to contain and conceal incontinence enables individuals to maintain their public identity as a "continent person" and to avoid the stigma associated with incontinence.

Selecting the best option is a challenge; there is a wide diversity of products, and comprehensive and current information is critical to reduce confusion and stress for both the layperson and the health care professional (Paterson et al., 2003). The intimate and stigmatized nature of incontinence means that issues relating to self-image may also affect user choices. Product success depends, in part, on the ability to conceal the problem (Shaw et al., 2001), but concealment may involve compromises. For example, the individual with high-volume leakage may need large capacity pads to prevent any leakage, but the size and bulkiness of the pad can create issues in terms of discretion and concealment. Fear of leakage may be especially marked in younger people, for whom body image may be particularly important and for whom effective management of incontinence may be essential to maintenance of social activities and interpersonal relationships (Hocking, 1999; Low, 1996). Finally, product accessibility may vary enormously between and within countries, depending on the funding available, health care policy, and the logistics of supply (Gibb & Wong, 1994; Paterson et al., 2003; Proudfoot et al., 1994).

Product Categories

Continence products may be divided into those that are intended to assist with toileting, manage urinary retention and/or incontinence, or provide containment and control.

The algorithm provided in Figure 12-1 provides guidance in determining which product or group of products is

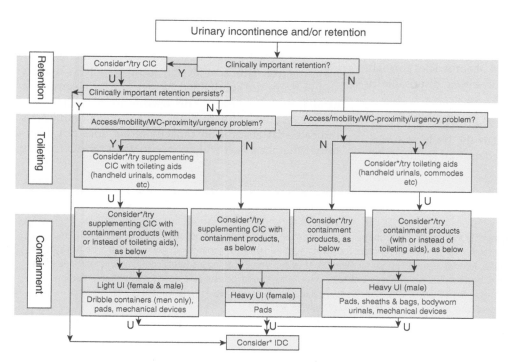

FIGURE 12-1. Algorithm to help identify the products most likely to help a patient with urinary incontinence and/or urinary retention. *Consideration should be based on assessment of the patient's physical characteristics, cognitive ability, and personal preferences, as well as the nature of their incontinence. (CIC, clean intermittent catheterization; IDC, indwelling catheter; N, no; U, unsatisfactory [considered and deemed unsuitable or tried and found not to work satisfactorily]; Y, yes.)

likely to be of benefit to a particular person. There are three main questions to be addressed:

1. Are there problems with toilet access (e.g., toilet proximity or toilet design or issues related to mobility and/or urgency)?
2. Is there urinary retention (with or without incontinence)?
3. If the goal is containment and control, is there urinary incontinence or fecal incontinence or both?

The answers to these questions help to identify the category(ies) of products most likely to help.

Patient Assessment Factors

Careful assessment is critical. Choice depends upon the resources, care available, user and caregiver preference, and client characteristics and needs (Gibb & Wong, 1994; Proudfoot et al., 1994). Assessment factors include the following:

- Physical characteristics such as anthropometrics
- Level of independence
- Mobility and dexterity
- Mental acuity
- The nature of the incontinence

The ability of the user to participate in product selection, apply the product correctly and easily, and understand specific instructions are key considerations in determining the best product (Hocking, 1999; Koch et al., 2001; McMillen & Soderberg, 2002; Phillips & Zhao, 1993). Correct use is critical to success and may be a simple matter of assuring correct fit and prompt changing of absorbent products or may involve more in-depth training (e.g., the ongoing management of a male condom catheter).

Main User Groups

Dividing users into major groups helps identify the category(ies) of products most likely to benefit them. Seven primary groups have been identified:

- People with urinary retention
- People who need help with toileting/toilet access
- Females with light urinary incontinence
- Males with light urinary incontinence
- Females with moderate/heavy urinary incontinence
- Males with moderate/heavy urinary incontinence
- People with fecal incontinence

An individual may belong to more than one group. Each group includes children and young people as well as adults, since the products available for children and adolescents are broadly similar to those for adults.

It is important to remember that the same product will not suit all people, even if assessment parameters are similar. Product preferences differ between people and priorities vary between users; some pad users will opt for a bulky and, therefore, less discreet product to achieve an acceptably low risk of leakage, while others will see the balance differently. It should also be noted that a mix of products from different categories may provide the best solution; for example, needs may vary between day/night and home/away situations. This mix may include absorbent products, urinals, male external catheters (also known as condom catheters or sheaths), and bedpans/commodes.

CLINICAL PEARL

The same product will not suit all people, even if they have the same clinical issue, because preferences and priorities differ from person to person.

Absorbent Products

Absorbent products (commonly known as pads) are marketed in a wide range of sizes and absorbencies for light to very heavy incontinence and in either disposable or reuseable forms.

Overview

Most are body worn (worn next to the body as underwear), but some are used on the bed or chair (underpads); in this section, the term "pad" refers to body-worn absorbent products. Absorbent products can be divided into two broad subgroups: light and moderate/heavy incontinence. Different design groups such as diapers and pull-ups are subdivided by size and/or absorbency, gender, and age group. This classification is shown in Table 12-1. Incidental findings from product evaluations indicate that absorption capacity alone does not determine whether a user will choose to use a product. Some

TABLE 12-1 Products and Devices for Urinary and Fecal Incontinence and Indicators for Patient Selection

People with urinary retention

Catheters for intermittent use	Optimum management method for urinary retention when surgery is not applicable or possible. Many advantages over an indwelling catheter. Insufficient evidence to recommend any particular type of catheter.
Indwelling urethral catheter	Avoid, or remove as soon as possible. High risk of asymptomatic bacteriuria (significant growth of bacteria in the urine without symptoms), which is inevitable after 1 month and increases the risk of symptomatic infection.
Indwelling suprapubic catheter	If a long-term catheter is essential, a suprapubic catheter may have some advantages over urethral catheters (comfort, ease of catheterization, sexual activity).

People who need help with toileting/toilet access

Commodes	Best to wheel patient over normal toilet (without commode pan). Privacy essential. Comfort, safety, trunk support, and pressure areas should be considered; therefore, do not use for long periods.
Male urinals	Offer for speedy toileting.
Female urinals	Offer for speedy toileting, wide range available, different urinals suit different women. Less successful if patient very disabled (i.e., unable to move to edge of chair or bed).

Females with light urinary incontinence

Absorbent products	Most commonly used products for this patient group. Small disposable pads are the most effective (least leaky) type of absorbent product, followed by menstrual pads, washable pants (with integral pad). Washable pads are least effective. Snug fit important to minimize leakage.
Mechanical devices	Seldom used. Intravaginal and intraurethral devices available to occlude urethra. Little evidence for efficacy and concerns about infection and trauma.

Males with light urinary incontinence

Absorbent products	Most commonly used products for this patient group. Male pad (pouch for penis/scrotum) better than standard absorbent pad and both are more effective (less leaky) than washable pants with integral pad. Snug fit important to minimize leakage.
Male devices	Male body-worn urinals and penile clamps are much less commonly used and require expert fitting.

Females with moderate/heavy urinary incontinence

Absorbent products	Preferred option for women. Women prefer "pull-up" designs or shaped pads worn with close-fitting pants. All-in-one (diaper designs) least preferred. Snug fit important to minimize leakage.
Urethral or suprapubic catheter	Avoid if possible. Risk of urinary infection is high and there is potential for trauma. Problems of leakage and blockage are common.

Males with moderate/heavy urinary incontinence

Absorbent products	Males are more likely to find all-in-one (diaper) pads more effective (leak less) than pads worn with pants. Pull-ups are difficult to change with trousers.
Sheath with leg bag	May be better/preferred to absorbent pads. Sizing and skilled fitting are important. Serious skin problems have been reported.
Other male devices	Male body-worn urinals used less commonly and require expert fitting.
Urethral or suprapubic catheter	Avoid if possible. Urinary infection is inevitable and there is potential for trauma. Problems of leakage and blockage are common.

People with fecal incontinence

Absorbent products	Most commonly used, particularly if urinary and fecal incontinence.
Anal plugs	Uncommonly used, reports of discomfort. May be most suitable for people with impaired sensation.
Fecal catheters and collection devices	Used for loose stool, and mainly confined to acute and critical care units.

From Cottenden et al. (2013).

users may have frequent, low flow loss of small volumes of urine ("dribble"), while others may be dry for days but then have a higher-volume, higher flow incontinence episode ("gush" or "flooding"). Both may prefer to use pads for light incontinence.

Mobile and independent community-dwelling women with all levels of incontinence generally prefer small pads and are often willing to change them more frequently rather than use larger products and change them less often (Fader et al., 1987). Conversely, less mobile individuals may prefer the security of larger products despite relatively low volumes of urine loss due to their dependence on others for pad changing. In one study, Cottenden et al. (1998) reported that men use pads less frequently than women, have little knowledge about purpose-built pads, are more likely to construct their own pads out of absorbent materials such as towels, and are less satisfied with pads than women. Another study indicated that men may prefer condom catheters rather than pads (Clarke-O'Neill et al., 2002). Recent advances in products specific for men may change these findings in the future.

> **CLINICAL PEARL**
>
> Absorbent products can be classified as either "body-worn" (pads, insert, briefs, pull-ups, and male pouches) or underpads and as either "light" or "moderate to heavy" in absorptive capacity.

Assessment Guidelines

Aspects of assessment that are particularly important regarding absorbent pads include the following:

- Frequency/severity of leakage
- Day/night incontinence
- Gender (some products are designed for, or are better for, men/women than others)
- Ability to change pad independently/need for carer and pad changing position (standing/lying)
- Laundry/drying facilities

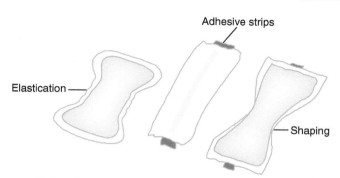

FIGURE 12-3. Disposable inserts for light incontinence.

- Individual priorities (e.g., need for discreetness)
- Personal preference for design/materials (washable/disposable)
- Lifestyle (at home, travel, work, etc.)

A key requirement is the ability of a product to hold urine without leakage. In addition, discreetness, containment of odor, ability to stay in place, comfort when wet, and ability to keep skin dry are all priorities for users of incontinence pads (or any continence product).

Body-Worn Products

Body-worn absorbent products can be divided into four main design groups: inserts, brief, pull-ups, and male pouches.

Inserts

Inserts (sometimes called liners or, in the case of small pads, shields) range between those for light to very heavy urinary incontinence and are held in place by close-fitting underwear or stretch mesh briefs (Fig. 12-2). Many disposable inserts (Figs. 12-3 and 12-4) have an adhesive strip on the back to help secure them to the underwear, and some have an indicator that changes color when the pad is wet to signal the need for a change. Longitudinal, elasticated gathers of hydrophobic mate-

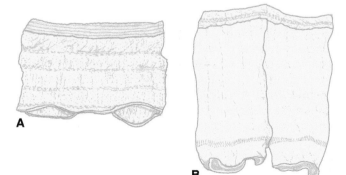

FIGURE 12-2. Mesh pants with **(B)** and without **(A)** legs, for securing incontinence pads in position.

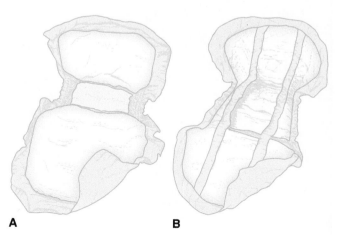

FIGURE 12-4. Disposable inserts with **(A)** and without **(B)** standing gathers, for moderate/heavy incontinence.

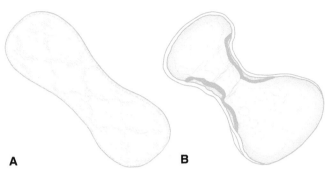

FIGURE 12-5. Reusable inserts for light **(A)** and moderate/heavy **(B)** incontinence.

rial help impede lateral leakage of urine and feces and usually fit snugly against the body. Washable inserts are usually more simply designed than disposable ones, with no elastication; they are typically either shaped or a simple rectangle (Fig. 12-5). For light fecal incontinence, the liner may be a small cotton gauze dressing placed against the anus and held in place by the cheeks of the buttocks (Fig. 12-6).

Briefs

Briefs (sometimes called all-in-ones or diapers) are adult-size versions of infant diapers. Disposable briefs (Fig. 12-7) usually have elasticated waist and legs and self-adhesive tabs (usually resealable); they may also provide a wetness indicator and standing gathers. More recently modified briefs have been introduced that fasten around the waist before the front is pulled into position and secured, which enables users to apply the brief while standing (Fig. 12-8). Washable briefs are usually elasticated at the waist and legs and are secured with Velcro or press studs (Fig. 12-9). Briefs are intended for moderate to very heavy incontinence.

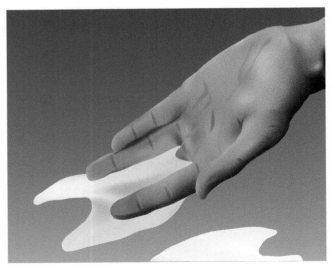

FIGURE 12-6. Liner for light fecal incontinence. It is positioned against the anus and held in place by the cheeks of the buttocks.

Inserts are pads or liners that are worn with snug underwear or mesh briefs; they range in absorptive capacity from light to very heavy. Briefs (also known as diapers) are intended for moderate to very heavy incontinence.

Pull-Ups

Pull-ups are similar in construction to trainer pants for toddlers. The absorbent material is built into a pull-up pant and is either limited to the crotch area or distributed throughout the pant (Figs. 12-10 and 12-11). Disposable pull-ups (Fig. 12-10) are usually elasticated throughout the pants to give a close fit. Both disposable and washable pull-ups have versions designed for different levels of incontinence. Washable pull-ups for light incontinence are often known as pants with integral pads (Fig. 12-11).

Male Pouches

Male pouches (sometimes called shields, guards, or leaves) for men with low-volume incontinence are designed to fit around the penis and sometimes the scrotum and typically have an adhesive back (Figs. 12-12 and 12-13). They are worn with close-fitting underwear or stretch mesh briefs.

Male pouches fit around the penis (and sometimes the scrotum); they are designed to be worn with snugly fitting underwear or stretch mesh briefs and are intended for low-volume leakage.

Underpads

Absorbent underpads are usually simple rectangles of different sizes designed to be used on the bed or chair (Fig. 12-14). Washable underpads (Fig. 12-15) may have a high friction backing or may have "wings" for tucking beneath the mattress of single beds to help keep them in place. Underpads vary widely in absorbency; less absorbent products may be used as "back-up" products (in conjunction with body-worn products), and more absorbent products may be used as sole protection on the bed at night.

Absorbent Product Materials

Concerns related to the environment and the cost of disposable products have led to an increase in the number of available products that are washable/reusable. An important consideration in the comparison of washable and disposable designs is the relative environmental cost, particularly disposal (landfill) costs of disposable designs versus energy costs associated with laundering the washables. A recent report on infant diapers concluded that there was no significant difference in environmental impact between three diaper systems (disposables, home, and commercially

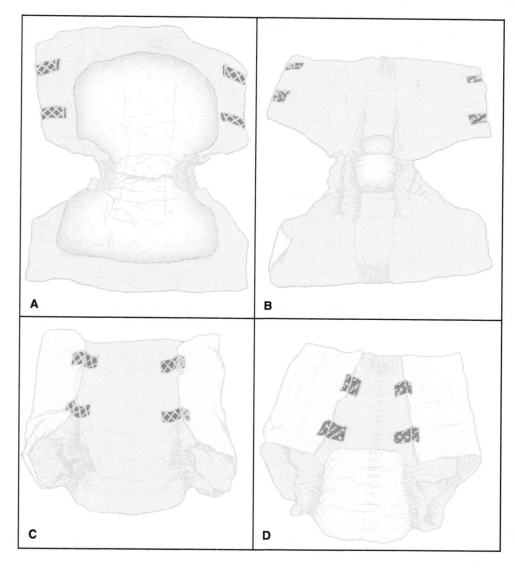

FIGURE 12-7. Disposable diapers with **(B, D)** and without **(A, C)** standing gathers, for moderate/heavy incontinence. Diapers are shown open **(A, B)** and with the tabs secured **(C, D)**.

laundered washables) although the type of impact did vary (Fader et al., 2000).

Absorbent Product Capacity

Pads come in a range of absorbencies to meet the needs of users with different levels of urinary incontinence;

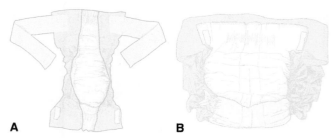

FIGURE 12-8. Modified (T-shaped) diaper. The waist band **(A)** is secured first and then the front pulled up and secured in position **(B)**.

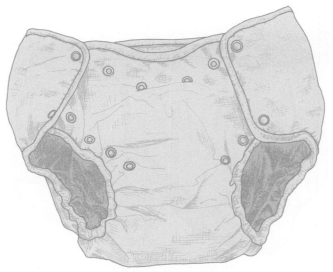

FIGURE 12-9. Reusable diaper.

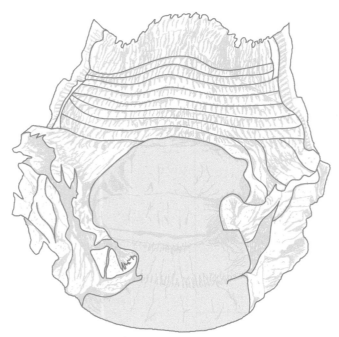

FIGURE 12-10.   Disposable pull-up.

understandably, purchasers wish to know how much urine the various pads will hold. Unfortunately, there is no simple answer; pads do not have a volume of urine below which they are guaranteed not to leak. Rather, the probability of success decreases as the volume of the urine increases and the position of the user changes. For example, a bed-bound individual places continuous pressure on the product, which increases the risk that they will "squeeze" urine out of the pad; in contrast, the same pad worn by a mobile individual will not leak. Body weight also affects pad capacity. However, for higher-absorbency pads, the performance falls away more slowly with increasing urine volume than it does for lower absorbency products.

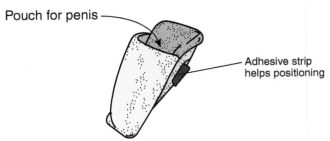

FIGURE 12-12.   Disposable pouch for men.

Absorbent Products for Women with Light Incontinence

The main product designs for women with light incontinence are disposable inserts, washable inserts, and washable pants. Menstrual pads are often used although they are not designed to hold urine. There is robust evidence that disposable inserts are more effective in terms of leakage and more acceptable than menstrual pads, washable pants, and washable inserts. However, menstrual pads are cheaper and washable pants are the least expensive option (on a per-use basis), and these products are acceptable to many, particularly those with lighter incontinence and particularly when used at home. Washable inserts are not acceptable to most women.

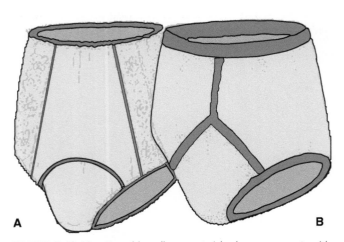

FIGURE 12-11.   Reusable pull-up pants (also known as pants with integral pad) for lightly incontinent women **(A)** and men **(B)**.

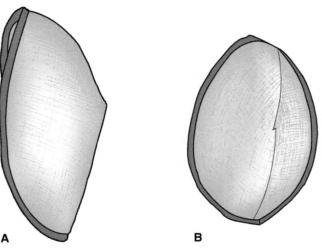

FIGURE 12-13.   Reusable pouches for men: side view **(A)** and front view **(B)**.

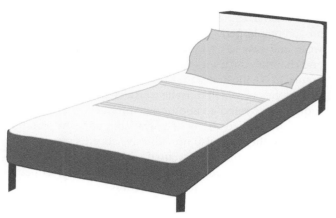

FIGURE 12-14. Disposable underpad.

Absorbent Products for Men with Light Incontinence

Product designs in this category include disposable and washable inserts, disposable and washable pouches, and washable pull-ups. However, disposable and washable insert pads are often unappealing to men as they are frequently marketed specifically for women and bear a strong resemblance to menstrual pads. Anatomical differences are also likely to mean that they are less effective for men. Pouch, shield, and leaf products (Figs. 12-12 and 12-13) are more suitable for men because they contain the penis or penis and scrotum. Disposable leafs (male pouches) are recommended as the most acceptable and effective design for men with light incontinence; simple insert pads are cheaper and may be acceptable to some men; and washable pants with integral pads are likely to be most suitable for men with very light incontinence who have difficulties keeping an insert or pouch in place.

CLINICAL PEARL

Insert pads are unappealing to most men with light incontinence because they are marketed to women and resemble menstrual pads; male pouches are usually a better recommendation.

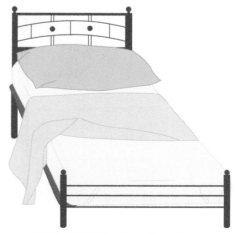

FIGURE 12-15. Reusable underpad.

Products for Moderate to Heavy Incontinence

For men and women with moderate–heavy urinary incontinence, there are at least 12 absorbent products. The most commonly used are disposable body-worn inserts and diapers (Figs. 12-3 to 12-8). Men leak substantially higher volumes of urine than women, and a brief is the most cost-effective design for men. For women, pull-ups are better overall than the other designs, though they are more expensive; the one exception is nighttime management of women living in nursing homes. There is evidence that pads containing superabsorbent polymers (SAP) leak less, are more comfortable, and keep the skin drier than those without.

CLINICAL PEARL

Men leak higher volumes of urine than women—a brief is the most cost-effective design for men. For women, pull-ups are the best design though they are more expensive.

Disposable Underpads

Disposable underpads such as "blue pads" are not designed for long-term management of incontinence, but have a useful role as temporary protection for chairs and beds during clinical procedures. They lack an absorbent filling and can allow pooling of urine on the thin plastic surface, placing the individual at risk for skin wetness and skin breakdown.

Washable Underpads

If washable underpads are the only absorbent product being used (i.e., without a body-worn product), the individual will need to be naked below the waist. Aspects of assessment that are particularly important regarding washable underpads are patient acceptability and preference, particularly with regard to willingness to be naked below the waist (if sole use intended) and availability of laundry and drying facilities. Provided an approved foul wash procedure is used, the risk of cross-infection between different users of bed pads is very low.

CLINICAL PEARL

Products containing SAP leak less, are more comfortable, and keep the skin drier.

Pads for Light Fecal Incontinence

There are very few quality products available for mild or moderate fecal incontinence; this is an area where improved products are desperately needed. For mild fecal incontinence (e.g., stool that remains trapped between the buttocks without soiling underwear), the only real option at this time is to place a soft pad or gauze between the buttocks.

Matching Products to People

As noted, the challenge is to create the best match between the product and the user. To choose the best product(s) for an individual, assessment must include the following:

- Frequency/severity of leakage (light, heavy, moderate)
- Day/night incontinence
- Gender (some products are better for men/women than others)
- Presence of retracted penis in men
- Ability to change pad independently/need for carer
- Pad changing position (standing/lying)
- Laundry/drying facilities
- Individual priorities (e.g., need for discreetness)
- Personal preference for design/materials (washable/disposable)
- Lifestyle (at home, travel, work, etc.) (see Table 12-1)

Male Condom Catheters

Condom catheters (also known as external catheters or sheaths) are typically used in combination with a urine drainage bag and are suitable for men experiencing moderate to heavy urine loss and for men who have limited mobility and are experiencing frequency and urgency; these devices may also be considered for use in combination with intermittent catheterization (IC). They are not recommended for those with cognitive impairment, men who are considered psychologically vulnerable, or men with decreased genital sensation (Golji, 1981; Pemberton et al.; Potter, 2007).

Proper size and fit of the condom catheter is critical to its effectiveness, and the care provider or user needs instruction in correct application of the device, followed by return demonstration of correct technique. Failure to follow the manufacturer's instructions may result in serious penile trauma, impaired penile skin integrity, and leakage. An effective male external catheter is one that stays securely in place for an acceptable period of time; is leak-free, comfortable to wear, and easy to apply and remove; avoids skin damage; and channels the urine effectively into a urine drainage bag. Figure 12-16 illustrates the principal design features of condom catheters, which must be considered when assisting an individual to select an appropriate product.

In addition to the widely available adhesive condom catheters, there are also nonadhesive sheaths secured with a strap, and penile cups secured with snugly fitting underwear. All of these devices require at least 1 inch of persistent penile protrusion for effectiveness.

CLINICAL PEARL

Proper size and fit of a condom catheter is critical to its effectiveness; sizing guides are available from manufacturers free of charge.

Features

Condom catheters vary in terms of material, size, adhesive design, availability of applicator, antitwist and antiblowoff features, connection features, durability, and appropriateness for use with a retracted penis.

Material

Condom catheters may be constructed of latex, silicone rubber, or other synthetic polymers. Some men are allergic to latex, and queries regarding allergies are an important component of assessment. In addition, regular users should be routinely checked as latex allergy status can change over time and with prolonged exposure.

Size

Most companies supply condom catheters in various lengths, with diameters ranging from about 20- to 40-mm, in 5- to 10-mm increments. It is critical for the product to

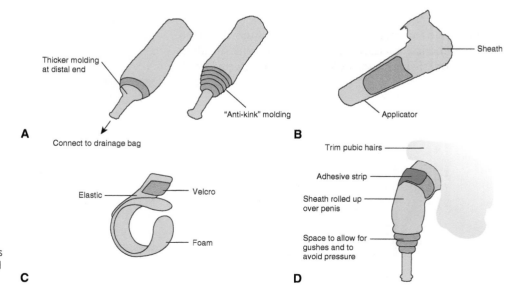

FIGURE 12-16. Various sheaths **(A, D)**, a sheath applicator **(B)**, and an external fixation strip **(C)**.

be accurately sized, and most companies provide simple and disposable sizing guides free of charge.

Adhesive

The adhesive may be integrated into the condom (one-piece systems) or may be provided as a separate strip or spray (two-piece systems). Some men are allergic to selected adhesives. Products with integral adhesive are popular and easier to apply than those with the separate adhesive strip.

Applicator

Some devices come with an applicator intended to help users and carers to put the sheath on.

Antikinking/Twisting Features

Some devices promote improved drainage by reducing kinking and twisting at the distal end, near the connection to the drainage bag tube. There is the risk of leakage (or urinary retention) if the condom twists or the external band is too tight, impairing drainage to the urine bag.

CLINICAL PEARL

Condom catheters come with an integrated adhesive feature (1-piece) or with an adhesive strip (2-piece); the 1-piece systems are easier to apply and generally preferred.

Antiblowoff/Falloff Feature

This feature is intended to reduce the likelihood of the external catheter coming off at high urine flow rates, for example, at the beginning of a void. This feature may involve a thickened and bulbous area at the distal end of the sheath that maintains sheath patency between voids.

Connection Features

Some condom catheters include features designed to increase the ease and security of connection to the drainage tube (e.g., a push ring or ridge at the end of the outlet tubing).

Retracted Penis Features

Some sheaths are designed with specific features intended to accommodate a retracted penis (e.g., a shorter sheath or a wider adhesive seal). In addition, there are selected products now available with hydrocolloid adhesive designed to safely adhere to the glans; these products are indicated for men with persistent or episodic retraction that prevents adherence of a condom catheter.

Durability

Some condom catheters are intended for use over a limited time period (e.g., 24 hours), while other (generally more robust) designs are intended for extended wear.

Transparency

Some condom catheters are transparent allowing for observation of the condition of the skin along the shaft and glans of the penis.

Tips for Effective Application and Management

Many nurses find use of condom catheters to be extremely frustrating due to frequent leaks; they may resort to absorbent products for management of incontinence. The following tips can be used to promote successful use:

- Prior to applying the sheath, ensure that any remaining adhesive or barrier cream is removed from the penis and that the skin is washed with soap and water and thoroughly dried.
- Trim long pubic hairs to prevent them being caught up in the adhesive.
- Protect the skin with liquid barrier film wipes and ensure that the skin has dried properly before applying the condom catheter.
- Leave a gap at the end of the sheath between the glans penis and the drainage tube to avoid trauma to the glans/prepuce. The gap should not be so large that kinking or twisting can occur.
- After the condom catheter has been applied and adhered, snip any reinforced ring or unrolled section at the base of the penis to eliminate the risk of a "tourniquet-like" constriction.
- Removal should not be rushed and is made easier by gently rolling off the device while bathing the penis in warm soapy water.
- Users should be monitored for skin health, tissue damage, and UTI.

Mechanical Devices for Men with Urinary Incontinence

Penile compression devices (penile clamps) are mechanical devices designed to prevent urine leakage by compressing the penis. Various designs are available but occlusion is usually achieved with either a clamp or a peripenile strap (Fig. 12-17). Such devices have the potential advantages of low cost and simplicity compared with a sheath

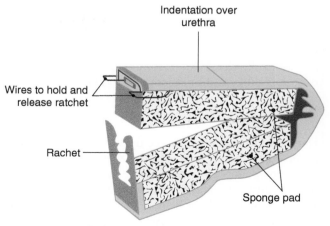

Indentation over urethra

Wires to hold and release ratchet

Rachet

Sponge pad

FIGURE 12-17. Penile clamp.

and drainage bag. However, there is potential for tissue damage and these devices should be used with caution.

These devices must be used with caution to prevent ischemic damage to the penis (due to restricted blood flow). Penile clamps should be fitted by a trained health professional and subject to regular review. Moore et al. (2004) evaluated three different devices (Timms C3 penile compression device; Cunningham clamp; and U-Tex male adjustable tension band) in a crossover study in which twelve men with stress urinary incontinence following radical prostatectomy tried each device in turn. Each of the devices significantly ($p < 0.05$) reduced mean urine loss (measured using 4-hour pad tests), as compared to baseline measurements of urine loss. There was some objective or subjective improvement in continence for each of the 12 men with at least one of the devices, although none completely eliminated urine loss when applied at a comfortable pressure.

Ten of the 12 men rated the Cunningham clamp positively; 2, the C3; and none, the U-Tex. However, the C3 and U-Tex maintained good cavernosal artery blood flow, while the Cunningham clamp caused a significant reduction in arterial flow. Overall, Moore and colleagues concluded that, used correctly, the Cunningham clamp can be an effective method of controlling urinary incontinence in men with stress urinary incontinence who are cognitively intact and aware of bladder filling and have normal genital sensation, intact penile skin, and sufficient manual dexterity to open and close the device. However, it should be noted that these devices do not totally eliminate leakage.

CLINICAL PEARL

Penile compression devices (penile clamps) should be used only for men with stress incontinence who are cognitively intact and aware of bladder filling and have intact sensation and the ability to open and close the device. Incorrect use can result in ischemic damage and penile loss.

Expert opinion and anecdotal reports suggest that penile clamps may be more successful when used for short periods (e.g., while attending meetings or engaging in activities such as swimming or jogging). Such activities may not only exacerbate incontinence but also preclude the use of bulky and/or absorbent products.

Handheld Urinals

Handheld urinals are portable devices designed to allow a person to empty their bladder when access to a toilet is not possible or convenient, due most commonly to mobility, hip abduction, or flexibility limitations. They can be especially helpful for those suffering from frequency and/or urgency. An effective handheld urinal must enable its user to empty the bladder in comfort,

require limited physical effort, and be easy to use with no spillage.

Before recommending a handheld urinal, the nurse should assess the potential user in terms of the following:

- User postures for voiding (in bed, on side of bed, back in chair, on edge of chair, standing/crouching/kneeling)
- Leg abduction
- Approach to urinal (from front, side, behind, above)
- Ability to initiate void
- Dexterity and ability to position and remove urinal
- Level and availability of assistance
- User preference

Female Handheld Urinals

Female handheld urinals come in various shapes and sizes (Fig. 12-18). Most are molded plastic, but they may be made from metal or single-use cardboard. Some are designed for use in particular postures, like standing, sitting, or lying down. Some have handles to facilitate grip and positioning, and some are designed for use with a drainage bag either during use or immediately after use.

Although female handheld urinals are often described and discussed in general nursing articles on continence products, they have only been the subject of one published crossover evaluation. Fader et al. (1999) carried out a multicenter study in which 37 community-based women (age range of 33 to 89 years; mean age of 61 years) were invited to evaluate all 13 products on the UK market in 1997. No product suited everybody, but each was successful for at least some of the subjects. The key requirements for success were that the user should be able to position the urinal easily and feel confident that it would catch urine without spilling. Many products were successful when used in the standing/crouching position or when sitting on the edge of a chair/bed/wheelchair. Fewer worked well for users sitting in a chair/wheelchair. Only one worked even reasonably well when users were lying/semilying (Suba-Seal). In general, subjects with higher levels of dependency found fewer suitable urinals. Future developments may include a powered urinal designed to pump urine into a reservoir (Macaulay et al., 2007).

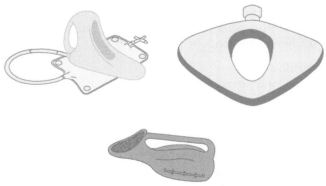

FIGURE 12-18. Various female handheld urinals.

Male Handheld Urinals

Most handheld urinals for men have a narrowed neck opening into which the penis is placed. Some products come with a detachable or integral nonspill adaptor containing a flutter valve to impede backflow of urine from the urinal. There are no published trials of such products.

Recommendations for selecting suitable urinals for men include flat bottom, which may be more stable (and less likely to spill) for those using a urinal in bed; soft plastic jug style or with a funnel for easier grip; lighter weight devices, especially for those with poor manual dexterity; and drainage bag attachment to simplify emptying the urinal for men living at home with limited support. Vickerman (2006) also suggests that homemade devices, such as empty wide-mouthed containers with a handle and lid (e.g., those used for clothes-washing liquid or conditioner) might be a practical (and inexpensive) option; however, care would be required to avoid sharp edges if modifying a plastic container. For those with a retracted penis, female urinals may be easier to use than male products.

Effective Use of Urinals

Successful use of urinals depends on many factors (Macaulay et al., 2006; McIntosh, 2001; Vickerman, 2003, 2006):

- Experimentation is often needed to find the optimum urinal. A "library" of urinals (i.e., a collection of different types of urinals to be lent out to users for experimentation) has therefore been recommended, but rigorous cleaning methods are needed.
- Clothing alterations can aid quick and easy use of a urinal. For men, extending the fly opening of trousers or replacing zippers with *Velcro* can be helpful, as can boxer shorts. For women, drop-front pants may be needed, particularly if mobility is limited.
- Disposable and reusable "travel" handheld urinals are available for both men and women. These urinals fold away to fit into a pocket and may therefore be more discreetly portable than conventional urinals. They are available at many camping suppliers.
- Some disposable urinals include superabsorbent polymer in their reservoirs, which turn urine into a gel and help to prevent spillage. Sachets of superabsorbent polymer may also be added to reusable urinals.
- Use of a urinal is not always free from leakage, and provision of absorbent chair or bed pads to protect bedding, clothes, and furniture (particularly when testing out urinals) may be necessary.
- The limited range of urinal options in acute settings, where often only bedpans are available, has been criticized, and the process of introducing handheld urinals to hospital services is recommended.
- When used by one individual in the home, urinals can be cleaned with soap and water between uses. If a library of urinals is used, then robust methods are

necessary and must be compliant with local infection control procedures.

Commodes and Bedpans

Toilet adaptations such as raised toilet seats, padded seats, and grab rails can be very helpful in enabling individuals with mobility issues to access the toilet easily and comfortably. Bottom wipers and bidets can also be useful. However, if access to the toilet is impossible, commodes and other toileting receptacles should be considered. Nurses should be aware that there are major defects in most of the current commode designs: poor aesthetics; poor trunk support; instability (i.e., a tendency to tip over easily); poor comfort; difficult cleansing; and poor pressure relief.

Defecation on a bedpan or other portable receptacle presents problems with safety and unacceptability to users and should be avoided if possible. A sani-chair/shower chair is usually preferable to a commode if direct transfer to a toilet is impossible or unsafe. The main user concerns about commodes and bedpans are lack of privacy; embarrassment related to noise and odor associated with stool and gas elimination, poor aesthetics, poor perineal cleansing accessibility, and inadequate facilities for cleaning the devices in the home.

If a commode is used, the nurse should assure that good trunk support is provided, the chair is stable, and methods are offered to manage concerns regarding noise and odor. Moreover, with commodes and sani-chairs/shower chairs, the user's buttocks should never be visible to others, and transportation to the toilet and use of the toilet or commode should be carried out with due regard to privacy and dignity. Patients at risk for pressure ulcers should not sit on a commode/sani-chair/shower chair for prolonged periods. The person should be provided privacy whenever possible and given a direct method of calling for assistance when left on the toilet/commode/sani-chair/shower chair. Cleaning of bedpans and commodes should be carried out after each use following local infection control policies (in institutional settings).

Urine Drainage Bags and Accessories

Urinary drainage bags are attached to an indwelling catheter or condom catheter to collect and store urine. Features of effective drainage bag systems include ease of operation of all components (connectors, taps, and support devices), comfort, and discreetness.

Aspects of assessment that are particularly important regarding urine drainage bags are patient/carer dexterity (Pomfret, 1996, 2006) and eyesight. Both are necessary to manage the drainage bag system, including the outlet tap used to empty the drainage bag. It is also important to assess the patient's preferred and usual mode of dress (Pomfret, 1996, 2006); for example, a male who prefers shorts will want a drainage system that is not visible and allows easy access for emptying,

Urine drainage bags fall into two major categories: leg/body-worn bags for daytime use; and large capacity body-free bags for nighttime use (night drainage bags), which are suspended from a stand or bed hook.

Leg/Body-Worn Bags

Leg/body-worn bags come with various features, of which the following are the most important.

Volume

Most bags have a volume in the range of 350 to 750 mL, but some are larger.

Material

Most bags are made from transparent PVC (polyvinyl chloride), but PVDF (polyvinylidene fluoride) bags are also available and are associated with less noise from rustling; polyethylene or rubber/latex may be used as well.

Sterility

Bags may or may not be supplied sterile.

Wear Position

Bags may be designed to be worn over the knee, across or down the thigh, down the calf, or against the abdomen.

CLINICAL PEARL

Urinary drainage bags are available in body-worn (leg bag) and bedside drainage versions; body-worn bags may be designed to be worn over the knee, down the thigh or calf, or against the abdomen.

Attachment/Suspension System

Most leg bags are attached to the leg with straps, which are usually made from latex or an elasticized fabric. Various hooks, loops, buttons/button holes, and Velcro may be used to secure straps and to attach bags to straps. Some bags are designed to be suspended around the waist. Some straps and suspension devices can be bought separately from bags, but they are generally not suitable for use with all bags (Fig. 12-19).

Connecting Tube

Leg bags come with various connecting tube lengths, which may impact on selection; for example, the length required for a bag to be worn on the calf will be greater than that for a bag to be worn on the thigh. Some tubes can be cut to the preferred length.

Drainage Tap

Drainage tap designs vary widely and can be easy or difficult to manage depending on cognition and manual dexterity (Fig. 12-20).

Sampling Port

Bags may or may not have a sampling port (for obtaining urine specimens).

Comfort Backing

Some leg bags have a fabric backing against the skin to reduce sweating and increase comfort.

Discretion

Some leg bags come with features intended to increase discretion—most commonly, internal welds/folds between the front and back faces to reduce bulging and/or noise caused by a large volume of liquid moving about as the user mobilizes.

Antikinking/Twisting Feature

Some bags come with features intended to improve drainage by reducing kinking and twisting in the connecting tube.

Infection Reduction Features

The risk of infection may be reduced with a nonreturn valve that reduces reflux of urine up the tubing when the bag is moved, a sampling port, and/or a tap with an outlet sleeve to allow attachment of the overnight bag to the body-worn bag. However, although convenient, there is no evidence that these features reduce UTI incidence. Presealed drainage systems to prevent breaking the closed system are also available, and these could be beneficial in reducing time to bacteriuria (Hooton et al., 2010).

Night Drainage Bags

These bags are also known as "bedside bags" and are usually attached to a suspension system on the bed frame (Fig. 12-21). They may be connected directly to the catheter, or they may be connected to the drainage tap of the

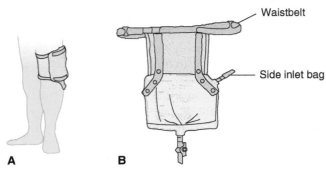

FIGURE 12-19. Body-worn urine drainage bags held in place using leg straps **(A)** and a waist band suspension system **(B)**.

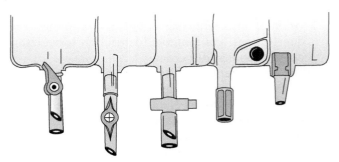

FIGURE 12-20. Various urine drainage bag tap designs.

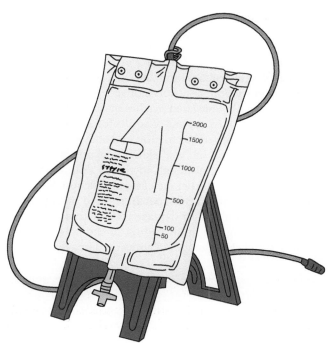

FIGURE 12-21. Night urine drainage bag on a stand.

leg/body-worn bag. They usually have a capacity of 2,000 to 4,000 mL and have various design features, many of which are similar to those for leg/body-worn bags. Night drainage bags are available without a tap (for single use) and with various drainage tap designs for emptying and reuse.

Current standard drainage tubing/bag designs may evacuate the bladder suboptimally, leading to residual urine. Outflow obstruction can be caused by the development of airlocks in the dependent curls or loops of tubing; thus, it is important to avoid dependent loops and to keep the tubing straight and patent in order to assure continuous drainage. Dependent loops permit pooling of urine and require increased bladder pressure to move urine into the drainage bag. In addition, there is no antireflux valve between the tubing and the bladder; if the drainage bag is lifted above the bladder, urine in the tubing will drain freely back into the bladder. New drainage tubing designs may incorporate a coiled downward-spiral-shaped configuration to eliminate airlock obstruction.

> **CLINICAL PEARL**
>
> Dependent loops of drainage tubing create outflow obstruction, and all caregivers must be taught to manage the tubing to prevent dependent loops.

There is little research to support the common practice of changing drainage bags every five to seven days (or any other particular change regime) and little to no guidance on solutions to clean the overnight bag except with soap and water (Royal College of Nursing). These practices appear to be based upon expert opinion, anecdotal evidence, and manufacturers' recommendations.

> **CLINICAL PEARL**
>
> The drainage bag should never be lifted above the level of the bladder as this permits urine to drain back into the bladder, increasing the risk of UTI.

Incontinence-Associated Dermatitis (IAD)

The skin of an incontinent individual will be regularly exposed to contact with urine and/or feces, which places the individual at high risk for skin damage. Most current knowledge about the effects of urine and feces on skin has been obtained from studies with pads or pad materials on animals, on healthy infants, or on body areas such as the forearm or back of adults. Where clinical trials have been conducted, they have usually been on infants and rarely on adults using pads. Skin irritation within the pad occlusion area is usually termed diaper dermatitis in infants. In adults, the term perineal dermatitis (PD) has been used in the past, but the more accurate and currently accepted term is *incontinence-associated dermatitis (IAD)*; this is a better term because the affected skin areas are not confined to the perineum (Gray et al., 2007) but frequently extend to involve the buttocks, hips, and sacrum. These areas are very high risk for damage because they are exposed to pressure, shear, and friction as well as stool and urine.

> **CLINICAL PEARL**
>
> The most accurate term for skin damage caused by prolonged or recurrent contact with stool and/or urine is *incontinence-associated dermatitis*.

Pathology of IAD

The mechanisms of skin damage in IAD include overhydration (maceration) of the skin, inflammation caused by irritants and enzymes, fungal or bacterial infections, and friction damage. Overhydration renders the skin vulnerable to penetration by pathogens and irritants and also increases the risk of friction damage and pressure ulcer development. Prolonged exposure to water alone has been shown to cause hydration dermatitis (Kligman, 1994; Tsai & Maibach, 1999), and prolonged occlusion of the skin (as within a continence product) reduces skin barrier function (Fluhr et al., 1999) and significantly increases microbial counts and pH (Aly et al., 1978; Faergemann et al., 1983). Repeated wetting and drying makes the skin more vulnerable to substances that are usually innocuous, for example, bile salts (Berg et al., 1986; Suskind & Ishihara, 1965). A product that keeps skin wet and occluded (even without the additional constituents of urine and feces) is therefore likely to cause skin irritation and increase skin permeability to other irritants.

> **CLINICAL PEARL**
>
> The mechanisms of damage in IAD include overhydration, friction, inflammation related to irritant penetration and enzymatic damage, and fungal or bacterial infection.

The role of feces in the etiology of IAD was evaluated in a laboratory setting using a hairless mouse model (Buckingham & Berg, 1986). Proteases and lipases were identified as the major irritants; fecal enzymes not only irritated the skin directly but also increased the susceptibility of the skin to other irritants such as bile salts. Skin damage appeared dependent on the concentration and length of exposure to the enzymes in feces (Andersen et al., 1994). From a clinical perspective, liquid stool has much higher levels of enzymes than solid stool and places the individual at higher risk for IAD than exposure to solid stool. Similarly, in considering the role of urine in the etiology of IAD, the irritant potential of urine by itself was minimal over short periods (48 hours); however, prolonged exposure (10 days) resulted in skin damage.

Buckingham and Berg also measured skin permeability and found that continuous exposure to urine increased skin permeability more than 15-fold as compared to occluded skin or skin exposed only to water. Not surprisingly, the combination of urine and feces caused significantly higher levels of irritation than urine or feces alone. The authors concluded that the presence of fecal urease results in the breakdown of urinary urea, causing an increase in pH; the elevated pH increases the activity of fecal proteases and lipases, which results in skin breakdown.

> **CLINICAL PEARL**
>
> Individuals with double (urinary and fecal) incontinence are at higher risk for IAD than those with fecal incontinence or urinary incontinence alone.

Microorganisms, which comprise approximately 50% of the solid component of feces, have also been hypothesized to play a role in the development of IAD; however, this issue remains unresolved. In one study, microorganisms on the skin of infants with and without diaper dermatitis were similar (Leyden, 1986). In contrast, Zimmerer et al. (1986) sampled the microflora of the skin in areas exposed to prewetted patches containing urine and found that the microbial counts were significantly higher for the wet patches relative to the dry patch controls. In an early study, it was shown that it is almost impossible to establish infection with the opportunistic organism *Candida albicans* on normal skin without complete occlusion of the site (Maibach & Kligman, 1962). Thus, it appears that bacterial or fungal infection is secondary to alterations in the skin barrier that occur with overhydration and that allow penetration of the microorganisms (Faria et al., 1996).

Another mechanism of injury associated with overhydrated skin is *friction damage* or an *abrasive type of injury* that occurs when vulnerable skin is rubbed against linens or another skin surface. Zimmerer et al. (1986) examined the role of skin wetness and the effects of wet and dry materials on friction, abrasion damage, permeability, and microbial growth. Prewetted patches of infant diapers were placed on the volar forearms of adults for 2 hours, and the skin was then subjected to friction and abrasion. The coefficient of friction for the "wet" skin was significantly higher than for "dry" skin, although increased fluid loading of wet patches did not further increase skin friction. Similarly, skin hydrated with a wet patch showed a significant increase in skin abrasion damage relative to a dry patch. Again, increasing the fluid loading of the patch did not produce significant changes in abrasion damage.

> **CLINICAL PEARL**
>
> Wet skin is much more vulnerable to friction damage and to invasion by fungal organisms such as *Candida albicans*.

It should be noted that the study conducted by Zimmerer and colleagues, as well as those conducted by other investigators into skin health, utilized the volar forearm, and this site may not be a valid model for the skin exposed to an incontinence pad, that is, buttocks and groins. Using transepidermal water loss (TEWL) to measure both skin barrier function and excess water in the skin from the volar forearm does not correlate with measures from the face (Schnetz et al., 1999), and it is likely that the volar forearm is not a valid test location for the buttocks and groin. Specifically, skin in the perianal area has been shown to be more sensitive to fecal irritation than that on the inner arm (Caplan, 1966).

The role of urinary and fecal incontinence in the development of pressure ulcers is unclear. It is generally agreed that both urinary and fecal incontinence are risk factors (Bergquist & Frantz, 1999; Brandeis et al., 1994; Maklebust & Magnan, 1994; Watret, 1999). Some studies have found that only fecal incontinence is a risk factor and that urinary incontinence alone is *not* a risk factor (Spector & Fortinsky, 1998; Theaker et al., 2000). Pressure ulcer risk assessment scales all have a subscale of incontinence or exposure to moisture, and the main mechanism whereby incontinence contributes to pressure ulcer development has been thought to be the increased friction coefficient, which increases the risk for shear damage if the patient slides down in bed or is dragged up in bed.

While IAD can potentially *contribute* to pressure ulcer development, the clinician must be aware that IAD lesions are moisture lesions rather than pressure ulcers, and they should not be classified or staged as pressure ulcers. Accurate classification of moisture lesions versus pressure ulcers remains a significant challenge for clinicians. In a study regarding the reliability of the European Pressure Ulcer Advisory Panel (EPUAP) staging system, the photographs used for the study included both "moisture lesions" (defined as lesions resulting from prolonged skin exposure to excessive fluid because of urinary or fecal incontinence, profuse sweating, or wound exudate) and pressure ulcers. A high degree of reliability for classification of moisture lesions was found among 44 pressure ulcer experts (Kappa = 0.80) (Defloor & Schoonhoven, 2004). However, interrater reliability was found to be much worse (Kappa = 0.37) when photographs were viewed by 473 nonexpert nurses (Defloor et al., 2006); similar results were obtained in a European study of 1,452 nonexpert nurses from five European countries (Kappa = 0.36). The authors concluded that better descriptors needed to be incorporated into the EPUAP system and more education was also needed.

> **CLINICAL PEARL**
>
> Accurate classification of pressure ulcers versus moisture lesions remains a clinical challenge.

Assessment of IAD

There is no widely available valid or reliable tool for the assessment of PD/IAD although four have been published (Borchert et al., 2010; Maklebust & Magnan, 1994; Nix 2002; Warshaw et al., 2002). One, the Perineal Assessment Tool, despite its name, is intended primarily for assessing the risk of IAD (vs. assessing skin health), and it has been described and used by its developer as such (Bliss et al., 2006a). Most researchers have reported ratings of color changes (degree of erythema) based on visual inspection, which may be confounded by the presence of reactive hyperemia in areas also exposed to pressure. A revised version of the incontinence-associated dermatitis and its severity instrument-D (IADS-D) for dark-toned skin was recently tested in 266 persons with excellent reliability and validity (Bliss et al., 2014).

Prevention and Management of IAD

Measures to maintain or restore skin health are a critical element of care for individuals with incontinence who require use of absorbent products. These measures include product selection, frequent hygienic care, and protective skin products.

Superabsorbent Polymers

In the 1980s, product manufacturers introduced diapers with SAP, which were designed to reduce skin wetness, buffer pH, and reduce skin contact with urine and stool. The effectiveness of SAP in reducing skin wetness (measured by TEWL), reducing pH, and reducing severity of diaper dermatitis was demonstrated in infants. Only one study, now 20 years old (Brown, 1993, 1994; Brown et al., 1995), has been conducted on adults with urinary incontinence. The authors reported better skin scores in those who were assigned to SAP products indicating skin health benefits of SAP. Further research with well-controlled studies is required to better understand the full benefit of SAP.

Frequent Checks and Prompt Change for Wet or Soiled Products

Prompt replacement of a wet or soiled product with a dry pad or diaper also reduces skin wetness and may therefore benefit skin health (Berg, 1987). In the inpatient setting, current recommendations also include leaving absorbent products open underneath the patient whenever he/she is in bed; this keeps the perineal skin cooler and drier and thus more resistant to both IAD and friction damage (Gray et al., 2012).

Preventive Skin Care

Effective management of the patient with urinary and/or fecal incontinence requires appropriate cleansing following each incontinent episode and routine use of moisturizers and moisture barriers to maintain skin health. Cleansing of soiled skin should occur as soon as possible and routine cleansing of the perineum is recommended (AHRQ, 1992; Gray et al., 2002, 2007; Lekan-Rutledge et al., 2003; Nix & Ermer-Seltun, 2004). Caregivers should be taught to cleanse the perineum from front to back, especially in women, in order to reduce the risk of fecal contamination of the urethral meatus; this may help to reduce the risk for UTI (Hurlow, 2006; Jackson, 2007; Leiner, 1995; Naish & Hallam, 2007; Stapleton & Stamm, 1997).

> **CLINICAL PEARL**
>
> Preventive skin care includes gentle cleansing with a no-rinse pH balanced cleanser, application of an emollient moisturizer to replace lost skin lipids, and use of a moisture barrier to prevent overhydration of the skin.

Appropriate cleansing includes attention to both the cleanser and the technique. While soap and water is still commonly used (Skewes, 1997), it is known that repeated exposure to anionic surfactants (common in soaps) results in skin irritation (Klein et al., 1992; Van der Valk & Maibach, 1990); in addition, most soaps are alkaline and adversely affect the pH of the skin. Thus, use of a no-rinse pH-balanced cleanser is recommended and is widely available in multiple forms (impregnated wipes, liquids, and foams). Caregivers must also be taught to use soft nonabrasive cloths and gentle technique in order to prevent mechanical damage to the stratum corneum (Bliss et al., 2006b; Cooper & Gray, 2001; Gray et al., 2007; Lekan-Rutledge et al., 2003).

Effective drying is also important, since damp skin is much more vulnerable to friction damage; however, the best approach to drying the skin remains controversial. There is some evidence that drying the skin by patting may be less effective than gentle towel drying or drying with a hair dryer (Voegeli, 2008), and anecdotal evidence supports use of a hair dryer on a cool setting for damaged skin. In addition to cleansing, moisturizers and moisture barriers should be routinely used to maintain the normal barrier function of the skin. The goal is to avoid both overhydration and dehydration (Tsai & Maibach, 1999).

Products labeled as "moisturizers" include emollients and humectants and are designed to prevent dehydration. Emollients are lipids that soften the skin, fill the gaps between the skin cells, and reduce TEWL; these products enhance the barrier function of the stratum corneum and are appropriately used for any incontinent patient. Emollient agents are typically ingredients in disposable cleansing wipes and are also available as stand-alone creams and as one component of combination moisturizer/moisture barrier products. In contrast, humectants are hygroscopic agents such as urea-based products that actually pull water into the skin; they are intended for use on very dry skin and would be *inappropriate* for use on overhydrated perineal skin.

> **CLINICAL PEARL**
>
> Humectant moisturizers are designed to pull water *into* the skin and are not appropriate for overhydrated fragile perineal skin.

Moisture barrier products are designed specifically to prevent penetration of urine and stool into the stratum corneum, thus reducing the risk of overhydration and IAD; the routine application of a moisture barrier is recommended on areas in contact with leaked urine and/or feces. For bed-bound and chair-bound patients, areas at risk typically include the buttocks, perianal area, groin, and inner thighs. For community-based patients who leak small amounts of stool and for hospitalized patients managed with internal bowel management systems, the "at-risk" area is the perianal skin.

Barrier products include liquid skin sealants containing polymers, dimethicone-based products, petrolatum-based products, zinc oxide-based products, and combination products. Some barrier products (e.g., dimethicone) allow TEWL while preventing penetration by external sources of moisture, while other barriers are occlusive and prevent TEWL (e.g., petrolatum). Currently, we lack data as to whether one type of barrier product is superior to another; studies done to date indicate that any standardized protocol that addresses the key elements of cleansing, moisturizing, and using barrier products is effective in significantly reducing the incidence of IAD (Gray et al., 2012). More research is needed to identify optimal strategies and products; in addition, there is a need for standardization of terms and definitions related to products used for perineal skin care.

> **CLINICAL PEARL**
>
> There is no data to indicate that one barrier product is superior to another; we *do* have data indicating that any standardized protocol that addresses the key elements of cleansing, moisturizing, and using barrier products significantly reduces the incidence of IAD.

Management of IAD

For patients with IAD resulting in skin loss, anecdotal evidence supports use of zinc oxide–based products or BCT ointments (products containing balsam of peru, castor oil, and trypsin); if zinc oxide products are used, it is critical to teach caregivers to use perineal cleansers and gentle technique for removal. For patients with candidiasis, antifungal products are recommended (such as a moisture barrier containing an azole agent or an antifungal powder followed by application of a moisture barrier ointment) (Gray et al., 2012).

 ## Conclusion

Evidence-based product choices remain problematic because of the lack of randomized controlled trials in the area. The challenge for researchers is that products are continually improved or modified so trial results can become outdated quickly. More important perhaps is the users evaluation of product designs—for example, in men, comparisons of penile clamps, condom catheters, and/or incontinence pads and exploring the subjective aspects of product use. A collaborative approach to choose the best product for the individual is required because choices differ between users, degree of incontinence, and length of use.

Teaching the individual or the caregiver about skin care is critical as IAD is a common problem among absorbent product users and skin wetness overhydrates skin, potentiates the effects of other irritants, and increases the risk of friction, abrasive damage, and pressure ulcer development. Those individuals with both urinary and fecal incontinence (especially liquid stool) are in a very high-risk group for skin issues since fecal matter is more irritating than urine and preventative measures must be taken to protect the vulnerable skin. Although most hospitals have a skin care protocol with appropriate products, individuals cared for at home may be using less optimal regimens, which may negatively affect skin health and pH. Caregivers and individuals with incontinence may require guidance on a regular and structured skin care regimen using appropriate cleansers, moisturizers, or barrier creams with a particular focus on skin folds and those areas of the perineum in direct contact with urine and stool. Product choices, patient teaching, and ongoing follow-up are critical to effective continence control and skin health in the care of an individual with urinary and fecal incontinence.

REFERENCES

Agency for Healthcare Research and Quality (AHRQ). (1992). Pressure ulcers in adults: Prediction and prevention (AHCPR publication no. 92-0047). Retrieved from http://www ncbi nlm nih gov/books/bv fcgi?rid=hstat2 section 4521

Aly, R., Shirley, C., Cunico, B., et al. (1978). Effect of prolonged occlusion on the microbial flora, pH, carbon dioxide and transepidermal water loss on human skin. *Journal of Investigative Dermatology, 71*(6), 378–381.

Andersen, P. H., Bucher, A. P., Saeed, I., et al. (1994). Faecal enzymes: In vivo human skin irritation. *Contact Dermatitis, 30*(3), 152–158.

Berg, R. W. (1987). Etiologic factors in diaper dermatitis: A model for development of improved diapers. *Pediatrician, 14*(1), 27–33.

Berg, R. W., Buckingham, K. W., & Stewart, R. L. (1986). Etiologic factors in diaper dermatitis: The role of urine. *Pediatric Dermatology, 3*(2), 102–106.

Bergquist, S., & Frantz, R. (1999). Pressure ulcers in community based older adults receiving home health care. Prevalence, incidence, and associated risk factors. *Advances in Wound Care, 12*(7), 339–351.

Bliss, D. Z., Hurlow, J., Cefalu, J., et al. (2014). Refinement of an instrument for assessing incontinent-associated dermatitis and its severity for use with darker-toned skin. *Journal of Wound Ostomy & Continence Nursing, 41*, 365–370.

Bliss, D. Z., Savik, K., Harms, S., et al. (2006a). Prevalence and correlates of perineal dermatitis in nursing home residents. *Nursing Research, 55*(4), 243–251.

Bliss, D. Z., Zehrer, C., Savik, K., et al. (2006b). Incontinence-associated skin damage in nursing home residents: A secondary analysis of a prospective, multicenter study. *Ostomy Wound Management, 52*(12), 46–55.

Borchert, K., Bliss, D. Z., Savik, K., et al. (2010). The incontinence-associated dermatitis and its severity instrument: Development and validation. *Journal of Wound Ostomy & Continence Nursing, 37*(5), 527–535. doi: 10.1097/WON.0b013e3181edac3e.

Brandeis, G., Ooi, W., Hossain, M., et al. (1994). A longitudinal study of risk factors associated with the formation of pressure ulcers in nursing homes. *Journal of the American Geriatrics Society, 42*(4), 388–393.

Brown, D. S. (1993). Perineal dermatitis: Can we measure it? *Ostomy Wound Management, 39*(7), 28–32.

Brown, D. S. (1994). Diapers and underpads, Part 1: Skin integrity outcomes. *Ostomy Wound Management, 40*(9), 20–22, 24–26, 28 passim.

Brown, D. S., Small, S., & Jones, D. (1995). Standardizing skin care across settings. *Ostomy Wound Management, 41*(10), 40–43.

Buckingham, K. W., & Berg, R. W. (1986). Etiologic factors in diaper dermatitis: The role of feces. *Pediatric Dermatology, 3*(2), 107–112.

Caplan, R. M. (1966). The irritant role of feces in the genesis of perianal itch. *Gastroenterology, 50*(1), 19–23.

Clarke-O'Neill, S., Fader, M. J., Pettersson, L., et al. (2002). *Disposable pads for light incontinence (Report no.: IN9)*. London, UK: Medical Devices Agency.

Cooper, P., & Gray, D. (2001). Comparison of two skin care regimes for incontinence. *British Journal of Nursing, 10*(6 Suppl), S6, S8, S10.

Cottenden, A. M., Fader, M. J., Pettersson, L., et al. (1998). *Disposable, shaped bodyworn pads with pants for heavy incontinence (Report no.: IN1.)*. London, UK: Medical Devices Agency.

Cottenden, A., Bliss, D., Buckley, B., et al. (2013). Management using continence products. In P. Abrams, L. Cardozo, S. Khoury, et al. (Eds.), *Incontinence: 5th International Consultation on Incontinence* (pp. 1651–1786). Arnheim, The Netherlands: ICUD-EAU Publishers.

Defloor, T., & Schoonhoven, L. (2004). Inter-rater reliability of the EPUAP pressure ulcer classification system using photographs. *Journal of Clinical Nursing, 13*(8), 952–959.

Defloor, T., Schoonhoven, L., Katrien, V., et al. (2006). Reliability of the European Pressure Ulcer Advisory Panel classification system. *Journal of Advanced Nursing, 54*(2), 189–198.

Fader, M., Barnes, E., Malone-Lee, J., et al. (1987). Continence. Choosing the right garment. *Nursing Times, 83*(15), 78–85.

Fader, M., Cottenden, A. M., & Getliffe, K. (2000). Absorbent products for light urinary incontinence in women. *Cochrane Database of Systematic Reviews, (2)*, CD001406, PMID: 10796783.

Fader, M., Pettersson, L., Dean, G., et al. (1999). The selection of female urinals: Results of a multicentre evaluation. *British Journal of Nursing, 8*(14), 918–5.

Faergemann, J., Aly, R., Wilson, D. R., et al. (1983). Skin occlusion: Effect on Pityrosporum orbiculare, skin PCO2, pH, transepidermal water loss, and water content. *Archives of Dermatological Research, 275*(6), 383–387.

Faria, D. T., Shwayder, T., & Krull, E. A. (1996). Perineal skin injury: Extrinsic environmental risk factors. *Ostomy Wound Manage, 42*(1), 28–4, 36.

Fluhr, J. W., Gloor, M., Lehmann, L., et al. (1999). Glycerol accelerates recovery of barrier function in vivo. *Acta Dermato-Venereologica, 79*(6), 418–421.

Fonda, D., & Abrams, P. (2006). Cure sometimes, help always—a "continence paradigm" for all ages and conditions. *Neurourology and Urodynamics, 25*(3), 290–292.

Gibb, H., & Wong, G. (1994). How to choose: Nurses' judgements of the effectiveness of a range of currently marketed continence aids. *Journal of Clinical Nursing, 3*(2), 77–86.

Golji, H. (1981). Complications of external condom drainage. *Paraplegia, 19*(3), 189–197.

Gray, M., Beeckman, D., Bliss, D. Z., et al. (2012). Incontinence-associated dermatitis: A comprehensive review and update. *Journal of Wound Ostomy & Continence Nursing, 39*(1), 61–74.

Gray, M., Bliss, D. Z., Doughty, D. B., et al. (2007). Incontinence-associated dermatitis: A consensus. *Journal of Wound, Ostomy, and Continence Nursing, 34*(1), 45–54.

Gray, M., Ratliff, C., & Donovan, A. (2002). Perineal skin care for the incontinent patient. *Advances in Skin & Wound Care, 15*(4), 170–175.

Hocking, C. (1999). Function or feelings: Factors in abandonment of assistive devices. *Technology and Disability, (11)*, 3–11.

Hooton, T. M., Bradley, S. F., Cardenas, D. D., et al.; Infection Diseases Society of America. (2010). Diagnosis, prevention, and treatment of catheter associated urinary tract infection in adults: 2009 International Clinical Practice Guidelines from the Infectious Diseases Society of America. *Clinical Infectious Diseases, 50*(5), 625–663.

Hurlow, J. (2006). Tag: F315: An opportunity for WOC nurses. *Journal of Wound, Ostomy, and Continence Nursing, 33*(3), 296–304.

Jackson, M. A. (2007). Evidence-based practice for evaluation and management of female urinary tract infection. *Urologic Nursing, 27*(2), 133–136.

Klein, G., Grubauer, G., & Fritsch, P. (1992). The influence of daily dishwashing with synthetic detergent on human skin. *British Journal of Dermatology, 127*(2), 131–137.

Kligman, A. M. (1994). Hydration injury to human skin. In: P. Elsner, E. Berardesca, & H. Maibach, (Eds.), *Bioengineering of the skin: Water and the stratum corneum*. Boca Raton, FL: CRC Press.

Koch, T., Kralik, D., Eastwood, S., et al. (2001). Breaking the silence: Women living with multiple sclerosis and urinary incontinence. *International Journal of Nursing Practice, 7*(1), 16–23.

Leiner, S. (1995). Recurrent urinary tract infections in otherwise healthy adult women. *Nurse Practitioner, 20*(2), 48–56.

Lekan-Rutledge, D., Doughty, D., Moore, K. N., et al. (2003). Promoting social continence: Products and devices in the management of urinary incontinence. *Urologic Nursing, 23*(6), 416–428, 458.

Leyden, J. J. (1986). Diaper dermatitis. *Dermatologic Clinics, 4*(1), 23–28.

Low, J. (1996). Negotiating identities, negotiating environments: An interpretation of the experiences of students with disabilities. *Disability and society, 11*(2), 235–248.

Macaulay, M., Clarke-O'Neill, S., Cottenden, A., et al. (2006). Female urinals for women with impaired mobility. *Nursing Times, 102*(42), 42–43, 45, 47.

Macaulay, M., van den, H. E., Jowitt, F., et al. (2007). A noninvasive continence management system: Development and evaluation of a novel toileting device for women. *Journal of Wound, Ostomy, & Continence Nursing, 34*(6), 641–8.

Maibach, H. I., & Kligman, A. M. (1962). The biology of experimental human cutaneous moniliasis (Candida albicans). *Archives of Dermatology, 85,* 233–257.

Maklebust, J., & Magnan, M. (1994). Risk factors associated with having a pressure ulcer: A secondary data analysis. *Advances in Wound Care, 7*(6), 25, 27–28, 31-4 passim.

McIntosh, J. (2001). A guide to female urinals. *Nursing Times, 97*(6), VII–VIX.

McMillen, A. -M., & Soderberg, S. (2002). Disabled persons' experience of dependence on assistive devices. *Scandinavian Journal of Occupational Therapy, 9*(4), 176–183.

Mitteness, L. S., & Barker, J. C. (1995). Stigmatizing a "normal" condition: Urinary incontinence in late life. *Medical Anthropology Quarterly, 9*(2), 188–210.

Moore, K. N., Schieman, S., Ackerman, T., et al. (2004). Assessing comfort, safety, and patient satisfaction with three commonly used penile compression devices. *Urology, 63*(1), 150–154.

Naish, W., & Hallam, M. (2007). Urinary tract infection: Diagnosis and management for nurses. *Nursing Standard, 21*(23), 50–57.

Nix, D. H. (2002). Validity and reliability of the perineal assessment tool. *Ostomy Wound Manage, 48*(2), 43–49.

Nix, D., & Ermer-Seltun, J. (2004). A review of perineal skin care protocols and skin barrier product use. *Ostomy Wound Management, 50*(12), 59–67.

Paterson, J. (2000). Stigma associated with post-prostatectomy urinary incontinence. *Journal of Wound, Ostomy & Continence Nursing, 27*(3), 168–173.

Paterson, J., Dunn, S., Kowanko, I., et al. (2003). Selection of continence products: Perspectives of people who have incontinence and their carers. *Disability and Rehabilitation, 25*(17), 955–963.

Pemberton, P., Brooks, A., Eriksen, C. M., et al. (2006). A comparative study of two types of urinary sheath. *Nursing Times, 102*(7), 36–41.

Phillips, B., & Zhao, H. (1993). Predictors of assistive technology abandonment. *Assistive Technology, 5*(1), 36–45.

Pomfret, I. J. (1996). Catheters: Design, selection and management. *British Journal of Nursing, 5*(4), 245–251.

Pomfret, I. (2006). Penile sheaths: A guide to selection and fitting. *Journal of Community Nursing, 20*(11), 14–18.

Potter, J. (2007). Male urinary incontinence-could penile sheaths be the answer? *Journal of Community Nursing, 21*(5), 4042.

Proudfoot, L. M., Farmer, E. S., & McIntosh, J. B. (1994). Testing incontinence pads using single-case research designs. *British Journal of Nursing, 3*(7), 316, 318–320, 322.

Schnetz, E., Kuss, O., Schmitt, J., et al. (1999). Intra-and inter-individual variations in transepidermal water loss on the face: Facial locations for bioengineering studies. *Contact Dermatitis, 40*(5), 243–247.

Shaw, C., Tansey, R., Jackson, C., et al. (2001). Barriers to help seeking in people with urinary symptoms. *Family Practice, 18*(1), 48–52.

Skewes, S. M. (1997). Bathing: It's a tough job! *Journal of Gerontological Nursing, 23*(5), 45–49.

Spector, W., & Fortinsky, R. (1998). Pressure ulcer prevalence in Ohio nursing homes: Clinical and facility correlates. *Journal of Aging and Health, 10*(1), 62–80.

Stapleton, A., & Stamm, W. E. (1997). Prevention of urinary tract infection. *Infectious Disease Clinics of North America, 11*(3), 719–733.

Suskind, R. R., & Ishihara, M. (1965). The effects of wetting on cutaneous vulnerability. *Archives of Environmental Health, 11*(4), 529–537.

Theaker, C., Mannan, M., Ives, N., et al. (2000). Risk factors for pressure sores in the critically ill. *Anaesthesia, 55*(3), 221–224.

Tsai, T. F., & Maibach, H. I. (1999). How irritant is water? An overview. *Contact Dermatitis, 41*(6), 311–314.

Van der Valk, P. G., & Maibach, H. I. (1990). A functional study of the skin barrier to evaporative water loss by means of repeated cellophane-tape stripping. *Clinical and Experimental Dermatology, 15*(3), 180–182.

Vickerman, J. (2003). The benefits of a lending library for female urinals. *Nursing Times, 99*(44), 56–57.

Vickerman, J. (2006). Selecting urinals for male patients. *Nursing Times, 102*(19), 47–48.

Voegeli, D. (2008). The effect of washing and drying practices on skin barrier function. *Journal of Wound Ostomy & Continence Nursing, 35*(1), 84–90.

Warshaw, E., Nix, D., Kula, J., et al. (2002). Clinical and cost effectiveness of a cleanser protectant lotion for treatment of perineal skin breakdown in low-risk patients with incontinence. *Ostomy Wound Manage, 48*(6), 44–51.

Watret, L. (1999). Using a case-mix-adjusted pressure sore incidence study in a surgical directorate to improve patient outcomes in pressure ulcer prevention. *Journal of Tissue Viability, 9*(4), 121–125.

Zimmerer, R. E., Lawson, K. D., & Calvert, C. J. (1986). The effects of wearing diapers on skin. *Pediatric Dermatology, 3*(2), 95–101.

QUESTIONS

1. A patient is experiencing urinary retention that persists after a trial of clean intermittent catheterization. What would be the next level of treatment to consider?
   A. Toileting aids
   B. Absorbent pads
   C. Indwelling catheter
   D. Surgical intervention

2. The continence nurse is considering a product to use for a female patient who has light incontinence. What would be an appropriate recommendation?
   A. Disposable insert
   B. Leaf product
   C. Disposable diapers
   D. Disposable underpants

3. A male patient complains of light fecal incontinence. What product would the incontinence nurse recommend for this patient?
A. Disposable underpants
B. Washable underpants
C. Absorbent disposable pad
D. Soft pad or gauze between the buttocks

4. For which patient experiencing heavy urine loss would a male condom catheter be the most appropriate continence product?
A. A patient who is cognitively impaired
B. A patient with limited mobility and who is experiencing frequency
C. A patient who is considered psychologically vulnerable
D. A patient with decreased genital sensation

5. The continence nurse is teaching a male patient how to apply and manage a condom catheter. Which of the following is an appropriate teaching point?
A. Protect the skin with liquid barrier film wipes and ensure that the skin has dried properly before applying condom catheter.
B. Make sure there is no gap at the end of the sheath between the glans penis and drainage tube.
C. Remove the condom catheter by quickly and forcefully rolling it off while sitting on the seat of a toilet.
D. Prior to applying the sheath, ensure that the penis and surrounding skin is washed thoroughly with an astringent cleanser.

6. The continence nurse orders a penile compression device for a male patient with incontinence. For what type of incontinence is this device generally recommended?
A. Stress incontinence
B. Overflow incontinence
C. Postvoid dribbling
D. Urge incontinence

7. The continence nurse is assisting a male patient who has urge incontinence to choose a handheld urinal. Which of the following is a recommended guideline?
A. Choose a urinal with a curved bottom.
B. Do not use a handheld urinal if penis is retracted.
C. Choose a lighter-weight urinal device.
D. Avoid using homemade urinal devices such as empty detergent bottles.

8. Which of the following is the primary user concern when using commodes and bedpans for defecation?
A. Safety
B. User friendliness
C. Device design
D. Lack of privacy

9. Which assessment parameter is particularly important when choosing to use a urine drainage bag for incontinence?
A. Patient preference
B. Patient/caregiver dexterity
C. Patient finances
D. Patient skin condition

10. The continence nurse is teaching a patient how to use a urinary drainage bag. Which teaching point follows recommended practice for use of this device?
A. Most bags have a volume in the range of 350 mL to 750 mL.
B. All drainage bags are supplied sterile.
C. Nonreturn valves on the devices are proven to reduce UTIs.
D. The drainage bag should be lifted above the level of the bladder.

11. Which statement accurately describes skin damage associated with incontinence?
A. Dry skin is more vulnerable to friction damage.
B. Individuals with fecal and urinary incontinence are at higher risk for IAD.
C. Underhydration is a mechanism of damage for IAD.
D. Pressure ulcers are easily distinguishable from moisture lesions.

12. The continence nurse is teaching a patient with incontinence how to avoid incontinence-associated dermatitis (IAD). Which teaching tip would the nurse include?
A. Vigorously scrub the perineal area with soap and water.
B. Never use a hair dryer to dry damaged perineal skin.
C. Use a no-rinse pH-balanced cleanser to clean the perineal area.
D. Use a humectant on overhydrated perineal skin.

ANSWERS: 1.**C**, 2.**A**, 3.**D**, 4.**B**, 5.**A**, 6.**A**, 7.**C**, 8.**D**, 9.**B**, 10.**A**, 11.**B**, 12.**C**

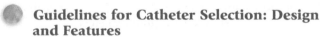

CHAPTER 13

Indwelling and Intermittent Catheterization

Katherine N. Moore and Lynette Franklin

OBJECTIVES

1. Identify indications and contraindications for use of indwelling catheters.
2. Describe guidelines for selection of an indwelling catheter, to include catheter material, catheter size, and balloon size.
3. Describe current guidelines for prevention and management of complications associated with indwelling catheter use: CAUTI, obstruction, and leakage/bypassing.
4. Discuss advantages and disadvantages of urethral versus suprapubic catheters.
5. Describe indications and guidelines for intermittent catheterization.

Topic Outline

Acatheter is a hollow flexible tube that is placed through the urethra or suprapubic space into the bladder to allow continuous flow of urine from the bladder into an external containment device. Bladder catheterization can be used for either short-term or long-term bladder management, such as for the critically ill patient who requires ongoing monitoring of urine output or for the patient with incomplete emptying (retention). Short-term catheterization is defined as insertion of a catheter for up to 2 to 4 weeks; long-term catheterization is generally accepted as use for 30 days or more (Smith & Rusnak, 1997).

This chapter will address indications and guidelines for use of indwelling urethral and suprapubic catheters and for intermittent catheterization (IC). As the names imply, indwelling *urethral catheters* are inserted into the bladder via the urethra; indwelling *suprapubic* catheters (SPCs) are placed into the bladder proximal to the suprapubic bone through the skin and an epithelialized track (see details of insertion in Chapter 6). Indwelling catheters are commonly known as Foley catheters, after a Boston-based American urologist, Dr. Frederic Foley. Although Dr. Foley never held the patent for the catheter (it remains with Davol Company), his design was adopted in the 1930s and manufactured by C.R. Bard, Inc. who named the prototypes in honor of Dr. Foley. While the materials used to construct indwelling catheters have evolved over the years, the original design of the catheter remains practically unchanged.

Catheters are not generally a good option for management of individuals with urinary incontinence; in fact, they should be considered as a last resort option for incontinence or retention not amenable to treatment by any other means.

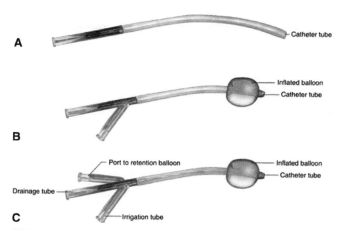

FIGURE 13-1. Types of urethral catheters. **A.** Intermittent (straight) catheter. **B.** Indwelling (Foley) catheter "two way." **C.** "Three-way" catheter used for irrigation and control of hemorrhage.

CLINICAL PEARL

Short-term catheterization is defined as insertion of a catheter for up to 2 weeks; long-term catheterization is generally accepted as use for 30 days or more.

Guidelines for Catheter Selection: Design and Features

Continence nurses should be knowledgeable regarding the various design features for indwelling (or intermittent) catheters, in order to select the best catheter for an individual patient. Features to be considered include balloon size, catheter tip, catheter size, and catheter material.

Catheter Balloon

The catheter is maintained within the bladder via an inflated balloon at the proximal end that is filled with sterile water. Saline should not be used to inflate the balloon because the fluid may crystallize in the balloon port, clogging it and preventing balloon deflation and catheter removal. Catheters have a double lumen, one for filling/inflation of the balloon and the other for drainage of urine (Fig. 13-1); they are occasionally referred to as "two-way catheters." Catheters used

for bladder irrigation postoperatively or in management of hemorrhage are called "three-way catheters" because they have an additional lumen to allow fluid influx; these catheters are only inserted urethrally. The usual balloon size on a standard "two-way catheter" is cited as 5 mL on the inflation end of most catheters; some indicate a balloon size of 10 mL. In clinical practice, all standard size balloons (both 5 mL and 10 mL) should be inflated with 10 mL of water, because the balloon itself requires 5 mL for symmetrical inflation, and 5 mL of water is retained along the filling channel, for a total of 10 mL. A larger balloon catheter should never be inserted for long-term bladder drainage because of the serious trauma on the bladder neck.

Catheter Tip

Catheter tips also vary depending on intended use. The most common is the straight tip; however, coudé-tipped catheters are frequently useful for men with prostatic hyperplasia and mild obstruction as they slip around the prostatic curve more readily than a straight catheter. Although the Foley catheter is most commonly used, on occasion other self-retaining catheters used in urology are a Malecot (for nephrostomy drainage) and Pezzer (suprapubic drainage). Figure 13-2 shows the various catheters.

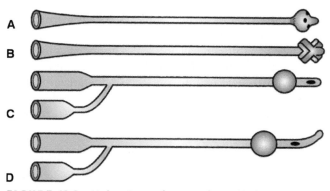

FIGURE 13-2. Various types of commonly used catheters. **A.** Mushroom or de Pezzer. **B.** Winged-tip or Malecot. **C.** Foley with inflated retention bag. **D.** Foley with coudé tip.

TABLE 13-1 Catheter Sizes

Age	Weight	French (Fr) Sizes
Premature		5–6
Newborn	Up to 9 kg	5–8
Toddler	10–30 kg	5–8
School-age child 11–12 y		8–10
Adult age >13 y		Female: 12–14 Male: 12–16
Adult: hematuria or clots		18
Adult: obstruction		20–24
Adult: with prostatic bleeding		30

From Wound, Ostomy & Continence Nurses Society. (2009). *Indwelling urinary catheters: Best practice for clinicians*. New Jersey: WOCN.

CLINICAL PEARL

Saline is not used to inflate the balloon because the fluid may crystallize in the balloon port, clogging it and preventing balloon deflation and catheter removal.

Catheter Size

Catheter size is measured by the outer diameter using a measurement scale known as the French scale. In adults, a 14 to 16 French size catheter is typically recommended, unless a larger or smaller catheter is indicated for specific urologic reasons. Table 13-1 shows the usual sizes for different age groups. Table 13-2 lists the various types of catheters and their use.

Catheter Construction (Material)

Indwelling catheters are manufactured from various materials, and the material used has significant implications for clinical use. Latex impregnated with polytef particles and hydrogel-coated latex catheters both reduce fluid absorption into the catheter surface and aid in a smooth insertion; uncoated latex is not used for urethral catheters as there is a high contact sensitivity to the material. Silastic catheters are silicone coated but latex based; in contrast, pure silicone catheters contain no latex and provide the advantage of a thinner wall and wider lumen as compared to latex-based catheters (Fig. 13-3). This is advantageous for individuals who require long-term catheterization and who are "mucous producing"; the wider lumen may maintain patency for longer periods than other catheter materials. Pure silicone catheters are also an important option for those with latex allergy.

The choice of catheter depends on the circumstances for use. In acute care and for short-term use, coated latex catheters are the norm (either polytef or hydrophilic/lubricious), while silastic or silicone catheters are more frequently used in long-term care. The cost of silicone catheters is higher than latex-based catheters, so another consideration is the length of time the catheter will remain patent. For example, if the individual "blocks" (obstructs) the catheter every 2 weeks, a silicone catheter may not be cost effective; in contrast, for the individual who only requires a catheter change monthly or less often, the silicone catheter could be an excellent choice. None of the catheters in this group are designed to reduce bacteriuria or catheter-associated urinary tract infection (CAUTI).

Antimicrobial Catheters

Two different catheters are available that are designed specifically to reduce the risk of CAUTI: antibiotic coated and silver alloy. There are two types of antibiotic-impregnated catheters that have been marketed, nitrofurantoin and a combination of minocycline and rifampicin. Current randomized control trial evidence suggests that the risk of bacteriuria is significantly reduced during the first week following insertion of the antibiotic-impregnated catheter; after that period, there is no apparent benefit (Pickard et al., 2012). For silver alloy catheters, the reduction in bacteriuria lasts up to 14 days (Lam et al., 2014). Because of the overall expense of the products, their use is generally recommended for high-risk individuals such as those in an ICU.

Parker et al. (2009) provided a comprehensive overview of the data available related to antimicrobial catheters, noting that at least four systematic reviews with meta-analysis had been conducted. Based on their summary of the current state of the science, it appears that antimicrobial catheters reduce bacteriuria and thus potentially reduce the risk of CAUTI but only for short periods of time (14 days or less); beyond that point, there is no benefit. Studies have yet to be conducted comparing antimicrobial catheters to standard indwelling catheters for long-term use (more than 30 days in situ).

CLINICAL PEARL

Antimicrobial catheters in situ for 14 days or less will reduce the incidence of bacteriuria and thus potentially reduce the risk of CAUTI; beyond 14 days, the benefit is no longer realized.

Catheter-Related Complications

Indwelling urinary catheters (IUC) are important adjuncts to patient care. When used on a short-term basis (i.e., for a few days), there are few complications apart from risk of urinary tract infection (UTI) or dislodgement. Conversely, when used on a long-term basis (over 30 days), both urethral and SPCs are associated with complications that can be serious. Foremost is CAUTI; additional potential complications include urethral erosion or tearing (iatrogenic hypospadias; Fig. 13-4), bladder neck injury (urethral catheters), bladder calculi, urinary leakage around the catheter, and epididymitis or orchitis. Risks specific to SPCs are skin irritation/breakdown at the

TABLE 13-2 **Catheter Types and Usage**

Material	Definition	Advantages	Disadvantages	Best Use
Silicone elastomer-coated latex	Coated chemically with bonded silicone adhered to a latex catheter	Reduces contact of latex to the urethra Reduces incidence of insertion trauma, urethritis, and encrustation Less expensive than 100% silicone For use with latex sensitivity	Flexibility: greater than 100% silicone; less flexible than 100% latex Elastic coating may dissolve over time exposing patient to latex Balloons may lose fluid filling over time as compared to 100% latex	Short-term usage Patients with latex sensitivity
Red rubber latex	A latex catheter that is soft and flexible Latex: natural product that is a yellowish brown in color	Flexibility; good for allowing for easy insertion especially for short-term usage Low cost Comfort	Contraindicated in patients with latex allergies Swells with absorption of fluid thereby decreasing diameter of lumen and increasing outside diameter Potential for toxicity with mucosal tissue resulting in stricture and inflammation Prone to encrustations	Short-term usage as in clean intermittent catheterization For patients without allergies to latex
PVC	A firm catheter made from a plastic polymer that has had plasticizer added to soften and increase flexibility.	Becomes soft and pliable with body temperature Has wide internal diameter	Limited utility as indwelling catheters, secondary to encrustation formation increased risk with >1 wk usage Has been debated as to safety with exposure to liquid over long periods of time, that is, may break down Uncomfortable due to stiffness Balloon may be made of latex	Short-term use
Silicone	An inert product that is clear or white in color	Thin-walled tube with larger lumen Catheters more compatible with lining of the urethra Latex free More lumen stability with bladder irrigation and aspiration	Stiff; uncomfortable for some Balloons tend to become "cuffed" when deflated thus making removal potentially traumatic Balloon has tendency to lose fluid filling over time requiring frequent evaluation and reinflation	Long-term usage, patients with allergies to other products Not recommended for SPT usage
Antimicrobial	Silver ions, bactericidal and nontoxic to humans, are used to coat the catheter on the outside, inner lumen, or both. Silver phosphate Nitrofurazone impregnated	Some evidence that catheter-related UTI (CAUTI) is reduced Potential reduction in the rate of asymptomatic bacteriuria with short-term use Reduces bacterial load for up to 14 d	More research needed to know full extent of CAUTI reduction Expensive Limited studies and benefit beyond 14 d Limited clinical studies May contain latex	Indwelling or SPT

From Wound, Ostomy & Continence Nurses Society. (2009). *Indwelling urinary catheters: Best practice for clinicians*. New Jersey: WOCN.

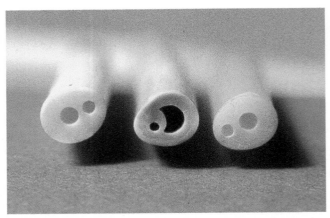

FIGURE 13-3. Comparison of a 16-French silicone catheter and 16-French latex-based catheter. Note the much larger lumen in the silicone (*blue*) catheter.

stoma site or dislodgement and track closure. In addition, SP catheter insertion has been associated with bowel perforation and bladder injury (Ahmed et al., 2004; Harrison et al., 2011). Long-term use of either a urethral or SP catheter also increases the risk of squamous cell bladder carcinoma (Groah et al., 2002; West et al., 1999).

CLINICAL PEARL

Risks specific to suprapubic catheters are skin irritation/breakdown at the stoma site or dislodgement and track closure.

Catheter-Associated Urinary Tract Infection

All individuals with catheters will develop significant microbial colonization within a few days, a condition known as asymptomatic bacteriuria (ASB); ASB does not produce symptoms and does not require treatment. ASB must be differentiated from CAUTI, which does produce symptoms and requires some type of intervention (Box 13-1). Much attention has been paid to infections

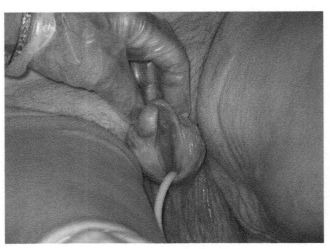

FIGURE 13-4. Latrogenic hypospadias from catheter trauma.

BOX 13-1. Signs and Symptoms of a Catheter-Associated Urinary Tract Infection

Symptoms may include
- Fever and/or chills
- Suprapubic or flank pain
- Hematuria
- Positive urine culture >10^5 CFU/mL
- Positive blood culture of the same organism as the urine culture
- Increased spasticity, autonomic dysreflexia, or "unease" (people with SCI)

Signs not directly associated with a CAUTI:
- Pyuria—not a good indicator as it is common in catheterized individuals
- Odor—the persistent bacteria in the urine of catheterized patients will produce odor

Possible signs in an elderly patient:
- Increased restlessness or altered mental status
- Change in health status not attributable to any other cause (pneumonia, medication side effects)

Treatment of CAUTI once diagnosis is established:
- If possible, remove the catheter and use alternate continence methods at least until the antibiotic course is completed.
- If not possible to leave the catheter out, change the catheter so that there is the least amount of biofilm present.
- Start antibiotics—typical course of antibiotics is 7 to 14 days, usually a fluoroquinolone.
- Chart symptom improvement.

Adapted from Hooton et al. (2010).

---

related to indwelling catheters (CAUTI), particularly since 2008; at that time, the Centers for Medicare and Medicaid Services (CMS) changed reimbursement regulations, calling CAUTI "preventable harm" and withholding payment for additional costs related to CAUTI treatment (Saint et al., 2009a).

Etiology of CAUTI

Biofilm development on the external and internal surfaces of the catheter occurs as early as 24 hours following insertion, and biofilm burden progressively increases the longer the catheter remains in situ (Stickler, 2008). Figure 13-5 illustrates the cycle of biofilm development, from initial microbial adherence to an anchored

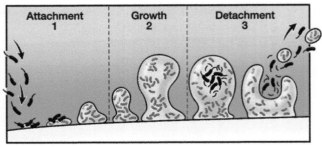

FIGURE 13-5. Biofilm life cycle. The three major stages in the life cycle of a biofilm: attachment, growth, and detachment.

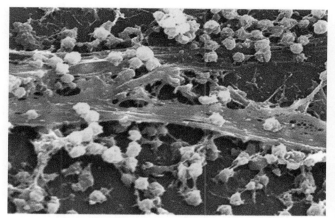

FIGURE 13-6. Electron micrograph depicting large numbers of *Staphylococcus aureus* bacteria, which were found on the luminal surface of an indwelling catheter. Of importance are the sticky-looking substances woven between the round cocci bacteria, which were composed of polysaccharides and are known as biofilm. This biofilm has been found to protect the bacteria that secrete the substance from attacks by antimicrobial agents such as antibiotics (magnified × 2,363).

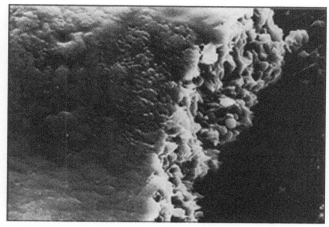

FIGURE 13-7. *Staphylococcus epidermidis* attached by its biofilm and growing on the surface of a catheter.

(sessile) community of organisms. The organisms within the sessile grouping are protected by a matrix of extracellular polymeric substances that, once established, are essentially impenetrable to antibiotics (Fig. 13-6) (Donlan & Costerton, 2002). Organisms comprising the biofilm typically originate from the periurethral area (and colonize the external surface of the catheter) or ascend via the catheter drainage tubing (and colonize the internal surface of the catheter); all organisms gain access to the bladder and new organisms are acquired at the rate of 3% to 7% a day (Nicolle, 2014). The most common infecting organism is *Escherichia coli*; *Enterococcus* spp. and *Candida* spp. along with other gram-negative and gram-positive organisms are also isolated in the urine of an infected patient, and many of these are resistant to antibiotics.

The microbiologic environment changes with long-term catheterization (more than 30 days); *Proteus mirabilis* is isolated in as many as 40% of samples from individuals requiring long-term catheter use. *Proteus mirabilis* is an important organism, because it is persistent and it produces copious amounts of biofilm, which can actually block the catheter; in addition, the bacteria in the biofilm can be extremely difficult to eradicate. *Proteus* is also a key urease-producing organism (Stickler et al., 1998). Urease alters the urine pH, which causes hydrolysis of the urea to free ammonia; this in turn raises the pH and promotes precipitation of minerals such as calcium phosphate and magnesium ammonium phosphate (struvite). These minerals deposit on the eyes and lumen of the catheter, forming a "gravel" of mineral encrustation (Fig. 13-7) (Donlan & Costerton, 2002; Getliffe & Mulhall, 1991).

There is no treatment for encrusted catheters except removal and replacement. Care must be taken during

removal, as large clumps of mineral deposits can form on the exterior of the catheter. In Figure 13-8, heavy mineral and mucous deposits have formed around a pubic hair, which was probably inserted (inadvertently) during catheterization.

Prevention of Biofilm and CAUTI Development

To date, research attempts to eradicate catheter biofilms have included flushing of catheters with acidic solutions, use of antibiotic meatal ointments, instillation of antibiotics into urine drainage bags, and antibiotic prophylaxis (Wilson et al., 2009), but none have been effective. Moreover, apart from antimicrobial catheters (which have a limited benefit), no catheter materials have demonstrated the ability to reduce biofilm development (Donlan & Costerton, 2002).

As Méndez-Probst et al. (2012) note, future research on catheter designs to reduce/prevent CAUTI "must include an improved understanding of biofilm formation and ways to avoid their occurrence. This knowledge along with improvements in biomaterials and in drug elution technology will pave the way for the next evolution in urologic device development" (p. 188).

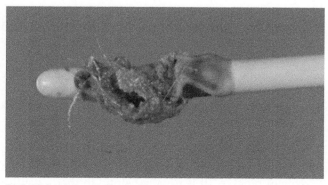

FIGURE 13-8. Biofilm buildup around a hair nidus at the tip of an indwelling catheter. Note that the eyes of the catheter are completely blocked.

Diagnosis of CAUTI

All individuals with long-term catheters will develop colonization (ASB), but urine cultures are not indicated unless the individual is symptomatic. Symptoms of CAUTI usually include fever, suprapubic or flank pain, hematuria, change in functional or cognitive status, and/or a positive blood culture that grows the same organism as the urine culture. However, especially in the elderly individual with cognitive impairment, CAUTI can be difficult to diagnose; this is because other disease processes can cause similar symptoms. Thus, diagnosis is usually one of exclusion. It is important for the continence nurse to realize that pyuria is not a good indicator of CAUTI because it is common even in the absence of symptoms and occurs because of the inflammatory reaction to the catheter as a foreign body (Box 13-1).

Obtaining a Urine Specimen

Before antibiotic therapy is initiated, urine for analysis is obtained via the specimen collection port of the catheter. A mature biofilm with multiple organisms will be established if the catheter has been in situ for longer than 14 days; urine specimens in this case should be obtained from a newly inserted catheter to increase the likelihood of culturing relevant organisms (Hooton et al., 2010).

Catheter Obstruction (Blockage)

Indwelling catheters may become blocked by blood or by precipitates and biofilm, and the management differs based on the obstructing substance. When the catheter is blocked or draining poorly due to blood clots (e.g., in patients post urologic surgery), catheter irrigation is indicated. This is typically done with a "three-way" catheter system and/or with gentle flushing of the catheter using normal saline and a 50-mL syringe. Irrigating in the situation of hemorrhage is an expert nursing practice skill.

In contrast, long-term indwelling catheters blocked by crystals, heavy mucus, or biofilm typically need to be removed and replaced (Fig. 13-9). In this situation, catheter irrigation provides no clear advantage even if done with specifically designed acidic catheter-washout solutions (Hagen et al., 2010). Rather than trying to unblock the catheter, which can be uncomfortable for the individual, time consuming for the nurse, and potentially traumatic to the bladder, the continence nurse should change the catheter and the drainage system. If the individual is a "frequent blocker," it is usually helpful to then establish an anticipatory change schedule; for example, changing every 10 days if blocking occurs by 12 days in situ. This approach can be very helpful in planning homecare visits

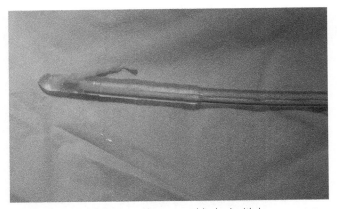

FIGURE 13-9. Silicone catheter eyes blocked with heavy mucus.

and in helping to reduce the risk of recurrent blockage and discomfort. The continence nurse should also consider a urology consultation to evaluate best options for long-term management.

Leakage Around the Urethral or Suprapubic Catheter

Pericatheter leakage is caused by the bladder forcing urine around the catheter. For individuals with urethral catheters, leakage places the perineal area at high risk for incontinence-associated dermatitis; for those with SPCs, in addition to urethral leakage, stoma leakage threatens skin integrity (Hunter et al., 2013). Possible causes include blockage of the drainage holes in the catheter from mucous or encrustations, kinked or crushed (caught in a bedrail) catheter drainage tubing, or blood clots. Leakage around the catheter should prompt the nurse to ask *"Is this catheter really necessary? Can it be removed and an alternate continence measure instituted?"*

If simple care measures are not effective, such as ensuring tube patency and proper catheter support, the catheter is probably blocked and the usual next step would be to change the catheter. If the problem continues, then further investigation may be indicated. For example, if ongoing "grit" or "gravel" is felt in the catheter or observed in the tubing or drainage bag, the individual may have a bladder calculus that will require urological intervention. As indicated earlier in this chapter, the practice of inserting a larger catheter or inflating the balloon with more fluid will not address the underlying problem and should not be done because of the risk of permanent bladder neck damage.

Occasionally, an antimuscarinic agent may be tried to reduce persistent leakage associated with overactive bladder, once reversible factors and tube anchoring have been addressed. If antimuscarinics are prescribed, the care plan must be updated to address the side effects of constipation and confusion and to include evaluation following 7 days of treatment. If there is no change in periurethral leakage after 7 days of antimuscarinic therapy, it should be discontinued as further improvement is unlikely; referral to a urologist should be considered.

> **CLINICAL PEARL**
>
> For individuals with urethral catheters, leakage places the perineal area at high risk for incontinence-associated dermatitis; for those with SPCs, in addition to urethral leakage, stoma leakage threatens skin integrity.

Prevention of Complications

Clearly, the most important prevention strategy is to avoid or remove the indwelling catheter and to consider alternate methods of management such as IC, condom catheter drainage, or incontinence pads and toileting.

Indwelling Catheter Use Restricted to Accepted "Indications"

Complication prevention begins with the decision to insert the catheter. The nurse should take into account the HICPAC CDC (Gould et al., 2009) guidelines for *appropriate catheter insertion*, which can serve as a checklist:

- To manage urinary retention or bladder outlet obstruction
- To provide accurate urine output measurements
- To manage bladder short term following select surgical procedures
- To assist in the healing of perineal wounds at risk of contamination by urine
- To improve comfort at the end of life

It is of note that incontinence is not a valid reason for insertion of an indwelling catheter unless there is a perineal wound that is being contaminated or the patient is at the end of life and wishes to have a catheter for comfort.

According to the guidelines, examples of *inappropriate* catheter insertion are

- To replace alternate continence strategies in care of an individual with incontinence
- To obtain a urine specimen if the individual is able to voluntarily void
- "For postoperative duration without appropriate indications (e.g., structural repair of urethra or contiguous structures, prolonged effect of epidural anesthesia)" (p. 11).

Despite the awareness of CAUTI and other catheter-associated complications, many catheters are inserted for unclear or inappropriate reasons. In one recent study (Murphy et al., 2014b), emergency room staff indicated high levels of uncertainty over when an IUC should be used, specifically citing concerns about missing a patient in retention. Some stated that insertion of a catheter for monitoring urine output was often a routine decision;

some indicated that catheters should be inserted for skin protection, comfort, and dignity; and others stated that catheters should not be used to manage urinary incontinence in any circumstances, except end of life care.

Older people are a particularly vulnerable group in terms of inappropriate catheter insertion; in another emergency-based study (Ma et al., 2014), 63% of catheter insertions occurred in patients ≥65 years old, only 43% had a written order for the IUC, and only 5% had a documented reason for IUC. Using the current CDC guidelines, the research team concluded that only 41% of the catheter insertions were appropriate. Both studies highlight the challenges faced by clinicians in emergency departments when time is limited and decisions need to be made quickly.

> **CLINICAL PEARL**
>
> Prevention of problems starts with the decision to insert the catheter. The nurse should take into account the HICPAC CDC guidelines for appropriate catheter insertion.

Aseptic Technique for Insertion

It is of note that although aseptic insertion of a catheter is almost universally agreed upon as an important component of CAUTI prevention, there is no robust evidence that it prevents the onset of CAUTI (Wilson et al., 2009). Nevertheless, unless indications to the contrary arise, aseptic insertion is the standard of practice for catheter insertion in acute care. Because of chronic colonization in individuals with long-term indwelling catheters, clean technique may be appropriate (clean gloves, tap water cleansing, sterile catheter tray, and sterile catheter). In one study in rehabilitation, there was no difference in incidence of bacteriuria between individuals who received IC using aseptic technique and those who received catheterization using a sterile single-use PVC catheter along with clean gloves, clean urine catch container, and clean wipes (Moore et al., 2006).

> **CLINICAL PEARL**
>
> Despite the awareness of CAUTI and other catheter-associated complications, many catheters are inserted for unclear reasons; older people are particularly at risk of inappropriate catheter insertion.

Bowel Management and Constipation Prevention

In many studies, constipation is noted as a predictor of urinary incontinence and detrusor overactivity. In one comprehensive review of constipation and bladder function, the authors note that the majority of studies are small with varying outcome measures and most involve children and younger women; interestingly, none of the studies addressed the impact of constipation on catheter-related outcomes (Averbeck & Madersbacher, 2011). One urodynamic study reported that women with an artificially distended rectum had statistically significant lower bladder volumes at which first and strong desire to void was felt as well as a 26% reduction in bladder capacity, as compared to the group without distention (Panayi et al., 2012).

Consequences of severe impaction are illustrated in case studies involving major rectal impaction resulting in ureteric obstruction and bilateral hydronephrosis in patients with spinal cord injury (SCI) (Downs et al., 2012) or cancer (Gonzalez, 2010). In both situations, the reports indicate that relief of the impaction resulted in gradual resolution of the hydronephrosis.

Individuals at particular risk for constipation and impaction are the frail elderly, those with neurogenic bowel and bladder, those with cancer, and those receiving opioid medications. All care plans for individuals with catheters should include comprehensive bowel assessment and systematic management. Intervention studies on constipation and catheter-related problems are scarce, but clinical judgment would suggest that nonconstipated individuals are at lower risk for straining and therefore less likely to evacuate the catheter from the bladder during a bowel movement.

Strategies to Reduce Catheter Time In Situ

Reminders on charts or flags similar to those used for medication reminders and/or ongoing (daily) review of the patient's need for a catheter, coupled with prompt removal when the catheter is no longer necessary, are effective methods of promoting appropriate and limited use of indwelling catheters (Bernard et al., 2012). There is good evidence that institutions that establish a catheter care bundle of education, catheter insertion/management guidelines, and surveillance can reduce CAUTI (Carter et al., 2014).

One bladder bundle program, "engage and educate/execute and evaluate," was associated with demonstrated success in reducing catheter usage and duration. The authors emphasize the importance of a team effort supported by a champion who not only provides education but also provides follow-up and feedback (Saint et al., 2009b). In a recent systematic review of various strategies to minimize the use of indwelling catheters (Murphy et al., 2014a), the successful groups took into account cultural norms, organizational barriers (context), and practitioner values or beliefs about indwelling catheter use rather than simply implementing a "top-down" policy of change. For continence nurses wishing to implement a catheter surveillance program (or any new program), considering the principles of behavioral change will be important for success.

In addition to assuring ongoing surveillance and prompt removal of indwelling catheters, it may be helpful to consider nursing unit policies about time of removal. In a systematic review of the eight existing trials on nighttime versus morning catheter removal, findings suggest that midnight removal allows time for the bladder to fill and then provides time in the morning for the individual to try voiding (Joanna Briggs Institute, 2008).

CLINICAL PEARL

Successful programs for changes in catheter management policies took into account cultural norms, organizational barriers (context), and practitioner values or beliefs about indwelling catheter use.

Catheter and Balloon Size

Avoiding long-term catheterization is the ultimate preventative strategy, but if ongoing catheterization is required, the catheter size should not be more than 16 French. Larger catheters significantly increase the risk of injury to the urethra, bladder neck, and meatus in addition to compressing the periurethral glands and increasing the risk of urethral erosion. Large catheters and balloons are of particular significance for women requiring long-term urethral catheters. Persistent tension on the catheter and the increased weight of large retention balloons can render the bladder neck and sphincter incompetent and cause irreparable bladder neck damage that leaves the patient completely incontinent. Large catheters and large balloons also increase the risk of bladder spasms, which are painful, cause leakage, and may result in the catheter being expelled. The temptation to use a larger catheter and balloon to prevent catheter dislodgement must be avoided since a larger balloon, 30 mL, for example, weighs 30 g and is almost the size of a chicken egg.

For the patient experiencing bladder spasms and leakage around the catheter, treatment with an antimuscarinic agent is warranted once other causes of overactivity have been ruled out. Routine use of a catheter-stabilizing device and routine use of a small catheter and balloon will minimize the risk of bladder spasms, leakage, and bladder neck/urethral erosion. Figure 13-10 illustrates the points at which a catheter exerts pressure on the bladder neck and urethra in a male.

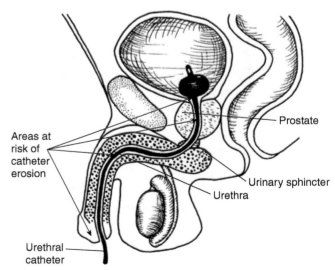

FIGURE 13-10. Pressure points at risk of injury from an indwelling catheter in a male: bladder neck, prostatic urethra, bulbous urethral, meatus.

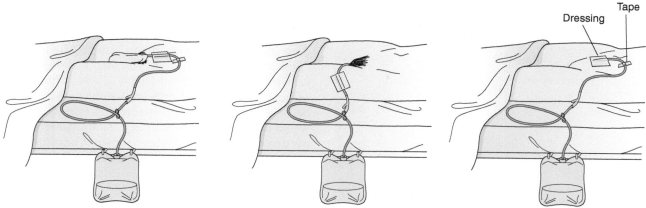

FIGURE 13-11. Properly supported urethral and suprapubic catheters in a male and female; note the ventral position of the penis to minimize tension and the drainage tubing with no dependent loops.

Catheter Support

Catheter support is critical for patient comfort and to prevent traction on the bladder neck as well as to optimize urine drainage. Catheters can be supported by medical adhesive tape or by commercial devices; the essential element to positive outcomes is elimination of tension on the catheter or the male urethral meatus (Figs. 13-11 and 13-12). Catheters for both men and women may be secured to the abdomen or thigh as long as tension on the catheter is minimal with both rest and activity. Figure 13-13

illustrates urethral trauma, edema, and dermatitis from an inadequately supported catheter and persistent leakage around the catheter in a man with reduced genital sensation as a result of stroke. Catheter support may also contribute to reduced movement of periurethral organisms, thereby delaying the onset of CAUTI, but only limited research has been conducted on the effects of catheter securement on reduction of UTI.

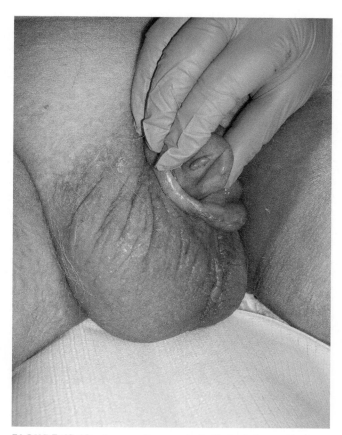

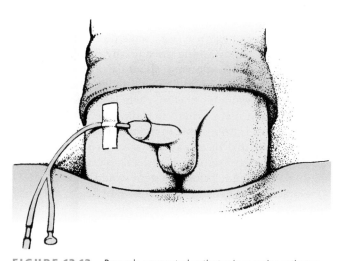

FIGURE 13-12. Properly supported catheter in a male: catheter attached to the thigh to straighten the angle of the penoscrotal junction, thus reducing pressure on the urethra.

FIGURE 13-13. Improperly supported catheter led to urethral injury, penile and scrotal edema, and incontinence-associated dermatitis in a long-term care patient.

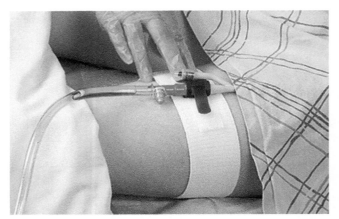

FIGURE 13-14. Catheter support on the upper thigh; note that the catheter is locked in the device at the Y junction to prevent slipping and movement of the catheter.

In a small study, Darouiche et al. (2006) examined the incidence of CAUTI in 118 adults with SCI or multiple sclerosis who were randomized to either a commercial securement device or usual care (preexisting practice such as adhesive tape, Velcro® straps, or no support). No significant differences were found between the groups, but the heterogeneity of the sample made it difficult to interpret the results; 30% of the participants had an SPC, some had no support and, for others, there was no description of the location of the support device.

The catheter can be secured to the leg or the abdomen. There are a variety of securement devices for ambulatory and bed-restricted individuals and include adhesive stays, straps, buttons, and hook and loop closure systems. The goal is to keep tension off the catheter and maintain the tubing and urine drainage bag in a dependent position so that urine will flow freely. Securing the tube at the Y-hub helps to decrease the incidence of bladder irritation and potential traumatic erosion (Fig. 13-14).

Prevention-Dependent Loops of Drainage Tubing

For an individual in bed, drainage tubing must be straight, without dependent loops (Fig. 13-11). In a laboratory study, it was found that dependent loops greatly increased the bladder pressure required to push urine through the tubing into the drainage bag, increased the length of time it took for urine to travel through the tubing, and increased the risk of backflow of urine into the bladder if the tubing and bag were raised above the bladder (Schwab et al., 2014).

CLINICAL PEARL

Dependent loops of tubing may increase bladder pressure required to push urine through the tubing into the drainage bag, increase the length of time for urine to travel through the tubing, and increase the risk of backflow of urine into the bladder if the tubing and bag are raised above the bladder.

Initial Drainage for Patient in Retention

Historically, if an individual was in urinary retention, nursing policies stated that bladder drainage should be done intermittently by inserting a catheter, draining a certain amount, typically 500 to 750 mL, then clamping the catheter for an unspecified length of time. These recommendations were based on fears that the individual could become hypotensive or that bleeding from the bladder would occur. Hematuria is, indeed, a known effect of bladder decompression but has been shown to be related to the degree of bladder damage that occurs prior to the obstruction event, rather than from the relief of obstruction or rate of emptying (Gould et al., 1976).

In a comprehensive review of the literature from 1920 to 1997, Nyman et al. (1997) found no evidence that gradual emptying improved outcomes or reduced side effects for patients in either acute or chronic retention. One source suggests that men in AUR should have clamping/unclamping over a ½ hour period but do not give a reference for this nor the amount of fluid to be drained at each interval (Méndez-Probst et al., 2012). Currently, evidence to support incremental bladder drainage is lacking, and nurses are advised to place the patient in a comfortable position, typically supine, and to fully drain the bladder (Christensen et al., 1987), unless institutional policy indicates otherwise.

CLINICAL PEARL

Evidence to support incremental bladder drainage is lacking, and nurses are advised to place the patient in a comfortable position, typically supine, and to fully drain the bladder.

Appropriate Management of Drainage Bag

A closed urinary drainage system with an integrated antireflux valve has long been recognized and is routinely recommended as an important measure in preventing early onset of CAUTI. Minimal disruption of the closed system should be allowed to reduce infection risk, especially in situations of short-term catheter use (e.g., acute care settings). Strict adherence to handwashing prior to any manipulation of the system (such as emptying) should also be maintained.

However, for active individuals living at home with long-term indwelling catheters, there is usually a need to change from a night system to a daytime leg bag, and a closed system is impossible to maintain. In this situation, given the fact that mature biofilms are present within 14 days of catheter insertion, it is debatable whether maintaining a continuous closed system would reduce CAUTI. One practice has been to connect a night bag to a leg bag, but there is no evidence to support this.

Most insurance companies provide a limited number of drainage bags per month, and thus, individuals need to clean their bags to control odor and remove debris. Although some research has been conducted on drainage bag cleaning with vinegar, soap and water, bleach, or

BOX 13-2.
Cleaning Drainage Bags

Drainage bags should be cleaned prior to reuse, such as after changing from leg to night drainage. Methods include the following steps:
1. Wash hands before and after bag cleansing with soap and water.
2. Disconnect bag from the catheter.
3. Run clear water through the system or use a soft squirt bottle to irrigate with water.
4. Irrigate with cleansing system with either a bleach solution *or* a vinegar solution.
   a. Bleach solution: 1 part bleach to 10 parts water
   b. Vinegar solution: 1 part vinegar to 3 parts water
5. Place solution in bag and tubing, irrigate for 30 seconds, and then drain.
6. Air-dry.
Be aware that bleach solution may discolor surfaces with which it comes in contact.

From Wound, Ostomy & Continence Nurses Society. (2009). *Indwelling urinary catheters: Best practice for clinicians.* New Jersey: WOCN.

hydrogen peroxide, there is no evidence that one solution is significantly better than another in controlling organisms and none that suggests CAUTI is reduced by a particular solution (Wilde et al., 2013). Cleaning is done primarily for control of odor and aesthetic purposes. Box 13-2 outlines WOCN recommendations for cleaning of leg bags when reuse is indicated.

Drainage bags vary in capacity, from 270 to 4,000 mL, and the capacity needed may vary based on situation and time of use. For example, larger systems are convenient for overnight use, while smaller leg bags may provide better discretion during the day.

Catheter Change Frequency

Traditionally, long-term indwelling catheters have been changed on a prescribed basis with the goal of preventing complications. Unfortunately, there is no specific catheter change interval that has been associated with reduced incidence of complications. For convenience, changing routines seem to be every 30 days, but there is no evidence that this improves patient outcomes. Some individuals require much more frequent changing, and others can manage for 2 months or longer. Why such variation occurs is not well understood although it appears partly related to the health of the individual, amount of fluid intake, and physical activity. Current clinical recommendations are to change the catheter when necessary rather than fixed intervals (Gould et al., 2009); however institutional/organizational policy may require changes every 30 days.

CLINICAL PEARL

Current recommendations are that the catheter is changed when necessary and not at fixed intervals.

Catheter Lubrication and Insertion

Indwelling catheter insertion requires lubrication for patient comfort as well as ease of insertion. The research is conflicting on whether topical anesthetic gel is effective for reducing the pain of catheter insertion. For females, water-soluble lubricant is typically used although at least one randomized trial has shown that females report significantly less discomfort with lignocaine gel versus water-soluble lubricant (Chan et al., 2014). In children, lignocaine gel applied topically or urethrally appears to reduce the pain of catheterization as compared to water-soluble gel (Mularoni et al., 2009). The authors note, however, that the pain was not fully controlled and that further investigation into best pain control for pediatric catheterization is required. For males, especially those in emergency in acute urinary retention, some trials have demonstrated reduced pain and ease of catheter insertion with lignocaine gel (Siderias et al., 2004); for cystoscopy, the difference in pain control is less clear (Schede & Thuroff, 2006; Tzortzis et al., 2009).

The usual recommendation is to instill the anesthetic gel slowly (over approximately 10 seconds) and to wait at least 2 minutes before proceeding with instrumentation. In one RCT comparing immediate instrumentation versus a 2-minute wait in men presenting to the emergency department in AUR or with a condition requiring urine output monitoring ($N = 22$), no difference was found in VAS pain score, which averaged 22 on a scale of 0 to 100, with 100 being the worst pain (Garbutt et al., 2008). However, the lack of a nonanesthetic gel control group makes it difficult to determine if it was the lubrication alone or the anesthetic gel that resulted in the low pain scores. It is possible that the primary benefit is the amount of intraurethral gel inserted, typically 10 to 20 mL, which then assists in dilating the urethra and allowing smoother insertion of the catheter. Until further research is undertaken, however, it is prudent for the clinician to follow manufacturers' instructions on use of the gel.

Suprapubic Catheters (see also Chapter 6)

There are some advantages to SPCs as compared to urethral catheters, especially for those who require long-term catheters. For short-term use, such as following gynecologic surgery, an SPC allows for a trial of voiding and may be a more acceptable alternative to IC for that group of patients. SPCs are an alternative to urethral catheters in patients with urethral/pelvic surgery or trauma, men with prostatic obstruction and urethral stricture, and those in whom it is difficult to insert a urethral catheter due to obstruction (Harrison et al., 2011).

In the longer term, an SPC provides protection of the bladder neck and urethra from trauma associated with urethral catheters. Although it has been suggested that UTI is lower with SPC, in long-term use, there appears to be no difference in UTI rates (Hunter et al., 2013). Moreover, SPCs offer protection to those individuals with a lack of urethral or perineal sensation or those who are sitting for

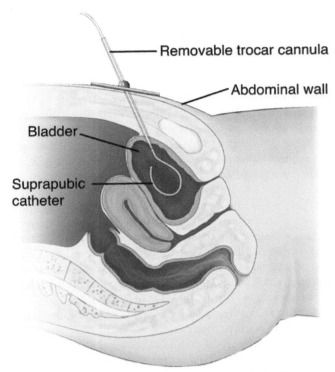

Removable trocar cannula

Abdominal wall

Bladder

Suprapubic catheter

FIGURE 13-15. Suprapubic catheter positioned in the bladder.

extended periods in a wheelchair, who are at risk for urethral or bladder neck injury caused by tension on the catheter or for pressure ulcers from sitting on the catheter tubing (Hunter et al., 2013). SPC may also be a better choice for individuals who wish to be sexually active or who experience urethral discomfort related to the urethral catheter (UC). Figure 13-15 shows an SPC in situ.

Care of the SPC is similar to that of a urethral catheter. The stoma site will need monitoring for skin irritation and urine leakage. Urethral leakage is also a possibility, and the continence nurse will need to ensure that good skin care, supportive user education about care and complications (Chapple et al., 2015) and appropriate continence containment products are available for the individual.

Contraindications to SPC use include pelvic radiotherapy or surgery resulting in adhesions or scarring, obesity, and hematuria requiring bladder irrigation. The frequency for changing an SPC is based on time frame to blockage (as with a urethral catheter). To remove the catheter, the nurse should gently rotate the catheter to loosen it. Once the balloon is deflated, if the catheter does not slip out with gentle traction, the nurse should reinsert some sterile water into the balloon to loosen any attached debris that may be preventing removal. Slight reinflation may also be beneficial for the individual who is being managed with an all-silicone catheter, as the walls of the balloon occasionally have irregularities that are smoothed out with slight reinflation. If, for some reason, the catheter cannot be removed, the patient should be referred to urology as there may be calcification involving the catheter and cystoscopy may be required for removal. If the SPC is

no longer required, the catheter should be removed and a gauze dressing should be placed over the stoma. Closure can occur within a few hours and should require no longer than 1 to 2 days.

Intermittent Catheterization

Intermittent catheterization (IC) is the act of inserting and then removing the catheter once urine has drained via the urethra or other catheterizable channel such as a Mitrofanoff continent urinary diversion. IC is an accepted method of bladder emptying for individuals with neurologic conditions that affect bladder function, such as SCI or multiple sclerosis, and for those with urinary retention. In acute care, IC is commonly used as an alternative to an indwelling catheter on orthopedic, neurology, and day surgery units (e.g., for the patient who is postherniorrhaphy). In addition to providing regular emptying of the bladder until voiding resumes, IC is used to

- Obtain urine sample in individuals who cannot provide a clean catch specimen
- Measure residual urine if portable ultrasound is not available
- Instill medication such as chemotherapy.

IC is not restricted by age; in fact, young children (such as those with spina bifida) may be able to self-catheterize by age four with parental supervision. Some older individuals may rely on their spouse or care giver to do IC where this is acceptable to both parties. Motivation and ability to understand and adhere to a catheterization routine are key success indicators. When assessing a patient for IC and preparing to teach him/her the procedure, the nurse must assure that the individual can adequately expose and access the urethra to safely insert the catheter; some individuals use visualization of the urethra to guide catheter insertion, while others use meatal palpation.

Individualized care plans should identify appropriate catheterization frequency; this decision is based on functional bladder capacity, postvoid residual urine volumes, the purpose and goals of the IC program, frequency–volume charts, and impact on quality of life. The number of catheterizations per day varies; a general rule for adults is to catheterize frequently enough to avoid a bladder urine volume greater than 500 mL, but clinical decisions must also take into account urodynamic findings, detrusor filling pressures, the presence of reflux, and renal function. For individuals with SCI who have high detrusor pressures or persistent incontinence due to detrusor overactivity, IC may be augmented with Botox or antimuscarinics. In one large study of people with SCI or MS who were using IC for bladder management, Rovner et al. (2013) reported that the most common adverse event was UTI and that complications were low across all treatment groups.

CLINICAL PEARL

Individualized care plans should identify appropriate catheterization frequency based on user goals, impact on quality of life, frequency–volume charts, functional bladder capacity, and postvoid residual urine.

Advantages

Advantages of IC over indwelling catheterization include the following:

- Increased potential for self-care and independence
- Reduced need for equipment and appliances, for example, drainage bag
- Greater freedom for expression of sexuality
- Reduced risk of symptomatic UTI compared to indwelling or condom catheters

Quality of life is a relative term and health care professionals must bear in mind and be sensitive to the fact that the individual who must self-catheterize may not perceive his/her quality of life as being "good." Post SCI, most individuals are discharged using IC; however, by 1-year follow-up, it is not uncommon for some to use other options, such as an indwelling catheter, citing personal preference, difficulty with caregiver catheterizing, incontinence, or urethral strictures as main reasons for discontinuing IC (Afsar et al., 2013). Perception depends, in part, on what type of bladder management the individual had prior to beginning IC as well as hand function, seating ability for catheterizing, continence status, and whether IC has actually improved the symptoms that precipitated the recommendation for IC (Yılmaz et al., 2014).

Another common concern is the lack of accessible toilets with a shelf on which to place equipment. Adherence to an IC program may require collaboration between the individual, nursing, occupational therapists, and physical therapists. Listening to the individual's concerns and providing accessible follow-up is a critical part of assisting people to adapt.

Catheters

Catheters for intermittent use come in a variety of designs, including plain uncoated; hydrophilic-coated; and nonhydrophilic-coated, prelubricated models.

Plain Uncoated Catheters

Plain uncoated catheters (typically clear plastic PVC or PVC-free) are packed singly in sterile packaging. As per industry standards, all disposable catheters are labeled for one-time use, and health care professionals recommend that catheters be used once only. Some individuals will reuse the catheter because of cost, limited insurance coverage, or concern about the environment. Most plain uncoated catheters are used with separate lubricant, although this is a matter of personal choice; some IC users prefer not to use lubricant or just to use water. Cleansing of the catheter varies from being washed with soap and water, boiled, soaked in disinfectant, or microwaved. Cleaned catheters are air-dried and then stored in a convenient container (often plastic containers or bags).

Hydrophilic-Coated Catheters

Hydrophilic-coated catheters are single use only (they may not be cleaned and reused) with an integral lubricated surface which may (according to manufacturers) reduce trauma and UTI. The most common coating is hydrophilic, which is either preactivated or requires the addition of water at the time of use to form a lubricious layer.

Nonhydrophilic, Prelubricated Catheters

Nonhydrophilic, prelubricated catheters are supplied prepacked with an integrated coating of water-soluble gel. There are also several prelubricated products with an integrated collection bag (all-in-one) which gives flexibility for the user and are efficient for hospital use.

Catheter length also varies and recent introductions on the market include small portable hydrophilic products that can be discreetly stored or carried in a handbag/backpack. These products are all single use and have been rated positively compared to the standard length hydrophilic catheters (Chartier-Kastler et al., 2013). Individuals vary in their preference of catheters for IC: some find the longer hydrophilic-coated products too slippery to handle, while others enjoy the prelubricated surface and single use. The more compact designs may reduce the difficulty with insertion. Others prefer PVC with added lubricant. People beginning an IC program should be offered a choice of products to determine the best fit for their lifestyle and personal goals for management.

Complications

The most common complication of IC is UTI. Other less common problems include urethral irritation, urethral stricture, and epididymitis/orchitis.

Urinary Tract Infection

UTI is the most frequent complication, and catheterization frequency and the avoidance of bladder overfilling are recognized as important prevention measures. Prophylactic antibiotics are indicated only for high-risk individuals such as children with high-grade reflux. It is unclear if single-use catheters reduce the incidence of UTI. A recent Cochrane review included 35 randomized trials on the topic and stated that evidence is inconclusive on one method versus another in community-dwelling individuals (Prieto et al., 2014). There is some evidence that in the short term in hospital, UTI onset may be delayed by the use of hydrophilic-coated catheters, but this benefit is not maintained over the long term (Cardenas et al., 2011; De Ridder et al., 2005).

Pyelonephritis

Pyelonephritis is a serious consequence of UTI and can cause renal scarring, hydronephrosis, and eventually renal failure. Individuals at risk are those with high-pressure bladders that are not easily controlled with routine IC. Close urology follow-up is necessary in these individuals, who may require Botox injections, neuromodulation, cystoplasty, or other more aggressive management.

Prostatitis

Prostatitis is an identified risk in men, but epididymitis and urethritis are relatively rare.

Trauma

Trauma secondary to catheterization, as measured by hematuria, is reported, but lasting effects appear limited. The recent introduction of hydrophilic-coated or gel-coated catheters is believed to reduce urethral trauma, and laboratory research measuring epithelial cells on coated or uncoated catheters supports this hypothesis. However, longitudinal research studies are required to assess the clinical significance for long-term catheter users. Continence nurses must teach individuals to lubricate their catheters well and to insert without pressure. At-risk people for urethral trauma are those with limited or no sensation. Observation of catheter insertion and assessment of the individual's understanding of insertion technique is critical in this group.

Urethral Strictures

Estimates of the prevalence of urethral strictures and false passages increase with longer use of IC and/or with traumatic catheterization. Campbell et al. (2004) reported on children with spina bifida who had used IC for at least 5 years. All used an uncoated PVC catheter plus water-soluble lubricant. The incidence of urethritis, false passages, or epididymitis was very low (and adherence to the protocol was excellent).

Based on clinical opinion, the most important preventative measures appear to be good education and ongoing support for all involved in IC, adherence to the catheterization protocol, healthy lifestyle, and bowel management/avoidance of constipation, although the level of evidence for these clinical opinions is weak (Wyndaele, 2002).

Patient Teaching

Beginning IC as an ongoing bladder management plan can be a necessary but difficult undertaking for people, and the continence nurse must be prepared to spend time and provide ongoing support and encouragement. Frequency of catheterization depends on patient history and the clinical reasons for initiating an IC program: for example, the individual with reflux and symptomatic UTI will require more frequent catheterization than the person who is using IC to manage leakage caused by incomplete emptying and who has no UTI symptoms. Women often panic when they view the vaginal and perineal area and cannot see the urethral meatus; men recoil at the thought of causing pain by putting something in their penis. Body size, ability to abduct the legs, hand dexterity and vision, mobility, motivation, and support from family/significant others all need to be taken into account. At times, the family member will be responsible for catheterizing; in this situation, all involved need to agree to the treatment plan. Teaching and support are not "one-time" events but require ongoing follow-up and encouragement from the continence nurse. This is particularly important for individuals with progressive diseases such as multiple sclerosis (Wyndaele, 2014).

CLINICAL PEARL

Initial steps in an IC program should include a bladder diary of fluid intake, voided volumes (if able to void), and postvoid catheterization amount.

Knowledge of cystometric bladder capacity and urodynamic results is helpful but not mandatory, depending on the individual's history. Initial assessment should include a bladder diary of fluid intake, voided volumes (if able to void), and postvoid catheterization amount. This will assist in planning the number of times a day for catheterizing as well as the best time—for example, early in the day, the individual may be able to void sufficiently to adequately empty the bladder but may be unable to void by evening. Thus, timing the catheterization(s) to coincide with the individual's personal schedule and clinical needs is a useful first step. In time, most individuals progress to catheterizing three to four times a day. Success in an IC program requires regular follow-up in person and by telephone.

It is not unusual for beginning IC users to develop a UTI. Teaching should include signs and symptoms of UTI and when to call the health care practitioner. Some clinicians start individuals with a short course of antibiotics, but a preferred approach is to treat only symptomatic infections and to base treatment on urine culture results.

If the insurance company provides enough catheters for single use, then people need advice on proper and safe disposal of products. If individuals are reusing their PVC catheters, then teaching on cleaning with soap and water, storage, and reuse will be important. Currently, there are no catheters for IC that can be flushed down the toilet.

Conclusion

Indwelling catheters are a necessary option for specific patient populations. Avoidance of long-term use, if possible, is recommended. Yet when unavoidable, staff and patients need to be educated to ensure that appropriate care and complication minimization is achieved for indwelling catheterization. Selection of equipment, patient education, and early recognition of problems will improve outcomes for this population.

REFERENCES

Afsar, S. I., Yemisci, O. U., Cosar, S. N. S., et al. (2013). Compliance with clean intermittent catheterization in spinal cord injury patients: A long-term follow up study. *Spinal Cord, 51*(8), 645–649.

Ahmed, S. J., Mehta, A., & Rimington, P. (2004). Delayed bowel perforation following suprapubic catheter insertion. *BMC Urology, 4*(16), 1–3. doi:10.1186/1471-2490-4-16.

Averbeck, M. A., & Madersbacher, H. (2011). Constipation and LUTS: How do they affect each other? *International Brazilian Journal of Urology, 37*(1), 16–28. doi:10.1590/S1677-55382011000100003.

Bernard, M. S., Hunter, K. F., & Moore, K. N. (2012). A review of strategies to decrease the duration of indwelling urethral catheters and potentially reduce the incidence of catheter associated urinary tract infections. *Urologic Nursing, 32*(1), 29–37.

Campbell, J. B., Moore, K. N., Voaklander, D. C., et al. (2004). Complications associated with clean intermittent catheterization in children with spina bifida. *Journal of Urology, 171*(6 Pt 1), 2420–2422.

Cardenas, D. D., Moore, K. N., Dannels-McClure, A., et al. (2011). Intermittent catheterization with a hydrophilic-coated catheter delays urinary tract infections in acute spinal injury: A prospective randomised, multicenter trial. *Physical Medicine and Rehabilitation, 3*(5), 408–417.

Carter, N. M., Reitmeier, L., & Goodloe, L. R. (2014). An evidence-based approach to the prevention of catheter-associated urinary tract infections. *Urologic Nursing, 34*(5), 238–245.

Chan, M. F., Tan, H. Y., Lian, X., et al. (2014). A randomized controlled study to compare the 2% lignocaine and aqueous lubricating gels for female urethral catheterization. *Pain Practice, 14*(2), 140–145. doi:10.1111/papr.12056.

Chapple, A., Prinjha, S., & Feneley, R. (2015). Comparing transurethral and suprapubic catheterization for long-term bladder drainage: A qualitative study of the patients' perspective. *Journal of Wound, Ostomy and Continence Nursing, 42*(2), 170–175. doi:10.1097/WON.0000000000000096.

Chartier-Kastler, E., Amarenco, G., Lindbo, L., et al. (2013). A prospective randomized crossover, multicenter study comparing quality of life using compact versus standard catheters for intermittent self-catheterization. *Journal of Urology, 190*(3), 942–947.

Christensen, J., Ostri, P., Frimodt-moller, C., et al. (1987). Intravesical pressure changes during bladder drainage in patients with acute urinary retention. *Urologia Internationalis, 42*(3), 181–184.

Darouiche, R. O., Goetz, L., Kaldis, T., et al. (2006). Impact of StatLock securing device on symptomatic catheter-related urinary tract infection: A prospective, randomized, multicenter clinical trial. *American Journal of Infection Control, 34*(9), 555–560.

De Ridder, D. J. M. K., Everaert, K., Fernandez, L. G., et al. (2005). Intermittent catheterisation with hydrophilic-coated catheters (SpeediCath) reduces the risk of clinical urinary tract infection in spinal cord injured patients: A prospective randomized parallel comparative trial. *European Urology, 48*(6), 991–995.

Donlan, R. M., & Costerton, J. W. (2002). Biofilms: Survival mechanisms of clinically relevant microorganisms. *Clinical Microbiology Reviews, 15*(2), 167–193. doi:10.1128/CMR.15.2.167-193.2002.

Downs, J., Wolfe, T., & Walker, H. (2012). Development of hydronephrosis secondary to poorly managed neurogenic bowel requiring surgical disimpaction in a patient with spinal cord injury: A case report. *Journal of Spinal Cord Medicine, 37*(6), 795–798.

Garbutt, R. B., Taylor, M. D., Lee, V., et al. (2008). Delayed versus immediate urethral catheterization following instillation of local anaesthetic gel. *Emergency Medicine Australasia, 20*(4), 328–332.

Getliffe, K. A., & Mulhall, A. B. (1991). The encrustation of indwelling catheters. *British Journal of Urology, 67*(4), 337–341.

Gonzalez, F. (2010). Obstructive uropathy caused by fecal impaction: Report of 2 cases and discussion. *American Journal of Hospice and Palliative Medicine, 27*(8), 557–559. doi:10.1177/1049909110367784.

Gould, C., Umscheid, C., Agarwal, R., et al.; Healthcare Infection Control Practices Advisory Committee (HICPAC). (2009). In *Guideline for prevention of catheter-associated urinary tract infections.* Atlanta, GA: Centers for Disease Control and Prevention (CDC). Retrieved from http://www.cdc.gov/hicpac/pdf/cauti/cautiguideline2009final.pdf

Gould, F., Cheng, C., & Lapides, J. (1976). Comparison of rapid versus slow decompression of the distended urinary bladder. *Investigative Urology, 14*(2), 156–158.

Groah, S. L., Weitzenkamp, D. A., Lammertse, D. P., et al. (2002). Excess risk of bladder cancer in spinal cord injury: Evidence for an association between indwelling catheter use and bladder cancer. *Archives of Physical Medicine and Rehabilitation, 83*(3), 346–351.

Hagen, S., Sinclair, L., Cross, S. (2010). Washout policies in long-term indwelling urinary catheterisation in adults. *Cochrane Database of Systematic Reviews,* (3), CD004012. doi:10.1002/14651858.CD004012.pub4.

Harrison, S. C. W., Lawrence, W. T., Morley, R., et al. (2011). British Association of Urological Surgeons' suprapubic catheter practice guidelines. *BJU International, 107*(1), 77–85.

Hooton, T., Bradley, S. F., Cardenas, D., et al. (2010). Diagnosis, prevention and treatment of catheter-associated urinary tract infection in adults: 2009 international clinical practice guidelines from the Infectious Diseases Society of America. *Clinical Infections Diseases, 50*(5), 625–663.

Hunter, K. F., Bharmal, B., & Moore, K. N. (2013). Long-term bladder drainage: Suprapubic catheter versus other methods: A scoping review. *Neurourology and Urodynamics, 32*(7), 944–951. doi:10.1002/nau.22356.

Joanna Briggs Institute. (2008). Removal of short-term indwelling urethral catheters. *Nursing Standard, 22*(22), 42–45.

Lam, T. B. L., Omar, M. I., Fisher, E., et al. (2014). Types of indwelling urethral catheters for short-term catheterisation in hospitalised adults. *Cochrane Database of Systematic Reviews,* (9), CD004013. doi:10.1002/14651858.CD004013.pub4.

Ma, A. Y., Hunter, K. F., Rowe, B., et al. (2014). Appropriateness of indwelling urethral catheter insertions in the emergency department (Abstract 317). *Neurourology and Urodynamics, 33*(6), 756–757.

Méndez-Probst, C. E., Razvi, H. R., & Denstedt, J. D. (2012). Fundamentals of instrumentation and urinary tract drainage. In A. J. Wein, L. R. Kavoussi, A. C. Novick, et al. (Eds.), *Campbell-Walsh urology* (pp. 177–191.e4). Philadelphia, PA: Elsevier.

Moore, K. N., Burt, J., & Voaklander, D. C. (2006). Intermittent catheterization in the rehabilitation setting: A comparison of clean and sterile technique. *Clinical Rehabilitation, 20*(6), 461–468.

Mularoni, P., Patrick, M. D., Cohen, L. L., et al. (2009). A randomized clinical trial of lidocaine gel for reducing infant distress during urethral catheterization. *Pediatric Emergency Care, 25*(7), 439–443.

Murphy, C., Fader, M., & Prieto, J. A. (2014). Interventions to minimise the initial use of indwelling urinary catheters in acute care: A systematic review. *International Journal of Nursing Studies, 51*(1), 4–13.

Murphy, C., Prieto, J., Fader, M. (2014). Understanding why clinicians make the decision to place a urinary catheter in acute medical care (Abstract 318). *Neurourology and Urodynamics, 33*(6), 755–756.

Nicolle, L. E. (2014) Catheter associated urinary tract infections. *Antimicrobial Resistance and Infection Control, 3*(23), 1–8. doi:10.1186/2047-2994-3-23.

Nyman, M. A., Schwenk, N. M., & Silverstein, M. D. (1997). Management of urinary retention: Rapid versus gradual decompression and risk of complications. *Mayo Clinic Proceedings, 72*(10), 951–956. doi:10.4065/72.10.951.

Panayi, D. D., Khullar, V., Digesu, G. A., et al. (2012). Rectal distention: The effect on bladder function. *Neurourology and Urodynamics, 30*(3), 344–347.

Parker, D., Callan, L., Harwood, J., et al. (2009). Nursing interventions to reduce the risk of catheter-associated urinary tract infection. *Journal of Wound, Ostomy and Continence Nursing, 36*(1), 23–34.

Pickard, R., Lam, T., Maclennan, G., et al. (2012). Types of urethral catheter for reducing symptomatic urinary tract infections in hospitalised adults requiring short-term catheterisation: Multicentre randomised controlled trial and economic evaluation of antimicrobial- and antiseptic impregnated urethral catheters (the CATHETER trial). *Health Technology Assessment, 16*(47), 1–197. doi:10.3310/hta16470.

Prieto, J., Murphy, C. L., Moore, K. N., et al. (2014). Intermittent catheterisation for long-term bladder management. *Cochrane Database of Systematic Reviews,* (9), CD006008. doi: 10.1002/14651858.CD006008.pub3.

Rovner, E., Dmochowski, R., Chapple, C., et al. (2013). OnabotulinumtoxinA improves urodynamic outcomes in patients with neurogenic detrusor overactivity. *Neurourology and Urodynamics, 32*(8), 1109–1115.

Saint, S., Meddings, J. A., Calfee, D., et al. (2009a). Catheter-associated urinary tract infection and the Medicare rule changes. *Annals of Internal Medicine, 150*(12), 877–884.

Saint, S. J., Olmsted, R. N., Forman, J., et al. (2009b). Translating health care–associated urinary tract infection prevention research into practice via the bladder bundle. *Joint Commission Journal on Quality and Patient Safety/Joint Commission Resources, 35*(9), 449–455.

Schede, J., & Thuroff, J. W. (2006). Effects of intra-urethral injection of anaesthetic gel for transurethral instrumentation. *BJU International, 97*(6), 1165–1167. doi:10.1111/j.1464-410X.2006.06199.x.

Schwab, W. K., Lizdas, D. E., Granvenstein, N., et al. (2014). Foley drainage tubing configuration affects bladder pressure: A bench model study. *Urologic Nursing, 34*(1), 33–37.

Siderias, J., Guadio, F., & Singer, A. J. (2004). Comparison of topical anesthetics and lubricants prior to urethral catheterization in males: A randomized controlled trial. *Academic Emergency Medicine, 11*(6), 703–706.

Smith, P. W., & Rusnak, P. G. (1997). Infection prevention and control in the long-term-care facility. SHEA Long-Term-Care Committee and APIC Guidelines Committee. *American Journal of Infection Control, 25*(6), 488–512.

Stickler, D. J. (2008). Bacterial biofilms in patients with indwelling urinary catheters. *Nature Clinical Practice Urology, 5*(11), 598–608.

Stickler, D., Morris, N., Moreno, M. C., et al. (1998). Studies on the formation of crystalline bacterial biofilms on urethral catheters. *European Journal of Clinical Microbiology and Infectious Diseases, 17*(9), 649–652.

Tzortzis, V., Gravas, S., Melekos, M. M., et al. (2009). Intraurethral lubricants: A critical literature review and recommendations. *Journal of Endourology, 23*(5), 821–826. doi:10.1089/end.2008.0650.

West, D. A., Cummings, J. M., Longo, W. E. E., et al. (1999). Role of chronic catheterization in the development of bladder cancer in patients with spinal cord injury. *Urology, 53*(2), 292–297.

Wilde, M. H., Fader, M., Ostaszkiewicz, J., et al. (2013). A systematic review of urinary bag decontamination for long-term use. *Journal of Wound, Ostomy, and Continence Nursing, 40*(3), 299–308. doi:10.1097/WON.0b013e3182800305.

Wilson, M., Wilde, M., Webb, M. L., et al. (2009). Nursing interventions to reduce the risk of catheter-associated urinary tract infection. Part 2: Staff education, monitoring, and care techniques. *Journal of Wound, Ostomy and Continence Nursing, 36*(2), 137–154.

Wyndaele, J. J. (2002). Complications of intermittent catheterization: Their prevention and treatment. *Spinal Cord, 40*(10), 536–541.

Wyndaele, J. J. (2014). Self-intermittent catheterization in multiple sclerosis. *Annals of Physical and Rehabilitation Medicine, 57*(5), 315–320.

Yılmaz, B., Akkoç, Y., Alaca, R., et al. (2014). Intermittent catheterization in patients with traumatic spinal cord injury: Obstacles, worries, level of satisfaction. *Spinal Cord, 52*(2), 826–830. doi:10.1038/sc.2014.134.

ADDITIONAL RESOURCES

Wound, Ostomy & Continence Nurses Society. (2011). *Suprapubic catheters: Best practice for clinicians.* New Jersey: WOCN.

Wound, Ostomy & Continence Nurses Society. (2009). *Indwelling urinary catheters: Best practice for clinicians.* New Jersey: WOCN.

QUESTIONS

1. For which patient would an indwelling catheter be considered an appropriate management measure?
   A. A patient who is diagnosed with incontinence
   B. A patient who is experiencing urinary retention for the first time
   C. A critically ill patient who requires ongoing monitoring of urine output
   D. Any postoperative patient until normal urinary functioning returns

2. The continence nurse is choosing a catheter for a patient who requires bladder irrigation postoperatively. Which catheter would be the best choice?
   A. Three-way catheter
   B. Two-way catheter
   C. One-piece catheter set
   D. Catheter with a balloon that is 30 mL or larger

3. The continence nurse chooses a coudé-tipped catheter for a patient. What is a usual condition warranting this choice of tips?
   A. Neurogenic bladder
   B. Condition resulting in "mucous production"
   C. Bladder infection
   D. Prostatic hypertrophy

4. The continence nurse is choosing a short-term catheter for a patient who is in an acute care unit. Which catheter is the norm?
   A. Coated latex
   B. Silicone
   C. Antibiotic coated
   D. Silicone coated (silastic)

5. Which potential complication is associated specifically with the use of a suprapubic catheter?
   A. CAUTI
   B. Track closure
   C. Bladder neck injury
   D. Bladder calculi

6. The continence nurse is caring for a patient who presents with asymptomatic bacteriuria (ASB). What treatment would the nurse recommend?
   A. Use of antibiotic meatal ointments.
   B. Flushing of the catheter with acidic solutions.
   C. Instillation of antibiotic into urine drainage bag.
   D. No treatment is required.

7. The continence nurse is caring for a patient whose indwelling catheter has become blocked with blood. What is the initial intervention recommended for this patient?
   A. Remove catheter and call primary care provider.
   B. Remove and replace catheter.
   C. Perform catheter irrigation.
   D. No intervention is required as blood clots pass spontaneously.

8. What question should be prompted when a continence nurse assesses leakage around the catheter?
   A. "Am I using the correct catheter?"
   B. "Is this catheter really necessary?"
   C. "Should this catheter be replaced on a regular schedule?"
   D. "Should this catheter be irrigated on a regular basis?"

9. Which of the following is a recommended guideline for inserting and changing indwelling catheters?
   A. Catheters should be changed as necessary, not at fixed intervals.
   B. Anesthetic gel is not effective for reducing the pain of catheter insertion.
   C. For an individual in bed, drainage tubing must contain dependent loops.
   D. Using a larger catheter helps prevent irreparable bladder neck damage.

10. For which patient would a suprapubic catheter be contraindicated?
    A. A patient with diabetes mellitus
    B. An obese patient
    C. An elderly patient
    D. A pediatric patient

11. What is the most common complication of intermittent catheterization?
    A. Pyelonephritis
    B. Prostatitis
    C. Trauma from catheterization
    D. Urinary tract infection

12. The continence nurse recommends an IC program for a patient choosing to use intermittent catheterization to manage leaking caused by incomplete emptying. What is the initial step when instituting an IC program?
    A. Teaching the patient clean technique
    B. Choosing a catheter size
    C. Keeping a bladder diary
    D. Learning cystometric bladder capacity and urodynamic results

ANSWERS: 1.**C**, 2.**A**, 3.**D**, 4.**A**, 5.**B**, 6.**D**, 7.**C**, 8.**B**, 9.**A**, 10.**B**, 11.**D**, 12.**C**

CHAPTER 14

Physiology of Normal Defecation

JoAnn Ermer-Seltun

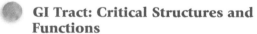
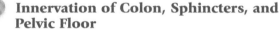
Fecal continence is defined as the ability to control stool elimination, that is, defecation that occurs at a socially appropriate place and time. In contrast, fecal *incontinence* refers to the accidental passage of formed or liquid stool (or gas) at an undesirable time or place. Functional bowel disorders, such as constipation, diarrhea, irritable bowel syndrome, fecal incontinence, or obstructed defecation syndrome, can all result in significant psychosocial morbidity and economic burden (Gorina et al., 2014). In order to properly evaluate and manage functional bowel disorders, the continence specialist must have a fundamental understanding of the anatomical structures and physiologic processes controlling bowel function and stool elimination. This chapter will provide an overview

of the basic structures and function of the small intestine, colon, anorectal unit, anal sphincters, and neural structures critical to normal function and continence and will also provide a discussion of environmental and social factors that impact on bowel function.

CLINICAL PEARL

To evaluate and manage functional bowel disorders, the continence specialist must have a fundamental understanding of the anatomical structures and physiologic processes controlling bowel function and fecal continence.

GI Tract: Critical Structures and Functions

Gastrointestinal tract function has a major impact on the volume and consistency of the stool and is therefore a critical determinant of bowel function and continence.

Small Intestine

The small intestine measures approximately 22 to 23 feet (6 to 7 m) and is subdivided into three functional segments: the duodenum, jejunum, and ileum (Doig & Huether, 2014). The primary function of the small bowel is to digest and absorb life-sustaining nutrients and fluids. It is noteworthy that the terminal ileum (distal 100 cm of ileum) is the only site in the bowel where bile salts and vitamin B_{12}–intrinsic factor complex can be reabsorbed.

Ileocecal Valve

The ileocecal valve is a one-way valve that is located at the junction of the ileum and cecum (the pouch-like structure that is the first segment of the colon and from which the appendix originates). The ileocecal valve controls passage of liquid stool from the small bowel into the colon and prevents retrograde (backward) flow of stool from the colon into the small intestine; this "one-way" flow pattern protects the small bowel against contamination with colonic bacteria (Doig & Huether, 2014).

Colon

The large intestine (colon) is much shorter than the small bowel, measuring approximately 4 to 5 feet or 1.2 to 1.5 m; anatomically, it is seen to "bracket" the small intestine. The colon is divided into the following sections: cecum with attached appendix, colon (ascending, transverse, descending, and sigmoid), rectum, and anal canal. Figures 14-1 and 14-7 depict the sections of the large intestine and its blood supply (Doig & Huether, 2014).

The cecum is located on the lower right side of the abdomen and is the entry point into the large intestine, accepting 500 to >1,000 mL daily from the ileum.

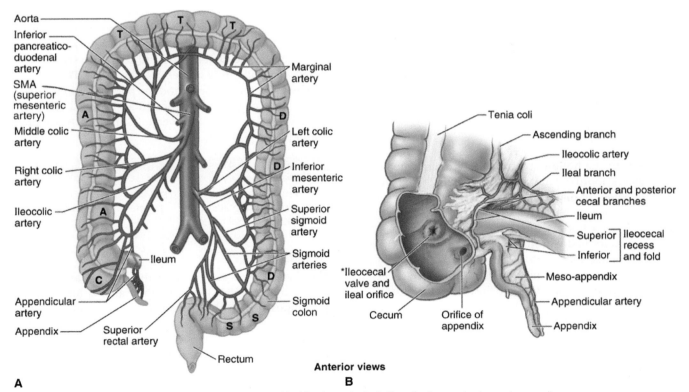

FIGURE 14-1. **A.** Colon and its blood supply. **B.** Orifices for ileocecal valve and appendix.

The cecum in turn drains into the ascending colon, which travels vertically upward on the right side of the abdomen to the hepatic flexure; the colon then makes a left turn to travel transversely across the abdomen along the inferior border of the liver, stomach, and spleen to the splenic flexure (transverse colon). The transverse colon is the primary site for mixing and storage of the fecal mass (Doig & Huether, 2014); the semifluid stool is reduced to a mush-like consistency. The transverse colon is very mobile because it has only two fixation points: one at the hepatic flexure and the other at the splenic flexure. The greater omentum (a vital, fatty intraperitoneal structure) hangs like an apron over the transverse colon and covers the intestinal surface down to the posterior abdominal wall. Once the transverse colon reaches the splenic flexure, it makes a sharp 180-degree turn down and backward to become the descending colon. This section of the colon begins just below the stomach and spleen and continues vertically down the left side of the abdomen until it reaches the level of the iliac crest; at this point, it becomes the sigmoid colon.

As the stool passes from the transverse colon to the sigmoid colon, it is converted from semimushy consistency to a more solid state. The sigmoid colon begins at the iliac crest and extends to the rectum. It resembles an "S-shaped" curvature because it bends more to the left at the distal portion and then curves back around to reach the rectum. This left curvature is the rationale for placing a patient on their left side for digital rectal or endoscopic exam and for giving an enema. Both the descending and sigmoid colon act as a conduit to deliver stool from the transverse colon to the rectum prior to defecation.

CLINICAL PEARL

The transverse colon is the primary site for mixing and storage of the fecal mass.

Rectum and Anal Canal

The rectum is a hollow, expandable, and angulated structure that is approximately 6 inches (15 cm) in length and slightly wider in diameter than the sigmoid colon, which allows it to accommodate stool for temporary storage. There are three folds of rectal mucosa, known as the *valves of Houston*, located within the rectum: the superior (left), middle (right), and inferior (left) rectal valves.

The rectum empties into the anal canal, which begins where the rectum passes through the levator ani muscle and ends at the anal verge (anus); the anal canal measures 1 to 1.5 inches (approximately 3 to 4 cm) in length. The anal canal is normally closed at rest in order to maintain fecal continence. This airtight seal is accomplished through the tonic activity of the anal sphincter complex (internal and external sphincters) and the compressive effect of the anal vascular cushions (venous hemorrhoidal plexus); these structures and their functions will be described in greater

detail later in the chapter. (See Fig. 14-2 for illustrations of the sphincters and venous hemorrhoidal plexus.) In addition, the puborectalis muscle loops around the anal canal and creates a 90-degree anorectal angle that assists in preservation of continence (Mahieu et al., 1984) (Fig. 14-3).

CLINICAL PEARL

The airtight seal characteristic of the anal canal (and critical to continence) is provided by contraction of the anal sphincters, the compressive effect of the anal vascular cushions (hemorrhoidal complex), and the 90-degree anorectal angle provided by the puborectalis muscle, which loops around the anal canal at the anorectal junction.

An important point of reference, the *dentate line*, is located at midpoint in the anal canal. To assist in identification of this midpoint, vertical folds of the mucosa create pillar-like structures called the columns of Morgagni that are located just above the dentate line. The significance of the dentate line is as follows: above this line, the anal canal is lined with columnar epithelium, and distal to the dentate line, it is lined with squamous epithelium, which is richly innervated with sensory receptors. The conversion from columnar to squamous epithelium occurs gradually in the area proximal to the dentate line, and this area is therefore known as the transitional zone. As noted, the squamous epithelium possesses a skin-like structure and sensory nerve fibers and is therefore very sensitive to pain, touch, hot, and cold. In addition, the sensory receptors in the distal anal canal permit differentiation between solid, liquid, and gaseous rectal contents, which is important to continence. This richly innervated area between the dentate line and the anal verge is often called the anoderm (Barleben & Mills, 2010). The dividing line between the anoderm and the perianal skin is known as the anal verge, which is located at the anus. The perianal skin begins at the anal verge (Gordon & Nivatvongs, 2007) (Fig. 14-4).

CLINICAL PEARL

The sensory receptors in the distal anal canal (also known as the anoderm) are able to differentiate between solid, liquid, and gaseous rectal contents.

Anal Sphincters

The anal canal is encircled by the internal and external anal sphincters (EAS). The internal anal sphincter (IAS) is composed of a thick band of smooth muscle within the anal canal that is actually an extension of the circular muscle layer of the rectum. It is about 2.5 to 5 cm long and encloses the anorectal junction and the upper 2 cm of the anal canal (Barleben & Mills, 2010). The IAS chiefly controls continence at rest and is best suited to this momentous task by its composition of slow-twitch, fatigue-resistant smooth muscle fibers (Palit et al., 2012).

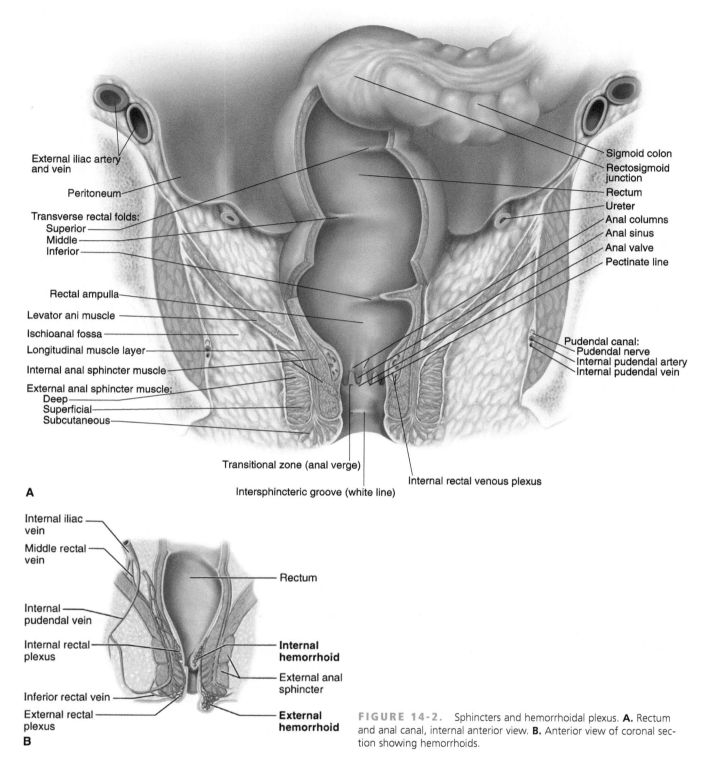

FIGURE 14-2. Sphincters and hemorrhoidal plexus. **A.** Rectum and anal canal, internal anterior view. **B.** Anterior view of coronal section showing hemorrhoids.

Because the IAS is a condensation of the circular muscle, it is primarily innervated by the myenteric plexus; it is also innervated by branches of the ANS and is therefore under involuntary control (Doig & Huether, 2014). In contrast, the EAS is composed of both striated skeletal and smooth muscle and overlaps the IAS. The longitudinal muscle of the rectum comprises the smooth muscle portion of the EAS, while the striated skeletal portion fuses with the puborectalis muscle to form a functional unit. The striated muscle of the EAS can be voluntarily contracted or relaxed; these fibers are innervated by the somatic fibers of the pudendal nerve, which exits the spinal cord at S2, S3, and S4 (Fig. 14-2).

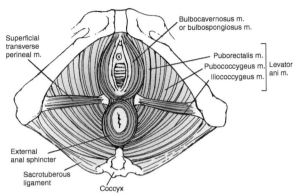

FIGURE 14-3. Puborectalis and levator ani.

CLINICAL PEARL

The internal anal sphincter is chiefly responsible for continence at rest and is well suited for this enormous task because it is composed of slow-twitch, fatigue-resistant muscle fibers.

Blood Supply

Blood supply to the cecum and the ascending and transverse colon is supplied by the superior mesenteric artery, while blood supply to the descending and sigmoid colon and proximal rectum is provided by the inferior mesenteric artery. Blood supply to the distal rectum is provided by the middle and inferior hemorrhoidal arteries. Venous drainage closely mirrors the arterial blood supply (Barleben & Mills, 2010; Doig & Huether, 2014) (Fig. 14-1).

Functions of Colon

The primary functions of the colon are (1) to absorb water, converting the liquid stool into a soft but solid fecal mass containing the waste products of digestion (food residue, unabsorbed GI secretions, shed epithelial cells, and bacteria) and (2) to serve as a reservoir for feces until a suitable time and place for elimination is found. Additional colonic functions are the responsibility of the colonic bacteria, which rise in concentration from the proximal colon to the distal colon. These bacteria play a vital role in functions such as metabolism of bile salts, estrogens, androgens, lipids, and various drugs, the conversion of unabsorbed carbohydrates to absorbable organic acids, and the synthesis of vitamin K and B vitamins (Doig & Huether, 2014).

The bacterial action on unabsorbed carbohydrates is the primary source of the odorous, flammable gas characteristic of the large bowel; swallowed air and the process of blood diffusion contribute lesser volumes of gas. Most of the gut flora are anaerobic bacteria (e.g., *Bacteroides* species and *Clostridium* species); *Escherichia coli* is a prominent gram-negative organism, and gram-positive bacteria

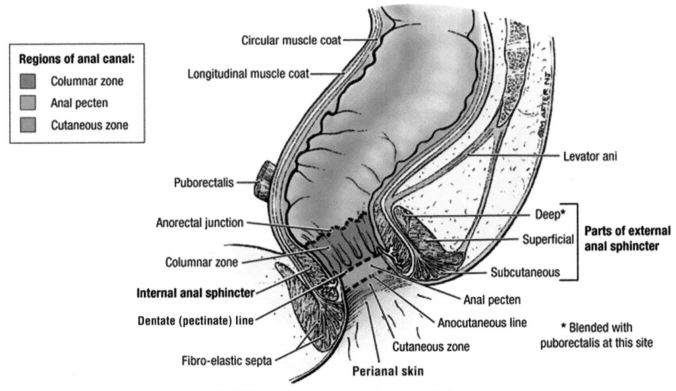

FIGURE 14-4. Rectal and anal mucosa/epithelium.

such as *Enterococcus faecalis, Bifidobacterium bifidum,* and *Staphylococcus aureus* are also present in large numbers (Todar, 2010).

> **CLINICAL PEARL**
>
> The primary functions of the colon are to convert the liquid stool to solid and to serve as a reservoir for feces until a suitable time and place for elimination are found.

Pelvic Floor

The pelvic floor consists of several muscle groups and ligaments that help support the pelvic viscera and promote anal sphincter function (Fig. 14-5); there are many descriptors given to these muscles by authors, which creates confusion even for the most savvy continence specialist. Basically, the pelvic floor is made up of three primary layers: (1) endopelvic fascia, (2) levator ani muscle, and (3) perineal membrane and EAS (Ashton-Miller & Delancey, 2007; Perucchini & DeLancey, 2008; Sampselle & DeLancey, 1998). For the purpose of this chapter, a brief discussion of the pelvic floor muscle as it relates to defecation and fecal continence is provided.

> **CLINICAL PEARL**
>
> The pelvic floor comprises connective tissue and muscles that support the pelvic organs and promote anal sphincter function.

Endopelvic Fascia

The pelvic floor layers must be anchored to the bony structures of the pelvis in order to provide optimal support. The first layer of the pelvic floor is the endopelvic fascia, which is unique in that it is composed of collagen, elastin, and smooth muscle. This fascial layer provides a confluent suspensory apparatus for the pelvic organs by connecting them to the bony pelvis. The endopelvic fascia is intimately linked with the pelvic viscera (soft organs within the pelvis) and with the second layer of the pelvic floor, which creates a secondary source of support for the cervix, vagina, and upper uterus plus indirect support for the bladder and rectum.

Levator Ani

The second layer and the principal source of support for the pelvic floor is the levator ani (Gray & Moore, 2009; Pradidarcheep et al., 2011; Sampselle & DeLancey, 1998). The levator ani is a group of smaller muscles including the iliococcygeus, pubovisceral (also known as the pubococcygeus), and puborectalis muscles, all of which function as a single unit (Figs. 14-3 and 14-5). The pubovisceral muscle is a thick U-shaped muscle that arises from the pubic bones, extends around the posterior rectum, and attaches to the lateral walls of the vagina and rectum. The puborectalis muscle blends with the upper end of the external sphincter and pubovisceral muscle and creates a U-shaped configuration around the anorectal junction (Bharucha, 2006).

The primary function of the pubovisceral and puborectalis muscles is to lift the anus, vagina, and urethra and to pull them forward; this anterior pull creates a compressive force against the lumen of these organs that promotes closure through increased intraurethral, intravaginal, and intra-anal pressures (Pradidarcheep et al., 2011; Sampselle & DeLancey, 1998). Some anatomists specifically label the section of the levator ani muscle complex that creates a U-shaped configuration around the anorectal junction as the puborectalis muscle. This muscle acts as a "sling" around the anorectal junction; at rest, the passive contraction of

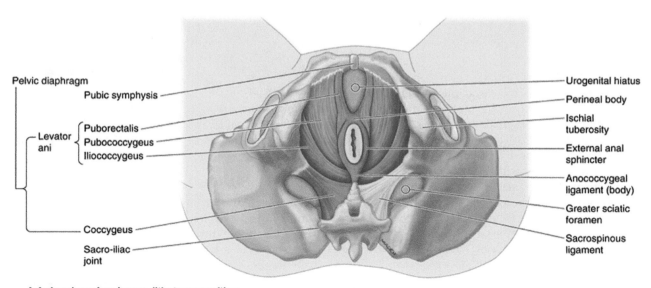

Pelvic diaphragm
Pubic symphysis
Levator ani — Puborectalis / Pubococcygeus / Iliococcygeus
Coccygeus
Sacro-iliac joint

Urogenital hiatus
Perineal body
Ischial tuberosity
External anal sphincter
Anococcygeal ligament (body)
Greater sciatic foramen
Sacrospinous ligament

Inferior view of perineum, lithotomy position

FIGURE 14-5. Structures of the pelvic floor.

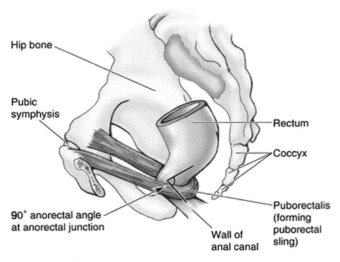

Hip bone

Pubic symphysis

Rectum

Coccyx

90° anorectal angle at anorectal junction

Puborectalis (forming puborectal sling)

Wall of anal canal

Medial view from left

FIGURE 14-6. The anorectal angle.

this muscle creates a 90-degree angle between the rectum and the anal canal that promotes continence (Fig. 14-6). However, with straining, this angle straightens to approximately 135 degrees to promote stool elimination. The iliococcygeus is a thinner muscle that attaches to the pelvic side walls (arcus tendineus) and covers the midplane of the pelvis with a sheet-like layer. In order for the levator ani to function normally and to provide optimal support for pelvic organs, there must be adequate attachment to the arcus tendineus and to the lateral walls of the vagina, rectum, and anus (Pradidarcheep et al., 2011; Sampselle & DeLancey, 1998).

> **CLINICAL PEARL**
>
> The primary support for the pelvic organs is the levator ani, which is actually a group of smaller muscles that function as a single unit.

The levator ani is innervated by the pudendal and levator ani nerve branches of the sacral plexus (Pradidarcheep et al., 2011); these nerves are prone to damage due to stretch injury during vaginal delivery or pelvic surgery (Pradidarcheep et al., 2011). The levator ani complex is composed of both type 1 (slow-twitch) and type 2 (fast-twitch) muscle fibers, with a predominance of Type 1 (70%). This predominance of Type 1 (slow-twitch) muscle fibers provides sustained muscle tone over prolonged periods of time, such as is needed by an individual in the standing position. In contrast, type 2 (fast-twitch) muscle fibers provide rapid, strong contractions of the pelvic muscles that are maintained for only a short period of time; these fibers provide the support needed to offset abrupt increases in intra-abdominal pressures that develop when an individual coughs, sneezes, or lifts something heavy.

Perineal Membrane

The perineal membrane and anal sphincter comprise the third supportive layer of the pelvic floor. The perineal membrane is a triangular fibrous structure that spans the anterior pelvis; the vagina and urethra pass through a central hole in this supportive membrane. The primary function of the perineal membrane is to limit descent of the pelvic organs by attaching the perineal body to the pubic bones. (The perineal body is a fascial/muscle structure that separates the distal vagina and rectum.) The perineal membrane provides secondary support by limiting descent of the perineal body and vagina when the levator ani is relaxed during the processes of defecation, urination, and birth (Sampselle & DeLancey, 1998).

● Histology of Colon Wall

The GI tract consists of four basic layers: mucosa, submucosa, muscularis, and serosa. It is innervated by nerve fibers from the intrinsic (also known as enteric, or within the intestine) and extrinsic (outside of the intestine) nervous systems. There are some unique differences between the histology of the small and large intestine. This chapter will focus on large intestinal histology as it relates more to the elimination process (Doig & Huether, 2014; Heitkemper, 2006) (Fig. 14-7).

Mucosa

The colonic mucosal layer is the innermost layer that comes in contact with fecal contents. It is composed of columnar epithelial cells, which assist in absorbing water, electrolytes (chloride and sodium), glucose, and urea. Intestinal glands known as Lieberkuhn's crypts extend into the deeper mucosa; along with goblet cells, these glands produce secretions that neutralize acids produced by bacteria, lubricate the feces to aid in transport, and protect the mucosa from injury by intraluminal substances. The pH of the stool is alkaline (approximately 7.8) due to the bicarbonate in these secretions. Of interest, stress and anxiety reduce mucus production while bacterial, mechanical, or chemical irritants increase secretion.

Submucosa

The submucosal layer aids in attachment of the muscularis to the mucosal layer. It contains blood and lymphatic vessels, connective tissue, and nerve fibers called Meissner's (or submucosal) plexus.

Muscularis

The muscularis consists of two types of smooth muscle: longitudinal and circular. The longitudinal muscle is gathered into three distinct bands known as the taeniae coli that begin in the ascending colon and continue through the descending colon; at the rectosigmoid junction, these muscle bands fan out to form a complete outer longitudinal layer. The taeniae coli produce a "gathered" appearance because the length of the muscle bands is shorter than the

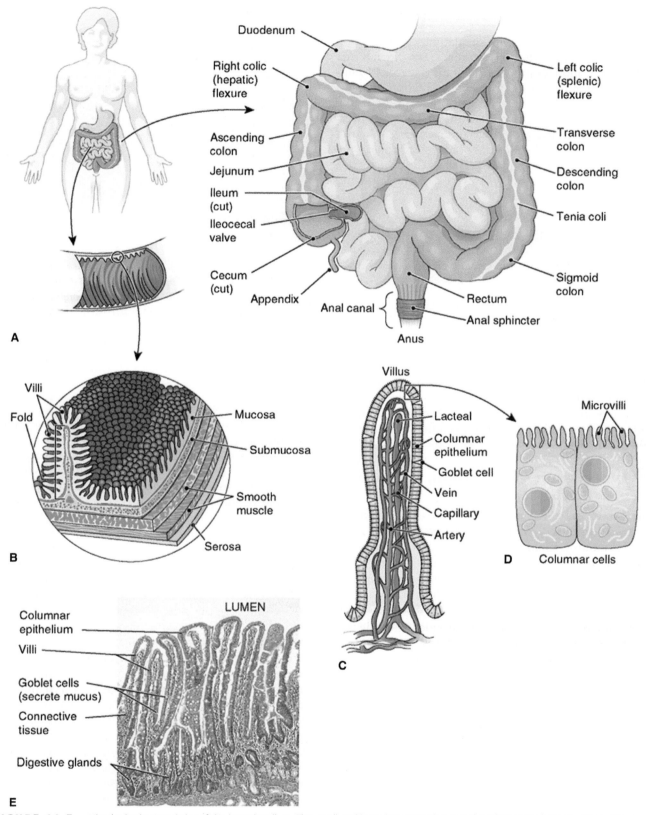

FIGURE 14-7. Histologic characteristics of the bowel wall. **A.** The small and large intestines showing the relationship between them. The small intestine has three sections: the duodenum, jejunum, and ileum. The colon is the main portion of the large intestine. **B.** The wall of the small intestine showing folds in the lining and multiple small villi. **C.** Drawing of a villus showing blood vessels, a lacteal of the lymphatic system, and goblet cells that secrete mucus. **D.** Columnar epithelial cells of the intestine with microvilli, folds of the plasma membrane. **E.** Micrograph of intestinal villi.

actual colon; the circular muscles act to separate the "gathers" and to create outpouchings called haustra. The haustra become more prominent with circular muscle contraction and less prominent during relaxation. The circular and longitudinal muscles produce rhythmic patterns of muscle contraction that promote mixing and fluid/electrolyte absorption as well as transport of stool from the cecum to the anal canal; mixing contractions are known as haustral contractions and propulsive contractions are known as peristaltic waves. The *Auerbach's* or myenteric plexus lies between the two muscle layers and plays the primary role in regulating colonic motility (Palit et al., 2012; Rodriguez et al., 2011).

CLINICAL PEARL

The circular and longitudinal muscle layers work together to mix and dehydrate the stool and to propel the stool distally; mixing contractions are known as haustral contractions and propulsive contractions are known as peristaltic waves.

Serosa

The outermost layer is the serosa. It is made of simple squamous epithelial tissue and is continuous with the mesentery and visceral peritoneum. It secretes a watery serous fluid to reduce friction between the visceral organs and the large intestine.

Innervation of the Colon, Sphincters, and Pelvic Floor

The bowel has three nervous systems that provide an extremely organized, complex, and integrated regulation of colonic motility, sphincter function, and fecal continence. Innervation involves the central nervous system (brain and spinal cord), the sympathetic and parasympathetic branches of the autonomic nervous system (ANS), and the enteric nervous system (ENS) (Fig. 14-8). In addition, the somatic system controls the voluntary muscles and thereby plays a vital role in maintenance of continence and normal defecation (Rodriguez et al., 2011).

CLINICAL PEARL

There are three nervous systems that work to provide integrated regulation of colonic motility, sphincter function, and fecal continence: the central nervous system, the enteric nervous system, and the autonomic nervous system.

Enteric Nervous System

The ENS and the ANS control sensory and motor function of the GI tract. The ENS is the intraintestinal (local)

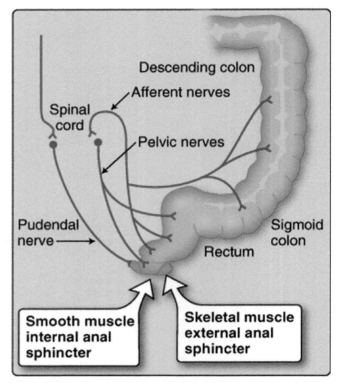

FIGURE 14-8. Innervation of colon, sphincters, and pelvic floor.

nervous system; it consists of sensory neurons, motor neurons, and interneurons that are situated in two primary plexuses: the submucosal (Meissner's) plexus and the myenteric (Auerbach's) plexus, located between the circular and longitudinal muscle layers. The primary function of the submucosal plexus is to detect intraluminal substances (such as irritants), control GI blood flow, and regulate epithelial cell function; the myenteric plexus exerts primary control over colonic motility. Nerve cell clusters or ganglia comprise these intramural nerve plexuses, which are interconnected to allow integration and processing of data and communication between the bowel wall and the ganglia along the entire length of the colon. Sensory neurons process thermal, chemical, osmotic, or mechanical stimuli transmitted by sensory receptors in the mucosa and muscle. For example, chemoreceptors respond to luminal contents by, in essence, "tasting" luminal substances; in contrast, mechanoreceptors within the muscle react to stretch and tension. Motor neurons control gut motility, secretion, and absorption by acting upon smooth muscle and secretory and endocrine cells. Interneurons provide a conduit between sensory neuron information and motor neurons; they "present" sensory information to motor neurons, which often leads to an action or response. For instance, messages from sensory receptors responding to stretch and tension within the bowel wall are relayed through the interneurons to motor neurons, which initiate smooth muscle contraction (peristalsis) (Palit et al., 2012).

Autonomic Nervous System

As stated, the ENS is the primary mediator for colonic motility (peristalsis), but it is augmented by the extrinsic ANS. The sympathetic and parasympathetic nerve fibers from the ANS terminate on the nerve cells of the myenteric and submucosal plexus to modulate colonic motility, by stimulating or inhibiting peristaltic activity. The sympathetic nervous system (SNS) arises from T10 to L2 of the spinal cord and acts to reduce intestinal secretion and motility. In contrast, the parasympathetic nervous system (PNS) arises primarily from S2 to S4 of the spinal cord and acts to promote peristaltic activity, especially in the descending and sigmoid colon (branches of the vagus nerve provide parasympathetic stimulation to the proximal colon, i.e., ascending and transverse colon).

Mass movements (series of peristaltic waves) propel stool into the sigmoid colon or rectum; when the amount of stool is sufficient to trigger rectal distention and the defecation reflex, the elevated intrarectal pressure stimulates reflexive contraction of the rectosigmoid, relaxation of the IAS, and contraction of the EAS. It is hypothesized that this reflexive activity is mediated by the sacral PNS and its outflow tracts. Increased pressure in the rectum stimulates afferent fibers to send messages *from* the rectum *to* the spinal cord and brain, which triggers parasympathetic efferent activity that sends messages *from* the brain *to* the distal bowel to stimulate reflex contractions in the sigmoid and rectum (Doig & Huether, 2014; Palit et al., 2012).

This reflex does not lead to the act of defecation in itself but produces a strong urge or "call to stool." This urge "to go" can be deferred with conscious contraction of the EAS and pelvic floor muscles, which interrupts peristalsis and causes rectal wall relaxation; this results in reduced intrarectal pressure and reduced sense of the need to defecate. The rectum may also displace the stool into the sigmoid by retrograde contraction until a more convenient time for elimination. Interestingly, pain or the fear of pain related to defecation (e.g., patient with fissures, hemorrhoids, or history of severe constipation) may also inhibit the defecation reflex (Doig & Huether, 2014).

Implications

Although the ENS is the primary mediator for colonic motility, the impact of ANS modulation should not be underestimated. For instance, the individual with an S2 spinal cord lesion loses not only their ability to sense rectal distention but also parasympathetic-induced peristalsis of the distal colon; this leads to profound constipation and increased risk for impaction. These individuals also lose voluntary control of the EAS, which is innervated by the pudendal nerve; however, they retain normal innervation of the IAS, which is controlled by the ENS, specifically the myenteric plexus. This is because the ENS is not affected by spinal cord injury.

Factors Affecting/Promoting Continence

Multiple factors may influence GI function, the evacuation process, and fecal continence. The most critical "control" factors include the following:

1. Colonic transit, stool volume, and consistency
2. Sensory awareness
3. Sphincter competence
4. Rectal compliance and capacity
5. Extrinsic factors, such as posture for defecation and cultural norms

Intrinsic factors such as age and comorbidities can also influence bowel function and continence.

Colonic Transit and Stool Volume and Consistency

Colonic transit time is defined as the amount of time it takes for food that enters the gut to be digested and absorbed and for the waste products to be evacuated through the anus. Stool transit time is determined by peristaltic activity, the coordinated colonic contractions that propel stool along the length of the colon and into the rectum; transit time profoundly impacts stool volume and consistency (Degen & Phillips,

1996a). Colonic motor activity demonstrates a predictable pattern: it increases after waking (Rao et al., 2001), is higher during the day than at night (Dinning et al., 2010; Narducci et al., 1987; Rao et al., 2001), and is significantly increased by eating (Bampton et al., 2001; Dinning et al., 2010; Rao et al., 2001), especially after a fatty meal (Rao et al., 2000; Renny et al., 1983). The upper limit for normal transit time is around 72 hours in adults (Spanish Group for the Study of Digestive Motility, 1998), whereas in children, it is faster, around 57 hours (Weaver, 1988). Of interest, transit time is reduced (i.e., faster) by coffee consumption (with effects equal to that of a meal) (Rao et al., 1998), fatty meals (Rao et al., 2000; Renny et al., 1983), and fecal contents with a high osmotic load (e.g., as occurs with bile salt malabsorption or lactose intolerance) (Rao, 2004), and increased (i.e., slower) with protein-rich meals (Battle et al., 1980; Wright et al., 1980) and alcohol (Berenson & Avner, 1981; Bouchoucha et al., 1991). Men have faster transit time than women (Stewart et al., 1999; Meier et al., 1995), and individuals over 65 usually have slower transit time and increased risk of constipation due to a multitude of factors (Chatoor & Emmnauel, 2009).

Intuitively, loose stools are usually associated with reduced (faster) transit time, due to the reduction in time for water absorption; this perception has been confirmed by some studies. In contrast, constipation is usually associated with slow gut motility and increased (slower) transit time; this provides increased time for water absorption, which results in smaller caliber and drier stools, both of which are risk factors for disordered defecation (Palit et al., 2012). Certainly, individuals with diarrhea have a greater potential for fecal incontinence since the rapid delivery of loose and large-volume stool may overwhelm the continence mechanism. However, frequency of stool elimination is poorly correlated with colonic transit time, possibly because individuals with constipation may make several attempts to evacuate stool (Dinning et al., 2011; Saad et al., 2010), passing only small amounts each time; in contrast, the individual with soft bulky stool may report less frequent but higher-volume bowel movements. Interestingly, Bannister et al. (1987a) demonstrated that stool size and the amount of time needed for stool evacuation are inversely related; more time and effort are required for defecation of small, hard stools (pellet-like) as compared to soft formed stools. Although not well studied, the postulated "ideal" stool for facilitation of defecation is about 2 cm in diameter and is formed but not dry (Heitkemper, 2006). In general, the frequency of normal defecation ranges anywhere from three stools per day to three stools per week as long as there is no discomfort and no excessive straining, and continence is preserved (Schaefer & Cheskin, 1998).

CLINICAL PEARL

The postulated "ideal stool" in terms of facilitated defecation is about 2 cm in diameter and is formed but not dry.

Sensory Awareness

The ability to recognize rectal filling promptly and to determine the type of rectal contents accurately is critical to the normal defecation process and the maintenance of continence. This perception of rectal distention and correct classification of rectal contents (gas, liquid, or solid) is provided by stretch receptors in the rectum and pelvic floor and sensory receptors in the anal canal. As previously discussed, colonic distention triggers afferent sensory (stretch) receptors in the rectum and pelvic floor muscles, which transmit the message to the spinal cord; it is then passed to the cerebral cortex, where it elicits conscious recognition of the distention and the "call to stool." The anal canal distal to the dentate line contains numerous epithelial sensory receptors that are able to distinguish between gas (flatus), liquid, and solid stool; this is known as the sampling reflex. (The sampling reflex occurs when rectal distention causes brief relaxation of the internal sphincter, which allows rectal contents to pass into the anal canal; the receptors in the distal anal canal then "sample" the contents and provide feedback to the individual as to type.)

Any damage to the stretch receptors, sensory receptors in the anoderm, neurologic pathways, or cognition will alter sensory awareness of rectal distention and type of contents and may compromise continence. For instance, if a person repeatedly defers the "call to stool," over time, their sensory awareness of rectal distention becomes blunted (limited). In fact, it may lead to a vicious cycle of chronic rectal distention (megarectum), constipation, and even fecal impaction. Habitually ignoring the urge "to go" may also alter or reduce cognitive processing of the urge sensation (Scott et al., 2011). This "conditioning" behavior can occur in children (as is seen in retentive encopresis) (see Chapter 17) as well as adults (Richards et al., 2010); the end results are reduced stool frequency and volume and increased rectosigmoid transit time. This supports the concept that constipation can be a "learned" behavior (Klauser et al., 1990). Other causes of reduced sensory awareness of the "call to stool" include neurologic conditions (e.g., diabetic neuropathy, MS, SCI, myelomeningocele), cognitive impairment (inability to appropriately interpret sensory messages to the CNS), and anorectal lesions (e.g., large hemorrhoids or rectal prolapse).

CLINICAL PEARL

Sensory awareness of rectal distention is provided by stretch receptors in the rectal wall and pelvic floor muscles; accurate differentiation among gas, liquid, and solid stool is provided by the sensory receptors in the anal canal.

Sphincter Competence: IAS and EAS

Normal sphincter function is essential to continence and involves both the IAS, which is under involuntary control, and the EAS, which can be voluntarily contracted.

Internal Anal Sphincter

The IAS is responsible for up to 85% of anal tone and predominantly responsible for continence at rest (Frenckner, 1975; Heitkemper, 2006). It is composed of slow-twitch, fatigue-resistant smooth muscle fibers, and "at rest," it is tonically contracted. The IAS relaxes in response to rectal distention. This involuntary, reflexive response is known as the rectoanal inhibitory reflex. This reflex also allows the sensory receptors in the anal canal to "sense" (or "taste") the rectal contents and to determine consistency (gas, liquid, or solid stool); this is called the sampling reflex, as already explained. In healthy individuals, it has been determined that the sampling reflex occurs seven times per hour (Miller et al., 1988b); it occurs less often in those who suffer from fecal incontinence (Miller et al., 1988a). The function of the IAS (and thus the sampling reflex) is primarily controlled by the ENS, specifically the myenteric plexus; as already explained, the branches of the ANS also contribute to innervation of the IAS. There is no sensorimotor innervation of the IAS; it is therefore under involuntary control (Doig & Huether, 2014; Frenckner, 1975; Meunier & Mollard, 1977). Sympathetic stimulation, which occurs via the hypogastric plexus that exits the cord at T10 to L2, causes release of norepinephrine and contraction of the IAS. In contrast, parasympathetic stimulation (via the pelvic plexus that exits the cord at S2 to S4) causes release of acetylcholine and reflexive relaxation of the IAS (Cook et al., 2001; Doig & Huether, 2014).

CLINICAL PEARL

The IAS relaxes in response to rectal distention (rectoanal inhibitory reflex); this permits contact between the anoderm and the rectal contents and the "sampling reflex."

External Anal Sphincter

The EAS is composed of both striated and smooth muscle and is innervated primarily by the somatic fibers of the pudendal nerve, which exits the spinal cord at S2, S3, and S4. A gentle stroke with a finger or cotton swab at the 3 and 9 o'clock position will elicit an observable quick contraction of the EAS, known as the "anal wink"; this assures pudendal innervation is intact. The EAS is also in a state of constant tonic contraction at rest, producing up to 30% of the resting anal tone (Lestar et al., 1989). The anal vascular cushions (hemorrhoidal plexus) also contribute to resting tone; more importantly, they provide the airtight seal that cannot be obtained by sphincteric tone alone (Lestar et al., 1989; Palit et al., 2012). One of the unique characteristics of the EAS is the tonic contraction provided by the sacral reflex. This sacral reflex activity is enhanced during activities that increase intra-abdominal and intrarectal pressure (e.g., coughing, lifting, and standing). In addition, the skeletal muscle components of the EAS can be voluntarily contracted, which doubles the anal canal pressure; this typically elevates anal canal pressure to a level that exceeds intrarectal

pressures, thus maintaining continence until the individual reaches an appropriate time and place for defecation. Maximum voluntary contraction of the EAS can be maintained for a limited time (1 to 3 minutes maximally); thus, adequate rectal capacity and compliance are required to maintain continence past the point at which the EAS begins to fatigue and anal canal pressures begin to decrease (Heitkemper, 2006). Because the EAS plays a critical role in maintaining continence during periods of rectal distention, any injury to the muscle itself or to the nerves innervating the muscle is likely to cause some level of fecal incontinence.

CLINICAL PEARL

The EAS has both reflex tone and voluntary contractility; strong contraction of the EAS and pelvic floor doubles the pressure in the anal canal and permits the individual to delay defecation until a socially appropriate time and place.

Impact of Sphincter Damage/Denervation

Damage to the IAS is likely to result in incontinence of gas and liquid stool, while injuries to or denervation of the EAS is commonly associated with "urge incontinence," that is, inability to maintain anal canal closure and continence during periods of rectal distention and fecal urgency. (Individuals with EAS damage or denervation report knowing when they have stool in the rectum, but being unable to "hold it," especially if the stool is mushy or liquid). If the EAS is severely denervated or totally disrupted, the individual may experience complete fecal incontinence, that is, involuntary passage of formed stool (Rao, 2004).

Rectal Capacity and Compliance

The rectum is a distensible organ that has the ability to act as a storage reservoir when defecation needs to be delayed. The reservoir is normally compliant, which enables it to store stool at relatively low pressure. Once the EAS returns to a resting state, the intrarectal pressure must drop to a level lower than that of the anal canal if continence is to be preserved; this requires both compliance (stretch) and capacity. The mechanisms responsible for normal compliance and capacity are complex and not well understood. Sensory awareness of rectal filling may occur at volumes as low as 11 to 68 mL, and rectal capacity usually ranges from 250 to 510 mL; once capacity is reached, intrarectal pressures rise significantly and defecation becomes imminent.

On average, rectal pressure begins to increase at about 300 mL; when capacity is approached and rectal pressures rise significantly, the defecation reflex is activated as explained previously (i.e., the IAS opens and there is increased peristaltic activity in the rectosigmoid that results in stool elimination unless the individual voluntarily contracts the EAS to delay defecation) (Heitkemper, 2006). Any increase or decrease in rectal capacity and compliance places the individual at risk for bowel dysfunction or fecal incontinence;

that is, increased rectal capacity and compliance are seen in those who habitually ignore the defecation urge, while reduced rectal capacity and compliance are experienced by those who suffer from inflammatory bowel disease or other inflammatory conditions of the anorectum. Individuals with inflammatory anorectal conditions experience intense fecal urgency and frequency and possibly incontinence due to loss of rectal capacity and compliance; they typically report that they can "hold it" only briefly and that if they cannot get to the bathroom quickly, they experience incontinence (Bharucha, 2006). Chapters 15 and 16 provide an in-depth discussion of bowel dysfunction and fecal incontinence.

> **CLINICAL PEARL**
>
> Normally, the rectum is a distensible compliant organ, allowing it to store stool at low intrarectal pressures.

Extrinsic and Intrinsic Factors

Additional factors that affect defecation and continence include posture, cultural norms, gender, and age (Palit et al., 2012). Posture is of particular importance and is determined primarily by cultural norms. To facilitate defecation, the anorectal angle must straighten from 90 to 135 degrees; this occurs when the sphincter and pelvic floor are voluntarily relaxed and the individual contracts the abdominal muscles via straining (Fig. 14-9). Research involving defecography (simulation of defecation with a stool-like substitute under fluoroscopic screening) has shown that a squat position facilitates straightening of the anorectal angle and promotes movement of stool from the rectum into the anal canal (Sikirov, 2003; Tagart, 1966). One could appreciate the importance of this position if asked to pass stool on a bed pan while in a supine position.

The position for defecation is most often dictated by cultural factors. For instance, in Africa and Asia, a squatting position is standard, because defecation occurs over a hole or low-lying receptacle on the floor; in contrast, in Western countries, sitting on a standard toilet/commode is the norm. In a study comparing a Western style commode to a standard toilet with a 10-cm footstool and to the squatting position, the squatting position offered the fastest and

most complete stool evacuation while the standard toilet without the stool provided the least optimal evacuation (Sikirov, 2003). Moreover, and not surprisingly, studies that compared defecation in a sitting to lying down position demonstrated better evacuation in the sitting position (Barnes & Lennard-Jones, 1985; Rao et al., 2006). Other extrinsic factors have been reported to affect bowel habits and GI function, including psychobehavioral factors such as psychological impairment (Dykes et al., 2001; Nehra et al., 2000; Wald et al., 1989), history of traumatic life events including sexual and physical abuse (Drossman et al., 1995; Leroi et al., 1995), coercive toilet training (Palit et al., 2012), stress and anxiety (Palit et al., 2012), lack of privacy or toilet substitute (Kamm, 2006), and dietary intake and pharmaceuticals that reduce gut motility.

> **CLINICAL PEARL**
>
> Squatting is reported to be the best posture for defecation because it promotes straightening of the anorectal angle and movement of stool from the rectum to the anal canal.

Intrinsic factors such as age and gender may also impact defecation and continence (Palit et al., 2012). Epidemiological studies report several spikes in the occurrence of constipation; the first occurs during infancy, with the transition from breast milk to formula, the second during early childhood (between 3 and 5 years of age) (Del Ciampo et al., 2002), and the third after the age of 60 to 65 (Sandler et al., 1990; Sonnenberg & Koch, 1989). Minimal functional changes have been documented within the GI tract as a result of aging; however, loss of tissue elasticity within the rectoanal unit (Bannister et al., 1987b), pelvic floor weakness and laxity (Ryhammer et al., 1996), prolonged intestinal transit time (Doig & Huether, 2014), increased occurrence of neuropathy (Bartolo et al., 1983), changes in mobility and/or cognition, and polypharmacy (Chatoor & Emmnauel, 2009) may negatively impact evacuation of stool.

With regard to gender, constipation is reported to be higher in women. It is postulated that this preponderance of female constipation may be related to slower colonic transit time in comparison to men (Degen & Phillips, 1996b; Meier et al., 1995), the influence of female hormones (Heaton et al., 1992) and the menstrual cycle (Celik et al., 2001; Fukuda et al., 2005), and the effects of pregnancy and childbirth on pelvic floor function (Kepenekci et al., 2011; Ryhammer et al., 1996; van Ginkel, et al., 2003). Of note, Gorina et al. (2014) studied fecal incontinence in noninstitutionalized individuals age 65 or over and found no statistical difference in the incidence of bowel leakage related to age, gender, or race.

Process of Normal Defecation

In the process of normal defecation (Fig. 14-10), the liquid stool that enters the cecum from the small bowel undergoes a gradual change to solid consistency as the

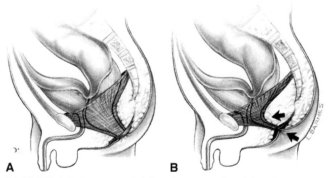

FIGURE 14-9. Normal defecation. **A.** During defecation. **B.** During sphincter contraction.

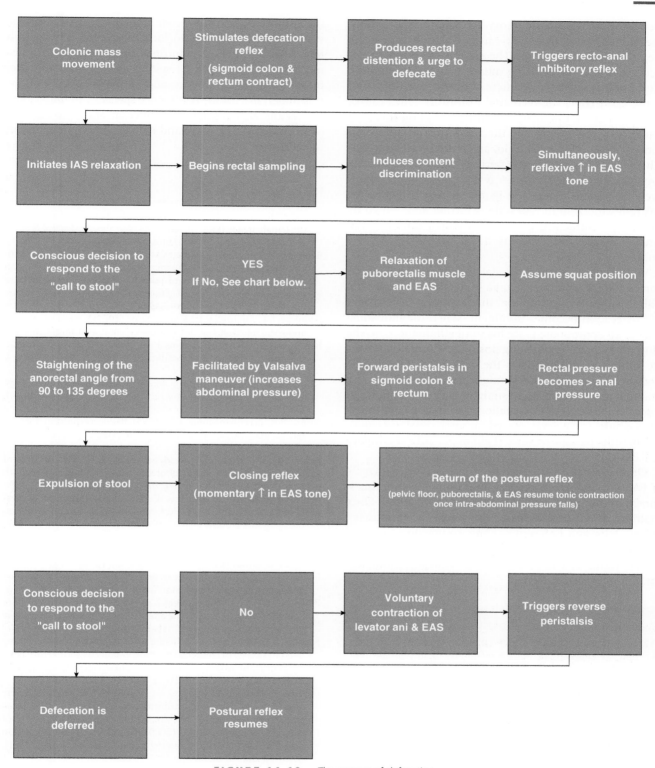

FIGURE 14-10. The process of defecation.

colonic contents are mixed and slowly propelled from the proximal to the distal colon. Complex colonic motility patterns facilitate this transition and transport; haustral contractions provide mixing and absorption of water, thus converting the stool from liquid to solid, and peristaltic waves provide progressive slow movement from the ascending to the transverse colon. As noted, stool is primarily stored in the transverse colon until just prior to defecation, at which point a series of peristaltic contractions known as mass movements rapidly propel the stool from the transverse colon to the rectum. The sudden rectal distention causes the urge to defecate (i.e., the "call to stool"). (The stretch receptors in the rectal wall and surrounding muscles are considered the source of this sensory awareness of the need to defecate.) At the same time, the rectoanal inhibitory reflex causes relaxation of the IAS, which permits "sampling" of rectal contents by the receptors in the anoderm and differentiation between gaseous, liquid, and solid rectal contents. While the IAS is relaxing to permit "sampling," there is a reflex increase in EAS tone; if the individual is cognitively intact and defecation is not socially appropriate, this reflex increase in EAS tone is further augmented by voluntary contraction of the EAS, which doubles anal canal pressure and prevents distal propulsion of the stool.

With limited levels of rectal distention, the relaxation of the IAS and intense urge to defecate are transient; with high levels of distention, the relaxation is persistent and defecation becomes imminent. When the individual reaches an appropriate place for stool elimination, he/she assumes a squatting or sitting position, voluntarily relaxes the sphincter, and contracts the abdominal muscles via straining (Valsalva). The sitting/squatting position and straining maneuver result in straightening of the anorectal angle, which facilitates evacuation, and increased intrarectal pressure (to a level exceeding anal canal pressure); this permits passage of stool (Palit et al., 2012; Rodriguez et al., 2011).

Once evacuation is complete, there is a brief increase in EAS activity, which triggers anal canal closure; this is known as the "closing reflex" (Brookes et al., 2009). Once straining and Valsalva cease, the pelvic floor muscles, puborectalis, and EAS resume tonic contraction (postural reflex), and the anorectal angle returns to 90 degrees; thus, the anorectal unit is returned to a "storage/continence" condition (Porter, 1962).

CLINICAL PEARL

Stool is stored in the transverse colon until just prior to defecation, at which point mass movements rapidly propel the stool into the rectum; this causes sudden distention, sensory awareness of the need to defecate, relaxation of the IAS, and contraction of the EAS.

Conclusion

Normal defecation and fecal continence require the integrated function of a variety of structures and processes. Specifically, the individual must have sensory awareness of rectal distention, the ability to control stool elimination via sphincter control, and the ability to store stool temporarily, which requires normal rectal capacity and compliance. These functions are orchestrated by voluntary and involuntary neural pathways that control peristalsis,

the sphincters, and the pelvic floor musculature; critical structures and pathways include the central nervous system, ANS, and ENS. Any intrinsic or extrinsic factor causing dysfunction of the GI system can dramatically alter bowel function, continence, and ultimately quality of life. It is imperative for the continence specialist to understand the factors affecting GI tract function and defecation in order to accurately assess and manage any dysfunction or incontinence.

REFERENCES

Ashton-Miller, J. A., & DeLancey, J. O. (2007). Functional anatomy of the female pelvic floor. *Annals of the New York Academy of Sciences 1101*, 266–296. doi: 10.1196/annals.1389.034

Bampton, P., Dinning, P., Kennedy, M., et al. (2001). Prolonged multipoint recording of colonic manometry in the unprepared human colon: Providing insight into potentially relevant pressure wave parameters. *American Journal of Gastroenterology, 96*(6), 1838–1848. doi: 10.1111/j.1572-0241.2001.03924.x

Bannister, J. J., Abouzekry, L., & Read, N. W. (1987a). Effect of aging on ano-rectal function. *Gut, 28*(3), 353–357. doi: 10.1136/gut.28.3.353

Bannister, J. J., Davison, P., Timms, J. M., et al. (1987b). Effect of stool size and consistency on defecation. *Gut, 28*(10), 1246–1250. doi: 10.1136/gut.28.10.1246

Barleben, A., & Mills, S. (2010). Anorectal anatomy and physiology. *Surgical Clinics of North America, 90*(1), 1–15. doi: 10.1016/j.suc.2009.09.001

Barnes, P. R., & Lennard-Jones, J. E. (1985). Balloon expulsion from the rectum in constipation of different types. *Gut, 26*(10), 1049–1052. doi: 10.1136/gut.26.10.1049

Bartolo, D. C., Jarratt, J. A., Read, M. G., et al. (1983). The role of partial denervation of the puborectalis in idiopathic fecal incontinence. *British Journal of Surgery, 70*(11), 664–667.

Battle, W. M., Cohen, S., & Snape, W. J., Jr. (1980). Inhibition of postprandial colonic motility after ingestion of an amino acid mixture. *Digestive Diseases and Sciences, 25*(9), 647–652. doi: 10.1007/BF01308322.

Berenson, M. M., & Avner, D. L. (1981). Alcohol inhibition of rectosigmoid motility in humans. *Digestion, 20*(4), 210–215.

Bharucha, A. E. (2006). Update of tests of colon and rectal structure and function. *Journal of Clinical Gastroenterology, 40*(2), 96–103.

Bouchoucha, M., Nalpas, B., Berger, M., et al. (1991). Recovery from disturbed colonic transit time after alcohol withdrawal. *Diseases of the Colon and Rectum, 34*(2), 111–114. doi: 10.1007/BF02049982

Brookes, S. J., Dinning, P. G., & Gladman, M. A. (2009). Neuroanatomy and physiology of colorectal function and defaecation: From basic science to human clinical studies. *Neurogastroenterology and Motility, 21*(Suppl 2), 9–19. doi: 10.1111/j.1365-2982.2009.01400.x

Celik, A. F., Turna, H., Pamuk, G. E., et al. (2001). How prevalent are alterations in bowel habits during menses? *Diseases of the Colon and Rectum, 44*(2), 300–301. doi: 10.1007/BF02234310

Chatoor, D., & Emmnauel, A. (2009). Constipation and evacuation disorders. *Best Practice & Research Clinical Gastroenterology, 23*(4), 517–530. doi: 10.1016/j.bpg.2009.05.001

Cook, T. A., Brading, A. F., & Mortensen, N. J. (2001). The pharmacology of the internal anal sphincter and new treatments of anorectal disorders. *Alimentary Pharmacology and Therapeutics, 15*(7), 887–898. doi: 10.1046/j.1365-2036.2001.00995.x

Degen, L. P., & Phillips, S. F. (1996a). How well does stool form reflect colonic transit? *Gut, 39*(1), 109–113. doi: 10.1136/gut.39.1.109

Degen, L. P., & Phillips, S. F. (1996b). Variability of gastrointestinal transit in healthy women and men. *Gut, 39*(2), 299–305. doi: 10.1136/gut.39.2.299

Del Ciampo, I. R., Galvao, L. C., Del Ciampo, L. A., et al. (2002). Prevalence of chronic constipation in children at a primary health care unit. *Jornal de Pediatria (Rio J), 78*(6), 497–502. doi: org/10.2223/JPED.906

Dinning, P. G., Hunt, L., Lubowski, D. Z., et al. (2011). The impact of laxative use upon symptoms in patients with proven slow transit constipation. *BMC Gastroenterology, 11*(1), 121–127. doi: 10.1186/1471-230X-11-121

Dinning, P. G., Zarate, N., Szczeniak, M. M., et al. (2010). Bowel preparation affects the amplitude and spatiotemporal organization of colonic propagating sequences. *Neurogastroenterology and Motility, 22*(6), 633–e176. doi: 10.1111/j.1365-2982.2010.01480.x

Doig, A. K., & Huether, S. E. (2014). Structure and function of the digestive system. In K. L. McCance, & S. E. Huether (Eds.), *Pathophysiology: The biologic basis for disease in adults and children* (7th ed., pp. 1393–1422). St. Louis, MO: Elsevier.

Drossman, D. A., Talley, N. J., Leserman, J., et al. (1995). Sexual and physical abuse and gastrointestinal illness. Review and recommendations. *Annals of Internal Medicine, 123*(10), 782–794.

Dykes, S., Smilgin-Humphreys, S., & Bass, C. (2001). Chronic idiopathic constipation: A psychological enquiry. *European Journal of Gastroenterology & Hepatology, 13*(1), 39–44.

Frenckner, B. (1975). Function of the anal sphincters in spinal man. *Gut, 16*(8), 638–644. doi: 10.1136/gut.16.8.638

Fukuda, S., Matsuzaka, M., Takahashi, I, et al. (2005). Bowel habits before and during menses in Japanese women of climacteric age: A population based study. *The Tohoku Journal of Experimental Medicine, 206*(2), 99–104. doi: 10.1620/tjem.206.99

Gordon, P. H., & Nivatvongs, S. (2007). *Principles and practice of surgery for the colon, rectum, and anus* (3rd ed.). New York, NY: Informa Healthcare.

Gorina, Y., Schappert, S., Bercovitz, A., et al. (2014). *Prevalence of incontinence among older Americans.* Vital Health Statistics. Series 3, # 36. Washington, DC: National Center for Health Statistics, Department of Health and Human Services.

Gray, M., & Moore, K. N. (2009). Atlas of genitourinary anatomy and physiology. In M. Gray & K. N. Moore (Eds.), *Urologic disorders: Adult and pediatric care* (pp. 12–43). St. Louis, MO: Mosby.

Heaton, K. W., Radvan, J., Cripps, H., et al. (1992). Defecation frequency and timing, and stool form in the general population: A prospective study. *Gut, 33*(6), 818–824. doi: 10.1136/gut.33.6.818

Heitkemper, M. M. (2006). Physiology of bowel function. In D. B. Doughty (Ed.), *Urinary & fecal incontinence: Current management concepts* (3rd ed., pp. 413–434). St. Louis, MO: Mosby.

Kamm, M. A. (2006). Clinical case: Chronic constipation. *Gastroenterology, 131*(1), 233–239. doi: 10.1053/j.gastro.2006.05.027

Kepenekci, I., Keskinkilic, B., Akinsu, F., et al. (2011). Prevalence of pelvic floor disorders in the female population and the impact of age, mode of delivery, and parity. *Diseases of the Colon & Rectum, 54*(1), 85–94.

Klauser, A. G., Voderholzer, W. A., Heinrich, C. A., et al. (1990). Behavioral modification of colonic function. Can constipation be learned? *Digestive Diseases and Sciences, 35*(10), 1271–1275. doi: 10.1007/BF01536418

Leroi, A. M., Bernier, C., Watier, A., et al. (1995). Prevalence of sexual abuse among patients with functional disorders of the lower gastrointestinal tract. *International Journal of Colorectal Disease, 10*(4), 200–206. doi: 10.1007/BF00346219

Lestar, B., Penninckx, F., & Kerremans, R. (1989). The composition of anal basal pressure. An in vivo and in vitro study in man. *International Journal of Colorectal Disease, 4*(2), 118–122. doi: 10.1007/BF01646870

Mahieu, P., Pringot, J., & Bodart, P. (1984). Defecography: I. Description of a new procedure and results in normal patients. *Gastrointestinal Radiology, 9*(3), 247–251. doi: 10.1007/BF01887845

Meier, R., Beglinger, C., Dederding, J., et al. (1995). Influence of age, gender, hormonal status and smoking habits on colonic transit time. *Neurogastroenterology and Motility, 7*(4), 235–238. doi: 10.1111/j.1365-2982.1995.tb00231.x

Meunier, P., & Mollard, P. (1977). Control of the internal anal sphincter (manometric study with human subjects). *Pflügers Archive: European Journal of Physiology, 370*(3), 233–239. doi: 10.1007/BF00585532

Miller, R., Bartolo, D. C., Cervero, F., et al. (1988a). Anorectal sampling: A comparison of normal and incontinent patients. *British Journal of Surgery, 75*(1), 44–47. doi: 10.1002/bjs.1800750116

Miller, R., Lewis, G. T., Bartolo, D. C., et al. (1988b). Sensory discrimination and dynamic activity in the anorectum: Evidence using a new ambulatory technique. *British Journal of Surgery, 75*(10), 1003–1007. doi: 10.1002/bjs.1800751018

Narducci, F., Bassotti, G., Gaburri, M., et al. (1987). Twenty four hour manometric recording of colonic motor activity in healthy man. *Gut, 28*(1), 17–25. doi: 10.1136/gut.28.1.17

Nehra, V., Bruce, B. K., Rath-Harvey, D. M., et al. (2000). Psychological disorders in patients with evacuation disorders and constipation in a tertiary practice. *American Journal of Gastroenterology, 95*(7), 1755–1758. doi: 10.1111/j.1572-0241.2000.02184.x

Palit, S., Lunniss, P. J., & Scott, S. M. (2012). The physiology of human defecation. *Digestive Diseases and Sciences, 57*(6), 1445–1464. doi: 10.1007/s10620-012-2071-1

Perucchini, D. & DeLancey, J. (2008). Functional anatomy of the pelvic floor and lower urinary tract. In K. Baessler, K. L. Burgio, P. A. Norton, B. Schüssler, K. H. Moore, & S. L. Stanton (Eds.), *Pelvic floor re-education* (2nd ed., pp. 3–21). London: Springer Verlag.

Porter, N. H. (1962). A physiological study of the pelvic floor in rectal prolapse. *Annals of the Royal College of Surgeons of England, 31*(6), 379–404.

Pradidarcheep, W., Wallner, C., Dabhoiwala, N. F., et al. (2011). Anatomy and histology of the lower urinary tract. In K. E. Andersson & M. C. Michel (Eds.), *Urinary tract, handbook of experimental pharmacology* (pp. 117–148). Berlin, Heidelberg, Germany: Springer-Verlag.

Rao, S. S. (2004). Pathophysiology of adult fecal incontinence. *Gastroenterology, 126*(1 Suppl 1), S14–S22. doi: 10.1053/j.gastro.2003.10.013

Rao, S. S., Kavlock, R., Beaty, J., et al. (2000). Effects of fat and carbohydrate meals on colonic motor response. *Gut, 46*(2), 205–211. doi: 10.1136/gut.46.2.205

Rao, S. S., Kavlock, R., & Rao, S. (2006). Influence of body position and stool characteristics on defecation in humans. *The American Journal of Gastroenterology, 101*(12), 2790–2796. doi: 10.1111/j.1572-0241.2006.00827.x

Rao, S. S., Sadeghi, P., Beaty, J., et al. (2001). Ambulatory 24-h colonic manometry in healthy humans. *American Journal of Physiology. Gastrointestinal and Liver Physiology, 280*(4), G629–G639.

Rao, S. S., Welcher, L., Zimmerman, B., et al. (1998). Is coffee a colonic stimulant? *European Journal of Gastroenterology & Hepatology, 10*(2), 113–118.

Renny, A., Snape, W. J. Jr., Sun, E. A., et al. (1983). Role of cholecystokinin in the gastrocolonic response to a fat meal. *Gastroenterology, 85*(1), 17–21.

Richards, M. M., Banez, G. A., Dohil, R., et al. (2010). Chronic constipation, atypical eating pattern, weight loss, and anxiety in a 19 year old youth. *Journal of Developmental and Behavioral Pediatrics, 31* (3 Suppl), S83–S85.

Rodriguez, G., King, J. C., & Stiens, S. A. (2011). Neurogenic bowel: Dysfunction and rehabilitation. In R. L. Braddom (Ed.), *Physical medicine and rehabilitation* (4th ed., pp. 619–640). Philadelphia, PA: Saunders.

Ryhammer, A. M., Laurberg, S., & Hermann, A. P. (1996). Long term effect of vaginal deliveries on anorectal function in normal perimenopausal women. *Diseases of the Colon & Rectum, 39*(8), 852–859. doi: 10.1007/BF02053982

Saad, R. J., Rao, S. S., Koch, K. L., et al. (2010). Do stool form and frequency correlate with whole-gut and colonic transit? Results from a multicenter study in constipated individuals and healthy controls. *The American Journal of Gastroenterology, 105*(2), 403–411. doi: 10.1038/ajg.2009.612

Sampselle, C. A., & DeLancey, O. L. (1998). Anatomy of female continence. *Journal of Wound, Ostomy, and Continence Nursing, 25*(2), 63–74.

Sandler, R. S., Jordan, M. C., & Shelton, B. J. (1990). Demographic and dietary determinants of constipation in the US population. *American Journal of Public Health, 80*(2), 185–189.

Schaefer, D. C., & Cheskin, L. J. (1998). Constipation in the elderly. *American Family Physician, 58*(4), 907–914.

Scott, S. M., van den Berg, M. M., & Benninga, M. A. (2011). Rectal sensorimotor dysfunction in constipation. *Best Practice & Research Clinical Gastroenterology, 25*(1), 103–118. doi: 10.1016/j.bpg.2011.01.001

Sikirov, D. (2003). Comparison of straining during defecation in three positions: Results and the implications for human health. *Digestive Diseases and Sciences, 48*(7), 1201–1205. doi: 10.1023/A:1024180319005

Sonnenberg, A., & Koch, T. R. (1989). Epidemiology of constipation in the United States. *Diseases of the Colon & Rectum, 32*(1), 1–8. doi: 10.1007/BF02554713

Spanish Group for the Study of Digestive Motility. (1998). Measurement of colonic transit time (total and segmental) with radiopaque markers. National reference values obtained in 192 subjects. *Gastroenterology and Hepatology, 21*(2), 71–75.

Stewart, W. F., Liberman, J. N., Sandler, R. S., et al. (1999). Epidemiology of constipation (EPOC) study in the United States: Relation of clinical subtypes to sociodemographic features. *American Journal of Gastroenterology, 94*(12), 3530–3540. doi: 10.1111/j.1572-0241.1999.01642.x

Tagart, R. E. (1966). The anal canal and rectum: Their varying relationship and its effect on anal continence. *Diseases of the Colon and Rectum, 9*(6), 449–452.

Todar, K. (2010). The normal bacterial flora of humans. In *Tudor's Online Textbook of Bacteriology*. Retrieved from http://textbookofbacteriology.net/normalflora.html

van Ginkel, R., Reitsma, J. B., Buller, H. A., et al. (2003). Childhood constipation: Longitudinal follow-up beyond puberty. *Gastroenterology, 125*(2), 357–363. doi: 10.1016/S0016-5085(03)00888-6

Wald, A., Hinds, J. P., & Caruana, B. J. (1989). Psychological and physiological characteristics of patients with severe idiopathic constipation. *Gastroenterology, 9*, 932–937.

Weaver, L. T. (1988). Bowel habit from birth to old age. *Journal of Pediatric Gastroenterology and Nutrition, 7*(5), 637–640.

Wright, S. H., Snape, W. J., Battle, W., et al. (1980). Effect of dietary components on gastrocolonic response. *American Journal of Physiology, 238*(3), G228–G232.

QUESTIONS

1. Which structure of the GI tract is responsible for the absorption of the vitamin B_{12}–intrinsic factor complex?
   A. Distal small intestine
   B. Ileocecal valve
   C. Colon
   D. Anal canal

2. What is the rationale for placing a patient on his or her left side for a digital rectal or endoscopic exam or for giving an enema?
   A. The location of the internal and external sphincter
   B. To better reference the *dentate line*
   C. To facilitate blood supply to the cecum
   D. To accommodate the left curvature of the sigmoid colon

3. Which structure of the GI tract is responsible for converting liquid stool to solid and serving as a reservoir for feces until it is expelled?
   A. Anal canal
   B. Colon
   C. Anal sphincters
   D. Pelvic floor

4. Which layer of the pelvic floor is the principal source of support for pelvic organs?
   A. Levator ani
   B. Endopelvic fascia
   C. Perineal membrane
   D. Anal sphincter

5. Which layer of the colon wall promotes mixing and peristalsis?
   A. Serosa
   B. Mucosa
   C. Muscularis
   D. Submucosa

6. Which nervous system is the primary mediator for colonic motility (peristalsis)?
   A. Central nervous system (CNS)
   B. Autonomic nervous system (ANS)
   C. Enteric nervous system (ENS)
   D. Somatic system

7. The continence nurse is counseling a patient with a sacral-level spinal cord injury. For what GI condition is this patient at risk?
   A. Constipation
   B. Diarrhea
   C. Flatulence
   D. Bowel perforation

8. Which of the following accurately describes a pattern seen in colonic motor activity?
   A. It decreases after walking.
   B. It is higher during the night than during the day.
   C. Men have faster transit times than women.
   D. Transit time is increased (slower evacuation) by coffee consumption.

9. Sensory awareness of rectal distention is provided by:
   A. Sensory receptors in the anal canal
   B. Sensorimotor innervation of the IAS
   C. Innervation of the somatic fibers of the pudendal nerve
   D. Stretch receptors in the rectal wall and pelvic floor muscles

10. A patient experiencing fecal incontinence complains that he "cannot get to the bathroom in time" when he feels the urge to defecate. Which structure helps delay defecation until a socially appropriate time and place?
    A. Rectum
    B. External anal sphincter (EAS) and pelvic floor
    C. Internal anal sphincter (IAS)
    D. Colon

11. Which position is the best posture for defecation?
    A. Squatting.
    B. Sitting.
    C. Supine.
    D. Position has no effect on defecation.

12. During the process of normal defecation, which action occurs following sensory awareness of the need to defecate?
    A. Stool is stored in the transverse colon.
    B. Mass movements propel the stool into the rectum.
    C. Relaxation of the IAS and contraction of the EAS occur.
    D. Distention of the rectum occurs.

ANSWERS: 1.**A**, 2.**D**, 3.**B**, 4.**A**, 5.**C**, 6.**C**, 7.**A**, 8.**C**, 9.**D**, 10.**B**, 11.**A**, 12.**C**

CHAPTER 15

Motility Disorders

Susan E. Steele, Claire Jungyoun Han, and Margaret Heitkemper

OBJECTIVES

1. Discuss the impact of bowel dysfunction or fecal incontinence on lifestyle and quality of life and implications for psychosocial support and counseling.

2. Explain how each of the following contributes to normal bowel function and fecal continence: normal peristalsis; sensory awareness of rectal distention and ability to distinguish between solid, liquid, and gaseous contents; internal anal sphincter function; external anal sphincter function; and rectal capacity and compliance.

3. Describe criteria and guidelines for use of anorectal pouching systems and internal drainage/bowel management systems.

4. Describe the etiology, pathology, clinical presentation, and management options for acute and chronic diarrhea.

5. Differentiate the pathology, presentation, and management of normal-transit constipation, slow-transit constipation, and obstructed defecation.

6. Describe the pathology and clinical presentation of irritable bowel syndrome.

7. Describe the critical components of assessment and management for the individual with irritable bowel syndrome.

Topic Outline

 Diarrhea
Definition
Epidemiology
Assessment
Classification of Diarrhea
Acute versus Chronic Diarrhea
Infectious versus Noninfectious Diarrhea
Characteristics of Stool

Treatment
Management Underlying Pathology
Supportive Care
Pharmacologic Therapy
Probiotic Therapy
Stool Containment
Hygiene and Skin Care

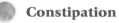 **Constipation**
Definition
Epidemiology
Assessment
History
Physical Examination
Types of Constipation
Simple Constipation
Functional Constipation
Obstructed Defecation
Treatment
Lifestyle Modifications
Laxatives and Enemas
Management of Fecal Impaction
Digital Removal of Feces
Alternative Therapies
Biofeedback
Sacral Neuromodulation
Surgical Treatment

Irritable Bowel Syndrome
Pathophysiology
Abnormalities in Gut Microflora
Diet
Pharmacologic Influences
Genetic Predisposition
Assessment and Diagnosis
Diagnostic Criteria
History and Physical Examination
Diagnostic Tests

Management
    Patient Education
    Dietary Modifications
    Exercise/Activity and Stress Management
    Pharmacologic Therapy

Conclusion

Bowel function disorders, such as diarrhea, constipation, and irritable bowel syndrome (IBS), cause considerable distress for both young and old. Transient episodes involving a change in stool consistency, frequency, or painful defecation are usually self-diagnosed and treated through dietary modification and over-the-counter (OTC) remedies. Persistent changes in bowel function, however, usually prompt consultation with a health care professional. Altered defecation patterns negatively affect quality of life due to the combination of physical symptoms, anxiety, and negative emotions arising from the symptoms (e.g., embarrassment). The emotional response to the physical symptoms may amplify the symptoms and cause further gastrointestinal (GI) distress (Brennan et al., 2011).

> **CLINICAL PEARL**
>
> Functional bowel disorders negatively affect quality of life due to the combination of physical symptoms, anxiety, and negative emotions such as embarrassment.

In this chapter, alterations in bowel motility are defined as a deviation from a "normal" pattern of regularly timed passage of soft, formed stools, without any difficulty or discomfort. Comprehensive management of bowel elimination problems by the continence nurse is described with a focus on reducing symptomatology and improving quality of life. Specific topics include pathology and clinical presentation of common motility disorders, guidelines for comprehensive nursing assessment, management options to include implications for patient-focused education and counseling, and indications and guidance for referrals to specialists.

A lack of clear definitions for terms such as *constipation* and *diarrhea* has hampered evidenced-based practice in the treatment of bowel irregularity. Client perceptions of bowel symptoms vary greatly; some individuals focus solely on stool consistency or frequency, while others are more concerned about associated symptoms, such as pain with defecation. Effective management of any disorder is dependent in large part on identifying and correcting the physiologic or structural source of the presenting symptoms; however, many common bowel problems are *functional* disorders, meaning that no structural or tissue abnormality can be detected that explains the symptoms (Longstreth et al., 2006).

> **CLINICAL PEARL**
>
> Many bowel problems are functional disorders, meaning that no structural or tissue abnormality can be detected that explains the symptoms.

Bowel motility may be conceptualized as a continuum as seen in Table 15-1. One extreme is severe slow-transit constipation, with marked reduction in peristaltic activity, while the other extreme is diarrhea, with rapid transit of stool and water through the colon. The definition of "normal" bowel function lacks precision and in fact "normal" function varies from person to person and is affected by that individual's perceptions of normal. For example, intermittent constipation with no additional symptoms is considered acceptable and normal by many, especially during events that disrupt normal daily routines, such as travel.

> **CLINICAL PEARL**
>
> The definition of normal bowel function lacks precision, and in fact normal function varies from person to person and is affected by that individual's perceptions of normal.

TABLE 15-1 **The Bowel Motility Continuum**

	No Go	**Slow-Go**	**Go**	**Go-Go-Go!**
Clinical condition	Obstructed defecation	Constipation IBS-C	"Normal" bowel pattern	Diarrhea IBS-D
Description	No bowel output	Stools hard, dry, difficult to pass without pain, strain, or discomfort. May be at less frequent intervals than usual bowel pattern	Stools soft, formed, passed at approximately regular intervals without pain, strain, or discomfort	Stools unformed or liquid, passed more frequently than normal bowel pattern (or >3 times/d) and often accompanied by cramping abdominal pain or tenesmus
Symbol	Stop Sign	Sloth	Clock	Road-runner

● Diarrhea

Diarrhea originated from the ancient Greek term *diarrhein*, meaning "flow through" (Oxford English Dictionary, 2014). For the individual suffering from diarrhea, it may indeed seem as though everything ingested flows immediately through the GI tract. Left untreated, diarrhea may result in dehydration, electrolyte imbalance, and death. It is frequently associated with perianal and perineal skin irritation that may range from mild erythema to epidermal erosion and ulceration. The previously toilet-trained child or adult client may experience fecal incontinence during an acute diarrheal illness, as the rapid filling of the rectum and large volume of stool may overwhelm rectal capacity and sphincter contractility and endurance.

Definition

Inconsistencies in both clinical and research literature demonstrate that there is no globally accepted definition for diarrhea. Although diarrhea is often operationally defined for research purposes as ≥3 loose or liquid stools within a 24-hour period or passage of greater than 200 g of stool in a 24-hour period, there are wide variations in individuals' normal stool volume and consistency. It should also be noted that research definitions disregard the impact of the symptom experience of diarrhea on the client (i.e., physical and emotional distress), when it is the symptom distress that usually prompts the individual to seek medical attention. In clinical practice, measurement of stool mass is rarely possible, and clinicians typically rely upon client reports regarding frequency and consistency of stooling and the impact of the diarrhea. Clinicians should also be alert to the fact that some individuals with fecal incontinence come to the provider with complaints of "diarrhea."

The World Health Organization (WHO) defines diarrhea as "the passage of three or more loose or liquid stools per day, or more frequently than is normal for the individual." NANDA International, Inc. simply defines diarrhea as "passage of loose, unformed stool (Herdman & Kamitsuru, 2014)." The Oncology Nursing Society has defined diarrhea as "an abnormal increase in stool liquidity and frequency that may be accompanied by abdominal cramping (Byar et al., 2011)." All of these definitions address stool consistency, and two include an increase in stool frequency; only one addresses related symptomatology, and none address symptom-related quality-of-life issues or distress.

In this chapter, diarrhea is defined as an alteration in bowel elimination characterized by an increase in both the frequency and volume of stools, and a decrease in the consistency of stools, as compared to the bowel elimination pattern that is normal for the individual. Diarrhea is often accompanied by abdominal cramping, a persistent sensation of stool in the rectum (tenesmus), and related psychosocial distress that may amplify the physical distress.

Epidemiology

The Agency for Healthcare Research and Quality (AHRQ) has estimated that, from 2008 to 2011, more than 400,000 U.S. emergency department admissions annually were due to a primary diagnosis of diarrhea, and pediatric cases (birth to age 17) comprised approximately 30% of the admissions. The WHO estimates that 1.7 billion cases of diarrhea occur globally each year (World Health Organization, 2013), and the most serious consequences are experienced by children under the age of 5. Estimates of disease burden due to diarrhea are difficult to determine due to lack of accurate surveillance and the variability in outcomes reported in epidemiologic studies (Arnold et al., 2011). However, a prospective study conducted in Asia and sub-Saharan Africa reported that children in these areas are 8.5 times more likely to die if they develop diarrhea before age 5 (Kotloff et al., 2013). More than half of these deaths are due to viral or bacterial infections (Lanata et al., 2013), which cannot be adequately treated without access to pure water and medical facilities.

CLINICAL PEARL

The most serious consequences of diarrhea are experienced by children under 5 years of age.

Assessment

Diarrhea should be considered both a symptom and a sign. Some clients use the term "diarrhea" to describe loose bowel movements, regardless of stool frequency. It is important to seek subjective information about associated symptoms such as cramping quality abdominal pain, tenesmus, bowel urgency, fecal incontinence, fatigue, and symptom distress when collecting assessment data for the client with complaints of diarrhea. Objective data collection should include inspection for perianal or peristomal skin breakdown and auscultation for hyperactive bowel sounds. Complaints of fatigue should trigger an assessment of functional status and safety, as well as clinical and laboratory assessment of fluid and electrolyte balance. In general, acute-onset diarrhea is caused by an infectious process, and workup includes a careful history to determine potential sources of exposure (e.g., travel history), clinical and laboratory assessment of fluid electrolyte balance, and stool analysis for bacteria, ova, and parasites. In contrast, chronic diarrhea is likely to be caused by an underlying disease process (e.g., malabsorption syndrome, motility disorder, or chronic inflammatory bowel condition); these individuals frequently require a gastroenterology referral and workup. Table 15-2 lists factors to include in a comprehensive assessment of bowel function.

TABLE 15-2 Comprehensive Collaborative Assessment of Diarrhea

Provider Level	Subjective Data	Objective Data

Specialist WOC Nurse	Focused History
	  Duration of diarrhea
	  Stool frequency
	  Stool form, using standardized pictorial tool
	  Stool color
	  Abdominal pain
	  Travel history
	  OTC and prescribed medications
	  Episodes of fecal incontinence
	  Associated symptoms
	    Bloating
	    Tenesmus
	    Change in stool odor
	  Distress
	    Anxiety/ hypervigilance
	    Fatigue
	    Fear of serious problems
	    Embarrassment
	    Loss of control
		Vital signs
		Presence of blood in stool
		Stool frequency
		Stool form, using standardized pictorial tool
		Stool color
		Stool odor
		Abdominal distention
		Bowel sounds
		Blood in stool
		Fluid balance
		  Skin turgor
		  Mucus membranes
		  Vital signs
		Perineal, perianal, or peristomal skin integrity

Advanced Registered Nurse Practitioner or Physician	Complete History
	  Recent travel
	  Self-care attempted
	    OTC drugs
	    Dietary changes
	    Alternative therapy
	  Diet recall
	  Antibiotic usage
	  Chronic illnesses (diabetes, HIV, hyperthyroidism)
	  Associated symptoms
	    Fever
	    Nausea
	    Vomiting
		Laboratory and Diagnostic Testing
		  Stool exams
		    Fecal leukocytes
		    Ova and parasites
		    Bacterial stool culture
		    Giardia antigen
		    C. difficile toxin
		    Fecal analysis, including occult blood and fecal fat
		  CBC
		  Hct and Hgb
		  Lactose tolerance
		  Flexible sigmoidoscopy or colonoscopy with intestinal biopsy
		  Flat plate of abdomen

CLINICAL PEARL

When assessing the individual with diarrhea, it is important to obtain information about cramping abdominal pain, tenesmus, fecal urgency, fecal frequency, episodes of incontinence, the presence of blood in the stool, and symptoms of fluid and electrolyte imbalance (such as fatigue).

The continence nurse can provide valuable contributions to the assessment data and may identify associated problems, such as skin irritation, that might be overlooked by the physician (or midlevel provider) focused primarily on identifying the underlying cause of diarrhea as a basis for medical and/or surgical treatment. In particular, the continence nurse can play a unique role in identifying the amount of GI distress (Brennan et al., 2011) experienced by the client and his/her specific concerns.

Classification of Diarrhea

Diarrhea is classified according to duration of illness, etiology and pathology (infectious vs. noninfectious), and characteristics of stool.

Acute versus Chronic Diarrhea

Acute diarrhea is that which lasts <14 days (Baldi et al., 2009; Barr & Smith, 2014; Deshpande et al., 2014). Diarrhea that has been present for 14 to 30 days is considered persistent (Deshpande et al., 2014), and diarrhea persisting longer than 30 days is termed chronic (Baldi et al., 2009; Deshpande et al., 2014).

Chronic diarrhea is usually noninfectious and may be caused by medications (such as those containing magnesium), artificial sweeteners such as sorbitol (an osmotic laxative), malabsorption syndromes (such as lactose intolerance or celiac disease), motility disorders (such as IBS), inflammatory conditions (such as Crohn's disease or ulcerative colitis), short bowel syndrome resulting from surgical resection of large portions of the small bowel, or bile salt–induced diarrhea caused by resection of the terminal ileum. Diarrhea may also occur following initiation of enteral feedings in individuals who have had very limited oral/enteral intake for a number of days, due to temporary flattening of the villi with resultant loss of absorptive surface.

Infectious versus Noninfectious Diarrhea

Acute diarrhea is most often caused by infectious disease via the fecal–oral route through contaminated food or water containing pathogens such as viruses, bacteria, and parasites. Infectious diarrhea is a leading cause of death in the developing world due to fluid and electrolyte imbalance. A systematic review of 22 papers from countries other than the United States revealed that, in the developing world, bacterial infections such as toxin-producing *Escherichia coli* and *Vibrio cholerae* are the primary organisms responsible for severe diarrhea requiring hospitalization (Walker et al., 2010). In contrast, less severe diarrhea managed in the outpatient setting was most commonly caused by the organisms *Salmonella* and *Shigella* and the parasite *Entamoeba histolytica* (Walker et al., 2010).

Within the United States, rotaviruses comprise the majority of infectious diarrhea in infants and children, while Norwalk virus (also known as Norovirus) comprise the majority of infectious diarrhea in adults. Foodborne illnesses play a significant role in acute infectious diarrhea and are continually monitored within the United States by the Centers for Disease Control and Prevention (CDC). Data from 2013 monitoring indicate that *Salmonella* infections have decreased slightly, while the rates of *Campylobacter*, *Vibrio*, and *E. coli* continue to rise (Centers for Disease Control and Prevention, 2014). Detailed information about surveillance procedures and data can be found at the CDC website http://www.cdc.gov/foodborneburden/trends-in-foodborne-illness.html.

CLINICAL PEARL

Acute episodes of diarrhea are usually caused by infectious processes, while chronic diarrhea is more commonly due to noninfectious factors such as medications, malabsorption syndromes, motility disorders, inflammatory bowel disease, or short bowel syndrome.

The term *traveler's diarrhea* is used to designate a nonspecific infectious diarrhea, typically bacterial, that occurs when an individual travels to a part of the world with poor sanitation. High-risk areas are Central and South America, Africa, and Asia (Baldi et al., 2009).

Of particular concern within health care organizations and group living facilities is diarrhea caused by the spore-forming bacterium *Clostridium difficile*. Although previously associated with advanced age, immunosuppression, and prior use of broad-spectrum antibiotics, recent outbreaks have involved more serious and possibly evolving strains that can affect previously healthy individuals (Cairns et al., 2012). Because *C. difficile* spores can survive in the environment for prolonged periods of time, person-to-person transmission can easily occur. Extremely virulent strains may result in a condition called pseudomembranous colitis, which is potentially fatal.

CLINICAL PEARL

Traveler's diarrhea is a nonspecific infectious diarrhea that occurs when an individual travels to an area with poor sanitation.

Characteristics of Stool

Diarrhea is also classified by type of stool. *Bloody stools* (hematochezia) are associated with inflammation; these patients commonly exhibit leukocytosis as well, due to the underlying inflammatory process. Bloody stools may result from an invasive infection, such as *C. difficile*, or may be the result of chronic inflammation, such as inflammatory bowel disease, cancer, or radiation proctitis. In all of these conditions, the intestinal mucosa is damaged, resulting in the visible blood within the diarrheal stools.

Fatty diarrhea occurs due to malabsorption. One of the most common causes is lactose intolerance, which frequently becomes a chronic condition requiring diet modification. Surgical procedures such as short bowel syndrome, bowel resection, and gastric bypass may be associated with malabsorption and fatty diarrhea, as is pancreatic disease. Various medications can also contribute to malabsorption, including orlistat and acarbose. Malabsorption is also the mechanism for diarrhea caused by the parasite *Giardia*.

Watery diarrhea is the most common type of diarrhea and is typically further classified as secretory, osmotic, or functional based on the underlying pathology. *Secretory* diarrhea occurs when the epithelial cells in the intestinal mucosa are damaged by an infectious organism or intestinal toxin, resulting in an inability to absorb water and electrolytes *from* the lumen of the bowel and abnormal secretion of fluid *into* the lumen of the bowel. Secretory diarrhea is usually high volume and unaffected by reduced oral/enteral intake. Irritant laxatives, serious enteric infections (such as *C. difficile*), and chemotherapy are potential causes of secretory diarrhea (Richardson & Dobish, 2007). In contrast, osmotic diarrhea is caused by the presence of high-osmolarity substances within the lumen of the bowel, which pull water from the blood stream into the gut. Osmotic diarrhea responds rapidly to reduced oral/enteral intake. Food additives, such as high-fructose corn syrup, sorbitol, and xylitol, osmotic laxatives (polyethylene glycol [PEG], milk of magnesia, lactulose), and celiac disease are associated with *osmotic diarrhea*. The final category, chronic watery diarrhea (also known as *functional diarrhea*), is typically due to a motility disorder such as IBS.

Treatment

Treatment for diarrhea is based upon management of the underlying etiology and supportive care to prevent complications.

Management of Underlying Pathology

Management of the underlying disease process is extremely variable, reflecting the wide variety of conditions causing diarrhea, but commonly involves antibiotic therapy (for infectious diarrhea), medical management of inflammatory conditions and motility disorders, and dietary modifications for individuals with malabsorption syndromes.

Supportive Care

Both adult and pediatric clients with diarrhea are at risk for fluid volume deficit and electrolyte imbalance, but the most vulnerable are the elderly and the very young (i.e., infants and young children). Nursing care involves careful monitoring of intake and output and monitoring for signs of dehydration. Dry mouth, decreased urinary output, skin tenting, hypotension, lethargy, tachycardia, and elevated temperature should arouse suspicion of dehydration with the potential for shock, especially in the pediatric client.

For clients who develop an actual fluid volume deficit, rehydration is essential. Oral rehydration is the route of choice, but intravenous fluids may be required for more rapid fluid resuscitation in the critically ill client. The WHO advocates making oral rehydration salts readily available, particularly in the developing world, so that early rehydration can be provided in the home setting. This is particularly important in management of diseases such as cholera, which can quickly cause mortality due to dehydration (Global Task Force on Cholera, 2014).

Dietary modifications are also frequently recommended. Although the BRAT diet (bananas, rice, applesauce, and toast) is frequently recommended by clinicians, there is little evidence to support this level of dietary restriction. Avoidance of highly spiced or fatty foods and increased intake of foods with significant amounts of soluble fiber are recommended and anecdotally reported as helpful. In an RCT of 80 children aged 1 to 28 months, with diarrhea lasting at least 14 days, ingestion of green plantain (50 g/L), as compared to a yogurt-based diet (not specified), resulted in a statistically significant decrease in stool frequency, volume, weight, and duration of diarrhea (Alvarez-Acosta et al., 2009); this suggests that green plantains may be a low-cost and effective dietary intervention. The WHO advocates zinc supplementation for young children with diarrhea at a rate of 10 mg/day for infants under 6 months and 20 mg/day for children over 6 months for a duration of 14 days (Khan & Sellen, 2011; Mazumder et al., 2010).

Pharmacologic Therapy

Antibiotics are typically prescribed for infectious diarrhea and should be based on identification of the specific organism and the agents to which it is sensitive (culture-based therapy). Antimotility agents are not recommended, because the goal is to eliminate the causative organism from the body as rapidly as possible. However, for diarrhea caused by chemotherapy, antimotility agents such as loperamide are frequently considered first-line therapy with progression to octreotide for persistent diarrhea (Shaw & Taylor, 2012). For traveler's diarrhea, bismuth subsalicylate is frequently recommended as a readily-available OTC remedy; however, persistent traveler's diarrhea is typically treated with a quinolone antibiotic. Chronic diarrhea in persons with radiation proctitis and short bowel syndrome may respond at least partially to use of psyllium fiber supplements to thicken the stool.

Probiotic Therapy

The use of probiotics has also received much attention in the research literature and has demonstrated some benefit in both the prevention and management of individuals with specific types of diarrhea. A meta-analysis of 16 studies involving more than 3,400 children suggests that probiotics, particularly *Lactobacillus rhamnosus* and *Saccharomyces boulardii*, can be beneficial in the prevention of antibiotic-associated diarrhea in otherwise healthy infants and children (Johnston et al., 2011). Meta-analysis of studies testing the effects of probiotics in the prevention of *C. difficile*–associated diarrhea in adults also identified benefit (Goldenberg et al., 2013; Johnston et al., 2012). A trial of a combination probiotic product containing *Lactobacillus acidophilus* and *Bifidobacterium longum* reduced daily number of stools, severity of diarrhea, and abdominal pain (Demers et al., 2014) in persons with diarrhea following pelvic radiation. A double-blind, randomized controlled trial of *S. boulardii* in children with acute diarrhea resulted in significantly shorter duration of diarrhea and decreased time until return of formed stools (Riaz et al., 2012). A meta-analysis of 63 studies involving both pediatric and adult subjects with acute infectious diarrhea demonstrated significant reduction in the duration of diarrheal symptoms as well as the frequency of stooling when probiotics were used in addition to oral rehydration therapy (Allen et al., 2010). Further research is needed to determine the specific agents, dosages, and indications for probiotic use in prevention and management of diarrhea.

> **CLINICAL PEARL**
>
> Early research suggests that probiotics may be of benefit in prevention and management of acute diarrheal syndromes; however, further study is needed to determine best agents and dosages.

Although research suggests benefit from probiotics in preventing and treating diarrhea due to acute problems, current meta-analytic results do not suggest a benefit for the induction or maintenance of remission in chronic diarrhea caused by ulcerative colitis (Mallon et al., 2007; Naidoo et al., 2011) or Crohn's disease (Butterworth et al., 2008; Rolfe et al., 2006).

Stool Containment

Containment of stool typically involves disposable absorbent diapers or pads; other products include reusable continence products (see Chapter 12), fecal pouches, or fecal containment systems. In the United States, the most common method of containment is disposable absorbent pads or diapers, which, in the case of infants and young children, raises infection control concerns in facilities such as daycare centers. Containment of stool is also a concern when an adult suffering from diarrhea is unable to toilet independently and is incontinent of stool. Diligent hygiene and skin care are critical, with regular checking of pads to reduce risk of skin erosion from fecal enzymes. Heavily contaminated disposable products used at home pose an additional economic burden related to both the initial purchase and safe disposal of the products. An in vitro study of briefs and pads for urinary incontinence (not fecal incontinence) suggested that briefs may be more cost-effective than pads (Yamasato et al., 2014). Further research is required to determine the best products for individuals with fecal incontinence. An in vitro study comparing fecal contamination among patients with *C. difficile* managed with underpads and those managed with a bowel management system documented spread of the pathogen with the underpad, indicating limited ability of absorbent products to contain infectious material (Jones et al., 2011). Further study is needed to determine the ability of perianal pouches and/or internal bowel management systems to reduce the risk of transmission by effectively containing the stool.

Stool containment pouches (perianal pouches) have been available for many years and are sometimes considered the "first-line" approach to stool containment, so long as the perianal skin is intact. These pouches are attached to a flexible pectin-based adhesive skin barrier designed to adhere to the perianal skin and inner buttocks of the individual. Their use is limited because they do not adhere

well to moist skin and are therefore ineffective when skin damage has already occurred. In addition, female clients may have inadequate tissue in the perineal bridge between the anal and vaginal openings for pouch adherence.

> **CLINICAL PEARL**
>
> Perianal pouches are considered the "first-line approach" to stool containment so long as the perianal skin is intact.

The use of a nasopharyngeal airway for containment of stool has been implemented for the management of incontinent liquid stool, particularly in critically ill adults. While limited clinical trials have demonstrated safety and effectiveness of these devices, more study is needed before definitive recommendations can be made (Pittman et al., 2011, 2012).

Fecal containment systems (or bowel management catheters) are devices that are inserted rectally and maintained in place by inflation of an internal balloon; they are most appropriate for patients who are bedbound with high-volume liquid stool. Three such devices are available commercially within the United States. Although similar in appearance and function, the three products differ somewhat in design features and in cuff pressures within the rectal vault (Marchetti et al., 2011). Because these devices involve insertion of tubing into the rectum and through the sphincter, they do not provide perfect containment; clinicians, patients, and families must be instructed to expect small amounts of leakage and resulting odor. In vitro research indicates that fecal containment systems may be effective in reducing the spread of *C. difficile*, but this has not yet been demonstrated in clinical practice (Gray, 2014; Jones et al., 2011) (Fig. 15-1).

> **CLINICAL PEARL**
>
> Internal fecal containment systems are most appropriate for patients who are bedbound with high-volume liquid stool.

Hygiene and Skin Care

Cleansing of skin wet with feces and/or urine should be provided using both a no-rinse perineal cleanser and soft disposable washcloth, or a disposable wipe impregnated with surfactants and moisturizers. The goal is effective cleansing with avoidance of trauma to the perineal and perianal skin. In some cases, a perineal bottle can be used to gently flush away the stool. The skin should be dried by gently rubbing with a soft absorbent cloth or by using a hair dryer on cool. ("Patting" the skin dry is not recommended; research on transepidermal water loss [TEWL] on the volar surface of the arm in healthy adults suggests that patting leaves the skin significantly wetter and at greater risk of frictional damage than gentle rubbing (Voegeli, 2008).) When the skin is dry, moisture barrier films, ointments, or pastes should be applied to protect the skin from the moisture and enzymes in the stool. If the skin is denuded, a product designed specifically for wet, weepy skin should be

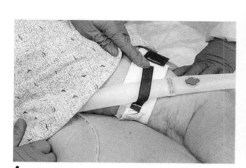

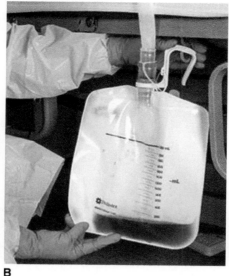

FIGURE 15-1. Internal fecal containment device. **A.** Tubing secured to leg by stabilization device. **B.** Drainage bag for fecal containment system.

applied, such as a pectin-based powder followed by a clear acrylate liquid barrier, or a zinc oxide–based ointment.

All caregivers must be taught the critical importance of correct application and removal of the zinc oxide–based product; a no-rinse perineal cleanser and soft cloth should be used to gently remove the soiled layers of zinc oxide without causing trauma. Additional ointment can then be applied. It may also be helpful to use fanfolded strips of zinc oxide–impregnated gauze (if available) to create a protective dressing; alternatively, a transparent adhesive dressing can be applied over the zinc oxide to prevent transfer of the ointment to the underpad or brief. Chapter 12 provides more detailed discussion on skin care and incontinence-associated dermatitis.

Constipation

Definition

Constipation can be defined as difficult defecation characterized by one or more of the following: (a) hard or dry stools, (b) decreased frequency of stooling, (c) a sensation of incomplete rectal evacuation following a bowel movement, and (d) pain or straining associated with stool elimination. Initial identification of constipation is usually based on a reduction in the frequency of stooling in comparison to an individual's normal bowel pattern. The National Digestive Diseases Information Clearinghouse (NIDDIC) uses the criterion of fewer than 3 bowel movements per week in its patient education materials (National Digestive Diseases Information Clearinghouse, 2013), a definition accepted by many clinicians. However, there is considerable variation among individuals in regard to the frequency of bowel movements, and the American Gastroenterology Society (AGS) recommends a focus on the signs and symptoms rather than fixed criteria related to frequency of bowel movements (Bharucha et al., 2013).

CLINICAL PEARL

Constipation can be defined as difficult defecation characterized by one or more of the following: hard dry stools; reduced frequency of defecation; sensation of incomplete evacuation; and/or pain or straining with defecation.

The NANDA International, Inc. and the American Gastroenterological Association (AGA) (Bharucha et al., 2013) identify constipation and perceived constipation as two separate conditions; constipation represents a genuine problem with stool elimination, whereas perceived constipation represents the perception that there is a problem when in fact bowel function is normal. Perceived constipation is actually a common problem, due to the widespread misconception that normal bowel function is defined by a bowel movement that occurs at the same time every day. Nurses can help to address this problem by providing accurate information regarding the characteristics of and variations in normal bowel elimination patterns. In addition to constipation and perceived constipation, NANDA also recognizes the nursing diagnosis "risk for constipation". Many of the interventions for persons at risk for constipation can be initiated by nurses independently, and early identification of at-risk individuals followed by implementation of a bowel management program can frequently prevent constipation, especially among hospitalized or institutionalized patients (e.g., individuals in long-term or rehabilitative care settings). Table 15-3 summarizes the differences between the three NANDA diagnostic categories related to constipation (Papatheodoridis et al., 2010).

CLINICAL PEARL

NANDA recognizes three nursing diagnoses related to constipation: constipation; perceived constipation; and risk for constipation.

TABLE 15-3 NANDA Definitions and Characteristics for Constipation, Perceived Constipation, and Risk for Constipation

Diagnostic Category	Key Elements of Definition	Characteristics

Constipation	Decreased stool frequency
	Difficult passage of stools
	Incomplete stool passage
	Excessively dry, hard stool
		Subjective:
		  Rectal fullness
		  Rectal pressure
		  Abdominal pain
		  Abdominal tenderness
		  Fatigue
		Objective:
		  Decreased stool volume
		  Abdominal distention
		  Hard, formed stools
		  Hyper-/hypoactive bowel sounds
		  Abdominal distention
		  Liquid stool

Perceived constipation	Self-diagnosed
	Laxative, enema, or suppository abuse
		Subjective:
		  Expectation of daily bowel movement
		  History of OTC medications to stimulate daily bowel movements
		Objective:
		  Absence of clinical signs of constipation

Risk for constipation	At risk for:
	  Difficult defecation
	  Passage of hard, dry stools
	  Incomplete stool passage
		Not applicable

Adapted from Doenges, M. E., Moorhouse, M. F., & Murr, A. C. (2013). *Nursing diagnosis manual: Planning, individualizing, and documenting client care.* Philadelphia, PA: F.A. Davis.

Epidemiology

In contrast to transient constipation, persistent constipation is a much more significant problem and the focus of most epidemiologic investigations. Within the United States, the prevalence of persistent constipation is estimated at 16% overall, and 33% among adults over age 65 (Bharucha et al., 2013). Interestingly, although constipation is more common in older adults, a recent cross-sectional study of adults with a primary diagnosis of constipation revealed that young and middle-aged clients reported constipation of longer duration and with higher prevalence of associated symptomatology such as abdominal pain, as compared to individuals over 65 (McCrea et al., 2010).

Prevalence of constipation reported in the literature varies among different populations. Studies of community-dwelling adults report prevalence rates ranging from 2.4% in Iran (Sorouri et al., 2010) to 15% in Greece (Papatheodoridis et al., 2010), and 25.8% in South Korea (Song, 2012). Two multinational studies based on reported laxative use identified prevalence rates of 2.5% to 26.3% among persons ≤age 29 and 11.2% to 27.3% in persons ≥age 60 (Wald et al., 2008, 2010). Not surprisingly, the rate of constipation among hospitalized and disabled individuals is higher. In a Danish study, the incidence of constipation among hospitalized individuals was 143 cases per 1,000 patient days, and in new admissions was 39% (Noiesen et al., 2014). Among children with disability due to cerebral

palsy, 57% had constipation and 55% used laxatives regularly (Noiesen et al., 2014). A meta-analysis of GI problems in children with autism spectrum disorder revealed more frequent complaints of constipation in these children as compared to normal children (McElhanon et al., 2014). In contrast, the 2004 to 2005 U.S. National Nursing Home Survey (NNHS) revealed a prevalence of only 10% for constipation among both male and female residents. This lower rate may be due to the increased emphasis on bowel management and constipation prevention in long-term care settings as compared to community or acute care settings.

The emotional consequences of persistent constipation cannot be overstated. Among children with chronic constipation, behavioral problems are much more common than among their peers without constipation (van Dijk et al., 2010). Iranian data indicate that anxiety and depression are much more prevalent in persons with chronic constipation (34.6% and 23.5%, respectively) than the general population (Hosseinzadeh et al., 2011). Constipation is also associated with a significant reduction in both physical and mental quality of life (Albiani et al., 2013; Wald et al., 2007), which may be due in part to the complex interaction between the brain and gut. In an international survey of individuals with reported constipation according to Rome II or III criteria and a matched nonconstipated cohort, those with constipation reported lower health-related quality of life (HRQOL) than in nonconstipated controls, as measured by the SF-36 and interview scores.

The results were similar to those reported in other studies involving participants with chronic diseases such as reflux, chronic obstructive lung disease, diabetes, or hypertension (Wald et al., 2007). Whether treatment of constipation would have a direct effect on improved HRQOL is unclear because of the multifactorial nature of chronic constipation.

> **CLINICAL PEARL**
>
> Chronic constipation is associated with a significant reduction in both physical and mental quality of life.

Assessment

A comprehensive history and physical exam are necessary for proper diagnosis and for development of an individualized treatment plan.

History

In addition to questions about medical and surgical history, focused questions should address the following:

- An individual's description of his/her constipation symptoms and his or her opinion regarding cause;
- Stool frequency, usual stool form/consistency, and presence/absence of blood in the stool
- Any straining or pain associated with bowel movements
- Measures previously and currently used to manage constipation and found to be successful, including use of laxatives, suppositories, enemas, manual maneuvers to facilitate stool elimination, and digital removal of stool
- "Red flag" signs and symptoms associated with colorectal cancer (Box 15-1). If present, these mandate referral for further workup (including colonoscopy)
- Previous investigations of the problem and outcomes

Use of a standardized instrument such as the Bristol Stool Scale (see Fig. 11-1, in Chapter 11) aids in the differentiation between true and perceived constipation and also

> **BOX 15-1.** **Red Flag Bowel Symptoms Requiring Colonoscopy**
>
> Recent onset of constipation
>
> Onset of symptoms occurring after age 50
>
> Age ≥50 years with no previous screening for colorectal cancer
>
> Visible or occult blood in stools
>
> Symptoms of bowel obstruction
>
> Family history of colorectal cancer in a first-degree relative
>
> Unintentional weight loss
>
> Narrowing of stool diameter
>
> Rectal prolapse

Data from Bharucha, A. E., Dorn, S. D., Lembo, A., et al. (2013). American Gastroenterological Association medical position statement on constipation. *Gastroenterology, 144*(1), 211–217. doi: 10.1053/j.gastro.2012.10.029; Gunnarsson, J., & Simrén, M. (2008). Efficient diagnosis of suspected functional bowel disorders. *Gastroenterology & Hepatology, 5,* 498–507; Jamshed, M., Lee, Z.-E., & Oldern, K. W. (2011). Diagnostic approach to chronic constipation in adults. *American Family Physician, 25,* 299–306.

provides an objective baseline measure for monitoring response to treatment. The Bristol Stool Scale correlates positively with stool transit time and has demonstrated acceptable sensitivity and specificity for predicting both colonic and whole gut transit time (Saad et al., 2010).

> **CLINICAL PEARL**
>
> Assessment of the individual with chronic constipation must include screening for alarm symptoms (blood in the stool, weight loss, change in stool caliber, family history of colorectal cancer, etc.); these symptoms require referral for workup.

In neonates and children, a history of progressively worsening constipation is commonly associated with congenital absence of bowel ganglia (Hirschsprung's disease), which results in a functional bowel obstruction. Neurogenic bowel dysfunction is a common cause of constipation in individuals with a history of neurologic lesions such as spina bifida, spinal cord injury, or back injury/surgery. Central nervous system diseases such as multiple sclerosis, Parkinson's disease, and Alzheimer's dementia are also associated with constipation, due in part to progressive loss of functional mobility as well as reduced dietary and fluid intake. Metabolic disorders, such as hypothyroidism and diabetic neuropathy, may also contribute, as can various medications (e.g., opioids and anticholinergics).

Further history should include questions about lifestyle such as exercise/activity and dietary and fluid intake. In many situations, it is lifestyle (and/or medications) that are the primary contributing factors to constipation, and correction of these is the first step in improvement of the problem. It is helpful to have the client describe his/her "usual day" and to conduct a 24-hour recall of food and fluid intake (or to have the client complete a food and fluid intake diary). In asking the client about lifestyle factors, the nurse can begin the process of education about normal bowel function and the factors contributing to constipation. The nurse should also be alert to indicators of anxiety or depression as there may be a relationship between HRQOL and constipation (Zhou et al., 2010).

It is imperative for nurses to recognize those at high risk for constipation and to initiate preventive measures. High-risk populations include individuals with decreased physical activity due to illness, injury, or surgery and those who require opioid analgesics for pain management, especially those with advanced cancer. Constipation among cancer patients is a common complication and has been shown to result in considerable distress and indecision regarding the continued use of opioids (Dhingra et al., 2013). Anticipatory education regarding fiber and fluid intake and judicious use of stool softeners and laxatives are essential to prevent severe constipation and possible fecal impaction.

Physical Examination

The focused physical examination should include an abdominal and anorectal examination and a perineal skin inspection. In women, a pelvic examination may be indicated to rule out enterocele and rectocele. The abdominal examination should include inspection for obvious distention or masses, palpation, and percussion; the nurse should percuss along the length of the colon to determine abnormal colon "loading" with stool (evidenced by a dull percussion note along the length of the colon, as opposed to the normal tympanic percussion note) and should palpate the abdomen to detect any masses, including evidence of retained stool in the sigmoid colon. Anorectal examination is done to assess sensation, determine presence of retained stool in the rectum, and assess the individual's ability to voluntarily contract and relax the sphincter on command. The perineal skin is inspected for dermatitis or ulceration.

Types of Constipation

As noted, there are different types of constipation based on the underlying etiology and reflected in clinical presentation and symptom severity. Table 15-4 provides a summary of the types of constipation, the underlying pathophysiologic process, and the signs and symptoms common to each type.

TABLE 15-4 Types of Constipation with Underlying Causes and Typical Data Presentation

Type of Constipation	Underlying Cause(s)	Signs and Symptoms

Transient	Dietary changes	Subjective:
		  Straining during defecation
		  Decreased stool frequency from baseline
		Objective:
		  Colonic tenderness on palpation
		  Palpable fecal mass in sigmoid colon

	Environmental and daily habit changes	Subjective:
		  Abdominal discomfort
		  Recent history of travel
		  Immobility
		  History of toilet training (children)
		  Decreased access to toilet facilities which are comfortable
		  Inability to achieve physiologic position for defecation
		Objective:
		  Abdominal distension
		  Irritability
		  Anorexia
		  Fecal soiling

	Pregnancy due to increase in progesterone (smooth muscle relaxant) and iron supplementation	Subjective:
		  Straining during defecation
		  Decreased stool frequency from baseline
		  Hard, dry stools
		Objective:
		  Dry, pellet-like stools
		  Hemorrhoids

	Pharmacologic side effects
	  Iron supplements
	  Calcium supplements
	  Opioid analgesics
	  Antacids
	  NSAIDS
	  Chronic laxative use
	  Calcium channel blockers
	  Antihistamines
	  Antipsychotics
		Subjective:
		  Medication history
		Objective:
		  Symptom improvement with medication discontinuation

	Painful anorectal condition with deliberate defecation delay
	  Hemorrhoids
	  Anal fissure
		Subjective:
		  Painful defecation
		  Hard, dry stools
		  Anal itching or pain
		Objective:
		  Blood on stools or toilet tissue with bowel movement
		  Visible fissure or hemorrhoid.
		  Pain with DRE

TABLE 15-4 Types of Constipation with Underlying Causes and Typical Data Presentation (*Continued*)

Type of Constipation	Underlying Cause(s)	Signs and Symptoms

Functional: normal transit	Persistent lifestyle deficits (fiber, fluids, and exercise)	Subjective:
		  Hard, dry stools
		  Straining at defecation
		  Sensation of incomplete evacuation or obstruction
		  <3 stools per week
		  Inadequate fluid or fiber intake
		  Limited exercise
		Objective:
		  Normal bowel sounds
		  Abdominal distention
		  Responds to laxative use
		  Responds to lifestyle changes (diet, fluids, exercise)

Functional: slow transit	Medical conditions
	  Diabetes mellitus
	  Depression
	  Hypothyroidism
	  Multiple sclerosis
	  Spinal cord injury
	  Parkinson's disease
		Subjective:
		  Massive, very infrequent stools
		  History of disease or condition affecting motility
		  Failed self-treatment with fiber, fluids, exercise or stimulant laxatives
		Objective:
		  Reduced transit time confirmed with diagnostic studies
		  Lack of anal wink (sacral nerve involvement)
		  Elevated TSH[a] (Hypothyroidism)

Obstructed defecation	Tumors	Subjective:
		  Thinning of stool diameter
		  Rectal discomfort
		  Blood in stool
		  Failed self-treatment with laxatives
		  History of unexplained weight loss
		  Bowel urgency
		Objective:
		  Abdominal distension
		  Positive fecal occult blood test
		  Palpable mass on DRE
		  Abnormal barium enema
		  Abnormal colonic biopsy
		  Rectal prolapse
		  Low hemoglobin

	Dyssynergia between pelvic floor and anal sphincter muscles	Subjective:
		  Difficulty passing even soft stools
		  Straining
		  Prolonged toileting
		  Sensation of incomplete evacuation
		  Rectal pain
		Objective:
		  Normal-transit time studies
		  Difficulty relaxing anal sphincter when bearing down
		  Abnormal pelvic muscle floor diagnostic testing

	Pelvic floor prolapse	Subjective:
		  Difficulty passing even soft stools
		  Straining
		  Prolonged toileting
		  Use of manual maneuvers to evacuate stool
		  Urinary incontinence
		Objective:
		  Rectal bleeding
		  Visible protraction of organs
		  Palpable protrusion of organs
		  Weak anal sphincter contraction

TABLE 15-5 Rome III Criteria for Diagnosis of Functional Constipation by Age Groups for Individuals Not Meeting Criteria for Irritable Bowel Syndrome (IBS)

Adult	Infant to 4 Years of Age	Developmental Age > 4 Years through Adolescent

Two or more of the following present:
  < 3 Stools per week
  Symptoms present ≥25% of defecations
    Straining
    Hard, lumpy stools
    Sensation that stool is still present in rectum
    Sensation that there is a blockage between the anus and rectum
In addition to these criteria, client does not meet the criteria for IBS, and rarely has loose stools unless a laxative is used.
	Two or more of the following present:
	  Two or fewer defecations per week
	  At least one episode/week of incontinence after the acquisition of toileting skills
	  History of excessive stool retention
	  History of painful or hard bowel movements
	  Presence of a large fecal mass in the rectum
	  History of large diameter stools which may obstruct the toilet
	  Associated symptoms that disappear following defecation:
	    Irritability
	    Decreased appetite, and/or early satiety
		Two or more of the following present:
		  Two or fewer defecations in the toilet per week
		  At least one episode of fecal incontinence per week
		  History of retentive posturing or excessive volitional stool retention
		  History of painful or hard bowel movements
		  Presence of a large fecal mass in the rectum
		  History of large diameter stools which may obstruct the toilet

Symptoms must be present for past 3 m with onset ≥6 mo	Symptoms must be present for at least 1 mo	Symptoms must be present for at least 2 mo

*Criteria fulfilled at least once per week for at least 2 mo prior to diagnosis.
Source: Rome III Disorders and Criteria. (2014). Retrieved from http://www.romecriteria.org/criteria/

Simple Constipation

Simple constipation is a transient problem, most often due to dietary or environmental issues, and is a common complaint among the elderly, pregnant women, or individuals whose normal routine has been disrupted by factors such as travel or even the use of public restrooms, where relaxation may be difficult. A low-fiber, "junk food" diet rich in simple carbohydrates is a common cause. A lack of exercise, such as the immobility associated with hospitalization, can exacerbate the problem by further reducing peristaltic stimuli. In children, simple constipation may be triggered by toilet training, changes in school, or use of unfamiliar toilet facilities. Simple constipation typically occurs sporadically and responds well to lifestyle changes, including dietary modifications and exercise.

> **CLINICAL PEARL**
>
> Simple constipation is a transient problem that responds well to lifestyle modifications, including dietary modifications and exercise.

Functional Constipation

Functional constipation is one of several functional bowel disorders, including IBS, for which diagnostic criteria have been established (i.e., the Rome III criteria). Constipation is considered functional when it is chronic and when no structural abnormality can be identified as a cause. However, this should not be interpreted to mean that there is no pathophysiologic basis for functional constipation. As Drossman (2006) notes: "the pathophysiological determinants of these (functional bowel) conditions are only beginning to be understood and relate to enteric dysfunction (abnormal motility and visceral hypersensitivity), mucosal immune alterations, and brain–gut dysregulation (altered CNS pain control and stress regulatory systems)" (p. 1172).

The diagnostic criteria include presence on ≥3 days/month during the preceding 3 months and onset of symptoms ≥6 months prior to seeking treatment. The diagnosis of functional constipation is based on the presence of at least two of the associated symptoms in the absence of bowel warning signs. The Rome III criteria for functional constipation differ by age group and are listed in Table 15-5.

> **CLINICAL PEARL**
>
> Constipation is considered functional when it is chronic and when no structural abnormality can be identified as a cause. It can be further classified as normal transit or slow transit.

Functional constipation includes two major subcategories: *normal-transit and slow-transit constipation.* Normal-transit constipation occurs in individuals who have a normal peristaltic response to stimuli such as colonic distention, but who do not have sufficient stimuli to activate the peristalsis. The problem is most commonly caused by inadequate fiber and fluid intake leading to small-caliber stools that do not cause colonic distention. Individuals with normal-transit constipation typically describe their stools as hard and pellet-like and may also describe associated complaints, such as straining to pass stool, abdominal pain, and bloating. Normal-transit constipation typically responds well to lifestyle changes designed to produce soft formed stool, because peristaltic activity is normal. Slow-transit constipation, in contrast, involves decreased frequency of both segmental and mass movements within the gut. Due to the marked reduction in peristaltic activity, the stool mass sits in the colon for prolonged periods, reabsorbing water and increasing in size. Defecation may not occur until the entire colon is filled with stool, at which point the colonic and rectal pressures exceed anal canal pressures and the stool is forced out. Many individuals with slow-transit constipation report very infrequent (and very large) bowel movements (1 to 4/month), with significant bloating. Slow-transit constipation does not respond well to fiber therapy, because the added fiber simply increases the size of the fecal mass but does not stimulate peristalsis. Response to stimulant laxatives is also poor, because those agents are designed to stimulate peristalsis. Stool softeners and osmotic agents may be more effective because they keep the stool soft and facilitate elimination. Slow-transit constipation is a very challenging disorder, and more research is desperately needed to guide treatment.

> **CLINICAL PEARL**
>
> In normal-transit constipation peristaltic function is normal; these individuals respond well to lifestyle changes that produce soft formed stool. Slow-transit constipation is associated with significant reduction in peristaltic activity and does not respond well to simple measures such as fiber therapy.

Transit time is the diagnostic tool used to objectively diagnose normal-transit constipation versus slow-transit constipation and can be measured with various different procedures. One approach is ingestion of wireless motility capsules that transmit signals regarding changes in pH associated with different portions of the GI tract and thus provide a clear record of time spent in each segment of the bowel (Rao et al., 2011). Video capsule endoscopy allows direct visualization of the bowel lumen as the capsule passes from stomach to small bowel to colon and rectum and evacuation (Rao et al., 2011). Orally ingested radio-opaque markers (Sitz markers) can be used in combination with serial radiographic exams to determine the time for markers to reach various segments of the bowel. Scintigraphy studies involve ingestion of either a radioactive meal or nonabsorbable charcoal that has been marked with radioisotopes.

Transit time studies are usually initiated in a physician's office or outpatient facility. Nursing education involves bowel preparation for capsule endoscopy and the need to wear a transmitter for 3 to 5 days with wireless remote procedures. Radio-opaque marker studies require frequent returns for x-rays and possible abdominal ultrasound procedures, and the patient may be asked to avoid use of any laxative agents until the study is complete. Neither wireless remote nor radiopaque marker studies require any type of bowel preparation.

> **CLINICAL PEARL**
>
> Transit time studies are used to differentiate between normal-transit and slow-transit constipation.

Obstructed Defecation

Obstructed defecation is best understood as dysfunctional defecation and may occur in people with normal stool consistency as well as those who have severe constipation (Ellis & Essani, 2012). Functional obstructed defecation is the result of defective pelvic floor function, specifically the inability to coordinate pelvic floor and sphincter relaxation with abdominal muscle contraction; the individual strains to pass the stool but is unable to empty the rectum effectively due to the functional obstruction created by persistent contraction of the anal sphincter (dyssynergia). Symptoms include prolonged toileting time, rectal pain, excessive straining followed by a sensation of incomplete emptying, and difficulty passing even soft stools (Ellis & Essani, 2012; Jamshed et al., 2011). Transit time through the colon is usually normal, as the pathology involves the pelvic floor and anorectal junction. Prolonged defecatory dysfunction leads to complications including chronic rectal distention (megarectum), pelvic floor muscle spasticity, weakening of the perineal musculature, and rectal ulcerations (Rosen, 2010). Various diagnostic tests can be used to confirm dyssynergic defecation: balloon expulsion, electromyography, anorectal manometry, and defecography, alone or in combination (Reiner et al., 2011).

> **CLINICAL PEARL**
>
> Obstructed defecation is characterized by extreme difficulty in elimination of stool and is caused by pathology involving the pelvic floor and anorectal junction, such as pelvic floor dyssynergia or pelvic organ prolapse.

Obstructed defecation can also occur due to mechanical causes such as rectal tumors, strictures following anal trauma, and rectoanal intussusception. Enterocele (herniation of the small bowel into the vagina) and rectocele (prolapse of the rectum into the vagina) make defecation extremely painful and difficult, and the patient may, if asked, acknowledge that she has to insert 1 to 2 fingers into the vagina to enable defecation (Ellis & Essani, 2012). Women with enterocele or rectocele may have coexisting symptoms including rectal bleeding and urinary incontinence (Ellis & Essani, 2012). Pelvic organ prolapse may result in obstructed defecation, requiring the woman to manually support the perineum to facilitate defecation. In obtaining the history of a patient with suspected obstructed defecation, it is essential to ask about manual maneuvers used to evacuate stool, because patients frequently do not volunteer this information due to embarrassment.

Some of the conditions resulting in obstructed defecation are evident either on visual inspection or on anorectal examination (e.g., tumors and strictures), and a preliminary assessment of pelvic floor dyssynergia can be made during anorectal examination by asking the patient to relax the sphincter and bear down as if trying to pass stool or gas. A normal response is visible relaxation of the anal sphincter accompanied by a downward push. The individual with pelvic floor dyssynergia will bear down but will be unable to relax the sphincter. However, some conditions can be identified only with defecography, a radiographic visualization of rectoanal function during attempted evacuation of contrast thickened to the consistency of stool. In the absence of symptoms or history suggesting risk of bowel cancer, colonoscopy is seldom indicated in the assessment of constipation.

Treatment

Treatment of constipation is based on the underlying cause. Although the initial care for simple constipation may be initiated independently either by the generalist or by the continence nurse, other types of constipation require interdisciplinary care that involves gastroenterologists, colorectal and general surgeons, diagnostic imaging professionals, and physical therapists or advanced practice nurses trained in biofeedback therapy. In addition to conventional medical and surgical care, clients may benefit from complementary therapy.

CLINICAL PEARL

Treatment of constipation is based on the specific type and underlying cause but typically involves lifestyle modifications to assure appropriate stool consistency and normal posture for defecation and selective use of laxatives and enemas.

Lifestyle Modifications

Lifestyle modifications can be taught to both adult clients and parents of children with simple constipation. The critical components of lifestyle modification include increased intake of fiber and fluid, increased activity, and elimination or reduction of constipating medications. Increased dietary fiber is recommended, but must be accompanied by an increase in fluid intake to prevent further constipation. The current recommendation for fiber intake in adults is about 14 g/1,000 calories. For females, this is 25 g/day and for adult males, 38 g/day (Food and Nutrition Board, 2005), balanced with sufficient fluid intake (approximately 1,500 to 2,500 mL/day). Fiber affects bowel function in several ways, including (a) increased moisture content and softening of stool; (b) increased stool bulk; (c) decreased colonic transit time; and (d) promotion of normal microbial balance through its role as a prebiotic; the normal flora add further bulk to the stool.

CLINICAL PEARL

The current recommendation for fiber intake in adults is 14 g/1,000 calories; fiber acts to soften the stool, increase stool bulk, reduce colonic transit time, and promote normal microbial balance.

Dietary fibers differ in their solubility in water, as well as their fermentability within the colon. These differences result in different clinical effects. *Soluble, highly fermentable* fiber substances do not reduce fecal transit time and primarily "work" through a mild laxative effect and by adding water and bulk to the stool; these fibers also contribute to microbial balance within the colon (Eswaran et al., 2013; Food and Nutrition Board, 2005). Included in this group are fructo-oligosaccharides (FOS), pectin, guar gum, and inulin. OTC fiber supplements in this category include Fiber Choice and Benefiber. Evidence suggests that in addition to their laxative benefits, oligosaccharides selectively support the proliferation of *Bifidobacteria*, an important species for colonic immunity. *Soluble fiber with reduced fermentation properties* is found in psyllium and β-glucans, such as oat bran. This type of fiber provides a much better laxative effect because it reduces transit time in addition to increasing stool bulk and retaining water to keep stool soft (Eswaran et al., 2013; Food and Nutrition Board, 2005). Various psyllium fiber supplements are available and include brand names such as Metamucil, Konsyl, Serutan, and Fiberall. Wheat bran, flax seed, whole grain cereals, quinoa, and vegetables are all good sources of *insoluble, partially fermentable fiber*. This type of fiber reduces fecal transit time and is therefore an effective laxative. Like soluble fibers that are only partially fermented in the colon, insoluble partially fermentable fibers provide an overall increase in bacterial species (Eswaran et al., 2013; Food and Nutrition Board, 2005). *Insoluble, nonfermentable fiber* is found in nuts, seeds, fruit and vegetable peels, and the food additive cellulose; these substances reduce transit time significantly and provide a strong laxative effect. Citrucel is an OTC supplement containing cellulose. High-fiber foods and supplements that are fermentable cause increased flatulence; thus, individuals are usually advised to begin with low-dose supplementation and to gradually increase the daily dose until the desired stool consistency is obtained (Eswaran et al., 2013). Increased activity is also recommended, because activity stimulates peristalsis and decreases transit time (time required for stool to pass through the bowel), resulting in softer stool. Finally, the nurse should collaborate with the patient and prescribing provider to reduce or eliminate constipating medications, such as those with anticholinergic effects.

Laxatives and Enemas

Although initial management of functional constipation usually includes lifestyle modifications (Jamshed et al., 2011), these measures may be insufficient in and of themselves. This is particularly true for patients with slow-transit constipation, for whom increased fiber intake may actually be contraindicated. Laxatives are usually a second line of treatment for both normal-transit and slow-transit constipation. Laxatives produce bowel movements through various physiologic mechanisms, including stool bulking, osmosis, and direct stimulation of peristalsis. Table 15-6 provides information regarding the mechanism of action for different laxative categories and key nursing administration issues. The only type of laxatives routinely recommended on a long-term basis are high-fiber foods or fiber supplements, such as psyllium.

Use of osmotic and stimulant agents for periods longer than 2 weeks should be supervised by an advanced practice nurse or physician. The continence nurse should realize that osmotic agents work by distending the bowel and *can* safely be used on a repetitive basis when needed, whereas stimulant laxatives activate the nerve cells within the bowel wall and are recommended for intermittent use only. Whenever any laxative is used, observation and documentation of stool frequency, form, color, and the ease or difficulty of stool elimination are important nursing assessments. Abdominal pain, nausea and/or vomiting, and fever all indicate possible peritoneal inflammation and are strict contraindications to laxative use.

TABLE 15-6 Commonly Prescribed Laxatives

Generic Name Brand Name(s)	Action	Nursing Actions
Fiber supplement Psyllium Metamucil Konsyl Fiber-all	Absorb water to add bulk to the stool, which promotes peristalsis	Encourage fluid intake 1,500 to 2,000 mL/d Assess regularly for bloating, distention, bowel sounds Withhold for constipation accompanied by abdominal pain, nausea, vomiting, especially if accompanied by fever
Osmotic agents Lactulose Polyethylene glycol (PEG) Miralax PEG with electrolytes Colyte Golytely	Draw water into the bowel lumen to increase water content of stool	Assess regularly for bloating, distention, bowel sounds Monitor for belching, flatulence, abdominal cramping Lactulose may increase glucose in diabetics PEG and lactulose not for use > 2 weeks PEG with electrolytes used only for bowel preparation; extreme caution with persons who do not have gag reflex
Hypertonic agents Phosphate/biphosphate Fleet enema Visicol Osmo-Prep	Inhibit water and electrolyte reabsorption in small intestine, causing water retention and increasing peristalsis	Assess regularly for bloating, distention, bowel sounds Often used as bowel preparation for procedures Caution with renal or cardiac disease due to electrolyte changes Administer early in day to avoid sleep pattern disturbance
Magnesium salts Milk of magnesia Citrate of magnesia Slo-Mag	Draw water into bowel lumen via osmosis	Assess regularly for bloating, distention, bowel sounds Caution in persons with renal insufficiency
Stimulants Bisacodyl Dulcolax Carter's Little Pills Feen-a-Mint Sennosides Ex-Lax Senokot Fletcher's Castoria	Stimulation of peristalsis through direct action on the colon to produce fluid accumulation	Assess regularly for bloating, distention, bowel sounds May decrease absorption of other oral medications Assess regularly for bloating, distention, bowel sounds May change urine color
Stool softeners Docusate sodium Colace Docusate calcium Surfak	Softens feces by absorption of water into stool	Assess regularly for bloating, distention, bowel sounds Administer with full glass of water or juice Do not administer within 2 h of other laxative, especially mineral oil due to risk of increased absorption

Data from Deglin, J. H., Vallerand, A. H., & Sanoski, C. (2013). *Davis's drug guide for nurses* (13th ed.). Philadelphia, PA: F.A. Davis.

Laxatives are most commonly used on an "as-needed" basis for treatment of simple constipation, or in combination with lifestyle changes for those with functional normal-transit constipation. For some individuals with functional slow-transit constipation, laxatives may be required on a routine basis. For on-going use, osmotic agents are generally considered the agent of choice, for two reasons: (1) these agents "work" by distending the bowel and softening the stool and may be more effective than stimulant agents in patients with reduced peristalsis; and (2) there are concerns that routine use of stimulant agents may adversely affect motility over the long term.

The continence nurse frequently needs to provide patient education regarding the safety of appropriately used laxative agents, because many people have been taught that long-term or routine use of *any* laxative is dangerous. While routine use of laxatives should not be used as a substitute for healthy lifestyle modifications, appropriate use of laxatives is an essential element of management for most individuals with slow-transit constipation, and patients should be counseled appropriately. A cross-sectional survey identified improved stool frequency and consistency with appropriate use of laxatives (Fosnes et al., 2011). Routine use of laxatives is also appropriate for management of constipation secondary to medication usage when the medication cannot be discontinued, such as the patient who requires opioid analgesics.

Persons with neurogenic bowel due to spinal cord injury, multiple sclerosis, or a progressive neurologic disease often require regular use of stool softeners combined with stimulant laxatives or suppositories. Establishment of a regularly scheduled time of day for bowel evacuation and use of digital stimulation and/or a suppository are often needed to prevent severe constipation, fecal impaction, and stool leakage. A RCT ($n = 68$) of individuals with long-standing SCI (mean 16 years) designed to reduce laxative use and digital stimulation with stepwise bowel interventions produced nonsignificant results and resulted in longer time for bowel care as compared to a standard care control group who used manual evacuation as needed (Coggrave & Norton, 2010). A Cochrane review revealed very little high-quality evidence to support any specific laxative or bowel management protocol for individuals with neurogenic bowel due to central nervous system disease or injury (Coggrave & Norton, 2013). See Chapter 16 for further discussion of neurogenic bowel management.

Enemas are often administered for treatment of short-term constipation. Small-volume prepackaged hypertonic enemas are designed to stimulate rapid evacuation, but they may cause electrolyte disturbances and must therefore be used with caution in patients with renal insufficiency and cardiac disease. Large-volume enemas are typically used for bowel cleansing, usually in preparation for a surgical or diagnostic procedure.

Management of Fecal Impaction

Fecal impaction is a potential complication of severe constipation and causes significant morbidity and patient distress; thus, the goal is prompt (and ideally painless) elimination of the obstructing fecal mass and measures to prevent recurrence. Whenever possible, the fecal mass is gently broken up by digital manipulation, and a cleansing enema is then administered to eliminate the retained stool. If the fecal mass is very hard, it may be necessary to first administer an oil-retention enema or a milk and molasses enema to soften the mass so that it can be broken up digitally. Once the mass has been broken up, a cleansing enema can be administered. (See Chapter 16 for further information on oil-retention and milk and molasses enemas.) An oral laxative may be given as well to assure effective colonic cleansing.

Digital Removal of Feces

Digital removal of feces is a procedure commonly included in fundamentals nursing textbooks. However, the procedure is not without risks, and there is little research evidence to guide the practice (Kyle et al., 2005; Solomons & Woodward, 2013). Although routine digital stimulation and/or evacuation are frequently required for individuals with neurogenic bowel conditions, the procedure should be considered a last resort for individuals with normal peristaltic function. Pain, bleeding, anal or rectal tears, and bradycardia due to vagal nerve stimulation are all potential complications of digital evacuation of stool. In the spinal cord–injured individual with a lesion at thoracic vertebra 6 or higher, autonomic dysreflexia is an additional risk. Thus, the priority in nursing management should be prompt identification of patients at risk for constipation and aggressive intervention to prevent severe constipation and fecal impaction. When manual disimpaction is required, the procedure should be carried out with extreme caution. The Royal College of Nursing guidelines advocate for client safety during digital removal of stool (Addison & Smith, 2000), and Kyle et al. (2005) provide a detailed procedure for digital removal.

Alternative Therapies

Various complementary and alternative therapies are described in the literature for treatment of constipation. Although some may be useful, there is a lack of high-quality research to recommend these therapies for wide adoption in practice. Two separate studies identified a desire for symptom relief and symptom distress as major reasons for the use of alternative medicine (Stake-Nilsson et al., 2012; van Tilburg et al., 2008).

Chinese herbal medicine has received a great deal of research, disseminated primarily in Chinese journals. Although there is some evidence that traditional Chinese herbs may benefit persons with functional constipation, many of the studies have methodological issues (Cheng et al., 2009). A systematic review of the effectiveness of abdominal massage revealed a similar problem with methodological rigor (Ernst, 1999). While complementary and alternative therapy may provide new directions for treatment of chronic constipation, more research, particularly well-designed clinical trials, must be conducted to measure their effectiveness.

Biofeedback

Biofeedback has been evaluated as a treatment for encopresis in children and obstructed defecation in both children and adults. A systematic review of 10 RCTs comparing biofeedback to other methods of treatment for constipation or encopresis did not find a significant difference between groups and concluded that there is insufficient evidence to recommend biofeedback as a treatment modality for these individuals (Coulter et al., 2002). However, given the paucity of treatment options and the fact that the modality is safe and provides at least modest benefit for some patients, it is an option to be considered when other strategies have failed, especially for treatment of obstructed defecation due to dyssynergia.

Evidence regarding biofeedback suffers from the same methodologic deficiencies as those affecting studies of complementary and alternative therapy. A systematic review of biofeedback studies found low-quality evidence in the 17 studies reviewed (Woodward et al., 2014). In a review focused on dyssynergic defecation, in which biofeedback was compared to Botox injection and surgery, the reviewers reported limited success with biofeedback, temporary success with injection, and the best outcomes with surgical treatment (Faried et al., 2010).

Sacral Neuromodulation

Sacral neuromodulation is a long-term treatment approach that uses implantable electrodes and a stimulation device to modulate colonic function. Candidates are screened for response to sacral neuromodulation before permanent implantation. Specifically, temporary leads are placed percutaneously and attached to an external stimulator; subjects then maintain a bowel diary for an average of 2 weeks. If there is a significant improvement in bowel function, the individual undergoes surgery to implant the electrodes and stimulation device. One prospective study demonstrated improvement in bowel function in 12/21 (57%) of persons with chronic constipation unrelieved by diet, laxatives, irrigation, or biofeedback who were treated with SNM (Sharma et al., 2011). Another retrospective study demonstrated a statistically significant reduction in constipation scores, increase in number of stools per week, and reduction in fecal incontinence in patients with incomplete spinal cord injury who had failed conservative approaches (Lombardi et al., 2010). While further study is needed, sacral neuromodulation appears to be a promising therapeutic option.

CLINICAL PEARL

Sacral neuromodulation appears to be a promising therapeutic option for patients with chronic constipation.

Surgical Treatment

Surgical approaches to the treatment of chronic constipation include procedures designed to address specific anatomic problems (such as resection of an acontractile section of bowel) and procedures that enhance management of the underlying functional issue.

For women with obstructed defecation due to pelvic organ prolapse, rectocele or enterocele, surgical intervention involves correction of the underlying problem. For persons with slow-transit constipation, surgical options include total colectomy with ileoanal anastomosis, low anterior resection, and anterior resection (Kumar et al., 2013). For children with Hirschsprung's disease, surgical treatment involves removal of aganglionic bowel, pulling the healthy bowel down, and connecting it to the anal opening (Kumar et al., 2013).

In contrast, the Malone antegrade continence enema (MACE procedure) is designed to enhance management of slow-transit constipation. Surgery involves creation of a small stoma connecting the abdominal wall to the proximal colon; to empty the bowel, the individual inserts a small catheter into the stoma and performs antegrade (proximal to distal) "washouts" every day or every other day. (See Fig. 17-5, in Chapter 17.) The MACE has been used widely for children with chronic constipation and neurogenic bowel and is also now used for adults. Long-term results indicate positive patient satisfaction, though some individuals require revision due to stomal complications (Ellison et al., 2013), and others require additional surgical procedures such as partial colectomy, total colectomy with ileal–anal anastomosis, or total colectomy with Brooke ileostomy (Meurette et al., 2010).

CLINICAL PEARL

The Malone Antegrade Continence Enema permits "top-down" irrigations for individuals with chronic constipation and/or compromised bowel control.

Irritable Bowel Syndrome

Functional GI disorders, including IBS, are among the most common and costly health care problems in the United States (Faresjo et al., 2007; Nyrop et al., 2007; Sandler, 1990; Schultz et al., 2009; Spiegel, 2009). Approximately 10% to 20% of adults experience chronic abdominal pain/discomfort and associated bowel changes (constipation and/or diarrhea) compatible with a diagnosis of IBS (Drossman et al., 2006; Rajilić-Stojanović, 2007). The public health impact is enormous with direct and indirect costs totaling approximately $1.35 billion/year (Inadomi et al., 2003); in addition, the symptom burden has a negative impact on quality of life (Bond et al., 2009; Heitkemper et al., 2011; Spiegel et al., 2008). In the United States as well as other Western countries, women seek health care services disproportionately more than men (Drossman, et al., 2006).

IBS is typified by the presence of abdominal pain or discomfort associated with bowel pattern changes and/or relieved by bowel movements, with patients usually suffering from diarrhea, constipation, or mixed diarrhea and constipation. Effective, targeted therapies are limited in part by the fact that there is tremendous variability in bowel symptoms ranging from diarrhea, constipation, or mixed defecation patterns, and symptom severity ranges from mild to severe, or even disabling. Box 15-2 lists the current diagnostic criteria for IBS.

CLINICAL PEARL

IBS is typified by the presence of abdominal pain or discomfort associated with bowel pattern changes and/or relieved by bowel movements, with patients usually suffering from diarrhea, constipation, or mixed diarrhea and constipation.

Pathophysiology

The underlying pathophysiologic mechanisms of IBS involve an interplay among multiple factors: increased GI permeability ("leaky gut"), abnormalities in the composition of the GI microbiota (bacteria, their genomes, and interaction with the host), altered immune responses,

---

BOX 15-2.   Diagnostic Criteria for Irritable Bowel Syndrome[a]

Irritable bowel syndrome is diagnosed by recurrent abdominal pain or discomfort (uncomfortable sensation not described as pain) at least 3 days/month in the past 3 months associated with two or more of the following:

Improvement with defecation

Onset associated with a change in frequency of stool

Onset associated with a change in form (appearance) of stool

---

[a]Criteria fulfilled for the past 3 months with symptom onset at least 6 months prior to diagnosis.

---

autonomic nervous system dysfunction, altered bile acid metabolism, and psychological distress (Alonso et al., 2008; Camilleri et al., 2012, 2014; Shankar et al., 2013). The role of psychological stress may be more significant than previously appreciated. Recent studies of prognostic markers suggest that IBS can develop from one or more of the following factors: adverse events and stress occurring early in life (Bradford et al., 2012), significant life events producing moderate stress in adults (Alonso et al., 2008), and/or luminal factors (e.g., infection or alterations in the GI microbiota that trigger immune activation) (Hughes et al., 2013). IBS is a complex and not well-understood disease. It remains unclear whether stress is a primary causative factor or a risk factor. In a recent survey of young adults who were diagnosed with functional abdominal pain as children, 41% met the Rome III criteria for IBS (Horst et al., 2014). The presence of extraintestinal somatic conditions and depressive symptoms at the time of initial pediatric diagnosis was most predictive of adulthood IBS.

CLINICAL PEARL

The underlying pathophysiologic mechanisms of IBS involve an interplay among multiple factors: increased GI permeability ("leaky gut"), abnormalities in the composition of the GI microbiota (bacteria, their genomes, and interaction with the host), altered immune responses, autonomic nervous system dysfunction, altered bile acid metabolism, and psychological distress.

Abnormalities in Gut Microflora

The largest microbial mass in the body is found in the GI tract, with estimates of $>10^{13}$ organisms present. Recent studies have identified novel associations between the gut microbiota and diverse diseases such as obesity, diabetes, rheumatoid arthritis, colorectal cancer, IBD, and IBS (Castellarin et al., 2012; Chassaing & Darfeuille-Michaud, 2011; Kostic et al., 2012; Rajilić-Stojanović et al., 2011; Sartor, 2008; Saulnier et al., 2011; Scher & Abramson, 2011; Thomazini et al., 2011; Turnbaugh et al., 2009; Walker et al., 2011; Willing et al., 2009). The microbiota affect immune and inflammatory responses within the GI tract itself, and research evidence suggests that the bacterial mix may also influence systemic inflammatory responses. For example, abnormal proportions of *Firmicutes* and *Bacteroides* have been identified in patients with type II diabetes (Larsen et al., 2010). These changes in the bacterial composition may induce a proinflammatory state as evidenced by elevated proinflammatory cytokine levels (Cani et al., 2008). A current hypothesis is that abnormalities in the bacterial mixture activate mucosal immune responses that increase epithelial barrier permeability, activate nociceptive (pain) pathways, and cause dysfunction of the enteric nervous system, thus adversely affecting normal peristaltic activity (Arumugam et al., 2011; Jeffery et al., 2012).

Diet

Although dietary intake and inflammatory bowel symptoms have long been linked, there are currently no data to prove a causal relationship between the two. While adults and children with IBS complain of subjective food intolerance more commonly than people without IBS (Hsueh et al., 2011; Jarrett et al., 2001; Walker et al., 1998), patients with IBS typically report dietary intake that is similar to their healthy counterparts. By convention, a patient with confirmed diet-related symptoms (e.g., celiac disease) is no longer considered to have IBS. Despite this, not only do the symptoms of IBS and celiac disease overlap but epidemiological studies also suggest a greater than by chance association (4- to 5-fold increased risk), especially in patients seeking health care (Verdu et al., 2009).

An alternative explanation for IBS symptoms is that bacterial breakdown of poorly digested (fermentable) carbohydrates (i.e., oligo-, di-, and monosaccharides and polyols [FODMAPs]) results in increased gas production and abdominal pain/discomfort. Interestingly, one study found that adults with IBS-like symptoms and fructose malabsorption, which probably alters the bacterial composition, had higher depression scores than those without malabsorption (Ledochowski et al., 2000), and exclusion of dietary fructose reduced depression scores by 65% (Ledochowski et al., 2000). The low-FODMAP diet has been shown to be effective in improving IBS symptoms in some patients (Muir & Gibson, 2013; Shepherd & Gibson, 2006).

Pharmacologic Influences

Various antibiotics alter bacterial balance by reducing bacterial diversity and creating a shift in bacteria genera; these changes occur within the first few days of therapy. One week after a course of antibiotics either the prior stable state (norm) is reestablished or an altered stable state may become the "new" norm (Dethlefsen & Relman, 2011). When the usual stable state and bacterial balance are altered, it can trigger changes in the immune response. For example, amoxicillin eradicates GI *Lactobacillus spp.* and alters levels of other aerobic and anaerobic bacteria; this can lead to increased mast cell protease expression and reduced immune response to specific antigens in the intestinal lumen. These changes in the bacterial balance and the immune response of the intestinal mucosa can increase the risk of GI infections (Buffie et al., 2012; Ubeda & Pamer, 2012; Ubeda et al., 2010). Proton pump inhibitors (PPIs) are another type of medication that can adversely affect the bacterial balance (through elevation of pH levels) (Bengmark, 2013).

Genetic Predisposition

Family and twin studies have demonstrated that genetic predisposition may play a role in IBS development (Haas et al., 2011; Lozupone et al., 2006). Genetic association approaches have been used to assess pathways involved in IBS symptoms and the comorbidity of psychiatric conditions and psychological distress (Saito et al., 2010). Serotonin (5-HT) is an important neurochemical mediator in the gut and brain, and genetic variants affecting 5-HT reuptake have been associated with higher vulnerability to psychological distress (Kumar et al., 2012; Lesch, 2011; Pata et al., 2002). Other studies have shown that genetic variations affecting 5-HT levels are associated with higher pain ratings; however, there is currently no conclusive evidence linking these variations to specific bowel symptoms (diarrhea, constipation) (Kumar, et al., 2012) or a diagnosis of IBS.

Assessment and Diagnosis

There is no widely accepted biomarker for diagnosis of IBS or assessment of disease activity nor is there an accepted single causative factor (Apweiler et al., 2009). The diagnosis and categorization of IBS are based on symptom-based Rome III criteria (Drossman et al., 2006). Although these criteria are accepted and used by most clinicians, they do not capture all of the pathology associated with IBS that may impact the individual's response to therapy (e.g., pain severity and level of psychological distress). Investigators are currently exploring diagnostic algorithms that incorporate GI symptom severity, pain, biomarkers such as bowel transit time, life impact, and psychological distress (Halpert, 2010). Some of these factors may be included in the Rome IV criteria, which are expected to be released in 2016.

Diagnostic Criteria

At present, the diagnosis of IBS is based on the Rome III criteria, coupled with the exclusion of organic disease via a careful history and physical examination and, when indicated, diagnostic procedures such as CT scan and endoscopy. The clinician should, however, be aware that many people with IBS experience symptoms other than those outlined in the Rome III criteria and should conduct a comprehensive interview designed to capture all factors contributing to the individual's distress; for example, many individuals report increased intestinal gas and fecal urgency. Patients should be encouraged to keep a symptom diary, and it is helpful to use a validated tool such as the Bristol Stool Chart to accurately determine usual stool consistency. (See Fig. 11-1 in Chapter 11.) As noted in the diagnostic criteria, alterations in bowel patterns range from diarrhea to constipation and can be mixed or alternating. Because of the variability in patterns, specific subtypes were designated by the Rome III criteria (Drossman, 2007) and are listed in Box 15-3.

> **CLINICAL PEARL**
>
> Diagnosis of IBS is based on the Rome III criteria, coupled with the exclusion of organic disease via a careful history and physical examination and, when indicated, diagnostic procedures such as CT scan and endoscopy.

History and Physical Examination

IBS can usually be diagnosed by a thorough history and physical examination, with a focus on the types of symptoms, symptom severity, and presence of any "alarm"

BOX 15-3.   Subtyping Irritable Bowel Syndrome by Predominant Stool Pattern

To subtype patients according to their bowel habit for research or clinical trials, the following subclassification may be used. The validity and stability of such subtypes over time are unknown and should be the subject of future research.

IBS with diarrhea (IBS-D)

Loose (mushy) or watery stools[a] at least 25% and hard or lumpy stools[b] <25% of bowel movements[c]

IBS with constipation (IBS-C)

Hard or lumpy stools[b] at least 25% and loose or watery stools <25% of bowel movements[c]

Mixed IBS (IBS-M)

Hard or lumpy stools[a] at least 25% and loose (mushy) or watery stools[b] at least 25% of bowel movements[c]

Unsubtyped IBS

Insufficient abnormality of stool consistency to meet criteria for IBS-C, D, or M

---

[a]Bristol Stool Form Scale 6–7 (Fluffy pieces with ragged edges, a mushy stool or watery, no solid pieces, entirely liquid).
[b]Bristol Stool Form Scale 1–2 (separate hard lumps like nuts "difficult to pass" or sausage shaped but lumpy).
[c]In absence of antidiarrheal or laxative use.

---

signs and symptoms. In addition to abdominal pain and discomfort associated with altered bowel function, patients with IBS often report various comorbid conditions, including headache with aura, chronic pelvic pain, temporomandibular joint syndrome, fibromyalgia, chronic fatigue, and, for women, menstrual discomfort. The clinician should be alert to any signs and symptoms that would suggest specific pathology and warrant further investigation; "alarm" signs and symptoms include fever, blood in the stool, anemia, weight loss, rectal bleeding, and increased levels of serum inflammatory markers.

The history should include queries as to the onset of symptoms, travel history (especially travel to areas where exposure to infectious enteric disease is likely), medication history to include OTC medications (with particular attention to recent intake of antibiotics), diet, and current and past stressors. Symptoms may begin in childhood or may be linked to a moderate-to-severe episode of enteritis or stress. The individual should be queried about any observed relationship between IBS symptoms and intake of foods containing gluten or complex fermentable carbohydrates (FODMAPs). Although the incidence of objectively proven celiac disease in the general population is quite low, some patients report that their symptoms improve with a gluten-free diet, and many report improved symptomatology with reduced intake of complex fermentable carbohydrates.

Diagnostic Tests

Diagnostic testing, in the absence of alarm symptoms, is usually limited to fecal occult blood testing and serum tests to rule out anemia and elevated levels of inflammatory

markers. Screening for celiac disease is recommended for patients with IBS-D and involves measurement of serum IgA antibody to tissue transglutaminase. Food allergy testing is rarely indicated in the diagnostic workup for IBS. Scanning and endoscopy are indicated only for patients with "alarm" symptoms.

Management

Management is symptom based and individualized and includes patient education, dietary modifications, routine exercise and stress management, and medications. A suggested algorithm is presented in Figure 15-2.

Patient Education

The first step in management of IBS, regardless of the predominant bowel pattern, is education. Individuals often have had symptoms for some time and may have consulted with other health care providers; many are very concerned that they have cancer or some other serious underlying condition. Developing a trusting relationship by actively listening to the history and concerns is foundational to effective management. Initial education should address the following points:

1. IBS is a common disorder that causes significant physical and emotional distress, but it is not life threatening and does not increase the risk for cancer.
2. At present, there is no known "cure" for IBS, but there are various treatment strategies that can significantly reduce symptoms and improve quality of life.
3. Determining the best treatment plan involves some trial and error and is unique for each individual.

As noted, there is currently no "cure" for IBS; thus, it is imperative for the clinician to work with the patient to establish realistic goals and strategies for self-management. A very helpful initial strategy is to have the patient maintain a 2-week symptom diary that includes a Bristol Stool Form chart, in which the patient can simultaneously track their bowel symptoms and stool elimination patterns. This information can then be reviewed by the care provider and individual at follow-up visits, and used as a baseline for assessment in improvement.

CLINICAL PEARL

Management of IBS is symptom based and individualized and includes patient education, dietary modifications, routine exercise and stress management, and medications.

Dietary Modifications

Although the link between diet and IBS is weak, modification in diet is typically the first step in self-management. Foods known to create gas and the sensation of bloating are a logical focus for trial elimination and include beans, onions, celery, carrots, raisins, bananas, apricots, prunes, and Brussels sprouts. Elimination or reduction of FODMAPs and

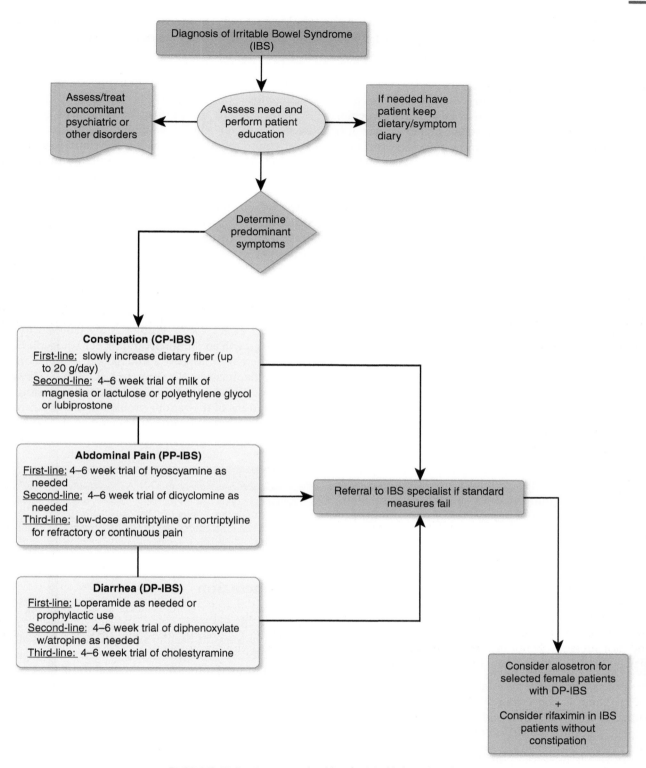

FIGURE 15-2. Treatment algorithm for irritable bowel syndrome.

lactose-containing foods has been shown to be effective for some patients with IBS (Gibson & Shepherd, 2010). A 2-week trial of dietary elimination is often recommended and should be sufficient to provide insight into any link between dietary intake and symptom severity. Identification of any foods that cause exacerbation of symptoms allows the patient to make her/his own decisions as to reduction, timing, or elimination; some individuals find long-term adherence to elimination of particular foods to be difficult and may elect selected intake as opposed to complete elimination.

Exercise/Activity and Stress Management

Physical activity may also help reduce symptoms. Limited research indicates that patients enrolled in an intervention trial experienced a reduction in symptoms following a 12-week exercise intervention program (Daley et al., 2008; Johannesson et al., 2011). Routine exercise may also help to reduce stress, which is known to be a trigger for symptom flares. Other stress management therapies may also be beneficial. For example, cognitively focused therapies such as cognitive–behavior therapy (CBT) may be helpful and can be delivered over the phone, web, or in person by a trained provider (Jarrett et al., 2009; Mahvi-Shirazi et al., 2012). However, the minimum number of sessions to deliver content related to relaxation and cognitive restructuring remains to be determined, and it can be challenging for patients to find providers who can provide this type of intervention.

Sleep disturbance can be regarded as one of the most important extraintestinal symptoms of IBS, which markedly affects quality of life and psychosocial well-being (Elsenbruch, 2005; Heitkemper et al., 2005). Mind–body therapy such as hypnosis and sleep hygiene may help decrease symptoms (Keefer & Keshavarzian, 2007).

Pharmacologic Therapy

The choice of medication(s) is based on the predominant bowel syndrome. For some patients, particularly those with IBS-C, the addition of psyllium/ispaghula improves stool bulk and intestinal transit time and reduces constipation (Ford et al., 2008). Soluble fiber, osmotic laxatives, and newer agents including lubiprostone and linaclotide may also be recommended for individuals with IBS-C. Osmotic laxatives, for example, PEG, are commonly prescribed when the addition of soluble fiber is insufficient to normalize stool consistency and elimination. While laxatives frequently correct the constipation, they do not decrease the abdominal pain/discomfort and are used only as needed for constipation management. Lubiprostone acts directly on the chloride channel activator to increase intestinal secretion and ultimately speed stool expulsion. Linaclotide is a guanylate cyclase agonist that stimulates intestinal secretion and peristalsis. While both are FDA approved for IBS-C, the long-term efficacy of these agents remains to be established. (Emmanuel et al., 2009). There is less evidence about selective serotonin reuptake inhibitors (SSRI) and serotonin norepinephrine reuptake inhibitors (SNRI) in the management of IBS. To date, clinical guidelines do suggest that SSRIs may be of more utility in IBS-C than IBS-D (Brandt et al., 2009; Wall et al., 2014).

People with IBS-D may be prescribed antidiarrheal agents for short-term use such as loperamide. While effective in reducing IBS diarrhea, it does not reduce the abdominal pain/discomfort, which is a limiting factor in its use. Another agent that may be tried when bile acid malabsorption is suspected is a bile acid sequestrant (e.g.,

cholestyramine). For individuals with severe diarrhea for whom other treatments are not effective after a 6-month period, the 5-HT$_3$ receptor antagonist alosetron (Lotronex) may be trialed. Of note, health care providers (e.g., doctors) who prescribe alosetron should be specially certified to prescribe (FDA, 2010).

Antispasmodic agents may be prescribed on an as-needed basis for relief of cramping abdominal pain; the most commonly used agents are dicyclomine and hyoscyamine, which are direct-acting GI smooth muscle relaxants. For patients with IBS-D or IBS-M in whom infectious enteritis is suspected, a trial of the nonabsorbable antibiotic rifaximin may be indicated. Antidepressants, in particular tricyclic agents, have been shown in randomized clinical trials to decrease symptoms such as abdominal pain and diarrhea in patients with IBS-D; in addition, they are associated with an improved sense of well-being. There is less evidence about SSRIs and SNRIs in the management of IBS.

Probiotics may be helpful for some patients with IBS (Guyonnet et al., 2007). Probiotics are believed to suppress the growth and luminal binding of pathogenic bacteria and thereby to improve epithelial barrier function and reduce inflammation (Guyonnet et al., 2007). However, clinical studies are needed to evaluate safety, dosing, and concentrations of the various probiotics and to determine optimal duration of treatment (Aragon et al., 2010; Ford et al., 2014).

CLINICAL PEARL

Probiotics may be helpful for some patients with IBS; however, clinical studies are needed to evaluate the dose and concentration of various agents as well as the optimal duration of treatment.

Conclusion

Functional bowel disorders such as constipation, diarrhea, and IBS are extremely common and exert a significant toll in terms of health care expenditures and quality of life. Effective management begins with a thorough history and focused physical examination to rule out "alarm symptoms" and to determine the specific disorder, associated symptomatology, and impact. Individuals with alarm symptoms must be promptly referred for further workup; individuals with no alarm symptoms can be managed symptomatically, with a focus on patient education, lifestyle modifications (e.g., fiber and fluid intake, dietary modifications, and exercise), and judicious use of pharmacologic agents (e.g., laxatives, antidiarrheals, and antispasmodic agents). A trusting patient/provider relationship is essential to effective management in all situations. Individuals with persistent diarrhea, slow-transit constipation, or obstructed defecation may require further workup and additional medical–surgical therapies.

CASE STUDIES

CASE STUDY: PATIENT WITH CONSTIPATION

An 87-year-old woman receiving in-home hospice care due to inoperable aortic stenosis complained of constipation. The client reported that she had managed her bowels with a daily dose of milk of magnesia for the past 7 years, a treatment that was no longer effective. She reported no bowel movement for the past 2 days, a sensation of rectal fullness, and inability to defecate. "The cardiologist told me I shouldn't strain because of my heart," she reported to the hospice nurse. The nurse noted that in addition to the cardiac problems, the client required fentanyl for management of chronic rheumatoid arthritis pain and was on fluid restriction for chronic renal insufficiency and congestive heart failure. Although still ambulatory, the client was unable to tolerate prolonged exercise without severe fatigue.

Diet recall for the previous 24 hours included the following: packet of instant oatmeal with milk, cup of coffee, ½ sandwich with ham, and a "t.v. dinner." When asked, the client admitted that she restricted her fluids much more than prescribed by her physicians so that she did not have to go to the bathroom so often.

Physical examination revealed abdominal distention, hypoactive bowel sounds, and left lower quadrant abdominal tenderness on palpation. After consultation with the cardiologist and obtaining permission from the client, a digital rectal examination (DRE) was performed. The DRE revealed an external hemorrhoid at the anal os and presence of a large, firm fecal mass in the rectal vault.

Because the etiology of constipation was complex, various nursing care measures were required:

Independent nursing actions:

1. Instruct client regarding the need to discontinue use of the stimulant laxative
2. Review a list of high-fiber foods with the client to determine which, if any, she might be willing and able to include in the diet.
3. Instruct the client in tracking fluid intake to achieve full daily fluid allowance.
4. Instruct the client in optimal toileting position and ensure availability of necessary assistive devices to achieve a physiologic defecation position
5. Provide simple bowel diary and stool form chart and instruct the client in completion between home visits

Dependent nursing actions:

1. Obtain prescription for daily stool softener.
2. Obtain prescription for oil-retention enema now and prn
3. Obtain prescription for prn PEG laxative

Interdependent nursing actions:

1. Monitor stool form and frequency with bowel diary.
2. Assess for flatulence, abdominal discomfort, or other complications of fiber therapy.

Response: Following administration of the oil-retention enema, the nurse was able to gently break up the fecal mass. The patient was instructed to take the PEG laxative and reported a normal bowel movement following this. The patient also increased her fluid and fiber intake and began taking the stool softener; 1 week following the initial visit, the patient reported soft formed stools every other day.

CASE STUDIES

CASE STUDY: PATIENTS WITH IBS-D

Common patient presentation: KS is a 25-year-old woman who was referred to a gastroenterologist for colonoscopy to evaluate a recent exacerbation of diarrhea with increased abdominal cramping. Currently, she is a graduate student at a large university. She describes her current life as stressful due to financial concerns. She reports a history of depression. Her abdominal symptoms started 2 years ago. She complains of lower abdominal pain, bloating, gas, and frequent, loose stools; she denies seeing any blood in the stool. Despite these symptoms, her weight has remained stable. For the last 6 months, her abdominal pain has been at least 3 days/month and is not associated with menstruation.

The pain is reduced with defecation. In addition, she reports feeling anxious, tired, and sleep deprived.

Basic workup: Her physical examination, vital signs, and body weight are within normal limits. There is no family history of organic GI disease. Her primary care provider orders a panel of laboratory tests (CBC, ESR, electrolytes, LFTs) and more stool studies (e.g., ova). These are WNL. Rectal examination revealed no hemorrhoids. No mucosal lesions were identified on colonoscopic examination, and random biopsies were taken from the descending and sigmoid colon. All findings were normal.

Individual management plan: The provider works with KS to establish a treatment plan. She is educated regarding the pathology and management of IBS and is reassured that the symptoms can be managed with lifestyle changes and medications if needed. KS is encouraged to keep a symptom and stool diary for 2 weeks. She is asked to reflect on her dietary intake and stress levels when she experiences symptoms and to make a note of these as well. The goal is to identify triggers that are associated with "flares" of symptoms. Nonpharmacological approaches such as relaxation, stress management, and sleep hygiene are initiated. In her diary, KS notes that on those days when she doesn't eat breakfast her symptoms are more intense. The clinic nurse provides education regarding the relationship of diet including the timing of meals and symptoms. Despite these nonpharmacological approaches, KS's symptoms persist and she is having difficulty continuing to attend school. Antidiarrheal and antispasmodic medications are prescribed, and KS reports that these are very beneficial in managing symptoms and that she is feeling better able to control her IBS and to complete her school assignments.

REFERENCES

Addison, R., & Smith, M. (2000). *Digital rectal examination and manual removal of faeces: Guidance for nurses.* London, UK: Royal College of Nursing.

Albiani, J. J., Hart, S. L., Katz, L., et al. (2013). Impact of depression and anxiety on the quality of life of constipated patients. *Journal of Clinical Psychology in Medical Settings, 20*(1), 123–132. doi: 10.1007/s10880-012-9306-3

Allen, S. J., Martinez, E. G., Gregorio, G. V., et al. (2010). Probiotics for treating acute infectious diarrhoea. *Cochrane Database of Systematic Reviews.* doi: 10.1002/14651858.CD003048.pub3

Alonso, C., Guilarte, M., Vicario, M., et al. (2008). Maladaptive intestinal epithelial responses to life stress may predispose healthy women to gut mucosal inflammation. *Gastroenterology, 135*(1), 163–172.e161. doi: 10.1053/j.gastro.2008.03.036

Alvarez-Acosta, T., León, C., Acosta-González, S., et al. (2009). Beneficial role of green plantain [*Musa paradisiaca*] in the management of persistent diarrhea: A prospective randomized trial. *Journal of the American College of Nutrition, 28*(2), 169–176.

Apweiler, R., Aslanidis, C., Deufel, T., et al. (2009). Approaching clinical proteomics: Current state and future fields of application in fluid proteomics. *Clinical Chemistry and Laboratory Medicine, 47*(6), 724–744.

Aragon, G., Graham, D. B., Borum, M., et al. (2010). Probiotic therapy for irritable bowel syndrome. *Gastroenterology & Hepatology, 6*(1), 39–44.

Arnold, B. F., Barreto, M. L., Boisson, S., et al. (2011). Epidemiological methods in diarrhoea studies—An update. *International Journal of Epidemiology, 40*, 1678–1692. doi: 10.1093/ije/dyr152

Arumugam, M., Raes, J., Pelletier, E., et al. (2011). Enterotypes of the human gut microbiome. *Nature, 473*(7346), 174–180. doi: nature09944 [pii]10.1038/nature09944

Baldi, F., Bianco, M. A., Nardone, G., et al. (2009). Focus on acute diarrhoeal disease. *World Journal of Gastroenterology, 15*(27), 3341–3348. doi: 10.3748/wjg.15.3341

Barr, W., & Smith, A. (2014). Acute diarrhea. *American Family Physician, 89*(5), 180–189.

Bengmark, S. (2013). Gut microbiota, immune development and function. *Pharmacological Research, 69*(1), 87–113. doi: 10.1016/j.phrs.2012.09.002

Bharucha, A. E., Dorn, S. D., Lembo, A., et al. (2013). American Gastroenterological Association medical position statement on constipation. *Gastroenterology, 144*(1), 211–217. doi: 10.1053/j.gastro.2012.10.029

Bond, B., Quinlan, J., Dukes, G. E., et al. (2009). Irritable bowel syndrome: More than abdominal pain and bowel habit abnormalities. *Clinical Gastroenterology and Hepatology, 7*(1), 73–79. doi: 10.1016/j.cgh.2008.08.011

Bradford, K., Shih, W., Videlock, E. J., et al. (2012). Association between early adverse life events and irritable bowel syndrome. *Clinical Gastroenterology and Hepatology, 10*(4), 385–390; e381–e383. doi: S1542-3565(11)01333-4 [pii]

Brandt, L. J., Chey, W. D., Foxx-Orenstein, A. E., et al. (2009). An evidence-based position statement on the management of irritable bowel syndrome. *American Journal of Gastroenterology, 104*(Suppl 1), S1–S35. doi: 10.1038/ajg.2008.122

Brennan, M. R., Spiegel, B. M. R., Khanna, D., et al. (2011). Understanding gastrointestiinal distress: A framework for clinical practice. *American Journal of Gastroenterology, 106*, 380–385. doi: 10.1038/ajg.2010.383

Buffie, C. G., Jarchum, I., Equinda, M., et al. (2012). Profound alterations of intestinal microbiota following a single dose of clindamycin results in sustained susceptibility to *Clostridium difficile*-induced colitis. *Infection and Immunity, 80*(1), 62–73. doi: 10.1128/iai.05496-11

Butterworth, A. D., Thomas, A. G., & Akobeng, A. K. (2008). Probiotics for induction of remission in Crohn's disease. *Cochrane Database of Systematic Reviews.* doi: 10.1002/14651858.CD006634.pub2

Byar, K. L., Davis, A. B., Kiker, E. S., et al. (2011). *Diarrhea.* Retrieved from https://www.ons.org/practice-resources/pep/diarrhea

Cairns, M. D., Stabler, R. A., Shetty, N., et al. (2012). The continually evolving *Clostridium difficile* species. *Future Microbiology, 7*(8), 945–957.

Camilleri, M., Busciglio, I., Acosta, A., et al. (2014). Effect of increased bile acid synthesis or fecal excretion in irritable bowel syndrome-diarrhea. *American Journal of Gastroenterology, 109*(10), 1621–1630. doi: 10.1038/ajg.2014.215

Camilleri, M., Lasch, K., & Zhou, W. (2012). Irritable bowel syndrome: Methods, mechanisms, and pathophysiology. The confluence of increased permeability, inflammation, and pain in irritable bowel syndrome. *American Journal of Physiology—Gastrointestinal and Liver Physiology, 303*(7), G775–G785. doi: 10.1152/ajpgi.00155.2012

Cani, P. D., Bibiloni, R., Knauf, C., et al. (2008). Changes in gut microbiota control metabolic endotoxemia-induced inflammation in high-fat diet-induced obesity and diabetes in mice. *Diabetes, 57*(6), 1470–1481. doi: 10.2337/db07-1403

Castellarin, M., Warren, R. L., Freeman, J. D., et al. (2012). *Fusobacterium nucleatum* infection is prevalent in human colorectal carcinoma. *Genome Research, 22*(2), 299–306. doi: 10.1101/gr.126516.111

Centers for Disease Control and Prevention. (2014). Trends in foodborne illness in the United States, 2013. Retrieved from http://www.cdc.gov/features/dsfoodsafetyreport/

Chassaing, B., & Darfeuille-Michaud, A. (2011). The commensal microbiota and enteropathogens in the pathogenesis of inflammatory bowel diseases. *Gastroenterology, 140*(6), 1720–1728. doi: 10.1053/j.gastro.2011.01.054

Cheng, C.-W., Bian, Z.-X., & Wu, T.-X. (2009). Systematic review of Chinese herbal medicine for functional constipation. *World Journal of Gastroenterology, 15*(39), 4886–4895.

Coggrave, M. J., & Norton, C. (2010). The need for manual evacuation and oral laxatives in the management of neurogenic bowel dysfunction after spinal cord injury: A randomized controlled trial of a stepwise protocol. *Spinal Cord, 48*, 504–510. doi: 10.1038/sc.2009.166

Coggrave, M., & Norton, C. (2013). Management of faecal incontinence and constipation in adults with central neurological diseases. *Cochrane Database of Systematic Reviews, 12*, CD002115. doi: 10.1002/14651858.CD002115.pub4

Coulter, I. D., Favreau, J. T., Hardy, M. L., et al. (2002). Biofeedback interventions for gastrointestinal conditions: A systematic review. *Alternative Therapies in Health and Medicine, 8*(3), 76–83.

Daley, A., Grimmett, C., Roberts, L., et al. (2008). The effects of exercise upon symptoms and quality of life in patients diagnosed with irritable bowel syndrome: A randomised controlled trial. *International Journal of Sports Medicine, 29*(9), 778–782.

Demers, M., Dagnault, A., & Desjardins, J. (2014). A randomized double-blind controlled trial: Impact of probiotics on diarrhea in patients treated with pelvic radiation. *Clinical Nutrition, 33*(5), 761–767. doi: 10.1016/j.clnu.2013.10.015

Deshpande, A., Lever, D. S., & Sofer, E. (2014). *Acute Diarrhea Disease Management Project*. Retrieved from Cleveland Clinic Foundation. Retrieved from http://www.clevelandclinicmeded.com/medicalpubs/diseasemanagement/gastroenterology/acute-diarrhea/

Dethlefsen, L., & Relman, D. A. (2011). Incomplete recovery and individualized responses of the human distal gut microbiota to repeated antibiotic perturbation. *Proceedings of the National Academy of Sciences of the United States of America, 108*(Suppl 1), 4554–4561. doi: 10.1073/pnas.1000087107.

Dhingra, L., Shuk, E., Grossman, B., et al. (2013). A qualitative study to explore psychological distress and illness burden associated with opioid-induced constipation in cancer patients with advanced disease. *Palliative Medicine, 27*(5), 447–456. doi: 10.1177/0269216312450358

Drossman, D. A. (2006). Functional versus organic: An inappropriate dichotomy for clinical care. *The American Journal of Gastroenterology, 101*(6), 1172–1175.

Drossman, D. (2007). Introduction. The Rome Foundation and Rome III. *Neurogastroenterology & Motility 19*(10), 783–786; *101*(6), 1172–1175.

Drossman, D. A., Corazziari, E., Delvaux, M., et al. (2006). *Rome III: The functional gastrointestinal disorders* (3rd ed.). McLean, VA: Degnon Associates, Inc.

Ellis, C. N., & Essani, R. (2012). Treatment of obstructed defecation. *Clinics of Colon and Rectal Surgery, 25*, 24–33. doi: 10.1055/s-0032-1301756

Ellison, J. S., Haraway, A. N., & Park, J. M. (2013). The distal left Malone antegrade continence enema—Is it better? *The Journal of Urology, 190*(4 Suppl), 1529–1533. doi: 10.1016/j.juro.2013.01.092

Elsenbruch, S. (2005). Melatonin: A novel treatment for IBS? *Gut, 54*(10), 1353–1354. doi: 10.1136/gut.2005.074377

Emmanuel, A., Tack, J., Quigley, E., et al. (2009). Pharmacological management of constipation. *Neurogastroenterology & Motility, 21*(s2), 41–54.

Ernst, E. (1999). Abdominal massage therapy for chronic constipation: A systematic review of controlled clinical trials. *Forschende Komplementärmedizin, 6*(3), 149–151.

Eswaran, S., Muir, J., & Chey, W. D. (2013). Fiber and functional gastrointestinal disorders. *American Journal of Gastroenterology, 108*, 718–727. doi: 10.1038/ajg.2013.63

Faresjo, A., Grodzinsky, E., Johansson, S., et al. (2007). A population-based case–control study of work and psychosocial problems in patients with irritable bowel syndrome—Women are more seriously affected than men. *American Journal of Gastroenterology, 102*(2), 371–379. doi: AJG1012 [pii]10.1111/j.1572-0241.2006.01012.x [doi]

Faried, M., El Nakeeb, A., Youssef, M., et al. (2010). Comparative study between surgical and non-surgical treatment of anismus in patients with symptoms of obstructed defecation: A prospective randomized study. *Journal of Gastrointestinal Surgery: Official Journal of The Society for Surgery of The Alimentary Tract, 14*(8), 1235–1243. doi: 10.1007/s11605-010-1229-4

FDA. (2010). *Medication Guide LOTRONEX®(LOW-trah-nex) Tablets (alosetron hydrochloride)*. Silver Spring, MD: Medication Guide.

Food and Nutrition Board, I. o. M. (2005). *Dietary, functional, and total fiberDRI: Dietary reference intakes for energy, carbohydrate, fiber, fat, fatty acids, cholesterol, protein, and amino acids*. Washington, DC:

National Academies Press. Retrieved from http://www.nal.usda.gov/fnic/DRI/DRI_Energy/energy_full_report.pdf

Ford, A. C., Quigley, E. M., Lacy, B. E., et al. (2014). Efficacy of prebiotics, probiotics, and symbiotics in irritable bowel syndrome and chronic idiopathic constipation: Systematic review and meta-analysis. *The American Journal of Gastroenterology, 109*(10), 1547–1561.

Ford, A. C., Talley, N. J., Spiegel, B. M. R., et al. (2008). Effect of fibre, antispasmodics, and peppermint oil in the treatment of irritable bowel syndrome: Systematic review and meta-analysis. *British Medical Journal, 337*, a2313.

Fosnes, G. S., Lydersen, S., & Farup, P. G. (2011). Effectiveness of laxatives in elderly—A cross sectional study in nursing homes. *BMC Geriatrics, 11*, 76. doi: 10.1186/1471-2318-11-76

Gibson, P. R., & Shepherd, S. J. (2010). Evidence-based dietary management of functional gastrointestinal symptoms: The FODMAP approach. *Journal of Gastroenterology and Hepatology, 25*(2), 252–258. doi: 10.1111/j.1440-1746.2009.06149.x

Global Task Force on Cholera. (2014). WHO position paper on oral rehydration salts to reduce mortality from cholera. Retrieved from http://www.who.int/cholera/technical/en/

Goldenberg, J. Z., Ma, S. S. Y., Saxton, J. D., et al. (2013). Probiotics for the prevention of *Clostridium difficile*-associated diarrhea in adults and children. doi: 10.1002/14651858.CD006095.pub3

Gray, M. (2014). Stool management systems for preventing environmental spread of *Clostridium difficile*: A comparative trial. *Journal of Wound, Ostomy, and Continence Nursing, 41*(5), 460–465.

Guyonnet, D., Chassany, O., Ducrotte, P., et al. (2007). Effect of a fermented milk containing *Bifidobacterium animalis* DN-173 010 on the health-related quality of life and symptoms in irritable bowel syndrome in adults in primary care: A multicentre, randomized, double-blind, controlled trial. *Alimentary Pharmacology and Therapeutics, 26*(3), 475–486. doi: 10.1111/j.1365-2036.2007.03362.x

Haas, B. J., Gevers, D., Earl, A. M., et al. (2011). Chimeric 16S rRNA sequence formation and detection in Sanger and 454-pyrosequenced PCR amplicons. *Genome Research, 21*(3), 494–504. doi: gr.112730.110 [pii]10.1101/gr.112730.110.

Halpert, A. D. (2010). Importance of early diagnosis in patients with irritable bowel syndrome. *Postgraduate Medical Journal, 122*(2), 102–111. doi: 10.3810/pgm.2010.03.2127

Heitkemper, M., Jarrett, M., Burr, R., et al. (2005). Subjective and objective sleep indices in women with irritable bowel syndrome. *Neurogastroenterology & Motility, 17*(4), 523–530.

Heitkemper, M., Cain, K. C., Shulman, R., et al. (2011). Subtypes of irritable bowel syndrome based on abdominal pain/discomfort severity and bowel pattern. *Digestive Diseases and Sciences, 56*(7), 2050–2058. doi: 10.1007/s10620-011-1567-4

Herdman, T. H., & Kamitsuru, S. (2014). *Diarrhea nursing diagnoses: Definitions & classifications, 2015–2017* (10th ed., pp. 200). Oxford, UK: Wiley Blackwell.

Horst, S., Shelby, G., Anderson, J., et al. (2014). Predicting persistence of functional abdominal pain from childhood into young adulthood. *Clinical Gastroenterology and Hepatology, 12*(12), 2026–2032. doi: 10.1016/j.cgh.2014.03.034

Hosseinzadeh, S. T., Poorsaadati, S., Radkani, B., et al. (2011). Psychological disorders in patients with chronic constipation. *Gastroenterology & Hepatology, 4*(3), 159–163.

Hsueh, H. F., Jarrett, M. E., Cain, K. C., et al. (2011). Does a self-management program change dietary intake in adults with irritable bowel syndrome? *Gastroenterology Nursing, 34*(2), 108–116. doi: 10.1097/SGA.0b013e31821092e8

Hughes, P. A., Zola, H., Penttila, I. A., et al. (2013). Immune activation in irritable bowel syndrome: Can neuroimmune interactions explain symptoms? *American Journal of Gastroenterology, 108*, 1066–1074. doi: 10.1038/ajg.2013.120

Inadomi, J. M., Fennerty, M. B., & Bjorkman, D. (2003). The economic impact of irritable bowel syndrome. *Alimentary Pharmacology & Therapeutics, 18*(7), 671–682.

Jamshed, M., Lee, Z.-E., & Oldern, K. W. (2011). Diagnostic approach to chronic constipation in adults. *American Family Physician, 25,* 299–306.

Jarrett, M. E., Cain, K. C., Burr, R. L., et al. (2009). Comprehensive self-management for irritable bowel syndrome: Randomized trial of in-person versus combined in-person and telephone sessions. *The American Journal of Gastroenterology, 104*(12), 3004–3014. doi: 10.1038/ajg.2009.479

Jarrett, M., Visser, R., & Heitkemper, M. (2001). Diet triggers symptoms in women with irritable bowel syndrome. The patient's perspective. *Gastroenterology Nursing, 24*(5), 246–252.

Jeffery, I. B., O'Toole, P. W., Ohman, L., et al. (2012). An irritable bowel syndrome subtype defined by species-specific alterations in faecal microbiota. *Gut, 61*(7), 997–1006. doi: 10.1136/gutjnl-2011-301501

Johannesson, E., Simren, M., Strid, H., et al. (2011). Physical activity improves symptoms in irritable bowel syndrome: A randomized controlled trial. *American Journal of Gastroenterology, 106*(5), 915–922.

Johnston, B. C., Goldenberg, J. Z., Vandvik, P. O., et al. (2011). Probiotics for the prevention of pediatric antibiotic-associated diarrhea. *Cochrane Database of Systematic Reviews,* (11), CD004877.

Johnston, B. C., Ma, S. S., Goldenberg, J. Z., et al. (2012). Probiotics for the prevention of *Clostridium difficile*-associated diarrhea: A systematic review and meta-analysis. *Annals of Internal Medicine, 157*(12), 878–888.

Jones, S., Towers, V., Welsby, S., et al. (2011). *Clostridium difficile* containment properties of a fecal management system: An in vitro investigation. *Ostomy Wound Management, 57*(10), 38–49.

Keefer, L., & Keshavarzian, A. (2007). Feasibility and acceptability of gut-directed hypnosis on inflammatory bowel disease: A brief communication. *International Journal of Clinical and Experimental Hypnosis, 55*(4), 457–466.

Khan, W. U., & Sellen, D. W. (2011). Zinc supplementation in the management of diarrhoea. *e-Library of Evidence for Nutrition Actions (eLENA).* Retrieved from http://www.who.int/elena/titles/bbc/zinc_diarrhoea/en/

Kostic, A. D., Gevers, D., Pedamallu, C. S., et al. (2012). Genomic analysis identifies association of *Fusobacterium* with colorectal carcinoma. *Genome Research, 22*(2), 292–298. doi: 10.1101/gr.126573.111

Kotloff, K. L., Nataro, J. P., Blackwelder, W. C., et al. (2013). Burden and aetiology of diarrhoeal disease in infants and young children in developing countries (the Global Enteric Multicenter Study, GEMS): A prospective, case–control study. *Lancet, 382*(9888), 209–222.

Kumar, A., Lokesh, H., & Ghoshal, U. C. (2013). Successful outcome of refractory chronic constipation by surgical treatment: A series of 34 patients. *Journal of Neurogastroenterology and Motility, 19*(1), 78–84. doi: 10.5056/jnm.2013.19.1.78

Kumar, S., Ranjan, P., Mittal, B., et al. (2012). Serotonin transporter gene (SLC6A4) polymorphism in patients with irritable bowel syndrome and healthy controls. *Journal of Gastrointestinal and Liver Disease, 21*(1), 31–38.

Kyle, G., Prynn, P., & Oliver, H. (2005). A procedure for the digital removal of faeces. *Nursing Standard, 19*(20), 33–39.

Lanata, C. F., Fischer-Walker, C. L., Olascoaga, A. C., et al. (2013). Global causes of diarrheal disease mortality in children <5 years of age: A systematic review. *PLoS ONE, 8*(9). doi: 10.1371/journal.pone.0072778

Larsen, N., Vogensen, F. K., van den Berg, F. W., et al. (2010). Gut microbiota in human adults with type 2 diabetes differs from non-diabetic adults. *PLoS ONE, 5*(2), e9085. doi: 10.1371/journal.pone.0009085

Ledochowski, M., Widner, B., Bair, H., et al. (2000). Fructose- and sorbitol-reduced diet improves mood and gastrointestinal disturbances in fructose malabsorbers. *Scandinavian Journal of Gastroenterology, 35*(10), 1048–1052.

Lesch, K. P. (2011). When the serotonin transporter gene meets adversity: The contribution of animal models to understanding epigenetic mechanisms in affective disorders and resilience. *Current Topics in Behavioral Neurosciences, 7,* 251–280. doi: 10.1007/7854_2010_109

Lombardi, G., Del Popolo, G., Cecconi, F., et al. (2010). Clinical outcome of sacral neuromodulation in incomplete spinal cord-injured patients suffering from neurogenic bowel dysfunctions. *Spinal Cord, 48*(2), 154–159. doi: 10.1038/sc.2009.101

Longstreth, G. F., Thompson, W. G., Chey, W. D., et al. (2006). Functional bowel disorders. *Gastroenterology, 130,* 1480–1491. doi: 10.1053/j.gastro.2005.11.061

Lozupone, C., Hamady, M., & Knight, R. (2006). UniFrac—An online tool for comparing microbial community diversity in a phylogenetic context. *BMC Bioinformatics, 7,* 371. doi: 1471-2105-7-371 [pii] 10.1186/1471-2105-7-371

Mahvi-Shirazi, M., Fathi-Ashtiani, A., Rasoolzade-Tabatabaei, S.-K., et al. (2012). Irritable bowel syndrome treatment: Cognitive behavioral therapy versus medical treatment. *Archives Medical Science, 8*(1), 123–129.

Mallon, P. T., McKay, D., Kirk, S. J., et al. (2007). Probiotics for induction of remission in ulcerative colitis. *Cochrane Database of Systematic Reviews.* doi: 10.1002/14651858.CD005573.pub2

Marchetti, F., Corallo Jr, J. P., Ritter, J., et al. (2011). Retention cuff pressure study of 3 indwelling stool management systems: Randomized study of 10 healthy subjects. *Journal of Wound, Ostomy, and Continence Nursing, 38*(5), 569–573. doi: 10.1097/WON.0b013e31822ad43c

Mazumder, S., Taneja, S., Bhandari, N., et al. (2010). Effectiveness of zinc supplementation plus oral rehydration salts for diarrhoea in infants aged less than 6 months in Haryana state, India. *Bulletin of the World Health Organization, 88,* 754–760. doi: 10.2471/BLT.10.075986

McCrea, G. L., Miaskowski, C., Stotts, N. A., et al. (2010). Age differences in patients evaluated for constipation: Constipation characteristics, symptoms, and bowel and dietary habits. *Journal of Wound, Ostomy, and Continence Nursing, 37*(6), 667–676. doi: 10.1097/WON.0b013e3181f91082

McElhanon, B. O., McCracken, C., Karpen, S., et al. (2014). Gastrointestinal symptoms in autism spectrum disorder: A meta-analysis. *Pediatrics, 133*(5), 872–883.

Meurette, G., Lehur, P. A., Coron, E., et al. (2010). Long-term results of Malone's procedure with antegrade irrigation for severe chronic constipation. *Gastroentérologie Clinique Et Biologique, 34*(3), 209–212. doi: 10.1016/j.gcb.2009.12.009

Muir, J. G., & Gibson, P. R. (2013). The Low FODMAP diet for treatment of irritable bowel syndrome and other gastrointestinal disorders. *Gastroenterology & Hepatology, 9*(7), 450.

Naidoo, K., Morris, G., Fagbemi, A. D., et al. (2011). Probiotics for the maintenance of remission in ulcerative colitis. *Cochrane Database of Systematic Reviews.* doi: 10.1002/14651858.CD007443.pub2

National Digestive Diseases Information Clearinghouse. (2013). Constipation. Retrieved from http://digestive.niddk.nih.gov/ddiseases/pubs/constipation/#what

Noiesen, E., Trosborg, I., Bager, L., et al. (2014). Constipation—Prevalence and incidence among medical patients acutely admitted to hospital with a medical condition. *Journal of Clinical Nursing, 23*(15/16), 2295–2302. doi: 10.1111/jocn.12511

Nyrop, K. A., Palsson, O. S., Levy, R. L., et al. (2007). Costs of health care for irritable bowel syndrome, chronic constipation, functional diarrhoea and functional abdominal pain. *Alimentary Pharmacology & Therapeutics, 26*(2), 237–248. doi: APT3370 [pii] 10.1111/j.1365-2036.2007.03370.x

Oxford English Dictionary. (2014). Oxford, UK: Oxford University Press. Retrieved from http://www.oxforddictionaries.com/us/definition/american_english/diarrhea

Papatheodoridis, G. V., Vlachogiannakos, J., Karaitianos, I., et al. (2010). A Greek survey of community prevalence and characteristics of constipation. *European Journal of Gastroenterology & Hepatology, 22*(3), 354–360. doi: 10.1097/MEG.0b013e32832bfdf0

Pata, C., Erdal, M. E., Derici, E., et al. (2002). Serotonin transporter gene polymorphism in irritable bowel syndrome. *American Journal of Gastroenterology, 97*(7), 1780–1784.

Pittman, J., Beeson, T., Schultz, M., et al. (2011). An interventional study of bowel management methods to decrease incontinence associated dermatitis. *Journal of Wound, Ostomy, and Continence Nursing, 38*(3S), S3–S4.

Pittman, J., Beeson, T., Terry, C., et al. (2012). Methods of bowel management in critical care: A randomized controlled trial. *Journal of Wound, Ostomy, and Continence Nursing, 39*(6), 633–639.

Rajilić-Stojanović, M. (2007). *Diversity of the human gastrointestinal microbiota: Novel perspectives from high throughput analyses.* Wageningen, The Netherlands: Wageningen Universiteit.

Rajilić-Stojanović, M., Biagi, E., Heilig, H. G., et al. (2011). Global and deep molecular analysis of microbiota signatures in fecal samples from patients with irritable bowel syndrome. *Gastroenterology, 141*(5), 1792–1801. doi: 10.1053/j.gastro.2011.07.043

Rao, S. S. C., Camilleri, M., Hasler, W. E., et al. (2011). Evaluation of gastrointestinal transit in clinical practice: Position paper of the American and European Neurogastroenterolgy and Motility Societies. *Neurogastroenterology & Motility, 23*, 8–23. doi: 10.1111/j.1365-2982.2010.0162.x

Reiner, C. S., Tutuian, R., Solopova, A. E., et al. (2011). MR defecography in patients with dyssynergic defecation: Spectrum of imaging findings and diagnostic value. *British Journal of Radiology, 84*, 136–144. doi: 10.1259/bjr/28989463

Riaz, M., Alam, S., Malik, A., et al. (2012). Efficacy and safety of *Saccharomyces boulardii* in acute childhood diarrhea: A double blind randomised controlled trial. *The Indian Journal of Pediatrics, 79*(4), 478–482. doi: 10.1007/s12098-011-0573-z

Richardson, G., & Dobish, R. (2007). Chemotherapy induced diarrhea. *Journal of Oncology Pharmacy Practice, 13*(4), 181–198.

Rolfe, V. E., Fortun, P. J., Hawkey, C. J., et al. (2006). Probiotics for maintenance of remission in Crohn's disease. *Cochrane Database of Systematic Reviews, (4)*, CD004826.

Rosen, A. (2010). Obstructed defecation syndrome: Diagnosis and therapeutic options, with special focus on the STARR procedure. *Israel Medical Association Journal, 12*, 104–106.

Saad, R. J., Rao, S. S. C., Koch, K. L., et al. (2010). Do stool form and frequency correlate with whole-gut and colonic transit? *American Journal of Gastroenterology, 105*(2), 403–411.

Saito, Y. A., Mitra, N., & Mayer, E. A. (2010). Genetic approaches to functional gastrointestinal disorders. *Gastroenterology, 138*(4), 1276–1285. doi: S0016-5085(10)00265-9 [pii] 10.1053/j.gastro.2010.02.037.

Sandler, R. S. (1990). Epidemiology of irritable bowel syndrome in the United States. *Gastroenterology, 99*(2), 409–415.

Sartor, R. B. (2008). Microbial influences in inflammatory bowel diseases. *Gastroenterology, 134*(2), 577–594. doi: 10.1053/j.gastro.2007.11.059

Saulnier, D. M., Riehle, K., Mistretta, T. A., et al. (2011). Gastrointestinal microbiome signatures of pediatric patients with irritable bowel syndrome. *Gastroenterology, 141*(5), 1782–1791. doi: S0016-5085(11)00922-X [pii]10.1053/j.gastro.2011.06.072

Scher, J. U., & Abramson, S. B. (2011). The microbiome and rheumatoid arthritis. *Nature Reviews Rheumatology, 7*(10), 569–578. doi: 10.1038/nrrheum.2011.121

Schultz, A. B., Chen, C.-Y., & Edington, D. W. (2009). The cost and impact of health conditions on presenteeism to employers. *PharmacoEconomics, 27*(5), 365–378.

Shankar, V., Agans, R., Holmes, B., et al. (2013). Do gut microbial communities differ in pediatric IBS and health? *Gut Microbes, 4*(4), 347–352.

Sharma, A., Liu, B., Waudby, P., et al. (2011). Sacral neuromodulation for the management of severe constipation: Development of a constipation treatment protocol. *International Journal of Colorectal Disease, 26*(12), 1583–1587. doi: 10.1007/s00384-011-1257-x

Shaw, C., & Taylor, L. (2012). Treatment-related diarrhea in patients with cancer. *Clinical Journal of Oncology Nursing, 16*(4), 413–417. doi: 10.1188/12.CJON.413-417

Shepherd, S. J., & Gibson, P. R. (2006). Fructose malabsorption and symptoms of irritable bowel syndrome: Guidelines for effective dietary management. *Journal of the American Dietetic Association, 106*(10), 1631–1639. doi: 10.1016/j.jada.2006.07.010

Solomons, J., & Woodward, S. (2013). Digital removal of faeces in the bowel management of patients with spinal cord injury: A review. *British Journal of Neuroscience Nursing, 9*(5), 216–222.

Song, H. J. (2012). Constipation in community-dwelling elders: Prevalence and associated factors. *Journal of Wound, Ostomy, and Continence Nursing, 39*(6), 640–645. doi: 10.1097/WON.0b013e31826a4b70

Sorouri, M., Pourhoseingholi, M., Vahedi, M., et al. (2010). Functional bowel disorders in Iranian population using Rome III criteria. *Saudi Journal of Gastroenterology, 16*(3), 154–160.

Spiegel, B. M. (2009). The burden of IBS: Looking at metrics. *Current Gastroenterology Reports, 11*(4), 265–269.

Spiegel, B., Strickland, A., Naliboff, B. D., et al. (2008). Predictors of patient-assessed illness severity in irritable bowel syndrome. *The American Journal of Gastroenterology, 103*(10), 2536–2543.

Stake-Nilsson, K., Hultcrantz, R., Unge, P., et al. (2012). Complementary and alternative medicine used by persons with functional gastrointestinal disorders to alleviate symptom distress. *Journal of Clinical Nursing, 21*(5–6), 800–808. doi: 10.1111/j.1365-2702.2011.03985.x

Thomazini, C. M., Samegima, D. A., Rodrigues, M. A., et al. (2011). High prevalence of aggregative adherent *Escherichia coli* strains in the mucosa-associated microbiota of patients with inflammatory bowel diseases. *International Journal of Medical Microbiology, 301*(6), 475–479. doi: 10.1016/j.ijmm.2011.04.015

Turnbaugh, P. J., Hamady, M., Yatsunenko, T., et al. (2009). A core gut microbiome in obese and lean twins. *Nature, 457*(7228), 480–484. doi: 10.1038/nature07540

Ubeda, C., & Pamer, E. G. (2012). Antibiotics, microbiota, and immune defense. *Trends in Immunology, 33*(9), 459–466. doi: 10.1016/j.it.2012.05.003

Ubeda, C., Taur, Y., Jenq, R. R., et al. (2010). Vancomycin-resistant *Enterococcus* domination of intestinal microbiota is enabled by antibiotic treatment in mice and precedes bloodstream invasion in humans. *Journal of Clinical Investigation, 120*(12), 4332–4341. doi: 10.1172/jci43918

van Dijk, M., Benninga, M. A., Grootenhuis, M. A., et al. (2010). Prevalence and associated clinical characteristics of behavior problems in constipated children. *Pediatrics, 125*(2), e309–e317. doi: 10.1542/peds.2008-3055

van Tilburg, M. A. L., Palsson, O. S., Levy, R. L., et al. (2008). Complementary and alternative medicine use and cost in functional bowel disorders: A six month prospective study in a large HMO. *BMC Complementary and Alternative Medicine, 8*, 46. doi: 10.1186/1472-6882-8-46

Verdu, E. F., Armstrong, D., & Murray, J. A. (2009). Between celiac disease and irritable bowel syndrome: The "No Man's Land" of gluten sensitivity. *The American Journal of Gastroenterology, 104*(6), 1587–1594. doi: 10.1038/ajg.2009.188

Voegeli, D. (2008). The effect of washing and drying practices on skin barrier function. *Journal of Wound, Ostomy, and Continence Nursing, 35*(1), 84–90. doi: 10.1097/01.WON.0000308623.68582.d7.

Wald, A., Mueller-Lissner, S., Kamm, M. A., et al. (2010). Survey of laxative use by adults with self-defined constipation in South America and Asia: A comparison of six countries. *Alimentary Pharmacology & Therapeutics, 31*(2), 274–284. doi: 10.1111/j.1365-2036.2009.04169.x

Wald, A., Scarpignato, C., Kamm, M. A., et al. (2007). The burden of constipation on quality of life: Results of a multinational survey. *Alimentary Pharmacology & Therapeutics, 26*(2), 227–236.

Wald, A., Scarpignato, C., Mueller-Lissner, S., et al. (2008). A multinational survey of prevalence and patterns of laxative use among adults with self-defined constipation. *Alimentary Pharmacology & Therapeutics, 28*(7), 917–930. doi: 10.1111/j.1365-2036.2008.03806.x

Walker, L. S., Guite, J. W., Duke, M., et al. (1998). Recurrent abdominal pain: A potential precursor of irritable bowel syndrome in adolescents and young adults. *Journal of Pediatrics, 132*(6), 1010–1015.

Walker, C. F., Sack, D., & Black, R. E. (2010). Etiology of diarrhea in older children, adolescents, and adults: A systematic review. *PloS Neglected Tropical Diseases, 4*(8). doi: 10.1371/journal.prntd.0000768

Walker, A. W., Sanderson, J. D., Churcher, C., et al. (2011). High-throughput clone library analysis of the mucosa-associated micro-biota reveals dysbiosis and differences between inflamed and non-inflamed regions of the intestine in inflammatory bowel disease. *BMC Microbiology, 11*, 7. doi: 10.1186/1471-2180-11-7

Wall, G. C., Bryant, G. A., Bottenberg, M. M., et al. (2014). Irritable bowel syndrome: A concise review of current treatment concepts. *World Journal of Gastroenterology, 20*(27), 8796–8806. doi: 10.3748/wjg.v20.i27.8796

Willing, B., Halfvarson, J., Dicksved, J., et al. (2009). Twin studies reveal specific imbalances in the mucosa-associated microbiota

of patients with ileal Crohn's disease. *Inflammatory Bowel Disease, 15*(5), 653–660. doi: 10.1002/ibd.20783

Woodward, S., Norton, C., & Chiarelli, P. (2014). Biofeedback for treatment of chronic idiopathic constipation in adults. *Cochrane Database of Systematic Reviews*, (3), CD008486.

World Health Organization. (2013). Diarrhoeal disease, Fact sheet number 330. Retrieved from http://www.who.int/mediacentre/factsheets/fs330/en/

Yamasato, K., Kaneshiro, B., & Oyama, I. A. (2014). A simulation comparing the cost-effectiveness of adult incontinence products. *Journal of Wound, Ostomy, and Continence Nursing, 41*(5), 467–472. doi: 10.1097/WON.0000000000000045

Zhou, L., Lin, Z., Lin, L., et al. (2010). Functional constipation: Implications for nursing interventions. *Journal of Clinical Nursing, 19*(13/14), 1838–1843. doi: 10.1111/j.1365-2702.2010.03246.x

QUESTIONS

1. A continence nurse is assessing a patient diagnosed with acute onset diarrhea. What is the usual cause of this condition?
   A. Malabsorption syndrome
   B. Infectious process
   C. Motility disorder
   D. Chronic inflammatory bowel condition

2. A continence nurse is assessing a patient diagnosed with "fatty diarrhea". What is one of the most common causes of this bowel alteration?
   A. *Clostridium difficile*
   B. Cancer
   C. Radiation proctitis
   D. Lactose intolerance

3. Which type of watery diarrhea is high volume and unaffected by oral intake?
   A. Osmotic
   B. Secretory
   C. Functional
   D. Dysfunctional

4. The continence nurse is monitoring an infant for dehydration related to chronic diarrhea. What sign should arouse the nurse's suspicion of this life-threatening complication?
   A. Skin tenting
   B. Increased urinary output
   C. Hypertension
   D. Bradycardia

5. For which patient would antimotility agents be considered first-line therapy?
   A. A patient with infectious diarrhea
   B. A patient with traveler's diarrhea
   C. A patient with diarrhea caused by chemotherapy
   D. A patient with osmotic diarrhea

6. A continence nurse is caring for a patient who is experiencing slow-transit constipation. What treatment measure is recommended?
   A. Fiber therapy
   B. Stimulant laxatives
   C. Osmotic laxatives
   D. Antibiotic therapy

7. A female patient explains to a continence nurse that she has to "insert her finger into her vagina to enable a bowel movement." What is the probable cause of this patient's bowel alteration?
   A. Rectal–anal intussusception
   B. Rectocele
   C. Rectal tumor
   D. Megarectum

8. How would the continence nurse explain the action of fiber in the diet to patients with bowel alterations?
   A. Fiber hardens the stool.
   B. Fiber decreases stool bulk.
   C. Fiber reduces colonic transit time.
   D. Fiber increases microbial activity.

9. Which agent is considered the agent of choice for ongoing use in patients with functional slow-transit constipation?
   A. Osmotic agents
   B. Stimulant laxatives
   C. Hypertonic enemas
   D. Stool bulking agents

10. The continence nurse is counseling a patient recently diagnosed with irritable bowel syndrome (IBS). What teaching point would the nurse include?
    A. "IBS is a life-threatening disease causing physical and emotional distress."
    B. "IBS increases the risk for cancer."
    C. "At present, there is no known cure for IBS."
    D. "Treatment plans for IBS are standardized according to age."

ANSWERS: 1.**B**, 2.**D**, 3.**B**, 4.**A**, 5.**C**, 6.**C**, 7.**B**, 8.**C**, 9.**A**, 10.**C**

CHAPTER 16

Fecal Incontinence
Pathology, Assessment, and Management

Laurie L. Callan and Midge Willson

OBJECTIVES

1. Discuss the impact of bowel dysfunction or fecal incontinence on lifestyle and quality of life and implications for psychosocial support and counseling.
2. Explain how each of the following contributes to normal bowel function and fecal continence: normal peristalsis; sensory awareness of rectal distention and ability to distinguish between solid, liquid, and gas; internal anal sphincter function; external anal sphincter function; and rectal capacity and compliance.
3. Relate the underlying pathology to management options for passive incontinence, urge incontinence, and seepage and soiling.
4. Describe data to be gathered during the interview and physical assessment that provide insight into peristaltic function, sensory awareness/sphincter function, and rectal capacity and compliance.
5. Synthesize data obtained during patient assessment to determine pattern of fecal incontinence and to develop appropriate management program.
6. Explain indications and guidelines for a colonic cleanout program, sphincter exercises, instruction in urge inhibition, biofeedback, and stimulated defecation program.
7. Identify options for the patient with refractory fecal incontinence.

Topic Outline

Conclusion

Fecal incontinence (FI) is a serious problem associated with significant physical and psychological morbidity. Incontinence itself is not a definitive diagnosis and the initial focus in management is to determine the cause of the problem. Once etiologic factors have been identified, management is directed toward correction of the causative factors and restoration of continence; when continence cannot be fully achieved, even with advanced medical and surgical interventions, containment products are available to help manage the problem and diversion should be considered (Findlay & Maxwell-Armstrong, 2010).

While FI can affect an individual at any age, older men and women are more likely to develop this problem (Pretlove et al., 2006). The negative social stigma that surrounds this condition tends to leave sufferers and caretakers to cope quietly with their feelings of embarrassment, humiliation, and social isolation (Farage et al., 2008); thus, sensitive and patient-focused nursing intervention is critical to positive outcomes and enhanced quality of life (QOL).

 Overview

Fecal continence is directly related to the individual's ability to sense rectal fullness and to control the urge to defecate or pas gas until an appropriate time and place (Halland & Talley, 2012; Van Koughnett & Wexner, 2013). It requires normal function of the gastrointestinal tract, intact sensory function and cognition, competence of the sphincters, and adequate rectal capacity and compliance and can be affected by various extrinsic and intrinsic factors, including comorbidities, medications, and diet.

> **CLINICAL PEARL**
>
> Fecal continence requires normal GI tract function, intact sensory function and cognition, competence of the sphincters, and adequate rectal capacity and compliance.

Definitions

FI is defined by some as an affirmative response to the question: "In the past year, have you had any loss of control of your bowels, even a small amount that stained the underwear?" (Goode et al., 2005). *FI* has also been defined as the involuntary loss of mucus, liquid, or solid bowel contents, a lack of control over defecation, or the inability to control the evacuation of stool at a socially acceptable location and time (Bellicini et al., 2008; Doherty, 2004; Dunberger et al., 2011; Findlay & Maxwell-Armstrong, 2010; Herbert, 2008; Mellgren, 2010; Northwood, 2013; Ostaszkiewicz et al., 2008). The involuntary loss of flatus, without loss of mucus or stool, is defined as *anal incontinence* (AI) (Northwood, 2013).

Urge bowel incontinence involves a sudden urgent need to defecate that results in incontinence when the individual is unable to reach a toilet in time (Sharpe & Read, 2010). In contrast, *passive fecal incontinence* involves the passage of stool or gas without any awareness on the part of the individual. *Encopresis* is the term used to describe voluntary or involuntary fecal soiling; retentive encopresis refers to involuntary fecal soiling, usually in children who have already been toilet trained and usually in response to subconscious withholding of stool. Encopresis will be discussed in greater detail in Chapter 17. Among adults, the leakage of small amounts of stool into undergarments is commonly labeled as *partial fecal incontinence*, fecal leakage, anal leakage, *fecal soiling*, or *fecal seepage*; FI or bowel incontinence is the term used to denote larger accidents or complete loss of rectal contents (Bartolo & Paterson, 2009; Doughty, 2000).

> **CLINICAL PEARL**
>
> Urge incontinence involves a sudden urgent need to defecate that results in incontinence when the individual is unable to reach a toilet promptly; in contrast, passive incontinence involves passage of stool or gas without any awareness on the part of the individual.

Prevalence and Incidence

Published FI incidence and prevalence rates vary and are generally believed to be inaccurate and low, based on evidence that FI is widely underreported (Rees & Sharpe, 2009). Throughout the literature, the overall prevalence rates of FI range between 1% and 21% and tend to increase with age (Mellgren, 2010; Roth, 2010). The prevalence of FI is reported as 0.5% to 1% for persons <65 years of age living in the community and 3% to 8% in those over 65 years of age (Eva et al., 2003; Mellgren, 2010). Prevalence reports for FI in women over 50 years of age are 15.2%, the prevalence of urinary incontinence (UI) is 48.4%, and the prevalence of both FI and UI is 9.4% (Farage et al., 2008). Although FI is more common in elderly female patients, it can also be seen in younger women, as a result of obstetric injury (Dudding et al., 2010; Gordon et al., 1999). There is limited data regarding the prevalence of FI in men, but the literature suggests that there may be a large number of symptomatic male patients who do not present to their medical practitioners despite the negative effect on QOL (Eva et al., 2003). Shamliyan et al. (2009) found cognitive impairment, poor general health, surgery, and radiation for prostate cancer to be associated with greater incidence of FI in community-dwelling men.

The prevalence rate of FI in nursing home residents has been reported as high as 47% to 50%; FI in these individuals is frequently associated with dementia and/ or immobility (Findlay & Maxwell-Armstrong, 2010; Roth, 2010). A higher incidence of FI is also found in patients with an acute illness and is often due to loose or liquid stools (Bliss et al., 2000). In acute care settings, the incidence range has been reported as 17% to 33% (Norton, 2009).

CLINICAL PEARL

Acute illness is associated with a higher incidence of FI and is often due to loose or liquid stools.

Impact

FI causes considerable distress and can have a devastating effect on QOL for individuals and often for their family members. Based on QOL surveys, 6% of patients with mild FI symptoms, 35% with moderate FI, and 82% with severe FI report a moderate to severe impact on their QOL (Bharucha et al., 2005; Hussain et al., 2014). The unpredictability of FI disrupts a patient's daily routine and affects every aspect of life including diet, skin health, sexuality, marriage, friendships, employment opportunities, and the ability to exercise (Crowell et al., 2007; Roth, 2010). FI leads to social stigmatization and isolation and is a common cause for institutionalization of the elderly

(Dunivan et al., 2010). FI is also a strong predictor of falls in the elderly.

Commonly reported psychological signs and symptoms related to FI include the following (Bellicini et al., 2008; Bliss et al., 2000; Crowell et al., 2007; Doherty, 2004; Eva et al., 2003; Farage et al., 2008; Palmieri et al., 2005; Roth, 2010; Whiteley, 2007):

- Reduced self-esteem and confidence
- Reluctance to share information about the FI problem with others, including health care providers
- Increased risk of anxiety and depression disorders
- Feelings of anger, grief, shame, embarrassment, fear, and frustration
- Dependence on others and isolation
- Poor self-perceived health

There are multiple assessment tools that have been developed for assessing FI. They can be classified based upon the parameters evaluated, that is, descriptive measures, severity measures, and impact measures (Hussain et al., 2014). The tools most commonly used in clinical practice are symptom severity questionnaires and health-related quality-of-life (HRQOL) impact scales. These tools can be very helpful to the clinician in more accurately assessing the impact of FI on the individual and family. However, not all assessment tools have been validated; thus, care must be taken if the tool is being used for research purposes. Some considerations when selecting a tool include ease of use by both the person and the practitioner, the parameters the tool is designed to measure, the tool's ability to detect a change in the person's condition, and the population for which it was designed. See Table 16-1 for a brief overview of currently available assessment tools specific to individuals with urinary and fecal incontinence.

Costs Associated with FI

FI is associated with increased hospital stays and an increased nursing workload to maintain patients' hygiene (McKenna et al., 2001). Therefore, FI is costly to the patient and to society, with specific costs including the following (Goode et al., 2005; Nix & Ermer-Seltun, 2004; Palmieri et al., 2005; Paterson et al., 2003): nursing time (labor), skin care products, containment products and protective pads, laundry costs, consultations, medical and pharmacy services, and long-term care services.

Incontinence-associated costs in the United States are estimated at $16.5 to $19.5 billion, and 9% of that is attributed to costs for absorbent products (Fader et al., 2009). Farage et al. (2008) reported similar estimates of costs at $16.4 billion per year for incontinence-related care and $1.1 billion for disposable products.

TABLE 16-1 Tools for Assessment of FI: Severity and Impact on Quality of Life

Abbreviation	Tool name	Description	Author(s)/Developer(s)	Reference Citation
Wexner or CCIS	Wexner Faecal Incontinence Symptom Severity Scoring System or the Cleveland Clinic Incontinence Score	Tool that uses five questions to score symptoms related to FI in terms of severity (1–20), frequency (1–4), and quality of life (QOL) impact. Has undergone psychometric evaluation	Steven D. Wexner, Cleveland Clinic	Thomas et al. (2006), Sansoni et al. (2013), Hussain et al. (2014)
FISI	Fecal Incontinence Severity Index	Tool developed by surgeons (with patient input) to assess severity of FI and AI independent of direct clinical assessment	Todd Rockwood, James Church, James Fleshman, Robert Kane, Constantinos Mavrantonis, Alan Thorson, Steven Wexner, Donna Bliss, Ann Lowry, Univ of Minnesota, Dept of Colon and Rectal Surgery	Rockwood et al. (1999), Northwood (2013)
BBUSQ-22	Birmingham Bowel and Urinary Symptom Questionnaire	22-item questionnaire covering a range of bowel and urinary symptoms in women; designed to evaluate the effects of pelvic surgery on FI and LUTS. Has undergone rigorous psychometric testing	L. Hiller, S Radley, C Mann, SC Radley, G Begum, SJ Pretlove, J Salaman	Hiller et al. (2002), Northwood (2013)
FIQoLS	Fecal Incontinence QOL Scale	29-item questionnaire addressing specific QOL indicators; measures the effect of FI treatment on HRQOL in adults. Has undergone psychometric evaluation	Todd Rockwood, James Church, James Fleshman, Robert Kane, Constantinos Mavrantonis, Alan Thorson, Steven Wexner, Donna Bliss, Ann Lowry, Univ of Minnesota, Dept of Colon and Rectal Surgery	Rockwood et al. (1999), Northwood (2013), Hussain et al. (2014)
MHQ	Manchester Health Questionnaire	31-item questionnaire that measures HRQOL in women with FI and AI. Has undergone psychometric evaluation	Bugg, G, Kiff, E, Hosker, G.	Northwood (2013)
RFIS	Revised Faecal Incontinence Scale	Scale designed to discriminate between different levels of incontinence severity. Has undergone psychometric testing	–	Sansoni et al. (2013)
SMIS	St. Mark's Incontinence Score	7-question questionnaire, with scores based on frequency (0–4) and severity (0–24) of symptoms; takes into consideration fecal urgency and management behaviors, along with QOL indicators. Has undergone psychometric evaluation	Vaizey, C, Carapeti, C, Cahill, J, Kamm, M.	Sansoni et al. (2013), Rusavy et al. (2014)
ICIQ-B	International Consultation on Incontinence Questionnaire-Bowels	QOL assessment tool that takes into account FI issues the patients identified as important	Cotterill, Norton, Avery, Abrams, Donovan	Hussain et al. (2014)

CCIS, Cleveland Clinic Incontinence Score; QOL, quality of life; FISI, Fecal Incontinence Severity Index; FI, fecal incontinence; AI, anal incontinence; BBUSQ, Birmingham Bowel and Urinary Symptom Questionnaire; LUTS, lower urinary tract symptoms; FIQoLS, Fecal Incontinence QOL Scale; HRQOL, health-related quality of life; MHQ, Manchester Health Questionnaire; RFIS, Revised Faecal Incontinence Scale; SMIS, St. Mark's Incontinence Score; ICIQ-B, International Consultation on Incontinence Questionnaire-Bowels.

Types and Pathology of FI

FI can be classified based on clinical presentation and on duration of the problem. Classification based on clinical presentation includes urge incontinence, passive incontinence, and fecal leakage or flatus incontinence.

Passive Incontinence

Passive incontinence involves the unrecognized leakage of mucus, fluid, or solid stool. FI that occurs with no awareness on the individual's part is most commonly caused by cognitive impairment (dementia) or sensorimotor dysfunction (e.g., incontinence in the patient with a neurologic lesion such as spinal cord injury); less commonly, this type of incontinence is caused by significant internal anal sphincter (IAS) dysfunction. Passive incontinence can range from mild soiling of the underwear to total evacuation of the bowel without warning (Bartolo & Paterson, 2009; Stevens et al., 2003).

CLINICAL PEARL

Passive incontinence can range from mild soiling to total evacuation of the bowel and is most commonly caused by cognitive impairment or sensorimotor dysfunction (neurogenic bowel).

Urge Incontinence

Urge incontinence is characterized by a sudden need to defecate and the inability to reach the toilet before defecation occurs, resulting in involuntary passage of mucus, gas, liquid, or solid stool. Urge incontinence may be caused by external anal sphincter (EAS) dysfunction (with an intact internal sphincter) (Bartolo & Paterson, 2009), a colorectal motility disorder, or reduced capacity and/or compliance of the rectal cavity.

CLINICAL PEARL

Urge incontinence may be caused by EAS dysfunction, a motility disorder, or diminished rectal capacity and compliance.

Flatus Incontinence

Flatus incontinence may be the first sign of FI. Fecal leakage, fecal soiling, and fecal seepage are minor degrees of FI and describe the incontinence of liquid stool, mucus, or very small amounts of solid stool. The leakage varies in severity, from staining, to soilage, to seepage, to small accidents in people who are continent and able to delay defecation the majority of the time (Bartolo & Paterson, 2009; Doughty, 2000). This pattern of incontinence may be caused by dysfunction of the IAS, which is normally responsible for preventing leakage of small volumes of stool or gas, or by sensory impairment that prevents prompt recognition of stool in the rectal vault.

Transient versus Chronic FI

Incontinence can also be classified based on duration; this classification includes transient and chronic FI. Transient FI refers to short-term (new-onset) incontinence caused by a change in stool consistency or sensory awareness; these individuals were continent until they became acutely ill, severely confused, or developed severe diarrhea. Management of these individuals is directed toward treatment of the underlying disease process, containment of the stool, and perianal skin protection. In contrast, chronic incontinence is a persistent or recurrent problem caused by chronic disease, injury to or denervation of the sphincter, cognitive impairment, or neurologic dysfunction (such as spinal cord injury); these individuals require a comprehensive management plan that is individualized based on the specific type and cause of the FI (Doughty, 2000; Wishin et al., 2008).

CLINICAL PEARL

Transient FI is usually caused by an acute diarrheal illness and/or alteration in mental status; management is focused on correction of the underlying disease process, containment of the stool, and perianal skin protection.

 Risk Factors for FI

There are multiple factors that predispose individuals to developing FI and multiple approaches to classifying those risk factors. In this text, we will categorize risk factors based on their impact on functional components of continence, because this approach provides the foundation for assessment and management of the individual with FI. Using this conceptual approach, the major risk factors can be grouped into the following categories: those related to gastrointestinal system function, bowel motility, and stool consistency, those related to neurologic control of defecation, those related to the integrity and innervation of the pelvic floor and anal sphincters, those affecting rectal capacity and compliance, and those affecting overall health status and mobility (Table 16-2). Other factors that have an impact on FI are age, gender, diet, and exercise (Mellgren, 2010; Roth, 2010; Shamliyan et al., 2009).

Conditions Affecting Bowel Motility and Stool Consistency

As explained in Chapter 14, one factor critical to continence is normal stool consistency; stool that is formed but soft is fairly easily retained even if the sphincter is somewhat weak, while high-volume liquid stool can overwhelm the strongest sphincter. Therefore, any condition producing liquid stool increases the risk of incontinence; the risk is further increased when the stool is high volume and/or in the individual with any degree of sphincter weakness.

TABLE 16-2 Risk Factors for Fecal Incontinence

Predisposing Factors	Reference Citation
1. Factors related to the integrity of the pelvic floor and anal sphincter(s)	
Obstetrical internal and/or external sphincter injury (due to forceps delivery, large head circumference, large birth weight, abnormal presentation at delivery)	Altman et al. (2007), Erekson et al. (2008), Groutz et al. (1999), Leung and Rao (2011), Mellgren (2010), Bartolo and Paterson (2009)
Pelvic organ prolapse. Rectal prolapse. Rectocele	Altman et al. (2007), Findlay and Maxwell-Armstrong (2010), Bartolo and Paterson (2009)
Vaginal parity	Erekson et al. (2008), Findlay and Maxwell-Armstrong (2010)
Trauma: Pelvic fractures, insertion of foreign bodies into anal canal, perineal lacerations. Sexual abuse. Anal intercourse	Roth (2010), Shamliyan et al. (2009)
2. Factors related to overall health status and mobility	
Obesity (e.g., altered transit, change in flora, significant difference in stool consistency). Pelvic floor weakness in morbidly obese prior to bariatric surgery contributes to FI after surgery.	Altman et al. (2007), Bharucha (2010), Gallagher (2005), Halland and Talley (2012), Pares et al. (2012)
Medications: a-blockers, calcium channel blockers, nitric oxide donors, diabetes meds, anticholinergics, antipsychotics (see additional list below)	Doherty (2004), Farage et al. (2008), Gallagher (2005), Leung and Schnelle (2008)
Hysterectomy	Altman et al. (2007)
Diabetes	Altman et al. (2007), Bartolo and Paterson (2009)
Postreconstructive: low anterior resection, pouch surgery	Bartolo and Paterson (2009), Doherty (2004), Erekson et al. (2008)
Radiation	
Hemorrhoidectomy, anorectal surgery	
Poor general health	Bellicini et al. (2008)
Prostate disease	Bellicini et al. (2008)
Enteral tube feedings	Bellicini et al. (2008)
Infectious: *Campylobacter*, *Salmonella*, *Shigellosis*, *Clostridium difficile/ perfringens*, pseudomembranous colitis, perianal sepsis, human papillomavirus, cytomegalovirus, lymphogranuloma venereum, etc.	Farage et al. (2008), Findlay and Maxwell-Armstrong (2010), Sabol and Friedenburg (1997), Wishin et al. (2008)
Malignancy: Paget's disease, Bowen's disease, lichen sclerosus, anal intraepithelial neoplasia	Findlay and Maxwell-Armstrong (2010), Bartolo and Paterson (2009)
Increased severity of illness	Bliss et al. (2000)
3. Factors related to neurological integrity	
Dementia, alteration in cognitive function	Farage et al. (2008), Leung and Schnelle (2008), Mellgren (2010)
Neurological/muscular impairment: stroke, parkinsonism, spinal cord injury, cauda equina injury, multiple sclerosis, spina bifida, muscular dystrophies, myasthenia gravis, muscular weakness, amyloidosis.	Bellicini et al. (2008), Coggrave (2007), Findlay and Maxwell-Armstrong (2010), Finne-Soveri et al. (2008), Formal et al. (1997), Mellgren (2010), Sharpe and Read (2010)
4. Factors related to bowel pattern or function	
Accelerated colonic transit, bowel resection, conditions resulting in diarrhea.	Bharucha (2010), McKenna et al. (2001), Stevens et al. (2003)
Loss of rectal wall compliance	
Alteration in intestinal and colonic bacterial flora after bariatric surgery	Bharucha (2010), Roberson et al. (2010)
Diarrhea. Fecal impaction	Bharucha (2010), Bliss et al. (2000), Erekson et al. (2008), McKenna et al. (2001), Mellgren (2010)
Cholecystectomy and fat malabsorption	Bharucha (2010)
Constipation, fecal impaction	Leung and Schnelle (2008)
Congenital anorectal anomalies, atresia	Bellicini et al. (2008)
Colorectal disease, inflammatory bowel diseases, acute diverticulitis, superior mesenteric bowel disease, venous thrombosis, ischemic bowel disease	Bellicini et al. (2008), Doherty (2004), McKenna et al. (2001), Sabol and Friedenburg (1997)
Anal sphincter dysfunction	Palmieri et al. (2005)
5. Factors related to the living situation	
Use of restraints	Leung and Schnelle (2008)
Lack of timely toileting assistance	Leung and Schnelle (2008)
Inability to toilet themselves	Leung and Schnelle (2008)
6. Factors related to mobility	
Impaired mobility, physical disability	Bellicini et al. (2008), Finne-Soveri et al. (2008), Gallagher (2005), Leung and Schnelle (2008), Wishin et al. (2008)
Overuse/misuse of absorbent pads and undergarments	Leung and Schnelle (2008)

TABLE 16-2 Risk Factors for Fecal Incontinence (*Continued*)

Predisposing Factors	Reference Citation
7. Other factors	
Older age	Bellicini et al. (2008), Bliss et al. (2000), Erekson et al. (2008), Farage et al. (2008)
Female gender	Bellicini et al. (2008)
Diet: lack of dietary fiber, high-fat diet	McKenna et al. (2001)
Lack of exercise	McKenna et al. (2001)
Smoking with chronic cough, increases intra-abdominal pressure	Halland and Talley (2012)

Conditions resulting in diarrheal stool include bacterial and viral infections (e.g., *Clostridium difficile*), malabsorption syndromes (e.g., lactose intolerance, fat malabsorption following cholecystectomy), surgical procedures resulting in reduced bowel length (e.g., major small bowel resection or colectomy), inflammatory conditions affecting bowel motility (e.g., Crohn's disease or ulcerative colitis), motility disorders (e.g., irritable bowel syndrome, diarrhea predominant), initiation of enteral feedings in a malnourished patient with flattening of the villi, and selected medications (e.g., antibiotics, prokinetic agents, magnesium-based antacids, sorbitol). Interestingly, severe constipation resulting in fecal impaction can also cause or contribute to FI, because a large bolus of stool in the rectum produces persistent relaxation of the IAS and permits leakage of liquid stool around the fecal bolus. (See Chapter 15 for an in-depth discussion of motility disorders.)

CLINICAL PEARL

One factor critical to continence is normal stool consistency; stool that is formed is fairly easily retained even if the sphincter is somewhat weak, whereas high-volume liquid stool can overwhelm the strongest sphincter.

Conditions Affecting Neural Control

The second group of risk factors includes conditions that affect neural control of defecation. As explained in Chapter 14, fecal continence is dependent on the individual's ability to recognize the presence of stool or gas in the rectum and to contract the external sphincter until he/she reaches a socially acceptable time and place to defecate. Thus, any condition that interferes with sensory recognition of rectal distention or with voluntary control of the sphincter places the individual at high risk for recurrent episodes of FI. The most common of these conditions include cerebrocortical dysfunction (e.g., acute delirium or advanced dementia) and spinal cord lesions (e.g., spinal cord injury, lower back syndrome, multiple myelitis, or multiple sclerosis). Altered mental status (delirium or dementia) alters the individual's ability to appropriately process and respond to the signals of rectal distention, and any spinal cord lesion prevents transmission of signals from the rectum and sphincters to the brain and vice versa.

CLINICAL PEARL

Any condition that compromises the individual's ability to recognize the presence of stool in the rectum and to voluntarily contract the sphincter places the individual at high risk for recurrent episodes of incontinence.

Sphincter Damage or Denervation

The third group of risk factors involves damage or denervation of the sphincters; any damage to the sphincter compromises squeeze pressure and the ability to retain stool in the rectum, especially when the stool is liquid and/or high volume. Conditions most commonly associated with damage or denervation of the sphincter include obstetric trauma, anorectal surgical procedures including hemorrhoidectomy, and anorectal trauma (e.g., impalement injuries, anal intercourse). Rectal prolapse can also compromise sphincter function.

CLINICAL PEARL

Damage or denervation of the anal sphincter is a common cause of chronic FI and is usually caused by obstetric trauma, anorectal surgery, or anal trauma.

Conditions Affecting Rectal Capacity or Compliance

The fourth group of risk factors includes conditions that alter rectal capacity or compliance; a fibrotic or inflamed rectum is unable to accommodate any volume of stool and is associated with severe urgency and urge incontinence. Conditions that alter rectal capacity and compliance include inflammatory conditions (e.g., ulcerative colitis, Crohn's proctocolitis, or radiation proctitis) and rectal fibrosis caused by radiation or repetitive inflammation. In addition, patients undergoing low anterior resection (removal of the rectum) are at risk for incontinence due to loss of the rectal reservoir; these individuals typically experience intense fecal frequency and urgency until the segment of colon immediately proximal to the anal canal distends to form a pouch-like structure that acts as a "pseudo rectum." Individuals undergoing ileal pouch anal anastomosis procedures are at risk for incontinence until the pouch has adapted (distended) sufficiently to provide an adequate reservoir.

> **CLINICAL PEARL**
>
> A fibrotic or inflamed rectum is unable to accommodate and "store" any volume of stool and is associated with severe urgency and urge incontinence.

In addition, any condition that causes severe debility or immobility can compromise the individual's ability to reach the toilet in a timely manner. Specific risk factors are listed in Table 16-2.

Assessment Guidelines

Accurate assessment of the patient with FI is critical to development of an appropriate individualized management plan. The novice practitioner will not be able to conduct the same level of expert assessment as an advanced practice continence nurse; however, the novice practitioner *can* use available tools and guidelines to conduct an effective baseline assessment including basic history and physical examination. For example, there are several tools available that assess the individual with FI in terms of symptom severity and impact on daily living and HRQOL; these questionnaires can be helpful to the affected individual as well as the nurse, because completion of the tool allows the person to articulate and quantify his or her symptoms, feelings, and experience. This is important because clinicians tend to underestimate symptom severity and impact on HRQOL. A table of available assessment tools was presented earlier in this chapter that can be of tremendous assistance to the clinician in determining the needs of their patients with FI.

> **CLINICAL PEARL**
>
> Use of structured tools to assess QOL is important, because clinicians tend to underestimate symptom severity and impact of FI on HRQOL.

Patient Interview

A comprehensive assessment of FI should include a thorough history, to include identification of risk factors, patterns of incontinence (i.e., urge FI vs. passive FI vs. minor leakage), symptom severity and impact on QOL (as discussed above), food and fluid intake, all medications taken, and goals for treatment. The initial interview should include a basic focused history; additional data can be gathered over time as indicated.

Review of Systems

In addition to obtaining information about the onset of the problem, type and severity of incontinence, current management approaches, goals for treatment, and food/fluid/medications, the nurse should query the patient about comorbid conditions and prior surgical procedures and should conduct a focused review of the following systems:

- Neurologic (to include history of stroke, spinal cord trauma or lesions, lower back problems or procedures, multiple sclerosis, cognitive status)
- Gastrointestinal (to include bowel resections, inflammatory bowel disease, irritable bowel syndrome, anorectal trauma, anorectal surgical procedures, anal intercourse)
- Obstetric/gynecologic (women) (number of vaginal deliveries, difficult deliveries, obstetric trauma, pelvic procedures)

> **CLINICAL PEARL**
>
> In addition to queries regarding duration and type of FI, impact on QOL and goals for treatment, dietary and fluid intake, and medications, the interview should include a brief review of the following systems: neurologic, gastrointestinal, and (for women) obstetric/gynecologic.

As noted, a complete list of all medications should be obtained and should include over-the-counter and herbal agents as well as prescription medications that could affect bowel function (Table 16-3).

Essential Questions

The nurse should also use the following questions and follow-up discussion to obtain insight into any derangements in bowel motility and stool consistency, sensory awareness and sphincter control, rectal capacity and compliance, and general ability to reach the bathroom in a timely manner:

1. How often do you have voluntary (controlled) bowel movements, and what is the consistency of the stool?
2. How often do you have involuntary leakage of stool, and what is the consistency of the stool?
3. Do you always know when there is stool or gas in your rectum? Can you differentiate between gas and liquid and solid?
4. If you get the urge to have a bowel movement, can you hold on to the stool at least briefly? For how long?

> **CLINICAL PEARL**
>
> The history should always include "key questions" related to stool frequency and consistency; sensory awareness; ability to differentiate between gas, liquid, and solid; and ability to delay defecation.

Contributing Factors

In conducting the interview and synthesizing the data, the continence nurse should be alert to the following potential contributing factors to the problems with FI (Doughty, 2000; Fader et al., 2010; Mellgren, 2010; Roth, 2010):

- Reversible risk factors: intestinal infections, fecal impaction, foods and medications affecting bowel motility (Tables 16-3 and 16-4), and initiation of enteral feedings

TABLE 16-3 Medications affecting bowel motility

Medication	Pharmacological Effect on Gastric/Colonic Motility	Reference Citation
Antidiarrheal Medications		
Codeine	Opioid agonist: Binds to opioid receptors, inhibiting peristalsis	Epocrates (2013)
Diphenoxylate hydrochloride and atropine sulfate (Lomotil, Pfizer, New York, NY)	Difenoxin binds gut wall opioid receptors, inhibiting peristalsis	Epocrates (2013)
Difenoxin/atropine sulfate (Motofen, Valeant Pharmaceuticals, Quebec, Canada)	Difenoxin binds gut wall opioid receptors, inhibiting peristalsis	Epocrates (2013)
Loperamide (Imodium, Janssen Pharmaceutical, Titusville, NJ)	Binds gut wall opioid receptors, inhibits peristalsis, increases anal sphincter tone	Epocrates (2013)
Octreotide acetate (Sandostatin, Novartis Pharmaceuticals, Basel, Switzerland)	Synthetic analog of somatostatin; reduces volume of intestinal secretions	Epocrates (2013)
Bismuth subsalicylate (Maalox, Novartis, Basel, Switzerland; Pepto-Bismol, Procter & Gamble, Cincinnati, OH; Kaopectate, Chattem, Inc., Chattanooga, TN)	Reduces secretions, possesses antimicrobial effects	Epocrates (2013)
Cholestyramine (Questran, Bristol-Myers Squibb, NY; Prevalite, Upsher-Smith Laboratories, Minneapolis, MN)	Binds intestinal bile acids, which have a promotility effect in the colon	Epocrates (2013)
Medications to Treat Constipation		
Bulk-forming laxatives Psyllium (Metamucil, Procter & Gamble, Cincinnati, OH) Methyl cellulose (Citrucel, GlaxoSmithKline, Brentford, Middlesex, UK) Calcium polycarbophil (FiberCon, Pfizer, New York, NY)	Increase bulk, increase water absorption, may take several days to work, require adequate fluid intake	Epocrates (2013), Marples (2011), Woodward (2012)
Osmotic laxatives Sodium phosphate, magnesium hydroxide, magnesium citrate, polyethylene glycol, lactulose Lubiprostone (Amitiza, Takeda Pharmaceuticals, Deerfield, Il.)	Pull fluid into the lumen of the bowel via osmosis, thus softening the stool and promoting peristalsis; decrease intestinal permeability*	Epocrates (2013), Marples (2011), Woodward (2012)
Stimulant laxatives Bisacodyl Castor oil Sennosides, senna	Increase peristalsis, increase water absorption from large intestine, can cause electrolyte imbalance in frail elderly	Epocrates (2013), Marples (2011), Woodward (2012)
Stool softeners Docusate calcium, docusate sodium Mineral oil	Soften stool; facilitate mixture of stool, fat, and water; make stool easier to pass; little evidence to support use	Epocrates (2013), Marples (2011), Woodward (2012)
Probiotics	May improve stool consistency and bowel regularity by normalizing intestinal flora (more data needed regarding specific agents and dosages)	Marples (2011), Woodward (2012)
Medications that Contribute to FI		
Anticholinergics Antihistamines Antispasmodics Tricyclic antidepressants Antipsychotics	Can contribute to constipation, possess anticholinergic properties, prolong colonic transit time, have antiemetic and sedative effects	Bliss et al. (2006), Epocrates (2013), Wuong (2012)
Cardiovascular medications Calcium channel blockers Beta-adrenergic antagonists Diuretics Antiarrhythmics	Can contribute to constipation	Bliss et al. (2006), Epocrates (2013)
Central nervous system depressants Anticonvulsants Antiparkinsonian drugs	Can contribute to constipation	Bliss et al. (2006), Epocrates (2013)
Narcotic analgesics Opiates Barbiturates Opioid derivatives (methadone, morphine, oxycodone)	Opioid agonists; bind to opioid receptors, inhibiting peristalsis	Bliss et al. (2006), Epocrates (2013)

(Continued)

TABLE 16-3 Medications affecting bowel motility (*Continued*)

Medication	Pharmacological Effect on Gastric/Colonic Motility	Reference Citation
Medications that Contribute to FI (*Continued*)		
Antineoplastics Vinca alkaloids	Can cause constipation and/or diarrhea as a side effect	Bliss et al. (2006), Epocrates (2013)
Cholestyramine	Bile acid–binding agent; used in treatment of diarrhea	Bliss et al. (2006), Marples (2011)
Nonsteroidal anti-inflammatory drugs Ibuprofen Naproxen	May cause constipation	Bliss et al. (2006), Epocrates (2013)
Oxybutynin	Constipation is common side effect due to anticholinergic effects.	Bliss et al. (2006), Epocrates (2013)
Medications that Cause Loose Stools/Diarrhea		
Oral hypoglycemics	May cause diarrhea as a side effect, delay or decrease intestinal absorption of glucose	Bliss et al. (2006), Epocrates (2013)
Alzheimer's disease medications Acetylcholinesterase inhibitors (donepezil)	Can cause diarrhea as a side effect; reversibly bind to and inactivate acetylcholinesterase, thus increasing levels of acetylcholine (which promotes peristalsis) (acetylcholinesterase inhibitor)	Bliss et al. (2006), Epocrates (2013)
Antibiotics Ampicillin Cefazolin, cephalexin, ceftriaxone, ceftazidime Ciprofloxacin Clindamycin, erythromycin	Alter intestinal mucosa and intestinal flora. Diarrhea is a common side effect.	Bliss et al. (2006), Epocrates (2013)

*Patient needs to have adequate fluid intake for these to be effective.

- Functional ability: mobility, dexterity, visual and mental acuity, and any issues with the living environment
- Bowel incontinence pattern: incontinence of gas, liquid, and/or solid stool; frequency of stools—voluntary and involuntary; description of stool; and awareness of rectal distention and incontinent episodes.
- Obstetric history: episiotomies, forceps, multiparity, and hysterectomy
- Surgical history: bowel resections, rectal prolapse, hemorrhoids, fissures, anorectal surgery or trauma, and malignancy
- Sexual history: anal sex or sex appliances that might cause dilation of anal sphincter
- CNS disorders, neuropathy, back injury, and dementia
- Chronic diseases: diabetes, Crohn's, ulcerative colitis, irritable bowel, arthritis, Parkinson's, and MS
- Medications (Table 16-3)

Focused Physical Examination

As is true of history taking, the physical examination can range from a basic examination to an extensive examination, depending on the individual's presenting symptoms and the examiner's level of expertise. A basic assessment should include an abdominal exam, an evaluation of anorectal anatomy, and a digital rectal examination to determine sphincter tone, presence of stool or masses, perineal sensation, and presence or absence of the anocutaneous reflex (i.e., anal wink sign).

CLINICAL PEARL

Basic physical assessment includes abdominal and anorectal examinations.

Abdominal Examination

Abdominal examination involves visual inspection for distention, percussion along the length of the bowel to assess for indicators of stool retention, and palpation of the lower quadrants to assess for evidence of stool retention. (An advanced practice nurse should also conduct a thorough abdominal examination to detect any masses.) Indicators of chronic constipation/stool retention include dull note to percussion along most of the colon, palpable nodules of stool in the left lower quadrant, and discomfort and resistance to palpation in the right lower quadrant. (Normally, the percussion note over most of the air-filled colon is tympanic or resonant, there is no palpable stool in the left lower quadrant, and palpation of the right lower quadrant is met with no resistance and no symptoms of pain or discomfort.)

Visual Anal Examination

A visual examination of the anus should be performed while the patient is at rest, during contraction, and while bearing down (Valsalva maneuver). The sphincter should be closed at rest; a patulous or gaping sphincter is indicative of a neurologic lesion causing denervation of the sphincter. The sphincter should visibly contract when the individual is instructed

TABLE 16-4 Foods affecting bowel motility

Food	Effect on Gastric/Colonic Motility	Reference Citation
Caffeine	Stimulates gastrointestinal motility; can cause diarrhea and FI; if taken in excess may contribute to dehydration and constipation	Crosswell et al. (2010), Hansen et al. (2006)
Alcohol	Stimulates gastrointestinal motility, increases risk of FI	Crosswell et al. (2010), Hansen et al. (2006)
Lactose	Intolerance and malabsorption of lactose results in diarrhea. FI is secondary to diarrhea.	Crosswell et al. (2010), Hansen et al. (2006)
Spicy foods	Increase gastrointestinal motility, increase FI secondary to loose stools	Crosswell et al. (2010)
Nuts (high in insoluble fiber)	Increase gastrointestinal motility	Hansen et al. (2006)
Foods high in insoluble fibers: Unprocessed bran, bran cereals, whole wheat fiber, popcorn, nuts, cabbage, green beans, wax beans, eggplant, apples, carrots	Increase stool bulk, but do not absorb water; can move through the GI system basically intact. Increased stool bulk contributes to distention of colon wall, which triggers peristaltic activity.	Hunter et al. (2002), Wisten and Messner (2005)
Foods high in soluble fibers (fruit fiber/pectin): Oats, dried beans, squash, pectin, apples, citrus fruits, psyllium	Absorb water and have high water retention, thicken stool, reduce bowel transit time, slow digestion, have a lubricating effect on the intestinal mucosa	Wisten and Messner (2005)
Chocolate	Increases gastrointestinal motility and risk of FI	Crosswell et al. (2010), Hansen et al. (2006)
Foods with both soluble and insoluble fiber: Onions, cabbage, Brussels sprouts, cauliflower, apricots	Cause flatus	Crosswell et al. (2010)
Greasy/fatty foods: Fast food, pizza, bacon, gravy, fried foods	Increase gastrointestinal motility and risk of FI	Crosswell et al. (2010)
Fruits: Fresh fruit (raisins), fruit juice (orange, prune)	Increase gastrointestinal motility and risk of FI	Crosswell et al. (2010)
Cheeses, dairy products	Increase risk of FI if lactose intolerant, can cause constipation if eaten in large amounts (taking place of high-fiber foods)	Crosswell et al. (2010), Woodward (2012), Wuong (2012)

FI, fecal incontinence.

to "tighten as if you are trying not to pass stool or gas," and there should be no visible defects. Inability to voluntarily contract the sphincter is evidence of a neurological problem or muscle deficit. Observation during bearing down may reveal the presence of rectal prolapse or pelvic organ prolapse. If the sphincter remains tightly contracted when the individual is instructed to "bear down, as if you are trying to eliminate stool or gas," it suggests compromised ability to coordinate pelvic floor and sphincter relaxation with abdominal muscle contraction (pelvic floor dyssynergia). Careful visual inspection may also reveal the presence of an anal fissure.

Digital Anorectal Examination
A digital anorectal examination should be done to assess for fecal impaction, hemorrhoids, masses, and the function of the pelvic floor musculature, including EAS and IAS tone and length. Normal anal resting tone is a closed sphincter. During digital exam, sphincter tone may vary; however, when the

individual is prompted to tighten the sphincter, normal function is evidenced by 360 degrees of symmetrical tension that is felt as a strong squeeze around the examining finger and a slight inward pull on the finger. Defects or gaps in the circumference of the external sphincter circumference can be palpated though it takes practice and experience to detect subtle abnormalities. During bearing down, a downward push should be felt, accompanied by sphincter relaxation; there should be no prolapse of the rectal vault (Doughty, 2000).

CLINICAL PEARL

When doing the anorectal exam, the examiner should instruct the individual to contract the sphincter as if "trying not to pass stool or gas"; normal response is evidenced by 360 degrees of symmetrical tension that is felt as a strong squeeze and slight inward pull.

Neurologic Examination

Neurologic examination is indicated in situations where a neurologic deficit is suspected and should include anal reflex and perianal sensory testing. The anal reflex is elicited by gently stroking the perianal skin with a finger or q-tip; normally, this causes the anus to quickly contract, the so-called anal "wink." No response may be indicative of neurological problems, though absence of the anal wink is not diagnostic in and of itself. Thus, the detection of any abnormalities during the physical examination warrants further anorectal physiologic testing, especially when there is additional evidence of denervation. Assessment of the patient's perineal skin is also necessary to evaluate skin injury and degree of discomfort as a result of the skin's contact with stool digestive enzymes and moisture (Bartolo & Paterson, 2009; Doughty, 2000; Nix & Haugen, 2010).

Bowel Diary

Bowel diaries provide objective information regarding the person's elimination patterns (Fig. 16-1). Bowel diaries allow the clinician to understand the patient's symptoms over time in order to determine the severity of the FI and the effectiveness of therapeutic procedures (Doughty 2000; Findlay & Maxwell-Armstrong, 2010). Examples of bowel diaries in the literature tend to evaluate both voluntary and involuntary stools for consistency, frequency of evacuation, volume and severity of incontinence, diet, discomfort, activity at time of incontinence, and/or presence of urgency.

Diagnostic Procedures

Additional diagnostic tests may be indicated for selected individuals, including those with persistent diarrhea of unknown etiology, indicators of sphincter dysfunction, suspected prolapse, and suspected malignancy.

CLINICAL PEARL

Additional diagnostic tests may be indicated for individuals with persistent diarrhea of unknown etiology, indicators of sphincter dysfunction, suspected prolapse, and suspected malignancy.

Date/time	Voluntary evacuation (amount and consistency)	Incontinent stool (amount and consistency)	Diet	Activity/ discomfort

FIGURE 16-1. Sample bowel diary. A bowel diary helps track changes in stool pattern over several days. Length of time depends, in part, on how often the individual has a bowel movement but should be recorded for at least a week. The bowel diary and Bristol Stool Chart should be used together to provide a complete record.

Diagnostic procedures for the individual with persistent diarrhea include stool testing for ova and parasites; stool cultures for *Salmonella*, *Shigella*, *Campylobacter*, *Escherichia coli*, *Entamoeba histolytica*, and *C. difficile*; blood work (e.g., CBC, electrolytes, calcium, phosphorus, and albumin); and malabsorption studies (e.g., hydrogen breath test or stool acidity test) (Sabol & Friedenburg, 1997).

Anal sphincter imaging and physiologic function studies are typically indicated when there is a suspected sphincter defect, such as a gap in the circumferential contraction of the sphincter on examination, or evidence of diminished contractility. The clinician should implement measures to correct motility disorders and other reversible factors prior to conducting studies of sphincter structure and function (Bellicini et al., 2008; Belmonte-Montes et al., 2001; Bharucha et al., 2010; Dudding et al., 2010; Roberson et al., 2010). Specific studies are discussed below.

Endoanal Ultrasound

Ultrasonography uses a transducer emitting sound waves to create an image of organ structure; it is used to determine anal anatomic integrity and to identify any structural abnormalities of the internal and/or external anal sphincter.

Anorectal Manometry

Anorectal manometry is used to assess sphincter function; it measures resting and squeeze pressures in the anal canal and also provides assessment of rectal vault distensibility. A catheter with three pressure-sensitive balloons is placed into the rectum and anal canal; the intrarectal balloon measures rectal pressures, the balloon positioned at the anorectal junction measures IAS pressures, and the balloon positioned midway down the anal canal measures EAS pressures. The intrarectal balloon is inflated to the point of sensory awareness and sensation of rectal fullness, which provides data regarding rectal capacity and sensory awareness of rectal distention. The response of the sphincters to rectal distention is evaluated simultaneously and should involve relaxation of the IAS and contraction of the EAS. Resting pressure reflects IAS function, and squeeze pressure reflects EAS function.

Electromyography

Electromyography is neurologic examination of the pelvic floor muscles and the nerves that control the anal and rectal muscles, using either surface electrodes or needle electrodes; the patient is instructed to contract the anal sphincter muscle and the electrodes measure the strength of the contraction. Needle electrodes provide more accurate data but the individual may experience discomfort or pain with insertion. EMG provides data regarding sphincter innervation and contractility.

Defecography

Defecography is used to diagnose functional problems with rectal evacuation, such as rectal prolapse, rectocele, or rectoanal intussusception. The rectum is filled with a radiopaque paste and imaging studies are obtained during rectal evacuation. It is a very difficult and embarrassing study for the patient and requires a skilled and empathetic examiner.

Proctosigmoidoscopy or Colonoscopy

Proctosigmoidoscopy or colonoscopy is indicated when there is any suspicion of malignancy (e.g., bleeding, change in bowel habits, and/or palpable rectal or abdominal mass); the examiner is able to directly visualize the intestinal mucosa and to obtain biopsies of any suspicious areas or lesions.

Magnetic Resonance Imaging

MRI uses radio waves and magnets to produce detailed pictures of internal organs and soft tissues without the use of x-rays. It may include the injection of contrast medium. It can provide detailed anatomic images of the IAS and EAS and is more accurate than ultrasound (US) in the diagnosis of sphincter defects and atrophy.

Data Synthesis

In summary, a thorough history and physical examination are required to identify the specific issues resulting in FI and to develop an appropriate management plan. All individuals require a basic history and physical examination; those with suspected sphincter defects, neurologic lesions, or persistent diarrhea may require additional studies. More advanced studies are also required for the patient who does not respond to basic management strategies.

In synthesizing the data and developing a management plan, the continence nurse should begin by answering the following questions.

Is the incontinence transient or chronic? If the FI is new onset and due to either high-volume liquid stool or altered mental status, the focus should be on treatment of the underlying medical conditions, containment of the stool, and protection of the perianal skin. For individuals with chronic FI, the continence nurse should review the assessment data to determine the following:

Is stool consistency normal (i.e., is stool soft and formed?)? Since stool consistency is a major determining factor for continence, the initial focus in management should be on correcting any abnormalities in stool consistency.

Is the individual cognitively intact, or does he/she have incontinent stools with no apparent cognitive awareness? The individual with incontinence due to dementia will require a routine toileting program and may require regular stimulated defecation (anal wash-out) *or* management with absorptive products.

Is sensory function intact, that is, does the individual always know when there is stool or gas in the rectum, and can the individual reliably discriminate between gas, liquid, and solid contents? If the individual usually senses stool in the rectum but sometimes leaks small volumes of stool without recognition, she/he should be referred for biofeedback to improve sensory function.

If the individual never senses rectal distention due to a neurologic lesion or process, she/he will require a stimulated defecation program.

Is sphincter function normal, or is there evidence of sphincter weakness or denervation? The individual with weak but contractile sphincter muscles will benefit from pelvic muscle exercises as initial management. The individual with total loss of sphincter contractility due to a neurologic lesion or process will require a stimulated defecation program.

Is there evidence of inadequate rectal capacity and compliance (i.e., persistent intense urgency and ability to delay defecation for only a short period of time)? These individuals should be evaluated by a gastroenterologist and possibly colorectal surgeon for management of the underlying disease process.

CLINICAL PEARL

Data synthesis is a critical step in determining appropriate management for an individual patient: factors to be addressed include differentiation between transient and acute FI, stool consistency, cognitive function, sensory awareness, sphincter function, and rectal capacity and compliance.

 Management of Fecal Incontinence

WOC nursing management of the patient with FI or AI will depend primarily on the underlying cause(s), the functional aspects of continence involved (as outlined in the section on data synthesis), and the specific care setting. Individualized and patient-focused management, protection of patient privacy, and maintenance of patient dignity are key nursing responsibilities in all settings. Initial treatment should focus on correcting the specific factors causing FI and on minimizing the physical and psychosocial impact (e.g., pain, skin damage, embarrassment) (Wishin et al., 2008). Implementation of measures to contain stool and control odor is essential in situations in which bowel control cannot be immediately achieved. In addition, protocols that assure effective management of diarrhea and constipation should be developed in all care environments (Fader et al., 2010; Leung & Schnelle, 2008; McKenna et al., 2001).

Management of Transient Incontinence

Transient incontinence due to acute diarrhea and/or acute alteration in mental status is common among hospitalized patients (Wishin et al., 2008); typical causes include infectious or acute inflammatory processes (e.g., certain strains of flu, *C. Difficile*, exacerbation of Crohn's or ulcerative colitis, antibiotic-associated diarrhea, medications with GI side effects, and radiation therapy or chemotherapy), heavy sedation, and/or delirium. Malnutrition or gluten sensitivity, protein deficiencies, and enteral feedings may also cause diarrhea (McKenna et al., 2001). While restoration of normal stool consistency and continence status is the ultimate goal for nursing management, stool containment and skin management may be the most immediate concerns, especially in critical care and acute care settings when there is high-volume liquid stool. An individualized program of management should be developed that includes skin cleansing with a mild agent and use of a pouching system or internal collection device to contain the effluent (Nix & Haugen, 2010; Wishin et al., 2008).

There are a variety of devices and products available for management of FI. These products can be divided into two major groups: (1) those designed to prevent fecal leakage onto the skin and (2) those designed to absorb the stool and protect the skin. Products that prevent leakage of stool onto the skin include fecal collection pouches, intra-anal devices, rectal tubes and trumpets, and internal bowel management systems. Absorbent pads and briefs are used for absorption and containment of the stool and must be used in conjunction with skin care products designed to prevent incontinence-associated dermatitis (Fader et al., 2010; Wishin et al., 2008).

CLINICAL PEARL

Effective containment of liquid stool is a key aspect of management for the individual with transient FI due to acute diarrheal illness; the best options are external fecal collection pouches and internal bowel management systems.

External Fecal Collection Pouches

External fecal pouches are products designed to collect and contain liquid fecal material in order to quantify the stool and protect the skin; they are recommended as the "first step" in management of large-volume liquid stool (see Fig. 16-2). An external pouching device adheres directly to the perianal skin and is replaced every 1 to 2 days and as needed for leakage. Benefits of external fecal pouches include the fact that they are noninvasive with no risk of damage to the sphincters or rectal tissue; they protect the perianal skin from breakdown; they are a closed system, which helps to prevent the spread of harmful organisms; they can be attached to ancillary drainage systems; they at least partially contain excrement and odor; and they help to reduce use of absorptive products and linens as well as nursing and caregiver time.

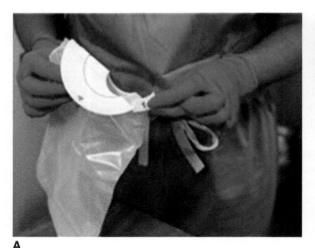

A

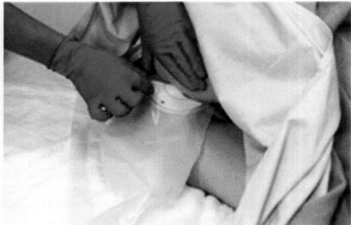

B

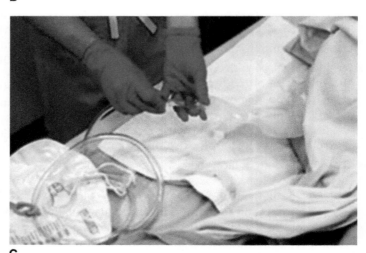

C

FIGURE 16-2. External fecal collection device. The fecal incontinence pouch is used to protect the skin when the client is having frequent liquid stools. **A.** The paper backing is removed from the pouch's adhesive. **B.** The pouch is applied covering the anal opening. **C.** The tube from the pouch is attached to the tubing of the collection bag, which is positioned below the level of the client's buttocks. It is secured to the bed in the same manner as the urine collection bag.

Disadvantages of fecal pouches include the following: their use is limited to nonambulatory patients who do not slide up and down in bed; it typically requires more than one caregiver to apply a rectal pouch (one to position the patient and one to apply the device); stool occasionally undermines the pouch and causes perianal skin breakdown if not changed in a timely manner (Wishin et al., 2008); rectal exams cannot be performed; and rectal medication cannot be administered with the pouch in place. A very significant disadvantage is the inability to use these devices effectively when there is perianal skin breakdown, because intact skin is required for a secure seal. In addition, removal from the patient with damaged skin carries the risk for additional skin breakdown (Wishin et al., 2008).

Internal Bowel Management Systems

Intended for use primarily in acute care settings, intra-anal management systems are designed to divert liquid stool away from the perianal skin and into a collection device, thus providing for both quantification of fecal output and protection of the perianal skin. The device includes soft silicone tubing connected to a low-pressure intrarectal balloon on one end and to a collection device on the other end (Fig. 16-3). The retention balloon is placed into the rectum and then inflated with air, water, or saline. While the catheter and intrarectal balloon can be left inside the patient for an extended period (29 days), the stool collection bags are detached when full and disposed of appropriately. Some intra-anal devices allow for fecal sampling and for medication administration and irrigation; in addition, some are equipped with an indicator that signals maximum inflation of the intrarectal balloon and actually prevents further inflation. Prior to placement of an intra-anal device, the nurse must carefully evaluate the patient to determine eligibility and to rule out contraindications (Page et al., 2008; Sparks et al., 2010). (See Box 16-1 for contraindications established by the manufacturers of these devices.)

Advantages of intra-anal devices include reduced risk of skin breakdown and discomfort; minimization of odor; enhanced patient dignity; protection of wounds, surgical sites, or burns from fecal contact; decreased exposure to

| BOX 16-1. | Contraindications to Use of Internal Bowel Management Systems |

Intra-anal devices should not be used in the following patients:

- Those known to be sensitive or allergic to any components within the system
- Those with clotting disorders
- Those who have had lower large bowel or rectal surgery in the last year
- Those with rectal or anal injury, severe rectal or anal stricture or stenosis (i.e., any patient if the distal rectum cannot accommodate the inflated cuff), confirmed rectal or anal tumor, severe hemorrhoids, or fecal impaction
- Those with suspected or confirmed rectal mucosa impairment (i.e., severe proctitis, ischemic proctitis, mucosal ulcerations)
- Those with indwelling rectal or anal devices in place, or who require enemas.

infectious microorganisms; more accurate measurement of output (measurements on any plastic collection device are approximate as the print may slip and slide during stamping); reduced risk of catheter-associated urinary tract infections; reduced soiling of linens; and reduced caregiver time required for hygienic care (Gray et al., 2014).

Disadvantages related to use of intra-anal devices include risk of bleeding, especially among patients receiving anticoagulants or antiplatelet medications or those sustaining inadvertent traumatic balloon removal, damage to the rectal mucosa, blockage of the tubing, expulsion of the tube, and stool leakage around the device (Echols et al., 2007; Kowal-Vern et al., 2009; Sparks et al., 2010; Padmanabhan et al., 2007; Page et al., 2008; Leung & Rao, 2011; Nix, 2006; Rees & Sharpe, 2009).

Strict adherence to the manufacturer's instructions for patient selection, application, and removal of the device is essential. Intra-anal devices should not be used for chronic diarrhea as the devices are not intended for use for more than 29 consecutive days. It is essential for caregivers to be competent in placement and management of intra-anal devices. Frequent routine patient and device assessments should be performed to ensure the tubing is not beneath the patient and that there is no tension on the device; in addition, care must be taken with patient transfers to prevent traumatic removal of the device.

There are some direct costs associated with an intra-anal management device, with some cost variations between manufacturers. However, the costs may be offset by the savings from reduced use of linens, lower laundry costs, reduction in nursing time required for care, and reduced incidence of skin problems (Kowal-Vern et al., 2009). Use of the devices has been linked to improved nursing assessment and documentation and better patient outcomes.

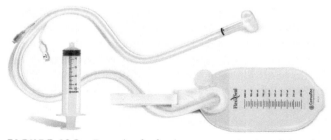

FIGURE 16-3. Example of a fecal management system: internal bowel management.

Rectal Trumpets

32-French nasopharyngeal airways have been used off-label for management of FI; the "trumpet" (flared end of the airway) is inserted into the rectum and the straight end of the tube is connected to a gravity drainage system. This device is not indicated for patients with leukopenia, perirectal abscess, or gastrointestinal bleeding. While very few studies have been done with these devices, the early outcomes have been positive (Wishin et al., 2008). The device should be changed every 2 days, and 1 hour of "rest time" should be provided before reinsertion. Use of a barrier cream around the anus helps protect the surrounding skin (Faller, 2005). The rectal trumpet device would not be effective or appropriate for the patient with severe colonic distention due to a high impaction and should be discontinued if the weight of the drainage collection device causes recurrent inadvertent removal of the trumpet from the rectum. Since newer fecal management systems with safety data are available, rectal trumpet use is not generally recommended (Beitz, 2006), and any use should be limited to short periods of time (days rather than weeks).

Rectal Tubes

Large lumen balloon-tipped indwelling catheters and rectal tubes have been used in the past for liquid stool diversion, gas reduction, or to administer medications or enemas. Rectal tubes are now considered unsafe and are *not recommended* as there is the potential for rectal necrosis, bowel perforation, and damage to the anal sphincter (Nix & Haugen, 2010; Rees & Sharpe, 2009).

Management of Chronic Fecal Incontinence

As noted, chronic FI may be due to alterations in stool consistency, dementia, impaired sensory function, compromised sphincter function, neurologic lesions causing total loss of sensory function and sphincter control, changes in rectal capacity and compliance, or functional issues such as immobility or restraints (Pares et al., 2012).

Restoration of normal controlled defecation is the goal for nursing management and begins with reversible factors, including elimination of any impacted stool and dietary, fluid, and medication modifications to normalize stool consistency; weight reduction, smoking cessation, and measures to improve mobility and functional status are also of benefit. Additional noninvasive interventions may include sphincter muscle exercises with or without biofeedback, bowel habit training, and stimulated defecation/transanal irrigation programs. For individuals who fail to respond to these noninvasive measures, surgical intervention should be considered; currently available surgical options include sphincter repair, stimulated graciloplasty, artificial anal sphincter, sacral nerve modulation, magnetic anal sphincter implantation, injectable bulking agents, the antegrade continence enema (ACE) procedure, and diversion (colostomy) (Halland & Talley, 2012; Mellgren, 2010; Van Koughnett & Wexner, 2013).

The principles of bowel management and knowledge of treatment options should be used to develop an individualized program for prevention or management of FI. For example, evidence suggests that individuals undergoing bariatric surgery are at risk for FI and that measures to normalize stool consistency and to improve pelvic floor muscle strength prior to surgery can reduce the incidence of FI in these individuals (Richter et al., 2005; Roberson et al., 2010).

> **CLINICAL PEARL**
>
> Evidence suggests that individuals undergoing bariatric surgery are at risk for FI and that measures to normalize stool consistency and to improve pelvic floor muscle strength prior to surgery can reduce the incidence of FI in these individuals.

Management of Fecal Impaction

Fecal impaction most commonly occurs as an acute exacerbation of chronic constipation; risk factors include routine use of laxatives (possibly due to the underlying motility issue triggering the need for laxatives), immobility, neurologic lesions or disease states, and constipating medications (e.g., anticholinergic, antidiarrheal, and narcotic agents). Fecal impaction creates a mechanical obstruction that prevents the elimination of stool proximal to the impaction. The hard mass of stool also causes persistent relaxation of the internal sphincter; this allows liquid stool to pass around the fecal mass and causes fecal leakage. Impactions most commonly occur at the level of the rectum but can also occur in the ascending or transverse colon (high impaction).

> **CLINICAL PEARL**
>
> Impactions most commonly occur at the level of the rectum but can also occur in the ascending or transverse colon; management is dependent on the level of impaction.

Rectal Impaction

When stool impaction is suspected, a digital rectal examination should be done; if there is a fecal mass in the rectum that is too hard and too large to evacuate, measures should be initiated to eliminate the fecal mass and to cleanse the proximal colon. Digital breakup should be attempted; if this is unsuccessful, lubricant and/or cathartic solutions should be administered rectally to soften the stool. Warm mineral oil enemas are frequently used to soften the stool and facilitate evacuation; they are typically given daily for 2 to 3 days, at which point the mass can usually be digitally broken up and removed. Anecdotal reports also support the use of a milk and molasses enema (typically a 1:1 mixture of molasses and milk, either powdered milk or cow's milk); the solution is warmed until it mixes thoroughly and then cooled for administration. Small volumes (60 to 90 mL) are instilled adjacent to the fecal mass, and the individual is asked to retain the mixture for about 30 minutes; digital breakup is then attempted. This procedure is repeated until the fecal mass can be broken up and removed.

Once the obstructing fecal mass has been removed, the proximal colon must be cleansed using suppositories, enemas, or laxatives. Oral polyethylene glycol or magnesium citrate solutions may be used to cleanse the proximal bowel so long as there are no contraindications (e.g., evidence of colonic distention or obstruction). Selection of a laxative must be made with any comorbidities in mind; for example, preparations containing magnesium, phosphate, or citrate should be avoided for individuals with heart failure or renal failure. Spontaneous evacuation of soft stool indicates that the bowel has been thoroughly cleansed (Stevens et al., 2003).

High Impaction

A high impaction occurs in the ascending or transverse colon and may be accompanied by nausea and vomiting, abdominal distention, and liquid stools. High impactions are treated with tap water or brand-name enemas to stimulate bowel movements; some clinicians recommend use of oral mineral oil to lubricate the fecal mass prior to enema administration. MD Anderson Cancer Center utilizes a protocol involving powdered milk and molasses enemas, as follows: 6 ounces of hot water are mixed with 3 ounces of powdered milk (not cow's milk); 4.5 ounces of molasses are added and the mixture is stirred until the solution color is even. The patient is positioned on his or her left side and the enema tube is inserted via the rectum about 12 inches (to reach the proximal descending and left transverse colon); the solution is instilled and then held for about 20 minutes. The procedure is repeated if needed with the patient in the left-side lying position and then with the patient in the right-side lying position. Once the fecal mass has been eliminated, oral laxatives are used to assure colonic cleansing, along with 2 L of fluid daily (Bisanz, 2011).

Prevention of Recurrent Impaction

Once the impaction has been cleared, the continence nurse must institute measures to prevent recurrence; this usually includes increased fiber and fluid intake, increased mobility as tolerated, and avoidance of constipating drugs (if possible); stool softeners may be needed if stools remain hard even after administration of adequate fiber and fluid. Osmotic laxatives can be given as needed, for example, whenever the individual has not had a bowel movement for 2 to 3 days despite use of fiber, fluids, and softeners. These agents "work" by pulling fluid into the lumen of the bowel, thus distending the bowel and promoting peristalsis; as a result, they can be used routinely if needed. In selecting an osmotic laxative, the nurse must always consider any contraindications to specific agents related to comorbid conditions.

Stimulant laxatives may be used when osmotic agents are ineffective; they work by stimulating the nerve cells within the bowel wall in addition to causing fluid secretion into the lumen of the bowel. Because they have direct effects on the nerve cells within the bowel wall, there are concerns that frequent repetitive use might have adverse effects on motility long term; thus, they are typically recommended for "PRN" use as opposed to routine use. For individuals with limited bowel control, enemas may be preferable to oral laxatives because the time frame for response is more predictable.

> **CLINICAL PEARL**
>
> Osmotic agents work by pulling fluid into the lumen of the bowel, thus distending the bowel and stimulating peristalsis; as a result, they can be used routinely if needed.

Measures to Normalize Stool Consistency and Bowel Function

Once any impacted stool has been removed, the continence nurse should focus on normalizing stool consistency and establishing a pattern for regular evacuation through dietary and fluid modifications to create soft formed stool and to reduce gas production, and use of medications as needed to assure normal stool consistency. Food intake patterns can also help to regulate bowel function. Individuals should be encouraged to eat at regular intervals every day and to avoid skipping meals. Weight loss should be encouraged for those who are overweight, since this has a favorable effect on bowel function (Crosswell et al., 2010; Hansen, et al. 2006; Wilde et al., 2014).

> **CLINICAL PEARL**
>
> Once any impacted stool has been removed, the continence nurse should focus on normalizing stool consistency and establishing a pattern for regular evacuation.

As explained previously, liquid stool may overwhelm the sphincters, and chronic constipation places the individual at risk for fecal impaction and subsequent leakage of liquid stool; thus, establishment of normal stool consistency is an essential element of management for most people with FI. Adequate hydration must be assured, watery to loose stools need to be thickened to decrease frequency and volume, and hard stools need to be softened. Both diarrhea and constipation may be positively affected by adequate fluid intake, dietary modifications, and use of fiber supplements. Medications may be recommended when these lifestyle measures provide insufficient effects or while waiting for advised fluid and dietary modifications to take effect (Hunter et al., 2002; Marples, 2011; Van Koughnett & Wexner, 2013).

Management of Diarrhea

This topic is addressed in Chapter 15, but the critical elements will be briefly highlighted here as well. All individuals with diarrhea should be counseled regarding the critical importance of fluid replacement, which should be initiated whenever there are frequent liquid stools. A simple and practical recommendation is to consume 8 ounces of liquid immediately following each loose stool in addition to their usual fluid intake; good choices include bouillon, broth-based soups, low-sugar sports drinks, herbal teas, gelatin (Jell-O), and water. Carbonated diet beverages, orange or prune juice, caffeinated beverages, alcoholic beverages, and chocolate should be avoided since they increase gastrointestinal motility and could worsen diarrhea. Liquids at room temperature may be better tolerated than those that are hot or cold. Milk should be limited or avoided altogether until diarrhea is no longer a problem, especially for those with known lactose intolerance; in contrast, yogurt with probiotics may help to restore normal colonic flora and thus to reduce diarrhea (Crosswell et al., 2010; Hansen et al., 2006).

Dietary modifications may also help to reduce diarrheal episodes. For example, greasy, deep-fried, and fatty foods such as bacon and pizza, some fast foods, and rich sauces and gravy may worsen diarrhea and increase the risk of FI. Foods and fluids with high sugar content, those sweetened with sorbitol, very spicy foods such as chili, and nuts and fruits (figs, plums, prunes, and oranges) may also be bothersome as they increase gastrointestinal motility. Products containing gluten (pasta, wheat flour, baked goods) can cause or worsen diarrhea, specifically in individuals who are gluten-sensitive (Hansen et al., 2006). Finally, foods that form gas can also cause diarrhea. Some of these gas-forming foods include onions, beans, cabbage, peas, broccoli, cauliflower, whole grain breads and cereals, nuts, and popcorn (Crosswell et al., 2010).

The BRAT diet is widely recommended for short-term relief of diarrhea: *Bananas, Rice, Apples* or *Applesauce*, and *Toast* (low-fiber or white bread) or *Tapioca*. Bananas may be more effective when they are green. See Table 16-4 for foods that slow motility.

Bulk-forming fiber supplements can also be used to thicken the stool. A teaspoon of methyl cellulose (Citrucel) or 3.4 g of psyllium (Metamucil) mixed with 2 ounces of water and ingested immediately before or after a meal may help to thicken small bowel contents and to slow motility through the bowel. No additional liquid should be taken for about 1 hour (Bisanz, 2011).

Management of Constipation

As noted previously, correction of constipation requires provision of adequate fiber and fluid, measures to increase mobility, elimination of constipating medications when feasible, and judicious use of stool softeners and laxatives as well as prompt response to the urge to defecate. Recommended fluid intake for adults is usually about 1.5 to 2.5 L of fluids or 30 mL/kg body weight/day up to 2.5 L. Factors to consider in making recommendations for a specific individual include weight, activity level, atmospheric temperature, and any conditions requiring fluid restriction, such as congestive heart failure. Liquids typically include water, tea, coffee, and fresh fruit juices, as well as foods with high water content, such as Jell-O or popsicles. Potentially dehydrating fluids, such as alcohol or caffeine in high volumes, should be avoided or limited, as should fluids with high sugar content.

Individuals on fluid restriction are at high risk for constipation because they are unable to consume adequate fiber and fluid. For these individuals, a combination of softener and stimulant (such as docusate + senna or docusate + bisacodyl) can help to prevent constipation, by keeping the stool soft and increasing peristaltic activity. Individuals should be instructed to follow manufacturers' guidelines in regard to dosage (Annels & Koch, 2003; Wilde et al., 2014).

Dietary measures to prevent constipation include reduced intake of high-fat and processed foods and increased intake of dietary fiber. High-fat foods slow motility and should be avoided or consumed in limited amounts; these include ice cream, cheese, whole milk, pizza, French fries, potato chips, and high-fat meats. Fast food should also be avoided or limited, because processing of fast food removes most of the beneficial dietary fiber; processed foods include all prepackaged foods, white or polished rice, refined sugars, refined white flour, doughnuts and pastries, and hotdog and hamburger buns.

Foods high in dietary fiber add bulk to the stool, thus promoting peristalsis and acting as natural stool-softening agents. Fresh fruits and raw vegetables are excellent choices of dietary fiber, as are high-fiber cereals and foods made with whole grains (Bisanz, 2011). Foods sweetened with sorbitol can help to relieve constipation because sorbitol is an osmotic laxative; licorice and green pumpkin seeds (pepitas) have also been reported to have natural laxative properties. Table 16-4 lists foods that promote soft stool and help to prevent constipation.

Various fiber supplements are available for individuals who are unable or unwilling to ingest a high-fiber diet. Medicinal fiber supplements can be divided into two categories: soluble and bulk-forming. Soluble fiber dissolves in water, remains gelatinous in the bowel, and slows peristalsis so that nutrients can be absorbed. Bananas contain natural inulin fiber, which has a softening effect but does not add bulk to the stool; Benefiber and Fiber Choice are manufactured products that also contain natural inulin. Bulk-forming fiber supplements work by absorbing water; with liquid stool, this results in thickening of the stool, and with hard stool, the fiber adds bulk to the stool, which attracts water and softens the stool. Examples of bulk-forming fiber supplements include psyllium (Metamucil) and methyl cellulose (Citrucel) (Bisanz, 2011). Individuals using fiber supplements are generally encouraged to take them daily, to titrate the dose to obtain appropriate stool consistency, and to assure adequate fluid intake. Adequate fluid intake is particularly important with bulk-forming agents. Individuals beginning fiber supplements should be informed that increased production of gas is common during the first few weeks of fiber therapy.

> **CLINICAL PEARL**
>
> Dietary modifications and use of fiber supplements can be beneficial in management of both constipation and diarrhea.

Medications are a common contributing factor to constipation; thus, management of the individual with constipation involves a thorough review of all medications being taken (including over-the-counter and herbal agents) and consultation with the prescribing provider regarding possible substitutions or dose modifications for medications known to cause constipation. If the patient requires continued use of the medication, constipation should be prevented through a program that includes adequate fiber and fluid intake (unless contraindicated), stool softeners, and osmotic and stimulant laxatives. See Table 16-3 for medications that commonly cause constipation.

> **CLINICAL PEARL**
>
> Medications are a common contributing factor to constipation; if the patient requires continued use of the medication (e.g., opioid analgesics), the patient should be placed on a program to prevent constipation (e.g., fiber supplements if tolerated, stool softeners, and laxatives as needed).

Various medications can be taken to promote peristalsis and relieve constipation, including suppositories, enemas, and oral laxatives. Enemas and suppositories should be avoided in individuals with low blood counts, due to the risk of bleeding or infection. Oral agents should be used only when there is no distal obstruction or impaction and should be selected based on any comorbid conditions, as noted earlier.

In general, fiber supplements and stool softeners are used to prevent constipation, and osmotic and stimulant laxatives are used to treat constipation. There are a wide variety of osmotic agents, including saline- and magnesium-based products, sorbitol, lactulose, and polyethylene glycol; all work by pulling fluid into the lumen of the bowel, which stimulates peristalsis and helps to soften the stool. The two stimulant laxatives widely used are senna and bisacodyl; both promote peristalsis through direct action on the nerves in the bowel wall. Softener–stimulant combinations have dual effects, as the classification suggests.

> **CLINICAL PEARL**
>
> In general, fiber supplements and stool softeners are used to prevent constipation, and osmotic and stimulant laxatives are used to treat constipation.

Medications should be titrated to maintain soft formed stools on a regular basis. Stool softeners, stimulant laxatives, and combination products can be purchased at drug and grocery stores without a prescription. Store-brand stimulant laxative/stool softeners should work as well as brand names and may cost less. Liquid forms of these medications are also available and may be prescribed by a physician.

Healthy Bowel Habits

Patients need to be taught the fundamentals of normal bowel function and bowel hygiene. Peristalsis creates an urge to defecate; if the individual responds promptly to this urge, she/he is working with their body and the stool is easily eliminated via the peristaltic activity. In contrast, if the individual suppresses the urge, peristaltic activity ceases and the rectum relaxes to provide fecal storage. When the individual voluntarily tries to eliminate the stored stool, she/he must use abdominal muscle contraction to force the stool out of the rectum. Thus, the patient with a tendency for constipation and irregularity should be instructed to do two things: (1) respond promptly to the urge to defecate whenever possible and (2) develop a consistent pattern for stool elimination about the same time every day. Since stool elimination is most likely to occur within 20 to 30 minutes following a meal (due to the gastroenteric reflex), the individual should be instructed to establish her/his time for attempted defecation immediately following a meal. Prerequisites to an effective bowel habit training program include elimination of retained stool (via enemas or laxatives) and establishment of soft formed stool via fiber, fluid, activity, and softeners if needed. Any known personal stimuli for defecation should be used, such as warm tea or coffee, prune juice, or yogurt with probiotics. The individual must also be taught the best posture for bowel evacuation, which is sitting upright on the commode with feet apart and flat on the floor. Some mild straining or abdominal muscle contraction might be necessary to increase intra-abdominal pressure.

> **CLINICAL PEARL**
>
> Healthy bowel habits include prompt response to the urge to defecate, use of any personal stimuli to defecation (such as warm tea, coffee, or prune juice), and correct posture for defecation (sitting upright with feet flat on floor or step stool).

Management of Flatus Incontinence

Passing gas is a natural elimination process that occurs on a daily basis; however, there are extreme variations among individuals in terms of daily volume. Factors affecting the volume of gas production include the amount of high-fiber foods and cruciferous vegetables ingested (vegetables with peels, cabbage and related vegetables, grains, high-fiber breads, beans, cereals, nuts, and seeds) and, to a much lesser extent, the amount of air that is swallowed.

Carbonated beverages, chewing gum, and drinking through straws increases the volume of swallowed air and may increase gas production in selected individuals; however, most swallowed air is absorbed prior to reaching the distal bowel. Individuals who report persistent high-volume gas production should be evaluated for an unrecognized malabsorption syndrome, such as lactose intolerance or gluten intolerance. Individuals who have flatus incontinence should be taught measures to reduce gas production and should also be taught sphincter strengthening exercises; if the flatus incontinence occurs without the individual's awareness of gaseous rectal distention, biofeedback may be indicated to improve sensory awareness. The most obvious strategy for reducing gas production is to reduce the intake of gas-producing foods. Additional measures include the use of simethicone and Beano. Simethicone breaks large gas bubbles into smaller bubbles so that it is more likely to be absorbed and less likely to cause distress. Beano is an enzyme that helps to break down complex carbohydrates to prevent bacterial action and gas production. Both of these products are readily available over the counter (Bisanz, 2011).

CLINICAL PEARL

Management of flatus incontinence includes measures to reduce gas production and instruction in sphincter strengthening exercises.

Pelvic Floor Muscle Exercises

Pelvic floor physiotherapy is an established mode of therapy for UI, but the technique is less well studied for FI. However, pelvic floor muscle exercises (PME) are of potential benefit to individuals who recognize rectal distention but have difficulty retaining stool due to weak or damaged sphincter muscles. The techniques for teaching and performing pelvic muscle exercises are essentially the same whether the individual has urinary, fecal, or mixed incontinence, but there is much less data available regarding the effectiveness of pelvic floor exercises for FI. The goal of sphincter exercises is to condition the external sphincter in terms of duration and speed of contraction in order to prevent fecal leakage, and the retraining may be used in conjunction with other conservative measures to improve fecal continence in patients with intact sensation, cognition, and volitional contraction of the sphincter (Wilde et al., 2014).

CLINICAL PEARL

The techniques for teaching and performing pelvic muscle exercises for individuals with FI are essentially the same as those for individuals with UI; the individual must be able to isolate and voluntarily contract the pelvic floor muscles without recruiting the abdominal muscles.

Wilde et al. (2014) describe the following steps in teaching PME: (1) assist the cognitively aware and compliant patient to identify and isolate the pelvic floor muscles; (2) teach the individual to contract the pelvic floor muscles without additionally contracting the abdominal muscles; and (3) establish an exercise program that specifies number of contractions and goal for duration of contraction. Isolating the pelvic floor muscles may initially be difficult for the individual. Sitting straight up in a chair with feet flat on the floor and pretending to "hold back flatus" may help the patient to identify the specific muscles. The clinician or therapist may also insert a gloved finger into the vagina or rectum and have the patient squeeze around the examining finger. Some clinicians have suggested the patient stop the flow of urine midstream to check that they are contracting the appropriate muscle group; this should be done only to assess muscle strength and not on a routine basis.

Once the patient can consistently isolate and contract the muscle, she/he is placed on an individualized exercise program to improve the strength, muscle coordination, and endurance of the muscles. Usually, a 12-week program is initiated in which the patient begins with a series of 10 pelvic floor muscle contractions at three different times during the day. The ultimate goal is that each individual contraction would last 10 seconds. However, the person with very weak muscles who is unable to hold the contraction for even 4 seconds may become discouraged; thus, an individualized goal should be established, for example, 3- to 5-second contractions at first, with gradual increase in duration to the sustained 10-second contraction. Once the patient is able to sustain 10-second contractions, the number of contractions may be increased as negotiated with the therapist. Although the exercises may be done lying, sitting, or standing, patients who have trouble isolating the pelvic floor muscles (and keeping the abdominal muscles relaxed) may be more successful if they perform the exercises while bending forward with arms pressed against a table or chair back or leaning forward with arms pressed against a wall. Biofeedback may also be a useful adjunct to standard pelvic muscle exercise therapy for some individuals.

The patient needs to be reminded that strength and endurance are built gradually over time, as is true with any exercise program. In addition, maintenance "toning" exercises should be continued throughout life. Another strategy to promote patient adherence and confidence in her/his progress is to have them keep a bowel diary to track FI episodes; this provides objective evidence of progress (reduced episodes of incontinence) that may serve to encourage and motivate the individual (Wilde et al., 2014).

Biofeedback

Biofeedback is a physical therapy modality considered to be a first-line treatment for mild to moderate incontinence (Leite et al., 2013). It can be used to improve sensory awareness, improve pelvic muscle strength and function, or improve coordination between abdominal and pelvic floor muscles. When coupled with pelvic floor exercises, biofeedback has been successful in improving continence for patients with FI refractory to lifestyle and medical treatment alone. Some sensation of rectal fullness and the ability to at least weakly contract the pelvic muscles must be present for biofeedback to be successful. Biofeedback may be used in conjunction with digital feedback, electrical stimulation, and manometric or US response monitoring (Stevens et al., 2003). Several different regimens have been defined and utilized in various studies; at present, there is insufficient data to support any one regimen as being superior (Leite et al., 2013). Biofeedback with adjunctive pelvic floor muscle exercises is suggested to be more effective than pelvic muscle exercises or biofeedback alone (Van Koughnett & Wexner, 2013).

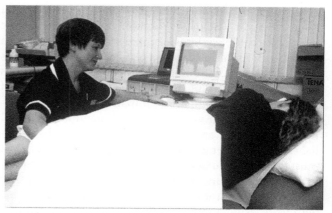

FIGURE 16-4. A patient and therapist during biofeedback treatment.

> **CLINICAL PEARL**
>
> Biofeedback can be used to improve sensory awareness, improve pelvic muscle strength and function, and/or improve coordination between abdominal and pelvic floor muscles.

Biofeedback can also be used to improve rectal sensation in individuals with blunted or delayed awareness of rectal filling; a balloon is placed into the rectum and gradually inflated to the point of awareness and then gradually deflated with the patient focusing on the sensation. Over time, the patient is "taught" to recognize lower levels of rectal distention and to immediately contract the sphincter in response to the sensation of fullness. As noted earlier, prompt recognition of stool in the rectum is an essential element of continence that prompts the individual to contract the EAS and to move to a toilet in a timely manner (Findlay & Maxwell-Armstrong, 2010). Therapy requires motivation (Mellgren, 2010) and a commitment between the therapist and patient for weeks, even months, to realize success. All candidates, especially the elderly, must be able to understand and comply with directions (Halland & Talley, 2012).

Biofeedback involves placement of a pressure-sensitive probe intravaginally or rectally. The probe detects and measures the strength and coordination of the sphincter and levator ani muscles at baseline and can be used to (Mellgren, 2010) monitor improvement over time. The patient can actually see the monitor screen as he or she is performing the contractions, which provides visual feedback that he or she is recruiting the appropriate muscles and that contractions are becoming stronger (Findlay & Maxwell-Armstrong, 2010) (Fig. 16-4). This visual feedback is helpful in supporting continued patient compliance with the treatment program. The frequency of in-clinic biofeedback therapy sessions is determined by the physical therapist and patient.

Electrical Stimulation

Electrical stimulation directly to the anal sphincter is another option for strengthening sphincter function and may be used in combination with biofeedback therapy. Sensors are placed intravaginally or intra-anally; alternatively, skin electrodes can be used with placement at specific points on the perineum. The stimulation device delivers a slight charge to the area, which causes the muscle to contract for the duration of the charge. The stimulation is said to feel like "pins and needles," similar to when your arm or foot "falls asleep." The charge is increased in strength and duration gradually over time. This therapy may be continued at home with a home unit; the individual should return to the clinic at regular intervals for evaluation of strength measurements and recalibration of the E-stim machine. At present, electrical stimulation is not widely used, due in part to the lack of substantial evidence regarding the technique and outcomes (Findlay & Maxwell-Armstrong, 2010). Better outcomes may be achieved among patients receiving E-stim as opposed to biofeedback; however, substantially more data is needed before E-stim can be widely recommended, and these data are also needed to obtain coverage by third-party payers. In addition, effective outcomes require a very skilled physical therapist as well as a compliant patient (Van Koughnett & Wexner, 2013).

As noted, third-party coverage for the cost of biofeedback and electrical stimulation is currently limited; however, this will probably improve once substantial data regarding efficacy can be provided. It should be noted that these advanced therapies are adjunctive to dietary and medication counseling and do not replace these basic interventions.

Neurogenic Bowel Management: Stimulated Defecation

By definition, neurogenic bowel involves loss of neural control of defecation; the individual with neurogenic bowel has absent or markedly reduced ability to sense rectal distention or to voluntarily contract the EAS, so stool elimination occurs whenever rectal pressures exceed anal canal pressures. The most common causes of neurogenic bowel are multiple sclerosis, spina bifida, and spinal cord injury; Parkinson's disease is a less common cause (Paris et al., 2011). Restoration of controlled defecation requires the individual to establish a schedule for elimination and to use peristaltic stimulants to initiate the evacuation process; prior to beginning the program, any impacted stool must be removed and soft formed stool must be established through dietary and fluid management. The bowel must then be stimulated to empty daily or every other day to avoid passive incontinence, which has an extremely detrimental psychological effect on the lives of people with neurogenic bowel. An effective bowel management/ stimulated defecation program typically requires 30 to 60 minutes a day devoted to thoroughly cleaning out the bowel (Norton & Chelvanayagam, 2010) and allows people to go on about their day without worrying about an accident.

CLINICAL PEARL

The individual with neurogenic bowel is unable to sense rectal distention and unable to voluntarily control the sphincter; restoration of controlled stool elimination requires establishment of a routine schedule for defecation and use of a peristaltic stimulus.

Oral laxatives are not routinely used for individuals with neurogenic bowel, due to the unpredictability of their results; constipation in these individuals is usually better managed with suppositories and enemas as well as dietary and fluid modification. Occasionally, low-dose laxative agents or softener–stimulant combinations may be used in the evening followed by a stimulated defecation program in the morning; however, the dose and timing must be carefully titrated to prevent fecal accidents.

Once any retained stool has been eliminated and normal stool consistency has been established, the individual should establish a schedule for elimination; stimulated defecation should be scheduled for the same time of day every day (or every other day) when the individual has the time to devote to stimulating the bowel and waiting for defecation to occur. Some patients may choose to lie in bed to administer the agent, followed by transfer to the toilet or commode chair; others may elect to administer the stimulus while seated on the toilet or commode chair or while seated on the shower chair or bench to save time with showering and personal cleanup after evacuation. For instance, the individual may use digital stimulation, a suppository, or a mini-enema to promote peristalsis and to move the fecal mass into the rectum. Choice of the agent is individual and may change over time with aging or changes in physical condition. How quickly the stimulant works also varies from person to person.

CLINICAL PEARL

In establishing a stimulated defecation program, the clinician and patient must work together to select the best stimulant for that individual; options include digital stimulation, suppositories, mini-enemas, and/or transanal irrigations/wash-outs.

Digital Stimulation

Digital stimulation is performed with a lubricated gloved finger inserted about an inch into the anal canal. Circular sweeps in the canal stimulate peristalsis as well as relaxation of the internal sphincter. Stimulation may need to be repeated for 5 to 10 minutes to initiate and prolong peristalsis. Usually, evacuation occurs in approximately 20 minutes. Performing digital stimulation depends on the person's ability to physically reach the anus and to maintain balance in a position to perform the finger movement. A wand-like device with a "finger" is commercially available. Some individuals rely on a caregiver to perform the procedure. This option is the most economical but does not necessarily provide effective results for everyone (Hammond & Burns, 2000).

Suppository

Use of a rectal suppository is another option for stimulation. Common choices include glycerin, bisacodyl, or carbon dioxide suppositories. Glycerin works by stimulating peristalsis and lubricating the rectum. Bisacodyl stimulates the nerves in the colon wall. Carbon dioxide produces carbon dioxide gas in the rectum, which expands the colon and stimulates peristalsis (Hammond & Burns, 2000).

Suppositories can be readily purchased and are not expensive; "trial and error" is typically needed to determine the type that is most effective for a particular individual. Devices for suppository insertion are available if needed. Over time, the suppository used initially may become less effective and the individual may need to use another type.

Mini-enemas

The third option for bowel stimulation is the use of small enemas. Mineral oil enemas lubricate the intestine, and mini-enemas stimulate the rectal lining and keep the stool soft (Hammond & Burns, 2000). Enemeez, Docu-Sol, and DocuSol Plus (with benzocaine) have snip off tops on flexible insertion tips. These mini-enemas usually work in 15 to 20 minutes. They are similarly priced at about $2.75 each.

Tap Water Enemas or Transanal Irrigation

A fourth option for stimulating defecation is use of warm tap water enemas or transanal irrigations; these options work by distending the bowel, which stimulates peristalsis. This option is used only when the individual gets inadequate results with digital stimulation and/or suppositories or mini-enemas. The enema should be administered through a balloon-tipped catheter inserted into the rectum, in order to provide adequate retention of the enema solution. The catheter is inserted into the rectum and the balloon is inflated; the enema tubing is then connected to the catheter and the fluid is allowed to flow into the rectum and distal bowel. Once the fluid has been instilled, the balloon can be deflated and the catheter can be removed. This option works by distending the bowel and activating the enteric nervous system; it is therefore sometimes effective for individuals with sacral-level lesions and loss of autonomic innervation.

Transanal irrigation is seen as a safe, conservative and effective neurogenic bowel management therapy that may be used when the individual does not respond well to simpler measures (Choi et al., 2013; Krassioukov et al., 2010; Preziosi et al., 2012; Preziosi & Emmanuel, 2009). The Peristeen Anal Irrigation System (Coloplast) received FDA approval in 2012 for use in the United States and is an easy-to-use system for transanal irrigation. The kit includes a hydrophilic-coated rectal balloon, a clear plastic water reservoir, and a handheld unit that allows the individual to inflate the balloon and to control water instillation into the bowel; the unit requires minimal hand strength for manipulation. One major advantage to this system as opposed to a standard "enema" unit is the rectal balloon, which comes with the unit and is designed specifically for intrarectal use; the other advantage is the delivery system for the water, which propels the fluid proximally to provide more effective evacuation. For most individuals, the time frame required for evacuation is only 20 to 30 minutes. This is a prescription item, and the patient must be trained in its use by a nurse or physician.

Oral Laxatives

Oral pharmacological agents may be used in conjunction with the stimulated defecation program to maximize effectiveness, but dose and timing must be carefully titrated to prevent incontinent episodes. Whatever the specific stimulus to defecation used by a specific individual, bowel evacuation is thought to be complete if no more stool is ejected after two digital stimulations or if mucus without stool is expelled.

Neurogenic Bowel Management: MACE Procedure

The Malone antegrade continence enema (MACE) is a procedure growing in popularity that was originally (and effectively) used in children with spina bifida. The reversed appendix (or narrowed tubular section of bowel) is implanted into the colon and connected to the abdominal surface as a small skin-level stoma; this permits the individual to intubate the stoma with a narrow lumen catheter and to administer antegrade (top-down) enemas through the catheter to flush the distal bowel while sitting on the toilet (see Fig. 17-5). In most situations, the appendix or tubular section of bowel is implanted into the cecum, ascending, or right transverse colon, though in some situations, it is implanted into the left transverse or descending colon. This procedure provides an alternative to stimulated defecation programs for individuals with neurogenic bowel and no voluntary control of defecation. In recent years, increasing numbers of spinal cord–injured individuals (especially women) are electing this procedure, both to regulate stool elimination and to eliminate chronic UTIs related to urethral contamination by stool. The daily or QOD enema usually involves tap water, though some individuals add small amounts of glycerin; the volume varies from individual to individual and is titrated to assure adequate colonic wash-out. Stoma complications, especially stenosis, are relatively common, and retrograde leakage can occur, especially if the colon becomes distended with stool (Ellison et al., 2013). This procedure is discussed in more detail in Chapter 17.

Effective management options for the individual with neurogenic bowel, such as the spinal cord–injured person, depend in part on whether the person has upper or lower motor neuron dysfunction. Lower motor neuron dysfunction is characterized by flaccid paralysis of the sphincter and frequent fecal leakage, whereas upper motor neuron dysfunction is characterized by increased sphincter tone. Stimulated defecation is more likely to be effective with individuals who have upper motor neuron dysfunction; the ACE procedure can be used with either type of dysfunction. The key elements of management for any patient with neurogenic bowel, as discussed above, are establishment of soft formed stool and a regular schedule for elimination. Elimination can then be managed either with stimulated defecation or with the ACE procedure, with the goal of producing daily or every other day bowel movements and no leakage in between movements (Krassioukov et al., 2010).

Neurogenic Bowel Management: Colostomy

An end colostomy is another option for individuals with neurogenic bowel who do not respond to conservative management. An end colostomy may improve QOL for the person who is spending considerable time on a bowel management program with variable or unsatisfactory results (Bleier & Kann, 2013). The colostomy can be managed with an odor proof pouch or through retrograde wash-outs (colostomy irrigation) performed daily or every other day.

CLINICAL PEARL

Surgical options for the individual with neurogenic bowel include the MACE procedure and fecal diversion (colostomy).

Surgical Management Options

Individuals who fail to respond to conservative measures should be referred for evaluation for possible surgical intervention. Surgical options currently available include sphincter repair, implantation of an artificial or magnetic sphincter, injection of bulking agents, neuromodulation (sacral nerve stimulation), MACE procedure, and fecal diversion. The MACE procedure and fecal diversion have already been described; the remaining options will be described briefly in terms of indications, contraindications, mechanism of action, and level of evidence to support use.

Sphincter Repair: Sphincteroplasty

Sphincteroplasty is the time-honored standard of care for management of FI for patients with EAS injury, but no neurologic deficit (Halland & Talley, 2012; Van Koughnett & Wexner, 2013). The most common procedure is the anterior overlapping sphincteroplasty; this procedure is generally successful in management of obstetric trauma involving the EAS so long as the IAS remains intact (Van Koughnett & Wexner, 2013). With a curvilinear incision on the perineum, the EAS is isolated. The ends of the sphincter are overlapped and sewn together creating more bulk to the sphincter (Mellgren, 2010). A diverting colostomy is not usually required to obtain optimal results (Van Koughnett & Wexner, 2013).

Sphincter Plication

Sphincter plication is uncommonly done due to the high incidence of recurrent FI; however, this may be the best approach to management of FI associated with an IAS that is anatomically intact, but functionally incompetent, which is a situation that may occur with a history of rectal prolapse. The plication procedure involves creation of a surgical "tuck" in the sphincter muscle that narrows the anorectal opening and thereby increases sphincter resistance. Plication is most successful among women with recent obstetrical defects and/or rectal prolapse, but there is a high risk for complications and a diverting ostomy is sometimes required if the nerves have been inadvertently damaged. Despite fairly good immediate results in about half of the patients, results are frequently not durable and continence may deteriorate over time (Mellgren, 2010).

Artificial Anal Sphincter

Initially developed for UI, artificial sphincters have been revised and altered for use with FI. The artificial sphincter is an approved treatment in the United States and usually reserved for such cases in which the only other alternative for extreme FI is a diverting colostomy (Mellgren, 2010). Using perineal entry, the silicone sphincter, or "cuff," is implanted around the existing sphincter. A channel is created to support an attached reservoir and hydraulic pump system that will control inflation and deflation of the cuff, which simulates contraction and relaxation of the sphincter. The reservoir is implanted in the groin, and the manually operated pump is placed in the scrotum or the labia majora.

About 4 to 6 weeks is required for healing following implantation before the device can be activated. When the device is activated, the fluid from the reservoir is used to fill the cuff, which compresses the anal canal and provides continence. When the individual feels the need to defecate, she/he uses the manually operated pump to transfer the fluid back into the reservoir, thereby deflating the cuff and opening the anal canal. Continence results are good, but there is a high rate of infection requiring reimplantation; reported rates of reoperation vary from 25% to 75%. Thus, further study and refinements are required before this procedure can be advocated for widespread use (Bleier & Kann, 2013; Mellgren, 2010).

Magnetic Artificial Sphincter

The magnetic artificial sphincter is an alternative to the artificial sphincter and involves surgical implantation of a ring of magnetic titanium beads into the anal sphincter; the magnets hold the anal canal closed until abdominal muscle contraction forces them open to permit defecation. Early results are positive, but more data are needed before definitive recommendations can be made (Andromanakos et al., 2013).

Complete patient understanding of either neosphincter procedure or the function of the device is essential. Having the procedure done at a facility that specializes in artificial sphincter placement is highly recommended (Mellgren, 2010).

Stimulated Graciloplasty

Another neosphincter procedure involves transfer of the gracilis muscle or the gluteus maximus muscle; the muscle segment is then wrapped around the anal sphincter and sutured into place to support the anal sphincter. The gracilis and gluteal muscles are the muscles of choice because of their immediate location adjacent to the anal area as well as the nerve innervation, which will tolerate the change in anatomic location. The gluteal muscle is a particularly good choice because this muscle spontaneously contracts when the individual contracts the pelvic floor muscles and sphincter to delay defecation (Van Koughnett & Wexner, 2013). Graciloplasty provides excellent results initially, but over time, the muscle deteriorates (Mellgren 2010).

Long-term results have been improved with surgical implantation of a stimulating device aimed at reducing muscle fatigue (Van Koughnett & Wexner, 2013). Nerve-stimulating leads are placed at the nerve origin and are then connected to a pacemaker-like generator. The pacemaker is placed in a surgically created subcutaneous pocket on the lower abdominal wall. The muscles that encircle the anal sphincter are held in a state of tonic contraction to prevent bowel evacuation. When the individual senses rectal distention and the urge to defecate, she/he passes a magnet over the pacemaker; this temporarily turns the generator off, which relaxes the sphincter and permits stool elimination. Stimulated graciloplasty is a very complex procedure that is done in very few centers and is not currently approved for use in the United States (Van Koughnett & Wexner, 2013).

Injectable Bulking Agents

Anal canal bulking agents have been developed based on some degree of success with urethral bulking agents for UI. In an outpatient setting, and without anesthesia, biomaterials are injected into the sphincter muscle or the submucosal tissues (Mellgren, 2010). Bulking agents may be comprised of collagen, silicone or carbon-coated beads, or dextranomer/hyaluronic acid (NASHA Dx) [Halland & Talley, 2012]. The aim is to supplement the function of the intact IAS. Based on the limited data available at present, injectables appear to provide modest improvement in incontinence scores, with limited durability of results; many individuals require repeat injections. Thus, some authors suggest that this therapy may be most effectively used for individuals with seepage and soiling as opposed to those with frank FI (Bleier & Kann, 2013). Zutshi et al. (2012) suggest that using a nonbiodegradable biological implant after surgery for sphincter repair provides better results over the long term compared to sphincter repair alone. More study that includes pre- and postanorectal testing and direction for procedural standardization is required before any definitive recommendations can be made regarding this procedure (Halland & Talley, 2012).

Sacral Nerve Stimulation

Sacral nerve stimulation was originally designed and tested for the management of UI but has been found to be very effective in the management of FI as well, with studies dating back to the mid-1990s (Bharucha & Rao, 2014). In May 2011, the FDA approved sacral nerve stimulation therapy for patients with FI who failed conservative therapy including dietary modifications, biofeedback, and medications (McNevin et al., 2014). Placement is a two-step process. Initially, an outpatient procedure is performed in which an electrode is passed through the foramina of S2–S4 and connected to an external temporary stimulator. The patient then undergoes a 2- to 3-week trial of pelvic nerve stimulation using the percutaneous wire electrodes and external stimulator; if there is significant improvement, a second procedure is performed in which the electrodes are permanently implanted and the permanent stimulator is implanted in the gluteal muscle area (Van Koughnett & Wexner, 2013). The exact mechanism of action is not specifically understood (Halland & Talley, 2012) but is thought to involve altered muscle function, improved sensory function, and altered motility.

Unlike artificial sphincter devices, sacral nerve stimulators do not have to be switched off (or deflated) to allow defecation (Roth, 2010). Sacral nerve stimulation appears to be effective for individuals with both external and internal sphincter injuries and is now often used as a first-line treatment when more conservative management has not been successful; 5-year success rates as high as 89% have been reported (Hollingshead et al., 2011). This therapy has also been shown to improve QOL scores for individuals struggling with both urinary and FI (Bleier & Kann, 2013; Faucheron et al., 2012; Bharucha & Rao, 2014).

Skin Care and Containment

Skin care for the individual who is incontinent of stool should be individualized. Thorough cleansing after each episode of leakage is essential. The need for skin protectants in addition to cleansing depends on the frequency of leakage, the viscosity and amount of stool, and whether the stool contains corrosive enzymes. For occasional seepage of small amounts of stool, cleansing alone may be adequate; perineal skin cleansers should be used as opposed to soap and water. However, if the frequency and volume is high, cleansing should be followed by use of a moisturizing and moisture barrier product; acceptable barrier products include liquid film barriers that do not wash off with cleansing, and moisture barrier ointments containing petrolatum, zinc oxide, and/or dimethicone.

Skin exposure to high-volume liquid stool with irritating enzymes requires a more aggressive approach to skin protection. Use of zinc oxide barriers is helpful, but the zinc oxide can be difficult to remove. Care should be taken not to forcefully scrub the fecal soiled areas; mineral oil or a perineal cleanser should be used to remove the soiled layers of the zinc oxide ointment, with the base layer left intact as long as it is not soiled (Beeckman et al., 2009; Gray, 2004). An alternative option is to use a product that contains both zinc oxide and petrolatum, which is easier to apply and to remove.

Fecal leakage has variable consistency and is not absorbed easily if at all by containment pads, diapers, or pads. In fact, their use may contribute to further skin irritation and even breakdown because of more prolonged exposure to the irritants in the stool. In addition, absorptive products do not effectively conceal odor, so the product should be changed as soon as possible following soiling. If an individual needs a containment product, the nurse must consider stool frequency, volume, and viscosity and whether the individual suffers with UI as well. The trend in inpatient care settings is to avoid use of diaper-type products unless the patient is ambulatory. The seal around the leg openings is usually snug enough to provide security while ambulating; the seal is also snug enough to mask odor for at least a short period of time.

Some garments are made specifically for those with minor FI for purposes of swimming or pool therapy. Small disposable pads are available for placement between the buttocks to absorb scant fecal seepage. Costs vary from product to product, and there is no third-party reimbursement for most absorptive and containment products. When recommending absorptive and containment products, the nurse must consider the patient's ability to use the products properly, the patient's preferences, and any financial concerns and limitations. At present, no products have been developed that effectively deal with odor or the noise related to flatus, which may occur independently or in combination with fecal leakage (Fader et al., 2010; Willson et al., 2014).

CLINICAL PEARL

We currently lack absorbent products designed to effectively contain stool and odor; products must be carefully selected based on stool volume and consistency, and skin care with routine use of moisture barrier products is essential.

Anal Plugs

The anal plug is an absorbent porous device that is positioned in the rectum to prevent accidental stool leakage; gas can pass through the device. It is a small white device similar to a tampon that is worn for up to 12 hours (Herbert, 2008); when activated by moisture, the plug expands into a "tulip"-shaped structure. The string on the plug is positioned between the buttocks and is used for plug removal. After removal, the plug should be disposed of in the waste bin, not flushed in the toilet.

Anal plugs are more appropriate for fecal seepage episodes versus large-volume FI. The device requires a prescription and is available in varying sizes and designs (Willson et al., 2014). An empty rectal vault is required to allow full expansion of the plug.

The anal plug is one of the few continence devices an individual may use independently. Thus, it is critical for the nurse to carefully evaluate the individual's dexterity and ability to correctly use the plug. It is also critical to provide sufficient education to assure that the patient can use the plug correctly and with confidence. Although the plugs have been found to be helpful in preventing stool leakage in some patients, the plugs can be difficult to tolerate (Deutekom & Dobben, 2012; Fader et al., 2010). At this time, anal plugs are not available in the United States.

Patient Education

FI is not necessarily a sign of aging, though the risk increases with age, and is more prevalent than imagined. Cultural taboos and embarrassment keep affected individuals from bringing the problem to the attention of a knowledgeable care provider. FI is usually related to conditions that can be reversed or remedied, and ongoing attention and self-care is key to effective management, as is true with other chronic conditions (Peden-McAlpine et al., 2008). Individualized dietary modifications, adequate hydration, and compliance with prescribed medications and bowel habit routine are the conservative measures initially employed to address FI

(Crosswell et al., 2010). Pelvic muscle exercises are recommended for individuals with compromised sphincter function, and stimulated defecation programs are the treatment of choice for those with neurogenic incontinence. In addition, there is a myriad of containment products in various sizes, absorbencies, and price ranges, although items specific for men are limited (Fader et al., 2010).

Qualified continence nurses should be able to assist in the selection of appropriate garments and skin protection agents for individual patients and in patient/caregiver education regarding their use. When FI is not responsive to conservative treatments, surgical interventions may be considered; individuals must be educated regarding options, advantages and disadvantages, and requirements for lifelong management (Roth, 2010).

CLINICAL PEARL

Ongoing patient education and support are essential to positive outcomes for the individual with FI.

Individualized education and support are required to assist patients with both conservative and advanced management and are essential to positive outcomes. While the continence nurse is most commonly involved in patient education regarding dietary and fluid modifications, appropriate use of medications, and pelvic floor strengthening exercises, the continence nurse should also be able to inform patients about other therapy options and should be able to make appropriate referrals. The continence nurse should consistently communicate to the individual her/his commitment to helping the individual identify and master strategies that reduce incontinent episodes and improve QOL (Halland & Talley, 2012).

Conclusion

FI is a devastating condition in terms of QOL; due to the embarrassment and stigma, individuals are reluctant to report the problem, even to their health care providers. Effective management begins with careful assessment to determine the contributing problems; most commonly, causative factors include alterations in GI tract function and stool consistency, sphincter damage or denervation, compromised sensory awareness or cognition, and/or altered rectal capacity and compliance. Management is directed toward the specific problems affecting the individual and includes elimination of impacted stool, measures to correct stool consistency and to normalize bowel function, sphincter strengthening exercises, biofeedback to improve sensory awareness and sphincter strength, and stimulated defecation programs for those with sensorimotor loss resulting in neurogenic bowel. Surgical options are available for those who fail to respond to primary measures; those with the greatest success to date include the MACE procedure and sacral nerve stimulation.

CASE STUDY

A 72-year-old female with a medical history of hypertension, diabetes, and high cholesterol lives in an assisted living center. She takes a beta blocker, metformin, and a statin medication. She feels well and has no physical symptoms, but she mentions she sometimes has accidents of stool during the day. Her obstetrical history consists of three vaginal births without complications. She reports occasional constipation and takes a stool softener and it helps. She denies diarrhea or abdominal pain. She admits this problem has been going on for many years and is one of the reasons she lives in an assisted living center. She reports her accidents occur frequently enough that she is afraid to go out and it has made a big difference in her lifestyle. She usually has family and friends come to visit her, and she avoids going anyplace where a bathroom is not readily available. She reports some sensation of urgency before the incontinence occurs but not always. She wears adult briefs all the time now. Her perineal area is slightly erythematous and tender; she states she uses diaper rash cream to try to protect her skin.

What predisposing factors does this patient have for FI? Vaginal births, age, possible mobility issues, diabetes, side effects of medications—beta blocker and metformin and possibly statin. Possibly diet and fluid intake

What other history is needed to help determine contributing factors? Usual frequency of defecation, accurate history of FI (frequency, consistency and volume of stool, any triggering events), usual consistency of stool with voluntary defecation, current management of constipation (to include use of stool softeners and laxatives), obstetric history to include episiotomy or change in continence after births, any other abdominal/intestinal/anorectal surgeries, history of any bowel disorders,

and ability to sense rectal distention and to accurately differentiate between gas, liquid, and solid

What would you ask about her diet and fluid intake? Usual daily fluid intake; any dehydrating fluids; usual caffeine intake; dietary fiber intake; any foods that cause increased flatus, dyspepsia, diarrhea, constipation, or GI irritability; foods usually eaten; and any food allergies

How do her medications contribute? May contribute to altered stool consistency (diarrhea or constipation)

What physical assessments should be performed to help determine underlying cause? Digital examination to assess sphincter tone and strength/endurance and assessment for retained stool in rectal vault, rectal masses, hemorrhoids, and perineal scars. Abdominal exam: inspection, percussion, and palpation to rule out retained stool. Functional status exam: mobility and cognitive status, ability to perform toileting on own, and dressing ability

What interventions have already been tried? Stool softener, adult briefs, skin barrier creams, dietary changes, moved into assisted living, and restricts her travel

What interventions can the nurse offer? Measures to normalize stool consistency (dietary modifications, fiber and fluid intake, medications as indicated); instruction in bowel hygiene (prompt response to "urge to go," correct posture, establishment routine time for attempted defecation); sphincter strengthening exercises; skin care; education regarding effects of chronic disease on bowel, effects of meds on bowel function, effects of diet and fluid choices on bowel function, and prevention and management of constipation; discussion about QOL issues and strategies to help her regain her ability to go out without fears; and education on containment products

REFERENCES

Altman, D., Falconer, C., Rossner, S., et al. (2007). The risk of anal incontinence in obese women. *International Urogynecology Journal and Pelvic Floor Dysfunction, 18*(11), 1283–1289.

Andromanakos, N., Filippou, D., Pinis, S., et al. (2013). Anorectal incontinence: A challenge in diagnostic and therapeutic approach. *European Journal of Gastroenterology and Hepatology, 25,* 1247–1256.

Annels, M., & Koch, T., (2003). Constipation and the preached trio: Diet, fluid intake, exercise. *International Journal of Nursing Studies, 40*(8), 843–852.

Bartolo, D., & Paterson, H. (2009). Anal incontinence. *Best Practice & Research. Clinical Gastroenterology, 23,* 505–515.

Beeckman, D., Schoonhoven, L., Verhaeghe, S., et al. (2009). Prevention and treatment of incontinence-associated dermatitis: Literature review. *Journal of Advanced Nursing, 65*(6), 1141–1154.

Beitz, J. (2006). Fecal incontinence in acutely and critically ill patients: Options in management. *Ostomy Wound Management, 52*(12), 56–58, 60, 62–66.

Bellicini, N., Molloy, P., Caushaj, P., et al. (2008). Fecal incontinence: A review. *Digestive Diseases and Sciences, 53*(1), 41–46. doi:10.1007/s10620-007-9819-z.

Belmonte-Montes, C., Hagerman, G., Vega-yepez, P., et al. (2001). Anal sphincter injury after vaginal delivery in primaparous females. *Diseases of the Colon and Rectum, 44*(9), 1244–1248. doi:10.1007/BF02234778.

Bharucha, A. (2010). Incontinence: An under appreciated problem in obesity and bariatric surgery. *Digestive Diseases and Sciences, 55,* 2428–2430. doi:10.1007/s10620-010-1288-0.

Bharucha, A., & Rao, S. (2014). An update on anorectal disorders for gastroenterologists. *Gastroenterology, 146*(1), 37–45.

Bharucha, A., Zinsmeister, A., Locke, G., et al. (2005). Prevalence and burden of fecal incontinence: A population-based study in women. *Gastroenterology, 129*(1), 42–49.

Bharucha, A., Zinsmeister, A., Schleck, C., et al. (2010). Bowel disturbances are the most important risk factors for late onset fecal incontinence: A population-based case-control study in women. *Gastroenterology, 139*(5), 1559–1566. doi:10.1053/j.gastro.2010.07.056.

Bisanz, A. (2011). *Bowel management: A guide for patients.* Houston, TX: The University of Texas, MD Anderson Cancer Center.

Bleier, J., & Kann, B. (2013). Surgical management of fecal incontinence. *Gastroenterology Clinics of North America, 42,* 815–836.

Bliss, D. Z., Doughty, D. B., & Heitkemper, M. M. (2006). Pathology and management of bowel dysfunction. In D. B. Doughty (Ed.), *Urinary & fecal incontinence: current management concepts* (3rd ed., pp. 425–452). St. Louis, MO: Mosby-Elsevier.

Bliss, D., Johnson, S., Savik, K., et al. (2000). Fecal incontinence in hospitalized patients who are acutely ill. *Nursing Research, 49*(2), 101–108.

Busija, L., Pausenberger, E., Haines, T., et al. (2011). Adult measures of general health and health-related quality of life. *Arthritis Care and Research, 63*(S11), S383–S412. doi:10.1002/acr.20541.

Choi, E., Shin, S., Im, Y., et al. (2013). The effects of transanal irrigation as a stepwise bowel management program on the quality of life of children with spina bifida and their caregivers. *Spinal Cord, 51*(5), 384–388.

Coggrave, M. (2007). Transanal irrigation after spinal cord injury. *Nursing Times, 103*(26), 47, 49.

Crosswell, E. B., Bliss, D. Z., & Savik, K. (2010). Diet and eating pattern modifications used by community-living adults to manage their fecal incontinence. *Journal of Wound, Ostomy, and Continence Nursing, 37*(6), 677–682.

Crowell, M., Schettler, V., Lacy, B., et al. (2007). Impact of anal incontinence on psychosocial function and health-related quality of life. *Digestive Diseases and Sciences, 52,* 1627–1631.

Deutekom, M., & Dobben, A. (2012). Plugs for containing faecal incontinence. *Cochrance Database of Systematic Reviews, 4,* CD005086.

Doherty, W. (2004). Managing faecal incontinence or leakage: The Peristeen anal plug. *British Journal of Nursing, 13*(21), 1293–1297.

Doughty, D. (2000). Chapter 13. Pathophysiology of bowel dysfunction and fecal incontinence, Chapter 14. Assessment and management of patients with bowel dysfunction and fecal incontinence. In D. Doughty (Ed.), *Urinary & fecal incontinence, nursing management* (2nd ed., pp. 325–383). St. Louis, MO: Mosby, Inc.

Dudding, T., Pares, D., Vaizey, C., et al. (2010). Sacral nerve stimulation for the treatment of faecal incontinence related to dysfunction of the internal anal sphincter. *International Journal of Colorectal Disease, 25,* 625–630. doi:10.1007/s00384-010-0880-2.

Dunberger, G., Lind, H., Steineck, G., et al. (2011). Loose stools lead to fecal incontinence among gynecological cancer survivors. *Acta Oncologica, 50*(2), 233–242.

Dunivan, G., Heymen, S., Palsson, O., et al. (2010). Fecal incontinence in primary care: Prevalence, diagnosis, and health care utilization. *American Journal of Obstetrics and Gynecology, 202*(5), 493. e1–e6.

Echols, J., Friedman, B., Mullins, R., et al. (2007). Clinical utility and economic impact of introducing a bowel management system. *Journal of Wound Ostomy Continence Nursing, 34*(6), 664–670.

Ellison, J., Haraway, N., & Park, J. (2013). The distal left Malone antegrade continence enema—is it better? *Journal of Urology, 190*(4 Suppl), 1529–1533.

Epocrates. (2013). Drugs: Gastrointestinal. Retrieved January 30, 2013, from Epocrates online: https://online.epocrates.com

Erekson, E., Sung, V., & Myers, D. (2008). Effect of body mass index on the risk of anal incontinence and defecatory dysfunction in women. *American Journal of Obstetrics and Gynecology, 198*(5), 596.e1–e4.

Eva, U., Gun, W., & Preben, K. (2003). Prevalence of urinary and fecal incontinence and symptoms of genital prolapse in women. *Acta Obstetricia et Gynecologica Scandinavica, 82*(3), 280–286.

Fader, M., Bliss, D., Cottenden, A., et al. (2010). Continence products: Research priorities to improve the lives of people living with urinary and/or fecal leakage. *Neurourology & Urodynamics, 29*(4), 640–644.

Fader, M., Cottenden, A., & Getliffe, K. (2009). Absorbent products for moderate-heavy urinary and/or faecal incontinence in women and men. *Cochrane Database of Systematic Reviews, 2008,* Issue 4. Art. No.: CD007408. doi:10.1002/14651858.CD007408

Faller, N. (2005). Diarrhea in acutely ill patients. *Journal of Wound Ostomy Continence Nursing, 32*(4), 217.

Farage, M., Miller, K., Berardesca, E., et al. (2008). Psychosocial and societal burden of incontinence in the aged population: A review. *Archives of Gynecology and Obstetrics, 277*(4), 285–290. epub November 20, 2007. doi:10.1007/s00404-007-0505-3.

Faucheron, J., Chodez, M., Boillot, B. (2012). Neuromodulation for fecal and urinary incontinence: Functional results in 57 consecutive patients from a single institution. *Diseases of Colon and Rectum, 55*(12), 1278–1283.

Findlay, J., & Maxwell-Armstrong, C. (2010). Current issues in the management of adult faecal incontinence. *British Journal of Hospital Medicine, 71*(6), 335–339.

Finne-Soveri, H., Sørbye, L., Jonsson, P., et al. (2008). Increased workload associated with faecal incontinence among home care patients in 11 European countries. *European Journal of Public Health, 18*(3), 323–328.

Formal, C., Cawley, M., & Stiens, S. (1997). Spinal cord injury rehabilitation. 3. Functional outcomes. *Archives of Physical Medicine and Rehabilitation, 78*(3 Suppl), S59–S64.

Gallagher, S. (2005). Challenges of obesity and skin Integrity. *The Nursing Clinics of North America, 40,* 325–335.

Goode, P., Burgio, K., Halli, A., et al. (2005). Prevalence and correlates of fecal incontinence in community-dwelling older adults. *Journal of the American Geriatrics Society, 53*(4), 629–635.

Gordon, D., Groutz, A., Goldman, G., et al. (1999). Anal incontinence: Prevalence among female patients attending a urogynecologic clinic. *Neurourology & Urodynamics, 18*(3), 199–204.

Gray, M. (2004). Preventing and managing perineal dermatitis: A shared goal for wound and continence care. *Journal of Wound Ostomy Continence Nursing, 31*(1 Suppl), S2–12.

Groutz, A., Fait, G., Lessing, J., et al. (1999). Incidence and obstetric risk factors of postpartum anal incontinence. *Scandinavian Journal of Gastroenterology, 34*(3), 315–318.

Gray, M., Omar, A., & Buziak, B. (2014). Stool management systems for preventing environmental spread of Clostridium difficile. *Journal of Wound, Ostomy, and Continence Nursing, 41*(5);460–465.

Halland, M., & Talley, N. (2012). Fecal incontinence mechanisms and management. *Current Opinion in Gastroenterology, 28*:57–62.

Hammond, M., & Burns, S. (2000). *Yes, you can! A guide to self-care for persons with spinal cord injury.* (3rd ed.) Washington, DC: Paralyzed Veterans of America.

Hansen, J. L., Bliss, D. Z., Peden-McAlpine, C. (2006). Diet strategies used by women to manage fecal incontinence. *Journal of Wound, Ostomy, and Continence Nursing, 33*(1), 52–61.

Herbert, J. (2008). Use of anal plugs in faecal incontinence management. *Nursing Times, 104*(13), 66–68.

Hiller, L., Radley, S., Mann, C., et al. (2002). Development and validation of a questionnaire for the assessment of bowel and lower urinary tract symptoms in women. *BJOG, 109*(4), 413–423.

Hollingshead, J., Dudding, T., Vaizey, C. (2011). Sacral nerve stimulation for faecal incontinence: Results from a single centre over a 10-year period. *Colorectal Disease, 13*(9), 1030–1034.

Hunt, S., McEwen, J., & McKenna, S. (1985). Measuring health status: A new tool for clinicians and epidemiologists. *The Journal of the Royal College of General Practitioners, 35*(273), 185–188.

Hunter, W., Jones, G. P., Devereux, H., et al. (2002). Constipation and diet in a community sample of older adults. *Nutrition & Dietetics, 59*(4), 253–259.

Hussain, Z., Lim, M., & Stojkovic, F. (2014). The test-retest reliability of fecal incontinence severity and quality-of-life assessment tools. *Diseases of the Colon and Rectum, 57*(5), 638–644.

Kowal-Vern, A., Poulakidas, S., Barnett, B., et al. (2009). Fecal containment in bedridden patients: economic impact of 2 commercial bowel catheter systems. *American Journal of Critical Care, 18*(3 Suppl), S2–15.

Krassioukov, A., Eng, J., Claxton, G., et al. (2010). Neurogenic bowel management after spinal cord injury: Systematic review of evidence. *Spinal Cord, 48*(10), 718–733.

Leite, F., Lima, M., & Lacerda-Filho, A. (2013). Early functional results of biofeedback and its impact on quality of life of patients with anal incontinence. *Arquivos de Gastroenterologia, 50*(3), 163–169.

Leung, F., & Rao, S. (2011). Approach to fecal incontinence and constipation in older hospitalized patients, *Hospital Practice (1995), 39*(1), 97–104. doi:10.3810/hp.2011.02.380.

Leung, F., & Schnelle, J., (2008). Urinary and fecal incontinence in nursing home residents. *Gastroenterology Clinics of North America, 37*(3), 697–707.

Marples, G. (2011). Diagnosis and management of slow transit constipation in adults. *Nursing Standard, 26*(8), 41–48.

McKenna, S., Wallis, M., Brannelly, A., et al. (2001). The nursing management of diarrhoea and constipation before and after the implementation of a bowel management protocol. *Australian Critical Care, 14*(1), 10–16.

McNevin, M., Moore, M., & Bax, T. (2014). Outcomes associated with Interstim therapy for medically refractory fecal incontinence. *American Journal of Surgery, 207*(5), 735–737.

Mellgren, A. (2010). Fecal incontinence. *The Surgical Clinics of North America, 90*(1), 185–194.

Nix, D. (2006). Prevention and treatment of perineal skin breakdown due to incontinence. *Ostomy Wound Management, 52*(4),26–28.

Nix, D., & Ermer-Seltun, J. (2004). A review of perineal skin care protocols and skin barrier product use. *Ostomy/Wound Management, 50*(12), 59–67.

Nix, D., & Haugen, V. (2010). Prevention and management of incontinence-associated dermatitis. *Drugs & Aging, 27*(6), 491–496.

Northwood, M. (2013). Fecal incontinence severity and Quality-of-Life instruments. *Journal of Wound, Ostomy, and Continence Nursing, 40*(1), 20–23.

Norton, C. (2009). Building the evidence base: The Zassi Bowel Management System. *British Journal of Nursing, 18*(6), S38, 40–42.

Norton, C., & Chelvanayagam, S. (2010). Bowel problems and coping strategies in people with multiple sclerosis. *British Journal of Nursing, 19*(4), 220–226.

Ostaszkiewicz, J., O'Connell, B., & Millar, L. (2008). Incontinence: Managed or mismanaged in hospital settings? *International Journal of Nursing Practice, 14*(6), 495–502. doi:10.1111/j.1440-172X.2008.00725.x.

Padmanabhan, A., Stern, M., Wishin, J., et al. (2007). Clinical evaluation of a flexible fecal incontinence management system. *American Journal of Critical Care, 16*(4), 384–393.

Page, B. P., Boyce, S. A., Deans, C., et al. (2008). Significant rectal bleeding as a complication of a fecal collecting device: A case report. *Diseases of Colon & Rectum, 51*(9), 1427–1429.

Palmieri, B., Benuzzi, G., & Bellini, N. (2005). The anal bag: A modern approach to fecal incontinence management. *Ostomy/Wound Management, 12*, 44–52.

Pares, D., Vallverdu, H., Monroy, G., et al. (2012). Bowel habits and fecal incontinence in patients with obesity undergoing evaluation for weight loss: The importance of stool consistency. *Diseases of the Colon & Rectum, 55*(5), 599–604.

Paris, G., Gourcerol, G., & Leroi, A. (2011). Management of neurogenic bowel dysfunction. *European Journal of Physical and Rehabilitation Medicine, 47*(4), 661–676.

Paterson, J., Dunn, S., Kowanko, I., et al. (2003). Selection of continence products: Perspectives of people who have incontinence and their carers. *Disability and Rehabilitation, 25*(17), 955–963.

Peden-McAlpine, C., Bliss, D., & Hill, J. (2008). The experience of community-living women managing fecal incontinence. *Western Journal of Nursing Research, 30*(7), 817–835.

Pretlove, S., Radley, S., Toozs-Hobson, P., et al. (2006). Prevalence of anal incontinence according to age and gender: A systematic review and meta-regression analysis. *International Urogynecology Journal and Pelvic Floor Dysfunction, 17*(4), 407–417. epub March 30, 2006.

Preziosi, G., & Emmanuel, A. (2009). Neurogenic bowel dysfunction: Pathology, clinical manifestations, and treatment. *Expert Reviews in Gastroenterology & Hepatology, 3*(4), 417–423.

Preziosi, G., Gosling, J., Raeburn, A., et al. (2012). Transanal irrigation for bowel symptoms in patients with multiple sclerosis. *Diseases of Colon & Rectum, 55*(10), 1066–1073.

Rees, J., & Sharpe, A. (2009). The use of bowel management systems in the high-dependency setting. *British Journal of Nursing, 18*(7), S19–20, 22, 24.

Richter, H., Burgio, K., Clements, R., et al. (2005). Urinary and fecal incontinence in morbidly obese women considering weight loss surgery. *Obstetrics & Gynecology, 106*(6), 1272–1277.

Roberson, E., Gould, J., & Wald, A. (2010). Urinary and fecal incontinence after bariatric surgery. *Digestive Diseases and Sciences, 55*(9), 2606–2613.

Rockwood, T., Church, J., Fleshman, J., et al. (1999). Patient and surgeon ranking of the severity of symptoms associated with fecal incontinence. *Diseases of the Colon and Rectum, 42*(12), 1525–1531.

Rockwood, T., Church, J., Fleshman, J., et al. (2000). Fecal incontinence quality of life scale. *Diseases of the Colon and Rectum, 43*(1), 9–16.

Roth, L. (2010). Fecal incontinence. *Medicine and Health, Rhode Island, 93*(11), 356–358.

Rusavy Z, Jansova, M., & Kalis, V. (2014). Anal incontinence severity assessment tools used worldwide. *International Journal of Gynaecology and Obstetrics, 126*, 146–150. Retrieved July 1, 2014 from http://dx.doi.org/10.1016/j.ijgo.2014.02.025. 0020-7292. International Federation of Gynecology and Obstetrics. Published by Elsevier Ireland Ltd.

Sabol, V., & Friedenburg, F. (1997). Diarrhea. *AACN Clinical Issues, 8*(3), 425–436.

Sansoni, J., Hawthorne, G., Fleming, G., et al. (2013). The revised faecal incontinence scale: A clinical validation of a new, short measure of assessment and outcomes evaluation. *Diseases of the Colon and Rectum, 56*(5), 652–659.

Shamliyan, T., Bliss, D., Du, J., et al. (2009). Prevalence and risk factors of fecal incontinence in community-dwelling men. *Reviews in Gastroenterological Disorders, 9*(4), E97–E110.

Sharpe, A., & Read A. (2010). Sacral nerve stimulation for the placement of faecal incontinence. *The British Journal of Nursing, 9*(7), 415–419.

Sparks, D., Chase, D., Heaton, B., et al. (2010). Rectal trauma and associated hemorrhage with use of ConvaTec Flexiseal fecal management system: Report of 3 cases. *Diseases of Colon & Rectum, 53*(3), 346–349.

Stevens, T., Soffer, E., & Palmer, R. (2003). Fecal incontinence in elderly patients: Common, treatable, yet undiagnosed. *Cleveland Clinic Journal of Medicine, 70*(5), 441–448.

Thomas, S., Nay, R., Moore, K., et al. (2006). *Continence Outcomes Measurement Suite Project (Final Report). Australian Government Department of Health and Ageing.* Retrieved March 2013, from http://www.bladderbowel.gov.au/assets/doc/ncms/Phase1-2InformationAndEvidence/11DevelopementofOutcomeMeasurementSuiteforContinenceConditions.pdf

Van Koughnett, J. A., & Wexner, S. (2013). Current management of fecal incontinence: choosing amongst treatment options to optimize outcomes. *World Journal of Gastroenterology, 19*(48), 9216–9230.

Whiteley, J. (2007). Effects of urinary & fecal incontinence on the skin. *Community Nursing, 21*(10), 26–29.

Wilde, M., Bliss, D., Booth, J., et al. (2014). Self-management of urinary and fecal incontinence. *American Journal of Nursing, 114*(1), 38–45.

Willson, M., Angyus, M., Beals, D., et al. (2014). Executive Summary: A quick reference guide for managing fecal incontinence. *Journal of Wound Ostomy Continence Nursing, 41*(1), 61–69.

Wishin, J., Gallagher, T., & McCann, E. (2008). Emerging options for the management of fecal incontinence in hospitalized patients. *Journal of Wound, Ostomy, and Continence Nursing, 35*(1), 104–110.

Wisten, A. M., & Messner, T. (2005). Fruit and fiber (Pajala porridge) in the prevention of constipation. *Scandinavian Journal of Caring Sciences, 19*(1), 71–76. Retrieved January 2013, from http://dx.doi.org/10.1111/j.1471-6712.2004.00308.x.

Woodward, S. (2012). Assessment and management of constipation in older people. *Nursing Older People, 24*(5), 21–26.

Wuong, S. (2012). Literature review: Management of constipation in people with Parkinson's disease. *The Australian and New Zealand Continence Journal, 18*(4), 112–118. Retrieved January 2013, from http://search.informit.com.au/documentSummary;dn=966388663074634;res=IELNZC

Zutshi, M., Ferreira, P., Hul,l T., et al., (2012). Biological implants in sphincter augmentation offer a good short-term outcome after a sphincter repair. *Colorectal Disease, 14*(7), 866–871.

QUESTIONS

1. A 75-year-old female patient confides to the continence nurse that she "frequently gets a sudden urge to move her bowels and sometimes has trouble getting to a bathroom in time." What is the label for this type of incontinence?
   A. Passive fecal incontinence
   B. Urge bowel incontinence
   C. Encopresis
   D. Fecal seepage

2. What is the usual cause of transient fecal incontinence (FI)?
   A. Acute diarrheal illness
   B. Chronic disease
   C. Injury to the sphincter
   D. Neurologic dysfunction

3. Which patient would the continence nurse place at higher risk for fecal incontinence related to sphincter denervation?
   A. A patient with irritable bowel syndrome
   B. A patient experiencing cerebrocortical dysfunction
   C. A patient with a malabsorption syndrome
   D. A patient who is postoperative anorectal surgery

4. Which technique would the continence nurse perform when conducting an abdominal examination on a person who reports fecal incontinence?
   A. Visual inspection for tumors
   B. Percussion to detect distention
   C. Palpation of the lower quadrants to assess for stool retention
   D. Auscultation for stool in the left lower quadrant

5. The continence nurse asks a patient to "bear down" during a visual examination of the anus. What bowel alteration might be assessed using this technique?
   A. Neurologic lesion
   B. Rectal prolapse
   C. Pelvic floor dyssynergia
   D. Rectal polyps

6. During an anorectal examination, the examiner elicits the "anal wink." No response to this test may be indicative of:
   A. Neurological problems
   B. Colon cancer
   C. Anal fissures
   D. Infection

7. A continence nurse suspects a patient is experiencing rectocele. What test is used to diagnose this functional bowel alteration?
   A. Electromyography
   B. Proctosigmoidoscopy
   C. Defecography
   D. Magnetic resonance imaging (MRI)

8. The continence nurse is caring for a patient with a fecal pouch. Which statement accurately describes an advantage/disadvantage associated with this device?
   A. It only takes one caregiver to apply the rectal pouch.
   B. Use of a fecal pouch is limited to nonambulatory patients.
   C. Rectal exams can be performed when using a fecal pouch.
   D. Fecal pouches are effective when there is perianal skin breakdown.

9. The continence nurse is providing teaching to a patient who is undergoing bariatric surgery. What intervention would the nurse recommend?
   A. Bowel habit training
   B. Stimulated defecation program
   C. Sphincter muscle exercises with biofeedback
   D. Pelvic floor strengthening exercises

10. The continence nurse is caring for a patient who has a high impaction. What initial intervention is recommended?
    A. Administer a tap water enema.
    B. Administer oral laxatives.
    C. Perform digital breakup.
    D. Administer mineral oil enema.

11. Which beverage would the continence nurse recommend to replace fluid for a patient experiencing diarrhea?
   A.   Hot chocolate
   B.   Orange juice
   C.   Broth-based soups
   D.   Ginger ale

12. What initial intervention would the continence nurse recommend for a patient who is experiencing acute constipation?
   A.   Fiber supplements
   B.   Osmotic laxative
   C.   Stool softener
   D.   Mineral oil enema

13. Which surgical procedure is approved for patients with fecal incontinence related to sphincter injuries who failed conservative therapy?
   A.   Injectable bulking agents
   B.   Sacral nerve stimulation
   C.   Stimulated graciloplasty
   D.   Magnetic artificial sphincter

ANSWERS: 1.**B**, 2.**A**, 3.**D**, 4.**C**, 5.**B**, 6.**A**, 7.**C**, 8.**B**, 9.**D**, 10.**A**, 11.**C**, 12.**B**, 13.**B**

CHAPTER 17

Bowel Dysfunction and Fecal Incontinence in the Pediatric Population

Anne Jinbo

The physiology of normal defecation and fecal continence has been covered in Chapter 14, and motility disorders and fecal incontinence in the adult population have been discussed in Chapters 15 and 16. This chapter focuses on types of bowel dysfunction and fecal incontinence unique to the pediatric population and the impact of developmental stage on management approaches.

Fetal Development of the Gastrointestinal System

Normal bowel function in the infant and child is dependent partly on normal fetal development of the gastrointestinal (GI) system. Although a detailed description of fetal GI tract development is beyond the scope of this text, a brief review of the critical aspects that are most likely to be involved in congenital anomalies is provided.

Development of Primitive Gut

Development of the gastrointestinal tract begins during the 4th week of fetal life, when the primitive gut arises from the dorsal part of the yolk sac. The primitive gut can be divided into three segments: the foregut, the midgut, and the hindgut. The foregut develops into the pharynx, lower respiratory system, esophagus, stomach, upper portion of the duodenum, liver, pancreas, and biliary system. The vascular supply for these bowel segments is provided by the forerunner to the celiac artery. The midgut evolves into the small bowel distal to the orifice of the bile duct, the cecum, appendix, ascending colon, and most of the transverse colon. The blood supply for the midgut is provided by the superior mesenteric artery, and these segments of bowel are attached to the posterior abdominal wall by the dorsal mesentery. The hindgut forms the left transverse colon, descending colon, sigmoid colon, rectum, and proximal portion of the anal canal. The inferior mesenteric artery provides the blood supply for the bowel segments arising from the hindgut (Mazier et al., 1995).

CLINICAL PEARL

Development of the gastrointestinal tract begins during the 4th week of fetal life.

Midgut Development/Rotational Anomalies

The midgut undergoes an interesting sequence of events during its development, and any defect in the normal sequence can produce congenital complications involving the small bowel and proximal colon. As the midgut lengthens and enlarges, it becomes too large for the developing fetal abdomen; as a result, the midgut herniates into the umbilical cord. When the fetal abdomen enlarges sufficiently to accommodate the midgut, these segments of bowel "return" to the abdominal cavity; however, they rotate in a counterclockwise position during their return.

The small bowel segment of the midgut is the first to return, and it passes into the abdominal cavity in a position that is posterior to the superior mesenteric artery. The ascending and transverse colon segments then return and assume a position anterior to the superior mesenteric artery. The mesentery for the midgut attaches to the posterior abdominal wall close to the duodenum and ascending colon, which causes these segments of the bowel to assume a retroperitoneal position. Abnormalities in rotation may produce obstructive syndromes in the neonatal period (Mazier et al., 1995).

Development of Patent Lumen

Another aspect of fetal development that is critical to normal gastrointestinal function after birth is the establishment of a patent lumen. Normal development of the gastrointestinal "tube" involves endodermal proliferation, which temporarily occludes the lumen of the gut. However, this period of occlusion is normally followed by recanalization. Failure to recanalize the lumen may result in atresia (complete obstruction of the lumen), stenosis, cysts, or intestinal duplication (Mazier et al., 1995; Walker et al., 1990).

Separation between Gastrointestinal and Genitourinary Systems

A final aspect of gastrointestinal development that is critical to normal function is the separation between the gastrointestinal and the genitourinary systems. In very early stages of fetal development, the rudimentary reproductive, urinary, and intestinal ducts terminate in a common hollow cavity known as the "cloaca." At about week 4, the urorectal septum begins to form. This sheet of connective tissue divides the cloacal cavity into two separate compartments: The anterior compartment develops into the lower genitourinary tract, and the posterior compartment develops into the rectum and anal canal. Congenital anorectal defects such as imperforate anus occur when this developmental sequence is interrupted or altered (Mazier et al., 1995).

Fecal Elimination in Children

Bowel function may be described in terms of stool frequency, stool consistency, and stool size (caliber). Unfortunately, it is difficult to define "normal" bowel habits among a healthy population because of the many variables that influence the frequency and consistency of fecal elimination. This variability is well documented among adult populations and is thought to be attributable in large part to differences in dietary intake; for example, studies among adults in Western societies reveal a variability in bowel movement frequency ranging from three times daily to three times weekly—bowel movement frequency fell within this range for 94% to 99% of the study population (Walker et al., 1990).

In infancy, normal stool frequency is much higher than among children and adults. For example, one study of newborn infants documented stool frequency ranging from one to nine stools daily during the first week of life (Walker et al., 1990). Infants between 2 and 20 weeks of age typically have one to seven stools daily, with significant reported differences between breast-fed and formula-fed infants; that is, breast-fed infants have fewer stools during the first week of life but a significantly higher number of stools thereafter as compared to formula-fed infants (Walker et al., 1990). These differences in stool frequency gradually diminish after 8 weeks; by 16 weeks of age, when many infants have been introduced to solid foods, there is no difference in stool frequency between the two groups (Walker et al., 1990).

CLINICAL PEARL

Infants between 2 and 20 weeks of age have about 1 to 7 stools daily; stool frequency in preschool children is comparable to that of adults.

Stool frequency among preschool children is reported to be comparable to stool frequency among adults, with significant variation reported among various populations. Individuals following high-fiber and vegetarian diets typically have a greater number of bowel movements than individuals following a meat-based, low-fiber diet.

Acquisition of Fecal Continence

Total control over bowel elimination is generally achieved by 4 years of age (O'Rorke, 1995), and most children achieve bowel and bladder control during *waking* hours by age 3. In order to achieve continence, the child must have functioning sphincters, normal rectal sensation, and normal rectosigmoid motility. In addition, the child must demonstrate both physiologic and developmental "readiness"; most children demonstrate "readiness" between 18 and 30 months of age (Christophersen, 1991). The two physiologic "readiness criteria" include *reflex sphincter control*, which can be demonstrated as early as 9 months of age, and *myelinization of the pyramidal tracts*, which is complete between 12 and 18 months of age. Some authors suggest that bladder control should be added to the list of readiness criteria; they define bladder control as the ability to empty the bladder completely with voiding and to stay dry for several hours (Christophersen, 1991). Psychological and cognitive "readiness" is equally critical but less predictable in terms of time frames for accomplishment.

Developmental criteria include motor skills such as walking to the bathroom, sitting on the toilet, clothing manipulation (such as pulling pants up and down), and flushing the toilet. Cognitive readiness is indicated by the child's ability to communicate impending urination or defecation, either through facial expressions or posturing, and instructional readiness. Instructional readiness includes both receptive language (such as words to describe voiding or defecation) and the ability to follow one-step or two-step commands. Some authors suggest that the most appropriate time frame for initiating toilet training for most children is between 24 and 30 months of age (Christophersen, 1991). O'Rorke summarizes a comprehensive approach that has been proven successful but notes that one approach may not be feasible for all parents (O'Rorke, 1995).

CLINICAL PEARL

Total control over bowel elimination is typically achieved by age 4; most children achieve bowel and bladder control during waking hours by age 3.

Bowel Dysfunction and Fecal Incontinence

Based on the previously cited time frames for "usual" acquisition of continence, one may consider a child who has not acquired bowel control by 4 years of age to be "fecally incontinent." There are several terms that are used to refer to bowel control problems among children, and these terms are defined as follows (Seth & Heyman, 1994):

- *Fecal incontinence:* Recurrent uncontrolled passage of fecal material for at least 1 month in an individual with a developmental age of at least 4 years
- *Fecal soiling.* Any amount of stool deposited in the underwear, regardless of the cause
- *Encopresis.* Fecal soiling usually associated with functional constipation; also used to refer to fecal incontinence not caused by an organic or anatomic lesion
- *Functional constipation.* Constipation not caused by organic or anatomic abnormalities *or* the requirement for medication to regulate bowel function after 4 years of age

CLINICAL PEARL

Encopresis is fecal soiling usually associated with functional constipation (constipation not caused by organic or anatomic abnormalities); functional constipation is constipation not caused by organic or anatomic abnormalities.

Children with fecal incontinence fall into four main groups: (1) children with functional fecal retention and overflow soiling (retentive encopresis), that is, fecal soiling caused by stool withholding behavior; (2) children with functional nonretentive fecal soiling (nonretentive encopresis), that is, fecal soiling without stool-withholding behavior; (3) children with anorectal malformations; and (4) children with neurologic lesions such as spina bifida. The pathophysiology of the dysfunction differs in each of these groups, and different management programs are required based on the underlying pathophysiology. Therefore, each of these groups will be addressed separately in terms of assessment/evaluation of each condition and treatment options.

Encopresis

It is estimated that the prevalence of constipation and/or encopresis among the pediatric population is as high as 5% to 10% and that 95% of childhood constipation is functional (Yousseff & Di Lorenzo, 2001). Encopresis accounts for 3% to 5% of visits to a general pediatric outpatient clinic and up to 25% of visits to pediatric gastroenterologists (Yousseff & Di Lorenzo, 2001). Encopresis is reportedly three to six times more common among males than females and is noted in 3% of 4-year-olds and 1.6% of 10-year-olds. Encopresis presents predominantly in children between 3 and 7 years of age; in one study, 35% of children with encopresis had experienced hard stools within the first 6 months of life, 40% had experienced delays in toilet training, and 60% had reported painful defecation during the first 3 years of life (Abi-Hanna & Lake, 1998).

Causative factors remain unclear; however, socioeconomic status, family size, ordinal position of the child within the family, and age of parents have not been found to correlate positively with incidence of encopresis. There *is* a correlation between enuresis (urinary incontinence) and encopresis; 25% of children with encopresis also have enuresis. This is thought to be due to the close proximity of the rectum and bladder; an overly full rectum can partially obstruct the bladder neck and urethra, resulting in incomplete emptying of the bladder and subsequent leakage. In addition, the nerves that supply the bladder and bowel originate from the same (sacral) area. If there are problems with innervation and coordination of the anal sphincter, there may be coexisting problems with innervation and coordination of the urethral sphincter, leading to dual bowel and urinary incontinence.

Classifications

Encopresis is sometimes classified as "primary" or "secondary" and as "retentive" or "nonretentive." Primary encopresis refers to the condition in a child who has reached 4 years of age and has never achieved sustained bowel control (i.e., fecal continence lasting for at least 1 year), whereas secondary encopresis is used to indicate the condition in a child who has been successfully toilet-trained and has maintained continence for at least 1 year and then "relapsed" in response to some secondary disorder (Steinberg, 2008; Stern et al., 1988). Approximately 50% to 60% of all encopretic children have secondary encopresis.

Retentive encopresis is the term used to refer to fecal incontinence clearly associated with constipation; these children retain stool and may even develop a megacolon. *Nonretentive encopresis* is defined as fecal incontinence in a child who has no evidence of constipation; it is usually additionally classified as primary nonretentive encopresis (incontinence in a child who has never acquired bowel control) and secondary nonretentive encopresis (incontinence in a child who successfully completes toilet training but later regresses) (Boon & Singh, 1991). It is generally thought that primary nonretentive encopresis may be caused either by an organic problem or by emotional stressors, whereas secondary nonretentive encopresis is almost always caused by psychological issues (Boon & Singh, 1991). Encopresis can also be classified as diurnal or nocturnal, but this classification is rarely used because nocturnal encopresis is quite uncommon.

> **CLINICAL PEARL**
>
> Fifty percent to 60% of children with encopresis have secondary encopresis, meaning that the child had attained continence and then "relapsed," usually as a result of psychological stress.

Etiology

Although the cause of encopresis is not well understood, Levine (1982) postulated that in many children, encopresis represents a functional bowel disorder that can be at least partly explained from a developmental perspective; he hypothesized that as children pass through critical developmental stages, the environment, people in their lives, or critical life events may contribute to a functional bowel disorder. This hypothesis is supported by evidence that the history of many children with encopresis is positive for several of these "risk" factors (Levine, 1982). Levine outlined the developmental stages and issues as follows:

Stage I: early experience and predisposition (infancy and toddler years). Children with a tendency toward constipation during this period, due either to genetics or to dietary factors, are at greater risk for the development of encopresis when they are older. The major risk factor during this stage is functional constipation, which may develop as a result of immature bowel function, surgical correction of congenital anomalies (such as imperforate anus), parental overreaction to toileting, or aggressive bowel management. These factors may lead to voluntary withholding of stool, in which defecation is perceived as a negative experience.

Stage II: training and autonomy (2 to 5 years of age). During this stage, the child is beginning to develop autonomy and independence, and potentiating factors for bowel dysfunction include psychosocial stressors (birth of sibling/sibling rivalry, mother returning to work, parental discord) during toilet training, coercive or extremely permissive toilet training, fears of toileting (such as monsters that bite when one sits down on the toilet), and painful or difficult defecation.

Stage III: extramural function (early school years). Extramural function refers to the time frame during which the child enters school. These children are faced with a new routine, which includes using the school bathroom or withholding stool until they return home. Dietary habits, such as excessive ingestion of milk and decreased intake of fruits, vegetables, and fiber, may contribute to constipation. Additional potential risk factors include frenetic lifestyles, psychosocial stressors that evolve with school relationships, and illness or injury that results in prolonged inactivity with a resulting change in bowel function.

Psychosocial stressors at any stage can cause enough distraction to prevent a child's full attention to the urge to defecate. Children with attention deficit hyperactivity disorder (ADHD) may be at greater risk due to their distractibility, difficulty linking actions to consequences, and inability to focus and sit still to finish a task. Improving their ability to attend is an essential first step in managing these children.

Cohen (2007) also suggested the possibility of a link between autism and changes in bowel function, as children with this condition seem to have more bowel symptoms than other children. For example, constipation, diarrhea, and gastroesophageal reflux are commonly seen among children with autism. From a developmental perspective, children with autism may have more problems related to food and feeding; selective eating is quite common among these children, which makes it difficult to ensure a healthy diet. As a result, these children may have harder stools, which causes discomfort during evacuation and can lead to stool withholding. Autistic children and other children with special needs may also require more patience with toilet training; however, Cohen emphasizes that stool withholding and toilet training are often two separate issues in the special needs population. In some cases, the health care provider is only able to successfully treat stool withholding and is not able to address toilet training issues; however, successful treatment of stool withholding will in and of itself have a great impact on the child's life. Health care providers have to also be alert to children and adolescents who have been physically or sexually abused as they may have developed a stool withholding pattern that can result in fecal soiling; in these cases, the emotional effects of the abuse are more often the cause of the soiling than the physical effects.

It is clear that the risk factors for each individual child are likely to be somewhat different; it is therefore critical to perform a comprehensive assessment as a basis for an individualized treatment plan (Levine, 1982).

CLINICAL PEARL

The risk/etiologic factors for each child with encopresis are likely to be somewhat different; therefore, a comprehensive assessment is required as the basis for an individualized management program.

Clinical Presentation

There seem to be three major clinical patterns among children with encopresis. In more than 95% of cases, encopresis is due to functional constipation. In this condition, retention of stool causes rectal distention, with resultant leakage of stool around the retained bolus. Because the rectum is chronically distended, the stretch receptors fail to signal the child that defecation is imminent. As a result, these children commonly have several fecal accidents per day as they are not capable of sensing rectal distention and the need to go to the bathroom. The stool size is usually small and the consistency of the stool is generally loose. These children are sometimes misdiagnosed as having diarrhea based on parental reports of odorous, thin, ribbon-like, or diarrheal stools.

CLINICAL PEARL

Ninety-five percent of children with encopresis have functional constipation, characterized by chronic stool retention and rectal distention; this causes loss of sensory awareness of the need to defecate and chronic relaxation of the internal anal sphincter, which permits leakage of stool around the fecal mass and resultant incontinence.

A much less common pattern of encopresis is the nonretentive pattern; children with this condition may experience stress-related diarrhea, which appears to be related to the disorder known as "irritable bowel syndrome" among adults, or may experience daily incontinence of stool that is of normal size and consistency.

The third and least common pattern is manipulative soiling, in which the child uses incontinent episodes to manipulate the environment (e.g., to avoid school or to passively display anger toward family members).

Almost all children with encopresis retain stool at least intermittently. Typically, the retention develops gradually over time. Some children with encopresis actually defecate daily but fail to effectively empty the lower bowel; because of this failure to empty, stool gradually amasses in the rectum and colon. The child may be asymptomatic or may complain of recurrent abdominal pain. Retained stool may be palpable on abdominal examination (if the child has significant colonic retention) or may be evident only on rectal examination (if the retained stool is confined to the rectum).

As rectal and colonic distention progress, sensory feedback from the bowel becomes impaired; that is, rectal distention no longer causes sensory awareness of the need to defecate. In addition, distention of the rectal wall overstretches the muscle fibers, which reduces contractile force. There is no awareness of the need to defecate and no propulsive force to eliminate the stool; as a result, stool continues to accumulate in the rectum, where continued water absorption creates a hard fecal mass. As the fecal mass becomes larger and harder, elimination becomes progressively more difficult and more painful; defecation may result in fissures or hemorrhoids. Painful defecation further contributes to the vicious cycle of stool retention.

Soiling occurs in the presence of retained stool because the retained stool causes sphincter dysfunction. The constant distention of the rectum causes persistent relaxation of the internal sphincter, mediated by the rectoanal inhibitory reflex. Relaxation of the internal sphincter permits liquid stool and mucus to seep around the impaction and into the anal canal. Continence past that point is dependent on external sphincter contraction; however, the child with chronic retention usually fails to sense rectal distention and fecal seepage into the anal canal and therefore does not voluntarily contract the external sphincter. Even if the child does recognize the leakage, he or she is able to contract the sphincter for only a short period of time. When the external sphincter returns to resting tone, the anal canal pressures are insufficient to prevent leakage, and soiling occurs. In addition, prolonged rectal distention and high intrarectal pressures can produce a "paradoxical" response of the sphincter; that is, increased rectal volume causes reduced sphincter muscle tone and increased risk of soiling, as compared to the normal response of increased sphincter tone.

Children with encopresis present with a wide range of associated symptoms. Children with recent onset of retention and incontinence typically complain of abdominal pain; in contrast, children with long-standing encopresis seldom complain of pain because they generally have developed tolerance to colonic distention. The presence of associated enuresis is also variable. In children who do present with enuresis, effective treatment of the stool retention may alleviate the child's problems with bladder control. Encopresis at night is relatively rare and seems to be associated with a poor prognosis (Levine, 1982).

Encopresis has a major effect on lifestyle and on self-esteem. The inability to control defecation is extremely humiliating to these children, who live in constant fear of discovery, exposure, ruthless teasing, bullying, and ridicule. In addition, these children are often punished and told that their problem with incontinence is an attention-getting act or a result of their own laziness. They may be told that they are negligent when they fail to change foul-smelling undergarments after an accident. Parents fail to realize that the sense of smell in these children (as in all people) accommodates to their own odors and that the child is frequently genuinely unaware of the accident and the offensive odor. Despite the fact that these children live with daily emotional trauma, acting-out behavior is not common; instead, these children are likely to isolate themselves to varying degrees and to show excessive dependence.

CLINICAL PEARL

Encopresis has a major negative effect on lifestyle and self-esteem and on family and social relationships.

Encopresis also has a tremendous influence on the other family members. Parents generally feel frustrated and possibly angry or guilty regarding their child's "failure to acquire continence." In addition, the fear of "accidents" may profoundly affect family activities; car trips, visits to friends, and even restaurants may be avoided because of the fear of embarrassment. Siblings may hesitate or refuse to invite friends over because of fecal odor or fear that the child could have an embarrassing accident. The stress generated by these limitations and adaptations may increase tension and conflict among family members and between various family members and the encopretic child. Thus, psychosocial factors should be an area of major concern when one is assessing and managing the child with encopresis.

Assessment

The assessment of a child with encopresis requires a thorough history (Table 17-1), a focused physical examination, and possibly radiographic studies or anorectal physiology testing (Stadtler, 1989). Laboratory tests are generally not beneficial in the evaluation of children with encopresis if medical conditions such as Hirschsprung's, cystic fibrosis, or hypothyroidism have been ruled out. An abdominal radiograph may be useful when the history is vague or the child is not cooperative with the examination. A barium enema may be considered when looking for medical causes of constipation such as Hirschsprung's. Abdominal and pelvic ultrasound studies can show if the child has stool retention or if other abnormalities exist. The ultrasound can also show whether a child empties their bladder; this is important because severe constipation and rectal distention can partially obstruct the bladder neck and urethra, resulting in incomplete emptying. It is not uncommon for children with severe constipation to report coexisting problems with urinary incontinence.

Lumbosacral spine films or magnetic resonance imaging may be needed if examination of the lower extremities indicates an abnormality or if there are any sacral abnormalities noted. However, the history and physical examination are usually the only diagnostic tools necessary to identify retentive encopresis and to rule out organic factors. Few cases of retentive encopresis and even fewer cases of nonretentive encopresis have an organic etiology.

Management: General Principles

Some years ago, Mikkelsen (2001) conducted a literature review and stated that there had been less progress in understanding the etiology and treatment of encopresis than enuresis. More recently, Reid and Bahar (2006) reviewed the literature on the management of encopresis; they noted a major emphasis on careful history taking, especially in regard to the psychoemotional aspects of the child's environment and on educating children and families about the condition. Frequently, constipation and subsequent hard stools lead to fecal retention due to the painful evacuation; thus, treatment must include measures to correct constipation, such as dietary modifications,

TABLE 17-1 History-Taking Guidelines for Children with Encopresis

Medical History

Medical treatment(s) or condition(s) that could lead to problems with constipation:

Anorectal anomalies such as imperforate anus or anorectal stenosis (treatment to date)

Hirschsprung's disease (aganglionic megacolon): age at diagnosis, management before and after diagnosis (usually managed by initial fecal diversion to "decompress" bowel, followed by resection or bypass of aganglionic segment or segments and anastomosis of proximal functioning bowel to anal canal)

Medications: anticholinergics, tricyclic antidepressants, sympathomimetics?

Chronic anal fissures or perineal dermatitis leading to painful defecation

Hypothyroidism (significant possibility only in child with delayed linear growth)*

Onset of encopresis

Present stooling and leakage pattern (frequency, amount, consistency of voluntary bowel movements and incontinent episodes; thorough description of encopretic episodes)

Past and current use of laxatives, enemas, and suppositories, and results obtained

Dietary intake with special focus on intake of fiber and fluid and foods and fluids known to be constipating (such as large amounts of milk or milk products)

History of urinary tract infections or daytime or nighttime wetting

Developmental History

Developmental stage at which problem with fecal elimination began

Age at which child was fully trained (if child was ever fully trained) and any evidence of encopresis during training period

Critical life events or transitions associated with onset of bowel dysfunction (such as entry into school)

Time frame for achievement of other developmental milestones (such as walking): normal or delayed?

Evidence of attention deficit problems (i.e., difficulty staying on task) that might interfere with ability to establish a normal bowel pattern?

Cognitive dysfunction or learning disability? (Note evidence that there is an increased incidence of learning disabilities among encopretic children.[†])

Overall academic performance and classroom behavior

Peer relationships: any identified problems?

Psychosocial Assessment

Psychosocial conditions in child's environment that could be contributing to the problem with encopresis (such as marital issues causing tension, problems with siblings)

Approach to discipline within family

Indications of deprivation or abnormal patterns of nurturance

Effect of encopresis on family: disagreement or disruption within family related to the problem? guilt and accusation related to the problem?

Parents' beliefs and understanding re: problem and cause; child's understanding and beliefs re: the problem and cause (if child is able to discuss the problem)

Past and present methods for handling the encopresis within the family, to include any punishment strategies (e.g., has child been spanked or had privileges withdrawn?); consistency (vs. variability) of response

Child's usual temperament style and general behavior at home; any evidence of depression?

Relationships with family members and friends; any social interactional difficulties?

Any evidence of secondary gains resulting from the encopresis?

*Datum from Boon RF, Singh N. (1991). A model for the treatment of encopresis. *Behavior Modification, 15*(3), 355–371.
[†]Datum from Stern HP, Lowitz G, Prince M., et al. (1988). The incidence of cognitive dysfunction in an encopretic population in children. *Neurotoxicology, 45*(3), 351–358.

that is, increased fiber and fluid intake. (See Table 17-2 for high-fiber diet and Fig. 17-1 for algorithm for the treatment of constipation). Loening-Baucke et al. (2004) reexamined the benefits of adding fiber to the diet and determined that fiber is of benefit in the treatment of constipation with or without encopresis. The use of laxatives is also a critical part of the treatment plan for these children (Table 17-3). Several centers currently recommend avoiding the use of enemas and/or suppositories as administering medication via the rectum can increase a child's aversion to defecation and can therefore increase their constipation problem. There have also been reports suggesting that repeated enemas can induce secondary anger,

complicating the original cause of encopresis. Currently, the majority of treatment programs emphasize dietary modifications with increased fiber and water, regular daily toileting, and a reward system.

Some centers have incorporated "treatment sessions" for the parent(s) and child and have documented cessation of soiling in 85% of those children who had been refractory to medical management alone. Reid and Bahar (2006) described a program involving intensive psychoanalytical therapy over a 3-year period for both the parent and child. These behavioral sessions addressed three themes that have been shown to result in anger or resentment: (1) parental conflict, (2) a newborn baby, and (3) tormenting

TABLE 17-2 High-Fiber Diet

General Guidelines

Dietary fiber is beneficial in that it adds bulk to the stool, reduces stool transit time, reduces intestinal intraluminal pressures, and slows gastric emptying.

Adequate fluid intake is essential when fiber is added to the diet. Fiber intake should be increased gradually to avoid unpleasant side effects.

A good approach is to use the following chart to identify high-fiber foods and to replace low-fiber foods in the diet with high-fiber foods until the desired "fiber intake goal" is reached.

Food	Serving Size	Fiber in Grams
Breads		
Cracked wheat	1 slice	2.1
Raisin	1 slice	0.4
Rye	1 slice	1.2
White	1 slice	0.8
Whole wheat	1 slice	2.1
Hamburger roll or bun	1 at 3½ inch diameter, 1½ inch height	1.2
Bagel, 100% whole wheat	1	5.4
Bagel, oat bran	1	7.7
Bran muffins made with		
Kellogg's All-Bran or Bran Buds cereal	1	3.2
Bran muffin made with Kellogg's 40% Bran Flakes cereal	1	1.3
Pancakes	1 at 4 inches diameter	0.5
Taco shell (tortilla)	1	0
Cereals		
Kellogg's All-Bran	⅓ cup (1 oz)	9.0
Kellogg's Bran Buds	⅓ cup (1 oz)	8.0
Kellogg's Cracklin' Bran	⅓ cup (1 oz)	4.0
Kellogg's Most	¾ cup (1 oz)	4.0
Bran flakes	1 cup	5.0 to 9.2
Fiber One	1 cup	27.5
Granola	1 cup	5.8 to 6.0
Grape Nuts	½ cup	5.4
Raisin Bran	1 cup	6 to 7.9
Oat bran, cooked	1 cup	6.4
Wheat germ toasted	½ cup	8.0
Macaroni, vegetable, tricolored	1 cup	5.8
Vegetables		
Avocado	Half	2.2
Asparagus (boiled, cut)	½ cup	1.1
Beans:		
Azuki bean, cooked	½ cup	5.8
Black, cooked	½ cup	7.5
Garbanzo, canned	1 cup	9.1
Kidney, canned	½ cup	5.9
Mung, boiled	½ cup	5.8
Pinto, cooked	½ cup	7.3
Bean sprouts	½ cup	1.6
Broccoli, steamed or stir fried	1 cup	5.0

TABLE 17-2 (Continued)

Food	Serving Size	Fiber in Grams
Brussels sprouts (boiled)	1 cup	7.2
Cabbage, shredded, boiled	½ cup	2.3
Carrots, drained, boiled	½ cup	2.3
Cauliflower, boiled	½ cup	1.1
Cucumber, raw	1 oz	0.1
Eggplant, peeled, drained	½ cup	2.5
Green beans, cut, boiled	½ cup	2.0
Green pepper	1 medium	0.8
Lentils, dry, boiled	1 cup	9.0
Lettuce	6 medium leaves	1.4
Mushrooms, raw	½ cup	0.9
Okra	½ cup	2.6
Peas, boiled, drained	½ cup	4.2
Radishes	10 medium	0.5
Spinach, boiled	½ cup	5.7
Squash, acorn, baked or mashed	½ cup	5.3
Tomato, raw	1 medium	2.0
Tomato, paste, canned	½ cup	5.4
Taro, sliced, cooked	1 cup	6.7
Turnips, boiled, mashed	½ cup	3.2
Fruits		
Apple with peel	1 medium	3.3
Apple, dried, rings	10 each	5.8
Applesauce, canned	½ cup	2.6
Apricots	2 medium	1.6
Apricots, dried halves	½ cup	5.0
Banana	½ small	1.6
Cantaloupe	¼ whole	1.6
Cherries, sweet	10 large	1.2
Dates, dried	5	3.1
Figs, dried	5	8.7
Grapefruit, fresh	½ whole	0.6
Grapes, seedless	12	0.3
Guava	2	9.7
Lemon, fresh	1 slice	0.3
Mango	1 cup	5.0
Nectarines	1 medium	3.0
Oranges	1 small	2.4
Peach, fresh	1 medium	1.4
Peach, dried halves	10	12.2
Pear, dried, halves	10	13.1
Pineapple, fresh	½ cup	0.9
Plums, fresh	2 medium	0.4
Pomegranate	1	5.5
Prunes, dried	10	7.8
Prunes, stewed	½ cup	7.0
Raisins	2 tablespoons	1.2
Strawberries	½ cup	1.7
Nuts and Seeds		
Almonds, dry roasted	½ cup	6.8
Coconut, fresh grated	1 cup	7.5
Coconut cream, canned	1 cup	6.5

(Continued)

TABLE 17-2 (Continued)

Food	Serving Size	Fiber in Grams
Coconut cream, raw	1 cup	5.3
Coconut milk, fresh, frozen	1 cup	5.3
Coconut milk, raw	1 cup	5.3
Macadamia, chopped	½ cup	5.1
Mixed, dry roasted with peanuts	½ cup	6.2
Peanuts, boiled without shell	1 cup	5.5
Peanuts, dry roasted	½ cup	5.0
Pistachio, dry roasted	½ cup	5.0

From Seth R, Heyman M. (1994). Management of constipation and encopresis in infants and children. *Gastroenterology Clinics of North America, 23*(4), 621–636, and Hawaii Dietetic Association, 1997.

older sibling(s). The children in this study were encouraged to play with a variety of age-appropriate toys. This facilitated the child's expression of feelings regarding the stressful situation(s) that had occurred in his/her family. Identification of the issue(s) of concern enabled the therapists to assist the parents in resolving the problems, which resulted in resolution or improved control of the bowel problem.

Newer treatment options being utilized include reflexotherapy for soiling, encopresis, and constipation. Bishop et al. (2003) provided six 30-minute sessions of reflexology to the child's feet with improvement in symptoms; specifically, they reported that six sessions of reflexology resulted in reduced incidence of soiling and increased frequency of bowel movement. However, this was a small study (n = 50), and the authors concluded that further study is needed before recommendations can be made. Chase and Shields (2011) conducted a review of the literature and concluded that the evidence for efficacy of nonpharmacological, nonsurgical, and nonbehavioral treatments of functional constipation is poor; the efficacy of chiropractic treatment, reflexology, acupuncture, and/or transcutaneous electrical stimulation (TENS) has not been established, though preliminary findings support further study. Acupuncture and TENS were the two more promising treatment options.

Biofeedback training may be used in conjunction with other behavioral measures. Biofeedback is based on reinforcement and is derived from psychological learning theory. It uses instrument-assisted exercises to improve physiologic control. Biofeedback has been used with children with constipation and/or encopresis to improve rectal sensation, strengthen and improve control of the external sphincter, and coordinate muscle contraction and relaxation to achieve continence. (In more than half of the children with constipation/encopresis, the anal sphincter contracts instead of relaxing during

defecation.) (DiLorenzo & Benninga, 2004). The role of biofeedback in the treatment of fecal incontinence must currently be considered to be unproven; more studies are urgently needed.

Management of the child with encopresis is variable, depending on the specific form of the encopresis (retentive vs. nonretentive) and on the unique characteristics of the individual patient and his or her family. Management of retentive and nonretentive encopresis is therefore discussed separately.

Management of Retentive Encopresis

Effective management of retentive encopresis requires a very comprehensive approach. A number of clinicians recommend beginning treatment with intensive psychoeducation, to demystify the shame and blame around the stool accidents. They emphasize the importance of reassuring the child and the parents that this is a common childhood problem and that it is no one's "fault" (Levine, 1982; Schonwald & Rappaport, 2004). The clinician should review the pathologic sequence of events leading to the current condition of a "stretched-out bowel," reduced sensory awareness of rectal filling, and reduced contractility of the colonic and rectal musculature. The overall principles of treatment are explained, and a specific treatment plan is developed with the child and parents. The importance of long-term follow-up care should also be addressed in this initial discussion regarding management.

CLINICAL PEARL

Management of retentive encopresis begins with education and reassurance for the child and parents, followed by "cleanout" (i.e., measures to eliminate all retained stool from the colon and rectum).

The next phase of treatment is the cleaning-out phase, the objective of which is to eliminate all retained stool from the colon and rectum. This may be accomplished by enemas, suppositories, laxatives, or combination therapy. In selecting a cleansing protocol, it is important to assess for impaction, since the use of laxatives and suppositories may be contraindicated in these children. Laxatives cannot eliminate a true impaction, and the increased peristaltic activity can cause severe cramping pain, which may lead to an emergency room visit. Suppositories are contraindicated because they are unable to break up the impaction or to facilitate elimination of a large fecal mass; in fact, they generally become imbedded in and contribute to the fecal mass and fail to aid in the cleansing objective (Schmitt & Mauro, 1992).

Several protocols have been recommended for the cleanout phase of treatment. Levine recommended using as many as four 3-day cycles as follows: day 1, two adult-sized Fleet enemas; day 2, bisacodyl suppository; and day 3, bisacodyl tablet. He found that many children required

CONSTIPATION, TREATMENT (PEDIATRIC)

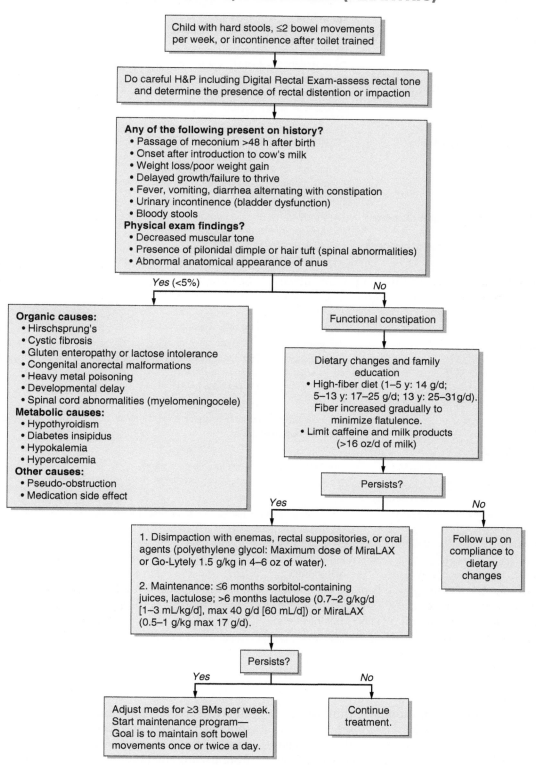

FIGURE 17-1. Algorithm for treatment of constipation in children.

TABLE 17-3 Dosage Guidelines for Stool Softeners and Stimulants[†]

Type of Agent	Guideline
Stool Softeners	
Mineral oil (plain)*	Age <1 year old: not recommended
	Disimpaction: 15–30 mL/y of age, up to 240 mL daily
	Maintenance: 1–3 mL/kg/d
Lactulose or sorbitol	1–3 mL/kg/d in divided doses
	(available as 70% solution)
Lavage	
Polyethylene glycol–electrolyte solution	For disimpaction: 25 mL/kg/h (to 1,000 mL/h) by nasogastric tube until clear
	or
	20 mL/kg/h for 4 h/d
	For maintenance: (older children): 5–10 mL/kg/d
Laxatives	
Barley Malt extract (Maltsupex) liquid or powder	2–10 mL/240 mL of milk or juice
	(Suitable for infants drinking from a bottle)
Magnesium hydroxide (Phillips' milk of magnesia or Haley's M-O)	1–3 mL/kg/d of 400 mg/5 mL
	(Available as liquid, 400 mg/5 mL, 800 mg/5mL and tablets)
Magnesium citrate	<6 y: 1–3 mL/kg/d
	6–12 y: 100–150 mL/d
	>12 y: 150–300 mL/d
	Single or divided doses
	(Available as liquid, 16.17% magnesium)
Senna preparation (Senokot)	2–6 years old: 2.5–7.5 mL/d
	6–12 years old: 5–15 mL/d (available as Senokot® syrup, 8.8 mg of sennosides/5 mL; also available as granules and tablets)
Bisacodyl (Dulcolax)	Age ≥3 y: 1–3 tablets per dose (available in 5-mg tablets)
Prokinetic	
Cisapride	0.2 mg/kg/dose, (available as suspension, 1 mg/mL and 5-, 10-, and 20-mg tablets) three or four times a day.
Rectal Suppositories	
Glycerin suppository	Use PRN (as needed) to stimulate defecation
Bisacodyl (Dulcolax) suppository	≥2 years old: 0.5–1 suppository (available in 10-mg suppositories)
Enemas	
‡Docusate sodium (Enemeez—minienema)	One unit rectally—to be used as an enema and not a suppository (available in bottles of 30 single-use, 5-mL tubes)
Mineral oil enema	2–11 y: 30–60 mL as a single dose
	Adolescents: as a retention enema, contents of one enema (range 60–150 mL)/d as a single dose
Sodium phosphate (Fleet) enema	<2 years old: to be avoided
	≥2 years old: 6 mL/kg up to 135 mL

*If mineral oil preparation is used, multivitamin supplementation recommended because of potential for reduced absorption of fat-soluble vitamins.
[†]From the medical position statement Baker S., et al. (1999). Constipation in infants and children: Evaluation and Treatment] of the North American Society for Pediatric Gastroenterology and Nutrition. *Journal of Pediatric Gastroenterology and Nutrition, 29,* 612–626.
[‡]Enemeez was the only medication not listed in the position statement.

four or even five cycles to obtain complete elimination of the retained stool (Levine, 1982).

Biggs and Dery (2006) reported on randomized controlled studies comparing methods of disimpaction. They reported that although enemas provide rapid rectal disimpaction, this approach is invasive and possibly traumatic for a child. They found that a common protocol for children 2 years or older is to administer a mineral oil enema followed by a phosphate enema. However, as noted, many clinicians recommend avoidance of enemas and suppositories if possible, and randomized studies have found varying doses of polyethylene glycol to be effective for disimpacting children, with reasonable acceptance by parents and children. Other oral medications utilized include mineral oil, senna, and magnesium citrate. Nurko et al. (2008) conducted a prospective, randomized, multicenter double-blinded, placebo-controlled study to determine dose ranges for PEG 3350 for children with functional constipation. The study confirmed the efficacy and safety of PEG 3350 for short-term treatment of children with functional constipation, with a recommended starting dose of 0.4 g/kg per day. An earlier study by Pashankar et al. (2003) found that long-term PEG therapy was effective for the treatment of chronic constipation with and without encopresis in children.

Other clinicians have tried variations of Levine's protocol; for example, Sprague-McRae reported success with the following adaptation: day 1, Fleet enema morning and evening; day 2, bisacodyl suppository morning and evening and Fleet enema in evening; and day 3, bisacodyl tablet taken orally in evening. This team recommends a pediatric-sized Fleet enema for children between 4 and 7 years of age or <50 pounds. and an adult-sized Fleet enema for children >7 years of age or >50 pounds. (Ingebo and Heyman, 1988).

In 1994, Seth and Heyman reported successful cleansing without the use of enemas. Their approach was to use mineral oil at a dose of 15 to 30 mL/kg/d, not to exceed 240 mL/d; this was used only for children >1 year of age. They documented initial cleansing within 3 or 4 days, with a 98% success rate and minimal side effects (one patient complained of abdominal cramps). Administration of mineral oil is facilitated by keeping it cold and mixing it in a 1:1 ratio with a fat-based substance such as pudding, yogurt, or chocolate syrup.

Other clinicians have also reported beneficial results with mineral oil; for example, Abrahamian and Lloyd-Still found that 47% of their pediatric population became completely asymptomatic after treatment with laxatives and mineral oil and an additional 36% were effectively controlled with laxatives after the original cleansing treatment (Howe & Walker, 1992). Clinicians selecting mineral oil for initial cleansing are cautioned to avoid its use in very young children and in children with gastroesophageal reflux or vomiting because of the potential for and danger of aspiration. In addition, it is generally recommended that the mineral oil be given 2 or 3 hours after meals or that a multivitamin tablet be given as part of the treatment because mineral oil inhibits absorption of fat-soluble vitamins (Howe & Walker, 1992).

Children with severe impactions usually require hospitalization and oral or nasogastric administration of a polyethylene glycol–electrolyte solution; this approach may also be required for children who are unresponsive to outpatient management or who cannot cooperate with the cathartic procedure (Boon & Singh, 1991; Gunn & Nechyba, 2002).

After successful colonic cleansing, a program is initiated to establish regular evacuation of soft formed stool and to eliminate withholding of stool and the evacuation of large stools. Components of the bowel retraining maintenance phase include medications and behavioral interventions. Mineral oil is one of the commonly recommended medications; the dose is titrated to produce soft formed stool and ranges from 2 tablespoons once daily

to 6 tablespoons twice daily. Polyethylene glycol without electrolytes is frequently used for children who cannot tolerate the taste of mineral oil. Again, the dose is titrated to maintain soft formed stool, but generally ranges from ½ cap to 1 cap daily (Schonwald & Rappaport, 2004).

> **CLINICAL PEARL**
>
> Following effective colonic cleansing, the child with encopresis is placed on a program to reestablish normal stool elimination; strategies used during this phase include routine toileting after meals and use of fiber supplements, fluids, and medications to keep the stool soft and to prevent recurrent stool retention.

Additional medications that may be used include lactulose, malt soup extract (Maltsupex), milk of magnesia, Haley's M-O, senna (Fletcher's Castoria), and bisacodyl (Dulcolax). Suppositories and enemas may be used to stimulate defecation on an as-needed basis. Table 17-3 provides dosage guidelines for each of the commonly used softener or stimulant agents based on the child's age and size.

Medications are generally used for at least 3 months and may be used for as long as 6 months. The goal is to prevent recurrent stool retention and to gradually restore the colon and rectum to normal size and function. Parents generally need to be reassured that laxatives are safe and not habit forming and that their child will have the laxatives tapered off once normal bowel function has been reestablished. Parents are also taught how to appropriately titrate the doses of mineral oil and any other medications and how to intervene if the child fails to have a bowel movement for 2 consecutive days.

> **CLINICAL PEARL**
>
> Parents of encopretic children need to be reassured that laxatives are safe and not habit forming and that they will be discontinued once normal bowel function has been reestablished.

In addition to using stool softeners and stimulants to normalize fecal elimination, the child's diet should be modified to eliminate constipating foods and fluids (such as excessive intake of milk and other dairy products) and to increase the intake of fiber. It is recommended that the transition to a high-fiber diet should be delayed until disimpaction has been completed (Smith, 1987). A dietary consultation may be helpful to the parents and child in determining ways to add fiber to the child's diet. The family should be provided with a list of fiber-containing foods (Table 17-2), and the child should be included in discussing ways by which to add fiber to the diet. It may be helpful to develop a sample meal plan so that the parents can see how to incorporate fiber-containing foods into daily menus.

In determining the fiber-intake goal for a particular child, the clinician should be aware that the American

Academy of Pediatrics has recommended 0.5 g of fiber per kilogram of body weight up to a maximum of 35 g daily. Another formula for estimating fiber intake needs in children over 3 years of age is as follows: "Child's age in years + 5 = desirable grams of fiber per day" (e.g., a 3-year-old child should receive 3 +5 g, or 8 g, of fiber daily). The clinician also needs to remember that high-fiber foods are more filling and lower in calories than low-fiber foods; with a child's small stomach, there is the potential for inadequate ingestion of calories when a high-fiber diet is begun. In addition, high-fiber foods can impede the absorption of minerals such as calcium, iron, copper, magnesium, phosphorus, and zinc; therefore, the child's weight should be monitored, and it is usually helpful to recommend a multivitamin–mineral compound daily.

In addition to measures to establish soft formed stool, the management program must include a toileting routine. It is not sufficient to teach the child to respond promptly to the urge to defecate, because the urge to defecate may not develop for 6 to 9 months following the initiation of treatment. Thus, it is essential to establish a regular schedule for sitting on the toilet and attempting defecation; this promotes appropriate elimination of stool into the toilet and helps to eliminate soiling. Having the child sit on the toilet for 5 to 10 minutes after breakfast and dinner will take advantage of the natural gastrocolic reflex, which increases the chance of successful defecation. In addition to encouraging the child to adhere to an established toileting routine, the entire family should be assisted to work on eliminating any negative issues regarding toileting that may have developed over time.

It is recommended that small rewards be used for positive reinforcement (e.g., stickers or special toys in the bathroom for preschoolers; stickers or handheld computer games for school-age children; and magazines and the assurance of privacy for adolescents). The "reward" should not be costly, and special age-appropriate rewards should be earned only by more advanced achievement, such as a certain number of days without soiling. The goal is to help the child accept responsibility for his or her actions and needs but to avoid any sense of punishment for an accident.

In establishing the medication and toileting schedule for any individual child, it is important to be flexible and creative and to assist the child and family to incorporate the care routine into their daily schedule with minimal disruption. It is also important to monitor the child's response and to taper the medications as the increased fiber and attention to toileting produce softer, more frequent stools. The goal is to wean the child from all medications once bowel function has normalized and the child has incorporated a high-fiber diet and routine toileting into his or her daily routine.

Management of Nonretentive Encopresis
As noted earlier, nonretentive encopresis is most commonly caused by psychological issues, though primary nonretentive encopresis may also be caused by organic problems. Therefore, it is essential to explore psychological issues when assessing the child and establishing a management plan.

The assessment of a child with *primary nonretentive encopresis* may reveal an organic cause of the encopresis but more commonly will reveal a history of coercive toilet training and the failure to achieve complete fecal continence. The parents may have been punitive in their approach to toilet training, and the child may have begun to use soiling as a way of getting back at them. Alternatively, the parents may have been controlling and intrusive though not punitive; in this case, the child may have reacted with anger and resentment. If the assessment reveals either a punitive or a controlling approach to toilet training and bowel management, the clinician should instruct the parents to stop trying to toilet train the child and to seek counseling and family therapy. The emphasis during counseling should be on development of positive parent–child relationships with appropriate use of positive reinforcement.

The history of a child with *secondary nonretentive encopresis* usually reveals psychosocial stressors in the home or the school environment that have caused the child to regress to an earlier developmental stage. Since the cause of the incontinence is psychological, the focus during treatment is on encouraging the child to identify and talk about the stressful situation that precipitated the regression. The child is reassured that he or she is not at fault for soiling and that there has been no change in the parents' unconditional love. This reassurance can help to eliminate or reduce guilt and blame. In planning and implementing treatment for a child with secondary nonretentive encopresis, it is important to provide the child with time to develop some control over the psychological crisis before introducing him or her to a bowel retraining program for correction of the fecal incontinence.

As noted above, the primary focus in treatment of the child with nonretentive encopresis is on resolution of the psychological issues that triggered the bowel dysfunction. Secondary management usually involves implementation of a comprehensive bowel management program, which typically includes many of the elements already described under management of retentive encopresis: medications when indicated, establishment of a routine toileting program, encouragement to respond promptly to defecatory urges, periodic underwear checks, and positive reinforcement for appropriate toileting. The child or family may also be under the care of a psychologist or psychiatrist, or the clinician may observe signs and symptoms that prompt a follow-up psychiatric/psychological consultation (such as conduct disorder, depression, or learning disabilities). Whenever the patient and family are under psychiatric or psychological care, it is critical for the continence nurse clinician to work in collaboration with the mental health professional. It may also be of tremendous benefit to enlist the cooperation of the staff at the child's school, preschool, or daycare setting.

Carefully monitored long-term follow-up care is critical for any child with encopresis. As explained, the initial goal is to establish regular voluntary elimination of soft formed stool and to eliminate withholding of stool and large fecal masses. Once an acceptable bowel elimination pattern has been in place for 4 to 6 months (such as two or three bowel movements per day), the child is gradually weaned off stool softeners. Data indicate that such a program results in complete and long-lasting remission in approximately 65% of the children, with an additional 30% reporting substantial improvement (Nolan & Oberklaid, 1993).

Children who continue to soil should have follow-up evaluation to determine the cause of the persistent problem; in some of these children, the problem may be paradoxical contraction of the external sphincter during attempted defecation (Nolan & Oberklaid, 1993). Benninga et al. evaluated the effectiveness of biofeedback retraining in 29 patients with chronic constipation and encopresis ranging in age from 5 to 16 years. Sixteen of these children exhibited inappropriate contraction of their external sphincters, and eight evidenced diminished rectal sensation. Biofeedback training was effective in teaching 26 of the children how to correctly relax the external anal sphincter and in normalizing rectal sensation in 18 (Seth & Heyman, 1994). Therefore, biofeedback should be considered for children with intact nerve pathways but attenuated rectal sensation or compromised ability to correctly contract and relax the pelvic floor and sphincter muscles.

The ultimate goal in treating encopresis is to restore the child to normal bowel function and a normal lifestyle and to prevent long-lasting psychological and emotional problems that may develop secondary to chronic fecal incontinence. Parents frequently report an overall improvement in the child's demeanor, appetite, and level of activity after successful treatment. The success of the treatment program is highly dependent on the child's willingness to address his or her problem with encopresis and on the parents' willingness to assist the child to remain compliant with the treatment program. As outlined, the treatment program is usually multifaceted and long term and must be carried out by the family members themselves, who are frequently juggling multiple other responsibilities and complex schedules. It is therefore essential for the health care clinician to establish rapport with the child and family and to work collaboratively with them to establish a workable treatment plan that incorporates the key elements of education, counseling, pharmacotherapy, and behavioral modification.

Neurogenic Bowel

Fecal incontinence is defined as the involuntary loss of stool (or rectal contents) at any time of life after toilet training. The term FI is used to indicate the involuntary passage of either solid or liquid stool at least once during the preceding 3 months; the term anal incontinence also includes the involuntary passage of flatus (Thomas & Chandler, 2007). Neurogenic bowel is described as a colonic dysfunction caused by neurologic dysfunction or damage; it is manifest by problems with storage and evacuation that result clinically in constipation and/or incontinence (Thomas & Chandler, 2007). Neurogenic bowel and fecal incontinence can be due to an organic or anatomic lesion, such as anorectal malformation, anal surgery, or trauma, or associated conditions such as meningomyelocele and other neuromuscular conditions. In pediatrics, there are several congenital conditions that can lead to fecal incontinence. The most common of these conditions include the following: short gut syndrome; imperforate anus; Hirschsprung's disease; meningomyelocele; and neuromuscular disorders, such as cerebral palsy, muscular dystrophy, and the various forms of hypotonia (Thomas & Chandler, 2007). Each of these conditions will be briefly described, as a basis for understanding treatment options.

Imperforate Anus

This condition includes several congenital anorectal malformations resulting from abnormal embryological development of the hindgut. The incidence rate is about 1 in 5,000 births in the United States. This anorectal anomaly may occur in isolation or as part of other conditions or syndromes such as VACTERL (vertebral, anorectal, cardiovascular, tracheoesophageal, renal and limb) syndrome. Imperforate anal lesions are divided into "high" or "low" lesions, depending on whether the distal end of the bowel terminates above or below the puborectal component of the levator ani complex (Jinbo, 2004). (See Table 17-4 for the Wing Spread Classification and Fig. 17-2 for illustration of imperforate anus.)

"Low defects" are characterized by complete formation of the distal bowel, including the anal canal, and descent of the anorectal junction and anal canal through the levator mechanism and the striated muscle complex; "low" defects involve anal stenosis or a "mismatch" between the anus and the perineal opening. Generally, low defects can be treated through simple dilatation or a minor perineal operation, and these children usually achieve normal continence (Jinbo, 2004).

TABLE 17-4 Wingspread Classification for Anorectal Anomalies

Female	Male
High Lesions	**High Lesions**
Anorectal agenesis	Anorectal agenesis
With rectovaginal fistula	With rectoprostatic urethral fistula
Without fistula	Without fistula
Rectal atresia	Rectal atresia
Intermediate Lesions	**Intermediate Lesions**
Anal agenesis with rectovestibular fistula	Anal agenesis with rectobulbar urethral fistula
Anal agenesis with rectovaginal fistula	Anal agenesis without fistula
Anal agenesis without fistula	
Low Lesions	**Low Lesions**
Anovestibular fistula	Anocutaneous fistula
Anocutaneous fistula	Anal stenosis
Anal stenosis	
Cloacal Malformations	**Cloacal Malformations**
Rare Malformations	**Rare Malformations**

With "intermediate-level defects," the distal bowel (rectum and anorectal junction) extends partially through the levator ani muscle but the anal canal and anus are missing; typically, a fistulous tract is present between the bowel and vagina in girls or between the distal bowel and rectobulbar urethra in boys. Plastic surgery is typically required to establish communication between the distal bowel and the perineum. Because the internal and external anal sphincters are intact, these children typically acquire continence with limited if any difficulty (Mazier et al., 1995).

In contrast, with "high defects," the distal bowel ends above the level of the levator ani muscle and the internal anal sphincter is usually absent, although there may be a slight thickening of the distal circular muscle at the end of the bowel. The external sphincter is almost always present—at least in part; in addition, the levator ani and puborectalis muscles are almost always present, although in these lesions, the puborectal muscle is quite small and tightly adherent to the urethra or vagina. Most of the higher lesions end with a fistula from the bowel to the bladder, urethra, or vagina. Often, there are associated anomalies in the genitourinary tract, spine, and/or heart. The high lesions are more common in boys, but there are no other known genetic factors (Walker et al., 1991). In girls, high lesions are usually associated with a high rectovaginal fistula. High defects require a temporary diverting colostomy and reconstructive surgery, known as a pull-through procedure, which is usually done between birth and 6 months of age. Once the

anastomosis and anoplasty are healed and necessary dilatations have been completed (Walker et al., 1991), the colostomy is closed.

CLINICAL PEARL

Imperforate anus refers to a spectrum of disorders involving fetal development of the distal bowel, anal canal, and sphincters; these abnormalities are usually classified as either "low" or "high" lesions, depending on whether the distal end of the bowel ends below or above the levator ani muscle complex.

Potential complications following the pull-through procedure include stricture of the anocutaneous anastomosis, recurrent rectourinary fistula, mucosal prolapse, anterior anal malposition, constipation and incontinence. Fecal incontinence is by far the most troublesome. The most important determinant of continence is the level of the initial lesion, and only a small number of those with high lesions achieve normal continence before school age. Most children continue to improve to the point of social continence by adolescence.

CLINICAL PEARL

The continence prognosis for children with "low" imperforate anus lesions is good, because the sphincters are intact. In contrast, the continence prognosis for children with "high" lesions is variable, because the internal anal sphincter is missing and the external sphincter may be incomplete.

Hirschsprung's Disease

Hirschsprung's disease is a congenital condition representing a failure of the cephalocaudal migration of neural crest cells into the hindgut, with subsequent lack of development of the autonomic ganglion cells in Meissner's and Auerbach's plexuses. The resultant loss of peristalsis causes a functional obstruction, followed by dilation of the proximal segment (Fig. 17-3). The proximal border of the defect is most often within the rectum or sigmoid colon (short-segment disease). In a smaller percentage of cases, longer segments of colon are involved (long-segment disease); in rare instances, the entire colon is aganglionic. Hirschsprung's disease accounts for a major proportion of cases of neonatal obstruction. Forty-six percent of all patients with Hirschsprung's disease are diagnosed in the neonatal period (Mazier et al., 1995).

CLINICAL PEARL

Hirschsprung's disease involves absence of ganglion (nerve) cells in the distal bowel; the affected bowel is unable to contract to propel stool distally, which creates a functional obstruction. Most children present with "short-segment disease," which means that the dysfunctional segments are the internal sphincter, rectum, and possibly part of the sigmoid colon.

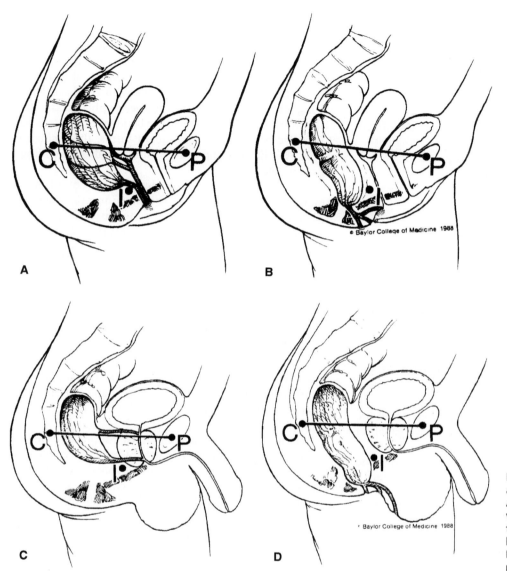

FIGURE 17-2. Imperforate anus in the female and male. **A.** High lesion with fistula to vagina. **B.** Low lesion with fistula to vestibule or perineum. **C.** High lesion with fistula to urethra. **D.** Low lesion with fistula to perineum or median raphe.

In a recent review of Hirschsprung's disease, Amiel et al. (2008) reported the incidence of Hirschsprung's disease as one in 5,000 live births; the male:female ratio is 4:1. The male:female ratio is higher for short-segment Hirschsprung's disease compared with long-segment Hirschsprung's disease. The incidence varies among ethnic groups, with rates of 1.0, 1.5, 2.1, and 2.8 per 10,000 live births in Hispanics, Caucasian Americans, African Americans, and Asians, respectively (Amiel et al., 2008). This disease occurs as an isolated trait in 70% of cases; a chromosomal abnormality is associated in 12% of cases and associated congenital anomalies in 18% (Amiel et al., 2008). There is also a genetic predisposition to Hirschsprung's disease.

Infants with short-segment disease may initially be diagnosed as "constipated"; if the diagnosis of Hirschsprung's disease is delayed, the affected child suffers from persistent constipation, with development of malodorous, ribbon-like stools and an enlarged abdomen with palpable fecal masses. The infant may present with intermittent bouts of intestinal obstruction from fecal impaction, hypochromic anemia, hypoproteinemia, and failure to thrive (Jinbo, 2004).

Assessment of the child with suspected Hirschsprung's disease involves a rectal examination, which typically reveals an absence of fecal material in the rectum and a narrow or snug rectum and anorectal junction during digital examination. A rectal biopsy is the most reliable method of diagnosis; histologic examination reveals an absence of ganglion cells. Manometric studies or pressure readings reveal failure of sphincter relaxation and absence of the rectoanal inhibitory reflex (RAIR), that is, failure of the internal sphincter to relax in response to rectal distention (Jinbo, 2004).

When the condition is diagnosed at birth, the functional (ganglionic) colon is anastomosed to the anal canal, and diversion may not be required. In contrast, when there is a

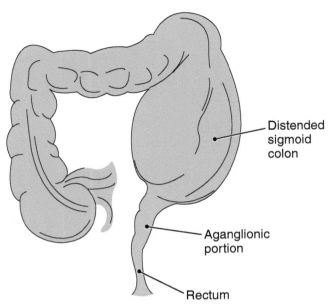

FIGURE 17-3. Hirschsprung's disease. Distal (aganglionic) bowel collapses due to absence of innervation and peristalsis; proximal (ganglionic) bowel becomes severely dilated.

delay in diagnosis, the functional obstruction results in significant dilation of the proximal bowel, and a temporary colostomy is required to decompress the dilated colon; the stoma is created in the dilated (functional) section of the colon (the distal point of bowel found to have ganglion cells on frozen section). Once the distended colon has been decompressed, the functional bowel is anastomosed to the anal canal, and the colostomy is closed (Doughty, 2006).

CLINICAL PEARL

Infants with short-segment Hirschsprung's disease may not be diagnosed in the early neonatal period, because the functional bowel is initially able to compensate and push stool through the dysfunctional segment. By the time these children are diagnosed, the proximal bowel is typically very dilated; therefore, a temporary colostomy is required to decompress the bowel, and the stoma is usually very large.

Potential postoperative complications include incomplete removal of the aganglionic section and abnormal spasticity of the internal sphincter, which can be corrected by performing a posterior sphincterotomy. In addition, postoperative incontinence may be a problem, and enterocolitis before or after surgery is an ominous complication that accounts for 30% of deaths in young infants (Roy & Alagille, 1995).

CLINICAL PEARL

Definitive management of Hirschsprung's disease requires a "pull-through" procedure, in which the functional (ganglionic) bowel is anastomosed to the anal canal.

Spina Bifida

Spina bifida is a syndrome caused by abnormal embryonic development of the neural tube and its surrounding structures (Molnar, 1985). The incidence of neural tube defects in the United States is about one in 1,000 live births. It is one of the leading causes of disability in children. There are higher incidence rates in some geographic areas, especially in the British Isles, where the incidence rate is 4.5 per 1,000 live births. With subsequent births, the incidence rate is 5% higher, rising to 10% after two affected siblings (Molnar, 1985).

One of the possible etiologies for this condition is low folic acid levels during the preconception period, which may cause failure of the neural tube to close completely; this closure normally occurs at 28 days of embryonic development. There are varying degrees of severity for this neural tube defect; the types of defects are as follows:

1. *Spina bifida occulta*—There is complete closure of the spinal column and no visible protrusion of the spinal cord or meninges; bowel and bladder dysfunction are rare.
2. *Meningocele*—there is a visible opening of the spinal column, with a visible sac that contains spinal fluid and meninges. The spinal cord is normal and is not in the sac. If repairs go well, bowel and bladder function may be normal.
3. *Myelomeningocele*—this is the most common of neural tube defects, where there is a visible opening of the spinal column with a sac that contains spinal fluid, meninges, and the spinal cord; the cord typically is damaged due to compression. Bowel and bladder dysfunction are common especially if the lesions are above the sacral area (Smith, 1991) (Fig. 17-4).

Thomas and Chandler (2007) reported that 78% of children with spina bifida have abnormal bowel function and 40% use digital stimulation to facilitate fecal evacuation.

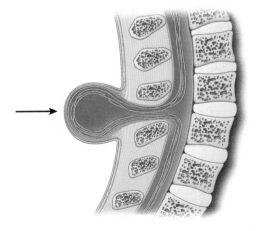

FIGURE 17-4. Spina bifida with myelomeningocele.

Neuromuscular Disorders

The list of locations and the neuromuscular conditions that could result in neurogenic bowel and bladder includes the following:

1. Cerebral cortex: cerebral palsy, degenerative CNS lesions, infections (meningitis)
2. Spinal cord: spinal muscular atrophies; infantile poliomyelitis, spinal cord injuries, tumors, or malformations; spina bifida with meningomyelocele
3. Neuromuscular junction: myasthenia gravis; botulism
4. Muscle diseases (dystrophy): Duchenne's muscular dystrophy; myotonic dystrophy

Collectively, children who require imperforate anus repairs or pull-through procedures for Hirschsprung's disease and children with meningomyelocele or spinal cord disorders who have bowel incontinence can be viewed as having some level of neurologic bowel impairment. Assessment and treatment of these children follow similar pathways, except for specific differences, which are emphasized among the various conditions.

Assessment of the Child with a Neurogenic Bowel

Children with neurogenic bowel conditions should have a comprehensive evaluation during each health care visit. Questions regarding health history and current care should be directed to the child with input from their parents/caregivers as needed. The initial encounter involves a thorough assessment including past medical history, developmental and psychosocial history, bowel management programs previously utilized, toileting behaviors, stooling patterns, diet, family lifestyle, and determination of the child's goals. With this in-depth assessment, the provider is equipped to monitor and alter plans based on the child's unique needs.

History

Box 17-1 provides guidelines for obtaining a comprehensive history from the child or adolescent with neurogenic bowel and fecal incontinence, to include developmental and psychosocial issues.

Physical Examination

The physical assessment is critical in determining the extent of stool retention and determining potential causes of lower bowel dysfunction, especially disorders affecting the lumbar sacral area. Provision of privacy is of utmost importance while examining an older child or adolescent.

Visual Inspection of Sacral Area

General inspection should include assessment of the sacral area for abnormalities, which would be indicative of potential neurologic lesions affecting the perianal, gluteal, and lower extremity regions. Physical signs of underlying disorders include flat buttocks (commonly seen in sacral agenesis) and a pilonidal dimple or tuft of hair, commonly seen in the individual with spina bifida occulta or an associated tethered cord. Motor and sensory function in the lower limbs and spinal area should also be assessed (Currie, 2000).

Abdominal Examination

During the physical examination, abdominal inspection, percussion, and palpation are done to assess for fecal retention as well as scars from prior surgeries. The presence and location of any type of urinary or bowel diversion and the stomal openings are also assessed. It may also be helpful to evaluate sexual maturity and to note any indicators of *precocious puberty*; it is not uncommon for children with meningomyelocele or hormonal imbalance to begin sexual development at a much younger age—commonly, less than 8 years of age (Steinberg, 2008).

Anal Inspection

Inspection of the anus should include anal placement, any visible indicators of sphincter muscle laxity (e.g., gaping or "patulous" anus), and perianal skin integrity (e.g., perianal fissures, rash, or incontinence-associated dermatitis). An anteriorly displaced anus (anterior ectopic anus) may cause constipation and straining with defecation in some individuals, although it is considered a normal finding in many patients. External examination of the anus should also include assessment for the anal wink and/or bulbocavernosus reflex (anal contraction in response to stroking of the perianal skin or to light compression of the glans penis or stroking of the clitoris); the presence of the anal

BOX 17-1.   History-Taking Guidelines for the Child with a Neurogenic Bowel

Current Bowel Patterns

- *Size and consistency of stools:* that is, "pellets," "balls," "logs," "ribbon-like" (obtain approximate length and diameter of stools if possible); liquid, mushy, soft, formed, hard, or variable consistency
- *Frequency and consistency of voluntary bowel movements (if applicable)*
- *Detailed description of stooling "accidents":* frequency (daily, multiple times weekly, etc.), any associated or precipitating events, volume of incontinent stools (smear, teaspoon, tablespoon, ½ cup, "diarrhea," etc.), number of underwear (or liners) soiled in 1 day, current management (is child aware that an accident has occurred? is child able to clean himself or herself up after an accident? does school or day care staff assist with management?)
- *Sensory awareness of rectal filling and defecation:* Can child sense rectal distention? Is child able to differentiate between gas, liquid, and solid? Is sensory awareness consistent or variable, and, if variable, how often is child able to recognize rectal distention?* (It is helpful to ask the child to point to where he or she feels the urge to have a bowel movement; many children with diminished or absent rectal sensation point to the left abdomen, indicating that their sensory awareness is related to peristaltic activity as opposed to rectal distention.)
- *Current bowel management program:* Has a bowel program been established? If so, what does it involve—digital stimulation? suppositories? enemas? regular toileting? medications? (If medications taken, determine strength, dose, and frequency.) Is child independent in bowel program and medication administration, or is assistance needed—if assistance is needed, how much assistance and who is providing it at present? What is the frequency of the current program; that is, how often are medications taken? stimulants used to initiate defecation? Routine toileting performed? Is the currently established bowel program effective? If not, what problems are associated with the current program?
- *Specific toileting behaviors:* What position does the child assume while toileting, that is, are his or her feet firmly positioned on the floor or in the air? Does the child have enough trunk stability to sit without having to support himself or herself? Is the child able to effectively do a Valsalva maneuver to "push the stool out"? (It may help to have the child demonstrate how he or she "pushes stool out.") If current bowel program includes routine toileting, how much encouragement does the child require to adhere to the program?
- *Dietary status:* Have any dietary modifications been made to address the problems with bowel function? If yes, what are they and what effect have they had? What types of high-fiber foods does the child eat and in what volume? What is the child's usual volume of liquid intake? Does the child have access to liquids in the school or day care setting? Is the child receiving any fiber supplementation, and, if so, what formula and in what volume? Is the child's dental status satisfactory, or are there dental problems contributing to inadequate fiber intake?
- *Goals and motivation:* What is the child's perception of the problem with fecal incontinence? What are the child's and parents' goals for management? How much assistance does the child require, and how much assistance and support are the parents able and willing to provide?

Medical History

The questions in this section are specific to the underlying cause of the neurogenic bowel dysfunction and are therefore grouped accordingly:

Imperforate Anus

- LEVEL OF ANOMALY, IF KNOWN: Was defect a "high" or a "low" defect, and what prognosis was given at the time of repair? Were any tests done to evaluate the potential for continence?
- SACRAL ANOMALIES: Was sacrum intact, or were abnormalities noted? (This is significant because children with imperforate anus combined with sacral anomalies are at greater risk for incontinence.)
- UROLOGIC PROBLEMS: Were any urologic defects or problems noted? Were any tests completed to evaluate the urologic system?
- CORRECTIVE SURGERIES: Number of corrective surgeries performed and any available data re the specific procedures
- MEDICAL–SURGICAL FOLLOW-UP STUDY AFTER REPAIR: Last checkup by surgeon? problems with constipation and overflow stooling? any studies done to rule out retained stool and dilatation of rectosigmoid colon?

Hirschsprung Disease

- EXTENT OF COLONIC INVOLVEMENT AND TYPE OF SURGERY DONE TO CORRECT THE PROBLEM (IF KNOWN): Any anal dilatations required postoperatively? If yes, when was last procedure done? It is important to carefully question the child or parents re: the caliber of stools; ribbon-like or pencil-thin stools may be indicative of anal stenosis, which is a common complication after surgical repair of Hirschsprung disease.
- HISTORY OF CONSTIPATION AFTER REPAIR: Current frequency and consistency of stools? Any use of softeners, stimulants, enemas, or suppositories? (These children are at significant risk for constipation caused by anal stenosis, dilatations causing an aversion to defecation, incomplete removal of the aganglionic bowel, or recurrent aganglionosis.†)
- HISTORY OF ENTEROCOLITIS (FEVER, ABDOMINAL PAIN, AND DIARRHEA): Treatment required.†

Myelomeningocele or Spinal Disorder

- LEVEL OF LESION: Children with lesions at or above the sacral cord usually present with a neurogenic bowel and bladder though some children have incomplete lesions with sparing of some of the sacral pathways (these children may retain some degree of bowel control)
- ANY ADDITIONAL NEUROLOGIC OR SPINAL CORD PROBLEMS, SUCH AS TETHERED CORD? If yes, effect on bowel and bladder function?
- MOBILITY AND INDEPENDENCE IN ADLs TO INCLUDE TOILETING: Is child able to ambulate with or without assistive devices? Is child able to self-toilet and to carry out own bowel program? If not, how much assistance is required, and who is available to provide the assistance needed to implement the program? Are assistive devices needed to facilitate the patient's transfer to the toilet and ability to maintain balance while on the toilet?
- UROLOGIC STATUS: Current bladder management (that is, spontaneous voiding versus Credé's maneuver versus clean intermittent catheterization); history of chronic UTIs and usual frequency of antibiotic therapy (there is a potential for antibiotic therapy to cause diarrhea and disrupt bowel program)

BOX 17-1.

History-Taking Guidelines for the Child with a Neurogenic Bowel (*Continued*)

Developmental Status
- TIME FRAME FOR ACHIEVEMENT OF DEVELOPMENTAL MILESTONES: Age at which toileting introduced and response to toileting. (The clinician should be aware that parents of children with congenital conditions sometimes tend to "excuse" the child from learning normal toileting behavior. The clinician should counsel the parents re: the importance of normalizing their child's life as much as possible and should explain that the child should be exposed to normal toileting by 3 years of age unless the child is cognitively impaired.)
- CURRENT CONTINENCE STATUS: Is child continent of urine but incontinent of stool? If child is managing bladder with clean intermittent catheterization (CIC), at what frequency does the child catheterize? If child is in school, how much distance is there between the classrooms and the bathroom facilities? Do the bathroom facilities provide privacy? Does the child have accidents at school? If so, how often and how are these handled?
- CURRENT ACADEMIC STATUS: Has the child been diagnosed with a specific disorder such as attention deficit disorder or developmental delay? Is the child in a regular classroom or a special

education program? (If the child is in a special education program, ask about the services provided. Some special education programs provide toileting assistance.) How is the child's attendance record in school?

Psychosocial Status
- BEHAVIORAL ISSUES: Is the child seeing a therapist for any behavioral or emotional problems?
- PEER RELATIONSHIPS: What is the child's peer group like? Are the child's friends aware of the problem, and, if so, what is their response? Are the child's peers able to detect any odor or problem with stool elimination?
- EXTRACURRICULAR ACTIVITIES: Does the child participate in school or extracurricular events? Does the child attend sleepovers or camps? Does the child participate in sports? How is the problem with bowel function handled in these settings?
- SCHOOL AND TEACHER SUPPORT: Are the school staff and the teacher aware of the child's medical needs and problems? Are they sensitive and supportive regarding the child's toileting needs?
- INCENTIVE PROGRAM: What type of incentive program is best suited for this child if a bowel program is implemented?

*Datum from MacLeod, J. (1988). *Endoscopy Review*, Nov–Dec, 45–56.
†Datum from Walker, W. A., Durie, P. R., Hamilton, J. R., et al. (1996) *Pediatric gastrointestinal disease, Vol. 2* , 2nd ed., (pp. 2077–2091). St. Louis, MO: Mosby.

wink and/or bulbocavernosus reflex indicates intact nerve pathways between the sacral cord and the perineum. It may also be helpful, especially in a child with a history of imperforate anus or spinal cord disorder, to assess sensation circumferentially around the anus; injury or denervation may cause loss of sensation. If no reflexes are elicited and the anus exhibits no tone, EMG studies can validate sphincter denervation and absence of sphincter contractility (Currie, 2000).

Rectal Examination

The rectal examination may be deferred until there is a trusting relationship established between the child and health care provider. Creating a trusting relationship is crucial, especially if the health care provider will be involved in providing biofeedback or in working with the child to establish compliance with a bowel management program. It may be helpful to ask the primary physician about the results of his/her rectal examination, to avoid repeated uncomfortable examinations (Jinbo, 2004).

If a rectal examination is performed, it is important to obtain the child's consent and cooperation and to perform the examination as gently as possible. During the examination, the nurse should note sphincter tone and any internal hemorrhoids, anal fissures, strictures, tenderness, or irregularities in the rectal vault. The nurse should note the amount and consistency of stool in the rectal ampulla and the size of the rectum and should then ask the child to contract the anal sphincter as if trying not to pass gas or stool and finally to "bear down" as if trying to expel stool.

These maneuvers allow the nurse to assess sphincter tone and contractility, as well as the child's ability to voluntarily control the sphincter, and to coordinate sphincter relaxation and abdominal muscle contraction (Currie, 2000). It also allows the nurse to assess for rectal prolapse, which sometimes is found in children or adolescents who have undergone anoplasty and in those with spinal disorders such as meningomyelocele. If rectal prolapse is present, the nurse should further assess for bleeding and tenderness and should refer any child or adolescent with significant prolapse for surgical evaluation (Currie, 2000).

CLINICAL PEARL

Once rapport has been established and the child/adolescent has given permission, a rectal examination should be performed; this examination permits the nurse to assess for retained stool, baseline sphincter tone, perineal hygiene, and the individual's ability to voluntarily contract the sphincter and to coordinate sphincter relaxation and abdominal muscle contraction.

During the rectal examination, it is also important to assess perineal hygiene. If the underwear is soiled or there is fecal material present due to inadequate cleansing, the nurse should determine the patient's awareness of the soiling and should specifically query the individual as to sensory awareness of rectal distention and of stool passage. The nurse should also be alert to the presence of rash or erythema and should discuss with the patient his/her hygiene and skin care routines (Currie, 2000).

Diagnostic Tests

Several tests play a valuable role in further assessing the pathophysiology of fecal incontinence and neurogenic bowel. Anorectal manometry, defecography, rectal compliance, and electromyography can all be helpful in the evaluation of rectal and sphincter function. A child with a spinal cord lesion such as myelomeningocele may benefit from anorectal manometry or defecography studies to assess their rectal sensation and ability to voluntarily control the sphincter (Currie, 2000). These children may also have problems with colonic motility, due to loss of autonomic innervation; if the individual reports persistent constipation, transit studies should be considered.

An abdominal x-ray may be helpful in assessing the amount of stool present in the colon, especially if there is a history of constipation. The presence of stool in various segments of the colon provides insight as to peristaltic activity and high versus low impaction (Jinbo, 2004).

An infant born with Hirschsprung's disease usually has a rectal biopsy and/or barium enema done at the time of diagnosis. If the child continues to have problems with defecation following the pull-through procedure, additional studies may be indicated and may include anorectal manometry, colonic transit studies, or colonic manometry in addition to possible repeat biopsy and barium enema (Jinbo, 2004).

If any individual with a neurogenic bowel exhibits signs and symptoms of neurological decompensation (e.g., increase in incontinence episodes, increased problems with gait or mobility, or back pain/discomfort), CT scans or MRI studies are usually indicated to evaluate the spinal cord. During growth spurts or periods of weight gain, these children and adolescents are at risk for developing a tethered cord and need to be monitored accordingly. In some instances, deterioration in bowel or bladder function is the first indication of a tethered cord or spinal problem. CT scans or MRI studies may also be ordered to evaluate the status of imperforate anus or Hirschsprung's disease repairs (Jinbo, 2004).

Treatment and Management of a Child with a Neurogenic Bowel

Due to the marked variations in the degree of neurological involvement, there is not one single treatment protocol for neurogenic bowel; rather, there are a variety of management options.

Behavioral Measures

Initially, as noted, the patient should be evaluated for evidence of stool retention; if the colon is filled with stool, a bowel cleanout is necessary to prevent overflow incontinence. The child will need to be given stool softeners and laxatives for cleanout and until bowel regularity is achieved (Table 17-3). If the child is unable (or unwilling) to take in enough dietary fiber, then fiber supplements should be offered, with the goal of establishing stool that is soft but formed and therefore both easily retained by a weak sphincter and also effectively eliminated with minimal straining. Behavioral therapy should include sitting on the toilet and attempting defecation two to three times a day (after meals) until a predictable pattern of elimination has been established. Careful observation is needed to ensure that the child is maintaining the optimal position for defecation and is allowing sufficient time for the stool to pass. The child's feet should be supported with a stool to ensure relaxation of the pelvic floor.

Biofeedback

It is inconclusive as to whether biofeedback is beneficial for these individuals; however, the incorporation of biofeedback into the program may help to improve sensory awareness and coordination of sphincter relaxation and abdominal muscle contraction. If the child has some external sphincter tone, biofeedback may optimize the degree of strength of the external sphincter.

Heymen et al. (2001) identified the following potential benefits of biofeedback: improved strength of the pelvic floor muscles in response to rectal filling, increase in the patient's ability to perceive distention of the rectum, or both. Thus, biofeedback treatment protocols can be designed to accomplish any of the following goals: (1) improve coordination of pelvic floor muscle contraction in response to rectal distention, (2) improve sensory awareness of rectal distention without strengthening pelvic floor muscles, or (3) strengthen the pelvic floor muscles without increasing sensory awareness of rectal distention (Heymen et al., 2001).

The data regarding use of biofeedback for treating children with imperforate anus are limited; however, Rao et al. (1996) and Leung et al. (2006) concluded that biofeedback training is an effective treatment for these children. Specifically, these investigators found that biofeedback helped children and adolescents to improve their squeeze pressure (external sphincter contractility) and their ability to maintain the sphincter contraction. Clinically, this enabled the participants to more effectively retain liquid in the rectum. They also found improved rectoanal coordination with a reduction in rectal pressure and an increase in the continence index. Used in combination with behavior modification, biofeedback has been found to be a clearly superior mode of treatment (Heymen et al., 2001). This author has also found, in treating this population of children, that several have developed paradoxical contractions; that is, when they Valsalva to defecate, there is an increase in external sphincter tone (as opposed to relaxation), which causes inadequate emptying of the rectal vault. Biofeedback has been helpful in teaching these children to relax the external sphincter muscle, which improves emptying of the rectal vault and decreases stooling accidents.

Peristaltic Stimuli (Stimulated Defecation)

If the child/adolescent cannot initiate a bowel movement, either with routine toileting or in response to some sensory awareness of the urge to defecate, use of a suppository or minienema can be helpful in stimulating peristalsis and evacuation. If the child does not respond to these stimuli, further studies are indicated to assess for a megarectosigmoid colon; if present, referral for surgical evaluation is indicated.

Management of Obstruction

All children and adolescents who have undergone pull-through procedures need to be carefully monitored for obstructive symptoms. If obstructive symptoms occur, it is important to determine the cause of the obstruction through diagnostic tests; management is then dependent on the specific causative factor. If anatomical problems, such as anal stenosis or strictures, are causing the obstruction, further dilatation or surgery may be indicated. If biopsy reveals recurrent aganglionosis in the child with Hirschsprung's disease, further surgery is required. If dysmotility is a problem, medications can be initiated to reduce transit time; if outlet problems are due to a hypertonic sphincter, a myectomy may be necessary. This author has also utilized biofeedback with a small number of children with Hirschsprung's disease to teach relaxation of the pelvic floor musculature, which reduces sphincter tone and improves evacuation.

Children and adolescents with outlet dysfunction need to be monitored for enterocolitis and require aggressive management to eliminate the obstruction; if dietary modifications (increased fiber and fluid intake), medications, and behavioral measures are insufficient, a myectomy may be required, as noted. If the child and caregiver are comfortable with digital stimulation, this can be introduced along with behavior management to enable them to defecate at a given time daily. Digital stimulation is an inexpensive way of eliciting rectal emptying but works only if the reflex arc is intact.

Anal Irrigation

Children with weak sphincters may find the use of enemas (anal irrigations or rectal "washouts") helpful in attaining continence. Utilizing a balloon-tipped catheter or bowel management tube allows the enema solution to be retained in a child with a weak anal sphincter. The bowel management tube is a silastic catheter with a balloon (30 to 50 mL) that is inflated to facilitate retention of the enema fluid; due to the possibility of latex allergies, especially in the spina bifida or meningomyelocele population, latex exposure should be minimized and silicone or silastic catheters should be used. Since proper volume and retention are difficult due to poor sphincter control, the balloon helps to "seal" the lower rectum as the enema solution is administered. "Cone enema" or a colostomy irrigation kit can also be utilized as a continence enema (Smith, 1991), or an anal irrigation system can be used, as described in Chapter 16. The child can then transfer to the toilet with the seal in place and expel the

contents of the colon when the balloon or cone is released. While this is usually an effective approach to controlled evacuation, children or adolescents with concomitant colonic dysmotility may prematurely expel the balloon or may experience incomplete evacuation despite administration of high-volume enemas; these individuals may experience increased incontinent episodes as the enema solution and stool is expelled slowly over a prolonged period of time. If this is a persistent problem, the enema/washout should be discontinued and another therapy approach should be explored.

> **CLINICAL PEARL**
>
> Management of the child/adolescent with neurogenic bowel must be individualized and includes strategies such as dietary modification and medications to establish soft formed stool, routine toileting, biofeedback, stimulated defecation programs, anal irrigations, and surgical intervention.

The balloon-tipped catheter can also be used as a biofeedback device, to help the child or adolescent learn to sense rectal filling. However, this is effective and appropriate only in children and adolescents who have normal cognitive function and some degree of innervation/sensory awareness.

Surgical Intervention (MACE or ACE Procedure)

In many instances when the anal sphincter is weak or denervated, successful administration of retrograde enemas is difficult. In addition, this approach to bowel regulation frequently limits the child or adolescent in achieving independence with care. If diet regulation, medication, enemas, and/or biofeedback fail to produce a positive response, other surgical interventions (e.g., a Malone antegrade continence enema (MACE) or antegrade continence enema (ACE) procedure or creation of a colostomy) may be indicated (Jinbo, 2004). In the late 1980s, the "MACE" or Malone antegrade continence enema was introduced. This new operative technique involved reimplanting the appendix in a nonrefluxing manner into the cecum with the other end brought out on the abdominal wall as a continent stoma (Churchill et al., 2001) (Fig. 17-5). (The stoma is normally continent of both stool and gas.) The "cecostomy button" technique is a variation of this procedure; a low profile device is placed into the tract between the abdominal wall and the bowel and is accessed daily for administration of the solution (Duel & Gonzalez, 1999; Lee et al., 2002). With each of these procedures, antegrade washouts are administered through the catheterizable channel or low profile device to produce colonic emptying. Many children and adolescents with neurogenic bowel, especially those with myelomeningocele, have benefited from this procedure and have found routine irrigations less invasive than having a colostomy or doing retrograde enemas.

In the past decade, there have been several modifications to the ACE procedure. When the appendix is not available

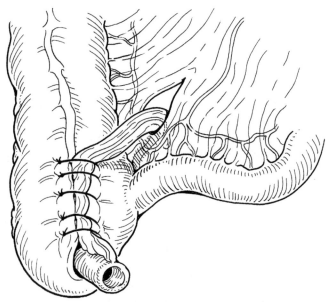

FIGURE 17-5. MACE procedure. The appendix is removed and reimplanted into the cecum (or transverse or descending colon); other end of appendix brought to abdominal wall as stoma. This permits antegrade "washouts" through the stoma.

or is unsuitable, a neoappendix can be created using the Monti technique. A segment of ileum or colon is detached from the GI tract while its blood supply is preserved. This segment of bowel is opened to form a rectangle and then reconfigured into a tube-like structure that is tunneled in an antireflux fashion into the bowel wall; it provides a continent, catheterizable conduit through which daily antegrade enemas can be administered (Jinbo, 2004).

More recently, Mitrofanoff has placed these antegrade continence enema conduits (and stomas) in the splenic flexure because the formed stool that needs to be expelled is stored in the left side of the colon (primarily left transverse and descending colon). There have even been modifications to this procedure where a Monti tube is created from the large bowel and placed at the splenic flexure (Heymen et al., 2001). The ACE procedure is also being done laparoscopically (Lynch et al., 1999).

The amount, frequency, and type of solutions vary and include normal saline, hypertonic phosphate, polyethylene glycol 3350 (Miralax), and tap water. Yerkes et al. (2001) studied the routine use of tap water as an irrigant, as there have been reported cases of hypernatremia with saline irrigations and electrolyte abnormalities with the use of hypertonic phosphate solutions. They found no significant hyponatremia or hypochloremia in any patient who used tap water for continence irrigations. However, although rare, electrolyte abnormalities with potential morbidity are a possible complication of tap water irrigation, and patients should therefore be monitored closely for any signs of electrolyte disturbances (Yerkes et al. 2001).

Kokoska et al. (2001) described their experience with irrigants and reported best results with normal saline and polyethylene glycol 3350; their third choice was a one-to-one

solution of glycerin and saline. Due to the potential for electrolyte imbalance with the various solutions, it is recommended that serum electrolyte studies be done to assess the child's tolerance to a solution (Kokoska et al., 2001; Yerkes et al., 2001). Graf et al. (1998) reviewed the literature on types and amounts of solutions utilized for irrigation. They found that the volume used varied from 80 mL to 1 L administered over 5 to 60 minutes. In the majority of patients, colonic evacuation occurred within 1 hour of enema administration. Enemas were given daily to once a week. They concluded that the type of solution, volume, and frequency must be individualized for each patient (Thies & McAllister, 2001).

> **CLINICAL PEARL**
>
> The MACE/ACE procedures permit antegrade washouts of the distal colon, and in general, children/adolescents and their families have been very satisfied with the results. However, the clinician must work with the individual child/adolescent to determine the optimal frequency of irrigation and the best volume and type of irrigant solution.

The MACE procedure and its variants have been performed for over a decade, and, in general, children and adolescents (and their families) have been very satisfied with the results. However, clinicians and patients must always be aware that there are potential complications, which include appendiceal and stomal necrosis; stomal stenosis; stomal leakage; difficulty catheterizing the stoma; pain with enema administration; wound infection; adhesions resulting in bowel obstruction; hypertrophic granulation tissue at the stoma site; mucus discharge and dermatitis around the stoma; cecal volvulus; nausea and dizziness during phosphate enema usage; and hyperphosphatemia with the use of phosphate solutions (Thies & McAllister, 2001). Positive outcomes with this procedure are dependent on patient/family motivation and on compliance with the enema regimen. Some centers believe that this procedure is more successful in children over 5 years of age as they are more motivated and have a better understanding of the care required (Graf et al., 1998; Thies & McAllister, 2001).

If all options for bowel management have been attempted without success, the child and their family should be given the option of having a colostomy created. Although this sounds like a dramatic option, the child with intractable fecal incontinence may find this quite rewarding, as they will actually regain "control" of defecation.

> **CLINICAL PEARL**
>
> If all options for management of neurogenic bowel have been trialed without success, the patient should be offered construction of a colostomy; while this may seem dramatic, it can provide significant improvement in quality of life.

The algorithm shown in Figure 17-6 depicts a common approach to managing a child with a neurogenic bowel;

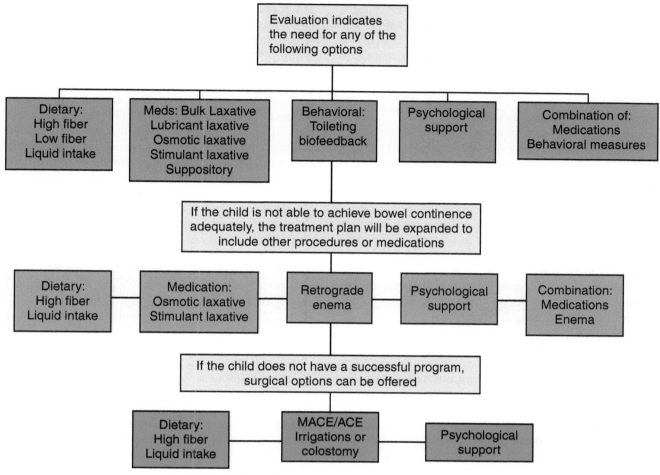

FIGURE 17-6. Algorithm for management of neurogenic bowel.

however, treatments are always individualized according to the child and his or her individual symptoms.

Key Concepts in the Management of the Individual with a Neurogenic Bowel

Ideally, it is hoped that adolescents with a neurogenic bowel have had ongoing monitoring and treatment for incontinence following the initial diagnosis. However, if an adolescent has had no prior treatment, there are several key concepts in working with a child and their caregiver.

Development of Rapport

The first concept for effective management of any adolescent with a chronic illness is the importance of a good rapport between the adolescent and health care provider. Due to the number of tests and examinations, many adolescents are suspicious of health care providers. It is especially important that trust be established if the health care provider needs to provide any type of therapy, such as biofeedback or electrical stimulation. These procedures can be seen as "invasive" or intimidating since leads or sensors are placed in or on the perineum. A good relationship also enables the adolescent to feel comfortable in discussing their feelings or reporting incontinence events. Caregivers need to be counseled regarding avoidance of punishment or blame for bowel incontinence and should be encouraged to assist with a positive reinforcement program, such as incentives for positive behaviors (Jinbo, 2004; Michaud et al., 2007).

Interdisciplinary Approach

A second key concept is an interdisciplinary team approach to management and care. An adolescent with fecal incontinence experiences many stressful emotional situations and would benefit from the counseling of a mental health professional (i.e., psychologist, psychiatrist, or counselor). The counselor or therapist can reinforce the treatment plan during therapy sessions with the adolescent and caregiver. It is a good proactive measure to routinely refer adolescents with multiple congenital problems and with long-standing incontinence for counseling, since many of these children are "suffering silently" and would benefit from ongoing counseling to help them deal with this problem as well as their disability (Jinbo, 2004). In school, a referral to the school health nurse is helpful so that the adolescent can be assisted in maintaining his/her bowel program, such as reminders to go to the toilet or access to private bathrooms. School nurses are also encouraged to incorporate activities of daily living (ADL) skills into the adolescent's Individualized Educational Plan (IEP) if there is a need to do procedures (such as catheterizations or behavior interventions) in the school setting (Michaud et al., 2007).

Patient and Caregiver Education

Education of the caregiver and adolescent is crucial, including a review of normal bowel function and a discussion of the causes of neurogenic bowel; it is also important to explain the options for management and to assure that the patient and family understand the treatment plan. This helps to promote cooperation and compliance. Information must be presented in a manner that is consistent with the adolescent's cognitive ability to understand the material. For example, instead of encouraging an adolescent with fecal incontinence to eat more fiber because these foods are healthier, it would be best to introduce the use of fiber to help bulk the stool and decrease weight and accidents (Michaud et al., 2007).

Developing a treatment plan in collaboration with the child and caregiver is helpful, as both parties can take ownership and responsibility for the various treatment options. Listening carefully to the adolescent is important in assuring adherence with the treatment plan. In many instances, the adolescent has experienced the use of various medications or treatments and may have preconceived ideas of how these treatments affect their bodies. The adolescent may also have employment or extracurricular activities that should be incorporated into the treatment plan. For example, if the adolescent has difficulty getting up in the morning, doing enemas in the morning may not be the optimal time for him or her. Trying to accommodate an adolescent's schedule into the treatment plan may necessitate administering an enema in the evening when the schedule is not as hectic. In middle adolescence, when there is a lot of effort at establishing identity, it is not uncommon for adolescents to have periods of rebellion when they feel that their lives are too tightly controlled; during this period, health care providers may need to compromise on different aspects of the adolescent's treatment plan. During late adolescence, there is more acceptance of their condition and there may be more instances where adolescents exhibit more control over their condition (Currie, 2000).

CLINICAL PEARL

Key concepts in effective management of the pediatric population include development of rapport, an interdisciplinary approach, patient and family education, and ongoing follow-up.

Follow-Up

Close follow-up with the adolescent and his or her family is essential during establishment and maintenance of a bowel management program. If the adolescent and their family/caregiver(s) are not able to return for follow-up appointments within the first week or two, a telephone follow-up should be done. The adolescent and family/caregiver(s) should be advised that each bowel management program is tailored individually to each child and that ongoing communication is essential in obtaining success. It is also helpful to emphasize that bowel control does not occur "overnight" and that finding the "right" treatment plan may take time. In addition, bowel management programs need to be maintained even when on vacation or admitted to a hospital, and the adolescent needs to understand that his or her bowel control will be affected by dietary changes as well as medications and illnesses. Keeping the adolescent focused and motivated during the process can be challenging; incentives can be utilized as a means of reinforcing positive behaviors and compliance with the bowel program. Sending reports and consultation notes to the primary physician, who may have referred the adolescent, is helpful in keeping all health care providers apprised of the situation and helping them be supportive of the interventions offered (Jinbo, 2004).

Figure 17-6 depicts the flow of patient management, based on assessment findings and response to treatment. Although treatment regimens differ based on the needs of the specific child, three typical cases are provided at the end of the chapter that illustrate management based on the underlying condition and severity of incontinence.

🔵 Diarrhea

As noted earlier, chronic constipation is a common contributor to incontinence in children. Diarrhea can also cause incontinence; it most frequently occurs as a response to an acute infectious process or as the result of a chronic condition or disease state.

Acute Diarrhea

"Acute diarrhea" is an increase in the number of stools and an alteration in stool consistency, as compared to the patient's normal stooling pattern. It is usually caused by viral, bacterial, or protozoal agents. In children, rotavirus and Norwalk-like virus are responsible for up to 50% of acute diarrheal cases during winter months (Jackson & Vessey, 2000). History will usually reveal a sudden onset of illness, and there may be other systemic symptoms, such as fever, cough, rash, or decreased activity level. With resolution of the infectious process, the diarrhea subsides as do the incontinent episodes.

Chronic Diarrhea

Chronic diarrhea is an increase in the frequency, fluidity, or volume of stool, compared to the child's normal pattern, for longer than 14 to 21 days. Stool output in excess of 10 g/kg/d in infants and >200 g/d in children is considered indicative of diarrhea (Jackson & Vessey, 2000). Disease states that commonly lead to diarrhea include short gut syndrome, Irritable Bowel Syndrome, Crohn's disease or ulcerative colitis, celiac disease, and cystic fibrosis. Children with peritoneal shunt infections commonly exhibit nausea, vomiting, and diarrhea as well as fever and abdominal pain. Children with congenital heart disease must be monitored closely during any episode of diarrhea, as it can be indicative of digoxin toxicity or worsening congestive heart failure (vs. an episode of acute gastroenteritis). Oncology patients may develop chemotherapy-induced diarrhea. Children with cerebral palsy who have limited mobility are frequently plagued with impactions that exhibit as constant diarrhea (because the liquid stool seeps around the impacted stool in the presence of persistent internal sphincter relaxation); it is critical to carefully balance fiber, liquid, and stool softeners in these children and to assess for impaction before treating episodes of "diarrhea." Any child with diarrhea requires careful assessment, since diarrhea in children is typically symptomatic of another condition that needs to be addressed. Once the underlying problem is corrected, the diarrhea and incontinence typically resolve.

Conclusion

Bowel management in the pediatric population is both challenging and rewarding. Fortunately, our society is moving toward a little more openness in discussion of elimination. There are more books for children and parents that explain problems with control of "poop" and "gas" and things that can be done to normalize and control their elimination patterns. Common problems include chronic constipation and encopresis; these problems are very responsive to management strategies including cleanout regimens, establishment of soft formed stool via increased fiber and fluid intake, and routine toileting. Neurogenic bowel is a less common but very difficult problem that is characterized by compromised sensory function and sphincter function. Management of these children requires in-depth assessment and individualized therapy; treatment strategies include correction of stool consistency, toileting programs, biofeedback, use of medications, use of peristaltic stimuli to regulate evacuation, and surgical options including antegrade continence enema procedures and colostomy formation.

Fundamental principles in working with children and adolescents include establishment of rapport, a multidisciplinary approach, ongoing education of the child and caregivers, and positive reinforcement. Ultimately, the goal is not only to normalize bowel function and provide continence but also to promote positive self-esteem; thus, the clinician must always remember:

The young child is dependent on adults for many things, but the most important is a sense of being cared for....
—Mally, T. (1974). *Montessori and your child.*
New York, NY: Schocken Books.

CASE STUDIES

MILD INCONTINENCE

Jasmine is a 13-year-old patient who just arrived in Hawaii from the Pacific Basin. Jasmine was born with an imperforate anus, and repair was done shortly after birth. According to her mother, Jasmine has been constipated several times a year and occasionally has been to the emergency room because of severe constipation. Jasmine is usually given an enema with good results and then discharged home.

Jasmine's mother states Jasmine is now having problems with very watery stools similar to diarrhea. Her mother also reports that Jasmine had a small amount of stool about 5 days ago. Jasmine stated it was five small balls of stool and added that she has not felt very hungry for the past 5 days.

Physical Examination

Constitutional: Jasmine is a well-developed, 13-year-old, ambulatory teen who is very alert and in no acute distress.

Weight: Jasmine weighs 104 pounds.

Abdomen: She has a distended abdomen, with palpable nodules of stool in the left lower quadrant, as well as along the transverse colon. No discomfort noted during palpation.

Perineum: Jasmine's anus had no signs of fissures, and her rectal vault was filled with small balls of stool. Sphincter tone was within a normal range. Perianal area was intact with no signs of any skin breakdown. Fecal staining noted on underwear.

X-ray: An abdominal x-ray revealed that Jasmine was impacted with stool throughout her colon.

Impression: Jasmine has a history of constipation and was currently impacted.

Plan

1. Cleanout with a full capful of Miralax in 8 ounces of fluid twice a day in addition to Senokot 2 tabs. Recommend a clear liquid diet during the cleanout.

2. Maintenance dose after cleanout: administer Senokot 1 tab daily with one capful of Miralax in 8 ounces of fluid. Resume diet for her current age after cleanout is complete.

3. Follow-up in 1 week.

CASE STUDIES

MODERATE INCONTINENCE

Sarah is a 12-year-old girl who was involved in a motor vehicle accident (MVA) that left her paralyzed from the waist down due to a partially severed spinal cord. She does have occasional sensations of rectal filling but is not able to consistently initiate a bowel movement. She has had a moderate amount of slightly firm stool over the past 2 days.

Physical examination

Constitutional: Sarah is a 12-year-old, thin but well-developed paraplegic, who sits in her wheelchair in no acute distress.

Chest: Sarah is developing breast buds.

Abdomen: Sarah's abdomen is flat, but she has palpable stool along the left lower quadrant.

Perineum: Her anus is closed, and she has a fairly high sphincter tone. Her rectal vault was full of stool.

Impression: She is status post-MVA with paraplegia and a neurogenic bowel.

Plan

1. Recommend use of Fleet enema × 1.
2. Start Miralax ½ capful daily in 4 ounces of fluid.
3. Recommend toileting after meals and utilize a glycerin suppository if no bowel movement × 1 day.
4. Will continue to monitor and if Sarah continues to have inadequate emptying, will recommend use of weekly Fleet enema.

CASE STUDIES

SEVERE INCONTINENCE

John is an 11-year-old who was born with S1–S2 spina bifida. Over the years, he, with the support of his parents, has tried a variety of oral medications, suppositories, and enemas with no success at achieving continence. John and his parents decided that he would do the ACE procedure in hopes of becoming continent. He is 6 weeks post-ACE procedure and has arrived with his parents for his second follow-up visit. Immediately post-op, John was doing well on daily 500 to 600 mL normal saline irrigations, evacuating his stool within 30 to 45 minutes. However, he and his mother noticed that after irrigating, he needs to sit on the toilet for 1.5 to 2 hours. He administers the irrigations shortly after dinner over a 5- to 10-minute period. Often, he will have a large accident 2 to 3 hours later. He is otherwise accident free. John is learning to catheterize and irrigate his stoma using a 10-French Coudé catheter.

Physical examination

Constitutional: John is a well-developed child who is ambulatory with braces.

Wt: 70 pounds

Abdomen: John's abdomen is fairly flat and soft with active bowel sounds. He has a flush stoma that is barely visible in his umbilicus. His peristomal skin is intact.

Perineum: He has a lax anal sphincter; however, perianal skin is clean; no rash noted.

Extremities: John wears braces on bilateral lower extremities.

Impression: John has a prolonged evacuation of ACE irrigation solution.

Plan

1. Discussed with John and his mother about increasing the volume of the saline solution to 700 to 800 mL of normal saline versus the use of two capfuls of Miralax in 500 mL of water. They decided to see if the increased volume of saline would expedite evacuation. If they continue to have a prolonged evacuation time, they will switch to the Miralax mixture.
2. They will follow up in the next 3 to 4 weeks.

REFERENCES

Abi-Hanna, A., & Lake, A. M. (1998). Constipation and encopresis in childhood. *Pediatrics in Review, 19,* 23–30.

Amiel, J., Sproat-Emison, E., Garcia-Barcelo, M., et al.; for the Hirschsprung Disease Consortium. (2008). Hirschsprung disease, associated syndromes and genetics: a review. *Journal of Medical Genetics, 45,* 1–4.

Biggs, W. S., & Dery, W. H. (2006). Evaluation and treatment of constipation in infants and children. *American Family Physician, 73*(3), 469–477.

Bishop, E., McKinnon E., Weir, E., et al. (2003). Reflexology in the management of encopresis and chronic constipation. *Pediatric Nursing, 15*(3), 20–21.

Blair, G. K., Djonlic K., Fraser G. C., et al. (1992). The bowel management tube: An effective means for controlling fecal incontinence. *Journal of Pediatric Surgery, 27*(10), 1260–1272.

Boon, R. F., & Singh, N. (1991). A model for the treatment of encopresis. *Behavior Modification, 15*(3), 355–371.

Chase, J., & Shields, N. (2011). A systematic review of the efficacy of non-pharmacological, non-surgical and non-behavioural treatments of functional chronic constipation in children. *The Australian and New Zealand Continence Journal, 17*(2), 40–50.

Christophersen, E. (1991). Toileting problems in children. *Pediatric Annals, 5*(20), 240–244.

Churchill, B. M., Abramson, R. P., & Wahl, E. F. (2001). Dysfunction of the lower urinary and distal gastrointestinal tracts in pediatric patients with known spinal cord problems. *Pediatric Clinics of North America, 48*(6), 2–51.

Cohen, A. (2007). *Constipation, withholding and your child.* Philadelphia, PA: Jessica Kingsley Publishers.

Currie, D. M. (2000). Bowel management in children with fecal incontinence. *Physical Medicine and Rehabilitation: State of the Art Reviews, 14*(2), 311–322.

DiLorenzo, C., & Benninga, M. A. (2004). Pathophysiology of pediatric fecal incontinence. *Gastroenterology, 126*, S33–S40.

Doughty, D. B. (2006). *Urinary and fecal incontinence: Nursing management* (3rd ed.). St. Louis, MO: Mosby, Inc.

Duel, B. P., & Gonzalez, R. (1999). The button cecostomy for management of fecal incontinence. *Pediatric Surgery International, 15*, 559–561.

Foster, E. (1995). Surgical options for managing chronic fecal incontinence in children. *Progressions, 7*(1), 13–21.

Graf, J. L., Strear, C., Bratton, B., et al. (1998). The antegrade continence enema procedure: A review of the literature. *Journal of Pediatric Surgery, 33*, 1294–1296.

Heymen, S., Jones, K. R., Ringel, Y., et al. (2001). Biofeedback treatment of rectal incontinence. *Diseases of the Colon and Rectum, 44*(5), 728–736.

Howe, A. C., & Walker, C. E. (1992). Behavioral management of toilet training, enuresis, and encopresis. *Pediatric Clinics of North America, 39*, 413–432.

Ingebo, K., & Heyman, M. (1998). Polyethylene glycol—electrolyte solution for intestinal clearance in children with refractory encopresis. *American Journal of Diseases of Children (1960), 142*, 340–342.

Jackson, P. L., & Vessey, J. (2000). *Primary care of the child with a chronic condition.* St. Louis, MO: Mosby.

Jinbo, A. K. (2004). The challenge of obtaining continence in a child with a neurogenic bowel disorder. *Journal of Wound, Ostomy, and Continence Nursing, 31*(6), 336–350.

Kokoska, E. R., Keller, M. S., & Weber, T. (2001). Outcome of the antegrade colonic enema procedure in children with chronic constipation. *American Journal of Surgery, 182*(6), 625–629.

Lee, S. L., DuBois, J. J., Montes-Garces, R. G., et al. (2002). Surgical management of chronic unremitting constipation and fecal incontinence associated with megarectum: A preliminary report. *Journal of Pediatric Surgery, 37*(1), 76–79.

Levine, M. (1982). Encopresis: Its potential, evaluation, and alleviation. *Pediatric Clinics of North America, 29*(2), 315–329.

Leung, M. W. Y., Wong, B. P. Y., Leung, A. K. P., et al. (2006). Electrical stimulation and biofeedback exercise of pelvic floor muscle for children with fecal incontinence after surgery for anorectal malformation. *Pediatric Surgery International, 22*, 975–978.

Loening-Baucke, V., Miele, E., & Staiano, A. (2004). Fiber (Glucomannan) is beneficial in the treatment of childhood constipation. *Pediatrics, 113*(3), e259–e264.

Ludman, L., & Spitz, L. (1996). Coping strategies of children with fecal incontinence. *Journal of Pediatric Surgery, 31*(4), 563–567.

Lynch, A. C., Beasley, S. W., Robertson, R. W., et al (1999). Comparison of results of laparoscopic and open antegrade continence enema procedures. *Pediatric Clinics of North America, 15*, 343–346.

MacLeod, J. (1998). Fecal incontinence: A practical program of management. *Endoscopy Review, 5*(Nov–Dec), 45–56.

Malone, P., Ransley, P., & Kiely, E. (1990). Preliminary report: The antegrade continence enema. *Lancet, 336*, 1217–1218.

Mazier, W., Levien, D., Luchtefeld, M., et al. (1995). *Surgery of the colon, rectum, and anus.* Philadelphia, PA: WB Saunders.

Michaud, P. A., Suris, J. C., & Viner, R. (2007). *The adolescent with a chronic condition.* (Discussion Paper.). Geneva, Switzerland: World Health Organization.

Mikkelsen, E. J. (2001). Enuresis and encopresis: Ten years of progress. *Journal of the American Academy of Child and Adolescent Psychiatry, 40*, 1146–1158.

Molnar, G. (1985). *Pediatric rehabilitation.* Baltimore, MD: Williams & Wilkins.

Nolan, T., & Oberklaid, F. (1993). New concepts in the management of encopresis. *Pediatrics in Review, 14*(11), 447–451.

Nurko, S., Youssef, N. N., Sabri, M., et al. (2008). PEG3350 in the treatment of childhood constipation: A multicenter, double-blinded, placebo-controlled trial. *The Journal of Pediatrics, 153*, 254–261.

O'Rorke, C. (1995). Helping children overcome fecal incontinence. *American Journal of Nursing, 95*, 16. A-B.

Pashankar, D. S., Bishop, W. P., & Loening-Baucke, V. (2003). Long-term efficacy of polyethylene glycol 3350 for the treatment of chronic constipation in children with and without encopresis. *Clinical Pediatrics, 42*, 815–819.

Poenaru, D., Roblin, N., Bird, M., et al. (1997). The pediatric bowel management clinic: Initial results of a multidisciplinary approach to functional constipation in children. *Journal of Pediatric Surgery, 32*(6), 843–848.

Rao, S. S. C., Welcher, K. D., & Happel, J. (1996). Can biofeedback therapy improve anorectal function in fecal incontinence? *The American Journal of Gastroenterology, 91*(11), 2360–2365.

Reid, H., Bahar, R. J. (2006). Treatment of encopresis and chronic constipation in young children: Clinical results from interactive parent–child guidance. *Clinical Pediatrics, 45*, 157–164.

Rowe, M., O'Neill, J., Grosfeld, J., et al. (1995). *Essentials of pediatric surgery.* St. Louis, MO: Mosby.

Roy, C., Silverman, A., & Alagille, D. (1995). *Pediatric clinical gastroenterology.* St. Louis, MO: Mosby.

Schmitt, B. D., & Mauro, R. (1992). 20 common errors in treating encopresis. *Contemporary Pediatrics, May*, 47–65.

Schonwald, A., & Rappaport, L. (2004). Encopresis: Assessment and management. *Pediatrics in Review, 25*(8), 278–283.

Seth, R., & Heyman, M. (1994). Management of constipation and encopresis in infants and children. *Gastroenterology Clinics of North America, 23*(4), 621–636.

Smith, E. (1987). The bath water needs changing, but don't throw out the baby: An overview of anorectal anomalies. *Journal of Pediatric Surgery, 22*(4), 335–348.

Smith, K. (1991). Myelomeningocele: Managing bowel and bladder dysfunction in the school-aged child. *Progressions, 3*(2), 3–11.

Sprague-McRae, J. M. (1990). Encopresis: Developmental, behavioral, and physiological considerations for treatment. *The Nurse Practitioner, 15*(6), 8–24.

Stadtler, A. (1989). Preventing encopresis. *Pediatric Nursing, 15*(3), 282–284.

Steinberg, L. (2008). *Adolescence* (8th ed.). New York, NY: McGraw-Hill.

Stern, P., Lowitz, G., Prince, M., et al. (1988). The incidence of cognitive dysfunction in an encopretic population in children. *Neurotoxicology, 9*(3), 351–358.

Thies, K. M., & McAllister, J. W. (2001). The health and education leadership project: A school initiative for children and adolescents with chronic health conditions. *The Journal of School Health, 71*(5), 167–172.

Thomas, R., & Chandler, B. (2007). Management of bowel dysfunction in neurological rehabilitation—A review. *Critical Review in Physical and Rehabilitation Medicine, 19*(4), 251–274.

Walker, W. A., Durie, P. R., Hamilton, J. R., et al. (1990) *Pediatric gastrointestinal disease, Vol.* (1st ed.). Philadelphia, PA: BC Decker.

Walker, W. A., Durie, P. R., Hamilton, J. R., et al. (1996). *Pediatric gastrointestinal disease, Vol. 2* (2nd ed.). St. Louis, MO: Mosby.

Yerkes, E. B., Rink, R. C., King, S., et al. (2001). Tap water and the Malone Antegrade Continence enema: A safe combination? *The Journal of Urology, 166*, 1476–1147.

Youseff, N. N., & Di Lorenzo, C. (2001). Childhood constipation evaluation and treatment. *Journal of Clinical Gastroenterology, 33*, 199–205.

QUESTIONS

1. A continence nurse is assessing an infant who is diagnosed with obstruction due to "failure to recanalize the lumen." Complete obstruction of the lumen is known as:
   A. Atresia
   B. Stenosis
   C. Cysts
   D. Intestinal duplication

2. Congenital anorectal defects such as imperforate anus occur when which developmental sequence is interrupted or altered?
   A. Development of patent lumen
   B. Development of the midgut
   C. Development of the hindgut
   D. Separation between the gastrointestinal and genitourinary systems

3. The continence nurse is counseling the parents of a 5-year-old male who has fecal incontinence not caused by an organic or anatomic lesion. What is the term for this condition?
   A. Chronic diarrhea
   B. Fecal soiling
   C. Encopresis
   D. Functional constipation

4. What test might the continence nurse order to determine whether a child who has functional constipation empties his bladder?
   A. Laboratory tests
   B. Ultrasound
   C. Barium enema
   D. Lumbosacral spine film

5. What is the primary goal for initial management of retentive encopresis?
   A. Finding the underlying cause
   B. Establishing a reward/punishment system
   C. Choosing a medication regimen
   D. Education followed by "cleanout"

6. The continence nurse is teaching the parents of a 6-year-old encopretic child how many grams of fiber the child should consume each day. What amount is recommended?
   A. 11 g
   B. 12 g
   C. 14 g
   D. 15 g

7. What is the primary focus when treating secondary nonretentive encopresis?
   A. Finding the organic problem causing the encopresis
   B. Adding fiber to the diet
   C. Resolving psychological issues that triggered encopresis
   D. Choosing a laxative that is effective

8. Which GI disorder results in loss of peristalsis causing a functional obstruction and dilation of the proximal segment?
   A. Hirschsprung's disease
   B. Imperforate anus
   C. Spina bifida
   D. Cerebral palsy

9. A continence nurse is assessing a child diagnosed with myasthenia gravis. What is the location of this neuromuscular disorder?
   A. Cerebral cortex
   B. Neuromuscular junction
   C. Spinal cord
   D. Muscles

10. The continence nurse examining an adolescent with neurogenic bowel notes "flat buttocks." What condition would the nurse suspect?
    A. Spina bifida
    B. Sacral agenesis
    C. Meningitis
    D. Meningomyelocele

11. The continence nurse documents "patulous" anus upon assessment of an adolescent with neurogenic bowel. What bowel disorder does this condition indicate?
    A. Perianal fissure
    B. Incontinence-associated dermatitis
    C. Internal hemorrhoids
    D. Sphincter muscle laxity

12. What test is usually performed at the time of diagnosis for Hirschsprung's disease in an infant?
    A. CT scans
    B. MRI studies
    C. Defecography
    D. Rectal biopsy and/or barium enema

13. An adolescent with a neurogenic bowel is scheduled for surgery to place a low-profile device into the tract between the abdominal wall and the bowel to administer antegrade washouts and produce colonic emptying. What is the name of this surgical technique?
    A. Pull-through procedure
    B. Bowel resection
    C. Cecostomy button
    D. Colostomy

ANSWERS: 1.**A**, 2.**D**, 3.**C**, 4.**B**, 5.**D**, 6.**A**, 7.**C**, 8.**A**, 9.**B**, 10.**B**, 11.**D**, 12.**D**, 13.**C**

ART CREDITS

Chapter 1

Figure 1-1. Tank, P. W., & Gest, T. R. (2009). *Lippincott Williams & Wilkins Atlas of anatomy.* Baltimore, MD: Wolters Kluwer Health.

Figures 1-2 and 1-3. Asset provided by Anatomical Chart Co.

Figure 1-4. Oatis, C. A. (2004). *Kinesiology—The mechanics and pathomechanics of human movement.* Baltimore, MD: Lippincott Williams & Wilkins.

Figure 1-5A. Premkumar, K. (2004). *The massage connection anatomy and physiology.* Baltimore, MD: Lippincott Williams & Wilkins.

Figure 1-5B. Ferri, F. F., & Fretwell, M. D. (1992). *Practical guide to the care of the geriatric patient* (2nd ed.). St. Louis, MO: CV Mosby; Andersson, K. E., & Wein, A. J. (2004). Pharmacology of the lower urinary tract: basis for current and future treatments of urinary incontinence. *Pharmacological Reviews, 56,* 581.

Chapter 4

Figure 4-1. Goroll, A. H., & Mulley, A. G. (2009). *Primary care medicine.* Philadelphia, PA: Lippincott Williams & Wilkins.

Figure 4-4. Frontera, W. R. (2010). *DeLisa's physical medicine and rehabilitation.* Philadelphia, PA: Lippincott Williams & Wilkins.

Figures 4-7, 4-8, 4-10, 4-11, 4-12, and 4-13. Courtesy of LABORIE.

Figure 4-14. Adapted from DeLancey, J. O. (1986). Correlative study of paraurethral anatomy. *Obstetrics and Gynecology, 68,* 91–97, with permission.

Figure 4-16. Berek, J. S. (2011). *Berek and Novak's gynecology.* Philadelphia, PA: Lippincott Williams & Wilkins.

Chapter 5

Figures 5-1 and 5-2. Reproduced with permission from 3rd ICI 2005.

Figure 5-3. Porth, C. (2010). *Essentials of pathophysiology.* Philadelphia, PA: Lippincott Williams & Wilkins.

Figures 5-4 and 5-5. Berek, J. S. (2011). *Berek and Novak's gynecology.* Philadelphia, PA: Lippincott Williams & Wilkins.

Figure 5-7. Nitti, V. W. (2006). Botulinum toxin for the treatment of idiopathic and neurogenic overactive bladder: State of the art. *Reviews in Urology, 8*(4), 198–208.

Figure 5-8A and B. Schrier, R. W. (2006). *Diseases of the kidney and urinary tract.* Philadelphia, PA: Lippincott Williams & Wilkins.

Figure 5-8C. Keighley, M. R. B., & Williams, N. S. (2008). *Surgery of the anus, rectum, and colon* (3rd ed.). Philadelphia, PA: W.B. Saunders, with permission.

Figure 5-9. After Sheldon, C. A., & Bukowski, T. (1995). Bladder function. In: M. I. Rowe, J. A. O'Neal, J. L. Grosfeld, et al. (Eds.), *Essentials of pediatric surgery.* St. Louis, MO: Mosby-Year Book, with permission.

Chapter 6

Figure 6-2. Anatomical Chart Company. Philadelphia, PA: Lippincott Williams & Wilkins, 2000.

Figure 6-3. Based on American Urological Association. (2003). *Guideline on the management of benign prostatic hyperplasia (BPH).* Linthicum, MD: American Urological Association Education and Research, Inc., with permission.

Figure 6-4. McConnell, T. H. (2013). *Nature of disease.* Philadelphia, PA: Lippincott Williams & Wilkins.

Figure 6-5. Schrier, R. W. (2006). *Diseases of the kidney and urinary tract.* Philadelphia, PA: Lippincott Williams & Wilkins.

Figures 6-7 and 6-8. Shiv Kumar Pandian and Marcus John Drake, Bristol Urological Institute.

Figure 6-9. Provenzale, J. M., Nelson, R. C., & Vinson, E. N. (2011). *Duke radiology case review.* Philadelphia, PA: Lippincott Williams & Wilkins.

Figure 6-10. Diepenbrock, N. H. (2011). *Quick reference to critical care.* Philadelphia, PA: Lippincott Williams & Wilkins.

Figure 6-11. Simon, R. R., Ross, C., Bowman, S. H., et al. (2011). *Cook county manual of emergency procedures.* Philadelphia, PA: Lippincott Williams & Wilkins.

Figure 6-12. Rosdahl, C. B., & Kowalski, M. T. (2011). *Textbook of basic nursing.* Philadelphia, PA: Lippincott Williams & Wilkins.

Chapter 7

Figure 7-1. Modified from McConnell, T. H., & Hull, K. L. (2010). *Human form, human function: Essentials of anatomy & physiology.* Philadelphia, PA: Lippincott Williams & Wilkins.

Chapter 8

Figure 8-1. Timby, B. K., & Smith, N. E. (2009). *Introductory medical-surgical nursing.* Philadelphia, PA: Lippincott Williams & Wilkins.

Figure 8-2. Agur, A. M., & Dalley, A. F. (2012). *Grant's atlas of anatomy.* Philadelphia, PA: Lippincott Williams & Wilkins.

Figure 8-3. LifeART image copyright (c) 2015. Lippincott Williams & Wilkins. All rights reserved.

Figure 8-4. Agur, A. M., & Dalley, A. F. (2009). *Grant's atlas of anatomy.* Philadelphia, PA: Lippincott Williams & Wilkins. (Figure taken from Gee, W. F., & Ansell, J. S. (1990). Pelvic and perineal pain of urologic origin. In: J. J. Bonica (Ed.), *The management of pain* (pp. 1368–1394). Philadelphia, PA: Lea & Febiger.)

Figure 8-5. LifeART image copyright (c) 2015. Lippincott Williams & Wilkins. All rights reserved.

Figure 8-6. Based on American Urological Association. (2003). *Guideline on the management of benign prostatic hyperplasia (BPH).* Linthicum, MD: American Urological Association Education and Research, Inc., with permission.

Figures 8-7 and 8-9. Arcangelo, V. P., & Peterson, A. M. (2011). *Pharmacotherapeutics for advanced practice.* Philadelphia, PA: Lippincott Williams & Wilkins.

Figure 8-8. *Stedman's medical terminology.* Philadelphia, PA: Lippincott Williams & Wilkins, 2010.

Figure 8-10. Kassirer, J. P., Wong, J. B., & Kopelman, R. I. (2009). *Learning clinical reasoning.* Philadelphia, PA: Lippincott Williams & Wilkins.

Figure 8-11. Adapted from Thompson, I. M., Pauler, D. K., Goodman, P. J., et al. (2004). Prevalence of prostate cancer among men with a prostate-specific antigen level < 4.0 ng per milliliter. *New England Journal of Medicine, 350,* 2239, with permission.

Figure 8-12. Washington University School of Medicine Department of Medicine; De Fer, T. M., Brisco, M. A., & Mullur, R. S. (2010). *Washington manual of outpatient internal medicine.* Philadelphia, PA: Lippincott Williams & Wilkins.

Figure 8-13. Willis, M. C., & CMA-AC. (2002). *Medical terminology: A programmed learning approach to the language of health care.* Baltimore, MD: Lippincott Williams & Wilkins.

Figure 8-14. Rubin, P., & Hansen, J. T. (2012). *TNM staging atlas with oncoanatomy.* Philadelphia, PA: Lippincott Williams & Wilkins.

Figure 8-15. Rubin, R., Strayer, D. S., & Rubin, E. (2011). *Rubin's pathology.* Philadelphia, PA: Lippincott Williams & Wilkins.

Figure 8-16. Rhoades, R. A., & Bell, D. R. (2012). *Medical physiology: Principles for clinical medicine* (4th ed.). Philadelphia, PA: Lippincott Williams & Wilkins.

Figure 8-17. Farrell, M., & Dempsey, J. (2010). *Smeltzer and Bare's textbook of medical-surgical nursing.* Philadelphia, PA: Lippincott Williams & Wilkins.

Chapter 9

Figure 9-1. Delancey, J. (1994). Structural support of the urethra as it relates to stress urinary incontinence: the hammock hypothesis. *American Journal of Obstetrics and Gynecology, 170,* 1718, with permission.

Figure 9-2. Brody, L. T. & Hall, C. M. (2010). *Therapeutic exercise.* Philadelphia, PA: Lippincott Williams & Wilkins.

Figure 9-3 and 9-5. Weber, J. R., & Kelley, J. H. (2013). *Health assessment in nursing.* Philadelphia, PA: Lippincott Williams & Wilkins.

Figure 9-4. LifeART image copyright (c) 2014. Lippincott Williams & Wilkins.

Figure 9-6. Stephenson, S. R. (2012). *Diagnostic medical sonography.* Philadelphia, PA: Lippincott Williams & Wilkins.

Figure 9-7. Brody, L. T., & Hall, C. M. (2010). *Therapeutic exercise.* Philadelphia, PA: Lippincott Williams & Wilkins.

Figure 9-8. Leyendecker, J. R., & Brown, J. J. (2004). *Practical guide to abdominal and pelvic MRI.* Philadelphia, PA: Lippincott Williams & Wilkins.

Figure 9-9. Gibbs, R. S., Karlan, B. Y., Haney, A. F., et al. (2008). *Danforth's obstetrics and gynecology.* Philadelphia, PA: Lippincott Williams & Wilkins.

Figures 9-10 and 9-17. Farrell, M., & Dempsey, J. (2010). *Smeltzer and Bare's textbook of medical-surgical nursing.* Philadelphia, PA: Lippincott Williams & Wilkins.

Figure 9-11. Robert Kovac, S. (2012). *Advances in reconstructive vaginal surgery.* Philadelphia, PA: Lippincott Williams & Wilkins.

Figure 9-12. Redrawn from original by Jasmine Tan.

Figure 9-13. Carter, P. J. (2011). *Lippincott textbook for nursing assistants.* Philadelphia, PA: Lippincott Williams & Wilkins.

Figure 9-14. Martius, H. R. (1956). *Martius' gynecological operations, with emphasis on topographic anatomy* (p. 173). Boston, MA: Little, Brown, and Company. Bolten, K. A., McCall, M. L., translators.

Figure 9-15. Bickley, L. S., & Szilagyi, P. (2003). *Bates' guide to physical examination and history taking* (8th ed.). Philadelphia, PA: Lippincott Williams & Wilkins.

Figure 9-16. Bump, R. C., Mattiason, A., Bo, K., et al. (1996). The standardization of terminology of female pelvic organ prolapse and pelvic floor dysfunction. *American Journal of Obstetrics and Gynecology, 175*, 12, with permission.

Chapter 10

Figure 10-1. Adapted from Administration on Aging, A Profile of Older Americans: 20132014, 06/24, http://www.aoa.gov/Aging_Statistics/Profile/Index.aspx

Figure 10-2. Adapted from Centers for Medicare and Medicaid Services.

Figure 10-3. Adapted from Wagg, A., Gibson, W., Ostaszkiewicz, J., et al. (2014). Urinary incontinence in frail elderly persons: Report from the 5th International Consultation on Incontinence. *Neurourology and Urodynamics*, Wiley Periodicals, Inc.

Chapter 11

Figure 11-1. Licensed under the Creative Commons Attribution-Share Alike 2.5 Generic, 2.0 Generic and 1.0 Generic license, Wikimedia Commons.

Figure 11-2. Courtesy of Paul S. Matz, MD.

Figures 11-3 and 11-6. Fleisher, G. R., & Ludwig. S. (2010). *Textbook of pediatric emergency medicine.* Philadelphia, PA: Lippincott Williams & Wilkins.

Figure 11-4. Farrell, M., & Dempsey, J. (2010). *Smeltzer and Bare's textbook of medical-surgical nursing.* Philadelphia, PA: Lippincott Williams & Wilkins.

Figure 11-5. Images A and B courtesy of Philips Medical Systems, Bothell, WA; Images C–F courtesy of Dr. Nakul Jerath, Falls Church, VA; Images G and H courtesy of Rechelle Nguyen, Columbus, OH.

Figure 11-7. Constipation Guideline Committee of the North American Society for Pediatric Gastroenterology, Hepatology and Nutrition. (2006). Evaluation and treatment of constipation in infants and children: Recommendations of the North American Society for Pediatric Gastroenterology, Hepatology and Nutrition. *Journal of Pediatric Gastroenterology and Nutrition, 43*(3), e1–e13.

Figure 11-8. From Saxton, H. M., Borzyskowski, M., & Robinson, L. B. (1992). Nonobstructive posterior urethral widening (spinning top urethra) in boys with bladder instability. *Radiology, 182*, 81, with permission.

Figure 11-9. Sweet, M. G., Schmidt-Dalton, T. A., Weiss, P. M., et al. (2012). Evaluation and management of abnormal uterine bleeding in premenopausal women. *American Family Physician, 85*, 35–43.

Figure 11-10. Berek, J. S. (2011). *Berek and Novak's gynecology.* Philadelphia, PA: Lippincott Williams & Wilkins.

Figure 11-11. Schrier, R. W. (2006). *Diseases of the kidney and urinary tract.* Philadelphia, PA: Lippincott Williams & Wilkins.

Chapter 13

Figure 13-1. Craven, R. F., Hirnle, C. J., & Jensen, S. (2012). *Fundamentals of nursing.* Philadelphia, PA: Lippincott Williams & Wilkins.

Figure 13-2. Diepenbrock, N. H. (2011). *Quick reference to critical care.* Philadelphia, PA: Lippincott Williams & Wilkins.

Figure 13-4. LeBlanc, K., & Christensen, D. (2005). *Journal of Wound, Ostomy, & Continence Nursing, 32*(2), 131–134.

Figure 13-5. Gehrig, J. S., & Willmann, D. E. (2011). *Foundations of periodontics for the dental hygienist.* Philadelphia, PA: Lippincott Williams & Wilkins.

Figure 13-6. Centers for Disease Control and Prevention Public Health Images Library. No. 7488. Courtesy of Rodney M. Donlan, Janice Carr.'

Figure 13-7. Harvey, R. A., & Cornelissen, C. N. (2012). *Microbiology.* Philadelphia, PA: Lippincott Williams & Wilkins.

Figure 13-8. Loiselle, C. G., Profetto-McGrath, J., Polit, D. F., et al. (2010). *Canadian essentials of nursing research.* Philadelphia, PA: Lippincott Williams & Wilkins.

Figure 13-10. Illustration by Janna Linsenmeyer.

Figure 13-11. Timby, B. K., & Smith, N. E. (2009). *Introductory medical-surgical nursing.* Philadelphia, PA: Lippincott Williams & Wilkins.

Figure 13-12. Nettina, S. M. (2001). *The Lippincott manual of nursing practice* (7th ed.). Philadelphia, PA: Lippincott Williams & Wilkins.

Figure 13-14. Lippincott Professional Development. Lippincott Williams & Wilkins, 2014.

Figure 13-15. Lynn, P. (2010). *Taylor's clinical nursing skills.* Philadelphia, PA: Lippincott Williams & Wilkins.

Chapter 14

Figures 14-1 and 14-2B. Moore, K. L., Agur, A. M., & Dalley, A. F. (2014). *Essential clinical anatomy.* Philadelphia, PA: Lippincott Williams & Wilkins.

Figure 14-2A. Tank, P. W., & Gest, T. R. (2009). *Lippincott Williams & Wilkins atlas of anatomy.* Baltimore, MD: Wolters Kluwer Health.

Figure 14-3. Pfeifer, S. M. (2011). *NMS obstetrics and gynecology.* Philadelphia, PA: Lippincott Williams & Wilkins.

Figure 14-4. Agur, A. M., & Dalley, A. F. (2012). *Grant's atlas of anatomy.* Philadelphia, PA: Lippincott Williams & Wilkins.

Figure 14-5. Moore, K. L., Agur, A. M. R., & Dalley, A. F. (2013). *Clinically oriented anatomy.* Philadelphia, PA: Lippincott Williams & Wilkins.

Figure 14-6. Moore, K. L., Dalley, A. F., & Agur, A. M. (2009). *Clinically oriented anatomy.* Philadelphia, PA: Lippincott Williams & Wilkins.

Figure 14-7. Reprinted with permission from Cormack, D. H. (2001). *Essential histology* (2nd ed.). Philadelphia, PA: Lippincott Williams & Wilkins.

Figure 14-8. Preston, R. R., & Wilson, T. (2012). *Physiology.* Philadelphia, PA: Lippincott Williams & Wilkins.

Figure 14-9. Corman, M., Nicholls, R. J., Fazio, V. W., et al. (2012). *Corman's colon and rectal surgery.* Philadelphia, PA: Lippincott Williams & Wilkins.

Chapter 15

Figure 15-2. American College of Gastroenterology Task Force on Irritable Bowel Syndrome, et al. (2009). An evidence-based position statement on the management of irritable bowel syndrome. *American Journal of Gastroenterology, 104*(Suppl 1), S1; Pimentel, M., et al.

(2011). Rifaximin therapy for patients with irritable bowel syndrome without constipation. *New England Journal of Medicine, 364,* 22.

Chapter 16

Figure 16-2. Evans-Smith, 2005.

Figure 16-3. Reprinted with permission from ConvaTec, Inc.

Figure 16-4. Corman, M., Nicholls, R. J., Fazio, V. W., et al. (2012). *Corman's colon and rectal surgery.* Philadelphia, PA: Lippincott Williams & Wilkins.

Chapter 17

Figure 17-1. Domino, F. J., Baldor, R. A., Grimes, J. A., et al. (2014). *5-Minute clinical consult standard 2015.* Philadelphia, PA: Lippincott Williams & Wilkins.

Figure 17-2. Crocetti, M., & Barone, M. A. (2004). *Oski's essential pediatrics.* Philadelphia, PA: Lippincott Williams & Wilkins.

Figure 17-3. Reproduced with permission from Pillitteri, A. (2003). *Maternal and child nursing* (4th ed.). Philadelphia, PA: Lippincott Williams & Wilkins.

Figure 17-4. Werner, R. (2012). *Massage therapist's guide to pathology.* Philadelphia, PA: Lippincott Williams & Wilkins.

Figure 17-5. Keighley, M. R. B., & Williams, N. S. (2008). *Surgery of the anus, rectum, and colon* (3rd ed.). Philadelphia, PA: W.B. Saunders, with permission.

GLOSSARY

Abdominal leak point pressure level of intra-abdominal pressure required to push urine through a partially closed sphincter; measurement obtained during filling cystometry by having patient perform various coughing or straining measures to determine abdominal pressure at which leakage occurs

Ablative techniques used for BPH and involve the use of lasers to vaporize prostatic tissue

Acetylcholine major parasympathetic neurotransmitter; mediates detrusor muscle contraction

Active surveillance conservative approach to management of localized prostate cancer in which active treatment is deferred and the patient undergoes routine monitoring for any evidence of disease progression, at which time treatment can be initiated (just in time treatment)

Acute diarrhea diarrheal episodes lasting <14 days

American Spinal Injury Association (ASIA) a system to classify the severity of the impairment associated with SCI; ASIA A SCI is a "complete injury" with no sensory or motor function below the level of the SCI; ASIA B SCI is defined as "sensory incomplete" with preservation of sensory but no motor function below the level of the injury

Acute/transient urinary incontinence newly occurring urinary incontinence of relatively sudden onset; typically <6 months in duration; caused by reversible factors

Acute urinary retention painful, palpable, or percussible bladder in patient who is unable to pass urine

Alpha-adrenergic agonists medications that increase tone in bladder neck and proximal urethra, thereby increasing bladder outlet resistance

Alpha-adrenergic antagonists medications that reduce tone in the bladder neck and proximal urethra, thus reducing bladder outlet resistance

Anal bulking agents biomaterials that can be injected into the sphincter muscle or submucosal tissue to supplement internal anal sphincter (IAS) function

Anal incontinence (flatus incontinence) involuntary loss of flatus without loss of mucus or stool

Anal verge dividing line between squamous epithelium of anal canal (anoderm) and perianal skin

Anal wink (anocutaneous reflex) reflex contraction of external anal sphincter (EAS) in response to stroking of perianal skin at 3 o'clock and 9 o'clock; indicates intact pudendal nerve pathways

Anorectal angle 90-degree angle between rectum and anal canal that is created by the "sling-like" effect of the puborectalis muscle and that promotes fecal continence; with straining, angle is increased to 135 degrees, which promotes stool elimination

Anorectal manometry diagnostic test that measures resting and squeeze pressures in anal canal as well as assessment of rectal capacity and distensibility

Antegrade continence enema (ACE) procedure (also known as Malone antegrade continence enema, or MACE procedure) surgical procedure in which small stoma is created between the abdominal wall and proximal colon; permits antegrade "washouts" that can be used to manage chronic refractory constipation or fecal incontinence due to neurogenic bowel

Anticholinergic/antimuscarinic medications that reduce urinary urgency and increase bladder storage capacity by blocking the activation of cholinergic/muscarinic receptors in the urothelium and detrusor

Artificial anal sphincter surgical placement of inflatable cuff around the anal sphincter; cuff connected to reservoir implanted in groin and manually operated pump placed in scrotum or labia. When cuff is inflated, anal canal is closed; when defecation is desired, the fluid is transferred to the reservoir via manual activation of the pump, which opens the anal canal

Atresia complete obstruction of bowel lumen

Atrophic urethritis/vaginitis thinning and drying of urethral and vaginal epithelium due to estrogen deficiency

Asymptomatic bacteriuria (ASB) all individuals with catheters will develop significant microbial colonization within a few days; ASB does not produce symptoms and does not require treatment

AUA symptom score (see IPSS)

Augmentation cystoplasty surgical procedure that uses segment of small bowel to enlarge bladder and increase bladder capacity

Balanced bladder one that empties completely and is not associated with recurring UTI or upper urinary tract distress; an imbalanced bladder does not empty completely and is associated with recurring UTI and/or upper urinary tract distress

Biofeedback use of visual or auditory feedback to improve awareness of physiologic activities; may be used in conjunction with pelvic muscle exercise program to improve sensory awareness, pelvic muscle strength and function, and/or coordination between abdominal and pelvic floor muscles

Bladder diary record of voiding and leakage episodes and associated symptoms; some diaries include record of fluid intake (type and amount)

Bladder retraining program behavioral therapy that involves gradual lengthening of voiding interval with the use of behavioral strategies to control urgency

Bladder–sphincter coordination sphincter relaxation prior to detrusor contraction; controlled by central nervous system and pontine micturition center

Bladder wall compliance the relationship between bladder volume and intravesical pressure during bladder filling/ storage; normal function is characterized by a distensible bladder that fills with minimal increase in intravesical pressure

Blue Pads disposable underpads used as temporary protection for chairs and beds during clinical procedures; they are not to be used as incontinence pads; lack an absorbent filling and can allow pooling of urine on the thin plastic surface, placing the individual at risk of skin wetness and skin breakdown

Bowel diary record of stool elimination that documents time, volume, and consistency of voluntary and involuntary stools, as well as associated symptoms (and possibly diet and fluid intake)

Brachytherapy a definitive treatment for Stage I prostate cancer that involves permanent placement of radioactive seeds into or near the tumor

BPH an increase in the size of the prostate due to unregulated proliferation of connective tissue, smooth muscle, and glandular epithelium. This mass effect is static and causes direct bladder outlet obstruction

Bulbocavernosus reflex (BCR) anal contraction in response to tapping of the clitoris or squeezing of the glans; one indication of intact neurologic pathways between the sacral cord and pelvic floor

C-fibers nerve fibers present in bladder wall that transmit signals of severe discomfort or pain; activated by extreme distention, inflammation of bladder wall, or noxious substances in urine

Chronic diarrhea diarrhea persisting >30 days

Chronic urinary incontinence urinary incontinence that lasts >6 months despite correction of reversible factors

Chronic urinary retention nonpainful bladder that remains palpable or percussible after the patient has passed urine

Closing reflex brief increase in external anal sphincter (EAS) activity that occurs following stool evacuation; triggers anal canal closure

Colonic transit time time required for liquid stool to pass through the colon and to be evacuated per anus

Compliance ability of bladder (or rectum) to distend with urine or stool while maintaining low intravesical (or intrarectal) pressures

Complete fecal incontinence involuntary passage of formed stool

Continent catheterizable stoma construction reconstructive procedure designed for persons who experience difficulty with CIC owing to urethral obstruction or prior urethral surgery, discomfort associated with catheterization, or the lack of mobility and dexterity required for urethral catheterization

Constipation difficult defecation characterized by one or more of the following: hard or dry stools; reduced frequency of stool elimination; sensation of incomplete evacuation following a bowel movement; or pain or straining associated with stool elimination

Coudé-tipped catheters have an angled tip and are useful for men with prostatic hypertrophy and mild obstruction as they slip around the prostatic curve more readily than a straight catheter

Defecography simulation of defecation using radiopaque stool substitute and fluoroscopic imaging

Delirium transient (reversible) alteration in mental status/cognition

Dementia irreversible decline in cognitive function

Dentate line midpoint of anal canal; above this point, anal canal is lined with columnar epithelium, and distal to this point, it is lined with squamous epithelium, which is richly innervated with sensory receptors (anoderm)

Detrusor smooth muscle of bladder

Detrusor overactivity involuntary contractions of detrusor muscle that occur during filling phase of urodynamic study

Detrusor sphincter dyssynergia failure of sphincter relaxation in response to detrusor contraction; creates significant risk for upper tract dysfunction

Detrusor underactivity weak and/or poorly sustained bladder muscle contraction resulting in prolonged flow of urine and possibly incomplete bladder emptying

Diarrhea alteration in bowel elimination characterized by increase in both frequency and volume of stools and reduced consistency of stool, as compared to individual's normal bowel elimination patterns

DIPPERS an acronym often used to help guide assessment of reversible factors contributing to urinary incontinence: delirium, infection, pharmaceuticals, psychological, excess urine output, mobility, stool impaction

Dysfunctional voiding abnormal voiding pattern characterized by intermittent flow pattern, intermittent detrusor contractions, and increased pelvic floor/ sphincter activity during voiding in neurologically intact individual

Dysfunctional Voiding Symptoms Score an assessment tool used to assess the impact of dysfunctional voiding on the individual's quality of life, and to track progress with treatment

Electromyography neurologic exam of pelvic floor nerve/muscle function using either surface electrodes or needle electrodes

Encopresis fecal soiling usually associated with functional constipation; fecal incontinence in children not caused by an organic or anatomic lesion. May be classified as "primary" (child >4 years of age who has never achieved bowel control) or "secondary" (child who was continent of stool for at least 1 year and has relapsed due to some secondary condition). Also classified as retentive and nonretentive

Enuresis categorized as monosymptomatic (no urinary symptoms and normal urinalysis) or nonmonosymptomatic (coexisting symptoms of lower urinary tract dysfunction)

Endoanal ultrasound use of transducer emitting sound waves to create image of anal sphincters and to identify any structural abnormalities

Endopelvic fascia layer of pelvic floor comprised of collagen, elastin, and smooth muscle that connects pelvic organs to bony pelvis

Enteric nervous system intraintestinal nervous system that consists of sensory receptors, motor neurons, and interneurons located in Meissner's and myenteric (Auerbach's) plexuses; mediates peristaltic activity in response to stretch and tension in bowel wall and intraluminal substances/irritants

External anal sphincter sphincter composed of both striated and smooth muscles that overlaps internal anal sphincter and terminates at anus; striated muscle component under voluntary control and permits individual to delay defecation; smooth muscle component controlled by enteric and autonomic nervous systems

External beam radiation therapy (EBRT) a curative treatment for Stage I prostate cancer that is generally recommended to men who are poor surgical candidates for radical prostatectomy

External urethral sphincter (rhabdosphincter) striated muscle located at midurethra in women and just distal to prostate gland in men innervated by branches of pudendal nerve and under voluntary control

Extraurethral incontinence urinary leakage through channels other than the urethra, usually due to a fistula or ectopic ureter

Fast-twitch muscle fibers muscle fibers that provide rapid strong contractions; comprise 1/3 of pelvic floor muscle fibers

Fatty diarrhea diarrhea caused by malabsorption syndrome (e.g., lactose intolerance), surgical procedure resulting in malabsorption (e.g., gastric bypass), medications causing malabsorption, or specific parasitic infections (e.g., Giardia)

Fecal continence ability to control stool elimination; defecation that occurs at socially appropriate place and time

Fecal incontinence accidental (involuntary) passage of stool or gas at undesirable time or place; inability to control evacuation of stool at socially appropriate place and time

Fiber (dietary fiber and fiber supplements) foods and supplements that promote normal microbial balance in colon, add water and bulk to stool, and may reduce transit time. Classified as soluble (fiber that dissolves in water) versus insoluble (fiber that does not dissolve in water) and fermentable (fiber that is broken down by bacteria and produces gas) versus nonfermentable (fiber that is not broken down by bacteria and does not produce gas)

Filling cystometry test that evaluates filling phase of micturition cycle and provides information re bladder capacity, sensory awareness, bladder wall compliance, and presence/absence of overactive bladder contractions. Involves placement of pressure-sensitive catheter into the bladder, followed by retrograde filling of the bladder

Frailty a medical syndrome with multiple causes and contributors that is characterized by diminished strength, endurance, and physiologic function and increases an individual's vulnerability for developing increased dependency and/or death

Functional bowel disorders disorders of bowel motility in which there is no structural or tissue abnormality to explain the symptoms; includes diarrhea, constipation, and irritable bowel syndrome

Functional constipation chronic constipation not caused by organic or anatomic abnormalities, or requirement for medication to regulate bowel function in child >4 years of age

Functional diarrhea diarrhea caused by motility disorder

Functional intervention training program in which caregivers incorporate musculoskeletal strengthening exercises into toileting routines

Functional urinary incontinence urinary leakage caused by factors outside the urinary tract that compromise the individual's ability to respond appropriately to signals of bladder filling (e.g., impaired mobility or cognitive impairment)

Gastrocolic reflex increase in peristaltic activity in response to food intake

Giggle incontinence a unique condition seen in girls where laughter triggers complete incontinence of urine

Gleason score index of prostate cancer aggressiveness, assigned by a pathologist grading each core sample on the 5-point Gleason scale that represents five histologic patterns of tumor gland formation and infiltration

Guarding reflex progressive "reflex" increase in outlet resistance in response to bladder filling

Habit retraining toileting program involving identification of the individual's toileting patterns via bladder diary, followed by establishment of toileting schedule based on that pattern

Hirschsprung's disease (aganglionic mega-colon) congenital absence of ganglion cells in bowel wall resulting in functional bowel obstruction due to absence of peristaltic activity in aganglionic section. Most cases are "short segment" (aganglionic segment limited to rectum or rectum and sigmoid); a small percentage involve greater lengths of the colon or, occasionally, the entire colon

Hostile bladder bladder outlet obstruction and risk to upper urinary tracts from elevated detrusor pressures and/or low bladder wall compliance in individuals with neurogenic bladder dysfunction

Ileocecal valve one-way valve located at the junction of the ileum and cecum that controls passage of stool from small bowel into colon and prevents retrograde flow of stool from colon into small intestine

Imperforate anus congenital anomaly involving distal colon/rectum and anal canal/sphincters; further classified as "high" or "low" lesion, depending on whether the distal end of the bowel terminates above or below the levator ani complex

Incontinence-associated dermatitis (IAD) skin damage caused by exposure to stool or urine

Infectious diarrhea diarrhea caused by pathogenic organisms (viruses, bacteria, parasites)

Intermittent catheterization (IC) the act of inserting and then removing the catheter once urine has drained via the urethra or other catheterizable channel such as a Mitrofanoff continent urinary diversion

Internal anal sphincter thick band of smooth muscle that is an extension of the circular muscle of the rectum; primary contributor to continence at rest; composed of slow-twitch muscle fibers innervated by enteric nervous system and autonomic nervous system; not under voluntary control

Internal bowel management system system designed to divert liquid stool away from perianal skin and into collection device; comprised of low-pressure intrarectal balloon, soft silicone tubing, and collection device

Internal urethral sphincter smooth muscle fibers within bladder neck that contribute to continence at rest; innervated by autonomic nervous system and not under voluntary control

International Prostate Symptom Score (IPSS) also known as the American Urologic Association score and one of the most common tools employed to assess LUTS in men

Irritable bowel syndrome (IBS) functional bowel disorder typified by abdominal pain or discomfort associated with alterations in bowel elimination and relieved by bowel movements; further classified as IBS-C (IBS associated with constipation); IBS-D (IBS associated with diarrhea); and IBS-M (IBS associated with alternating diarrhea and constipation)

Lamina propria suburothelial layer of bladder wall, located between urothelium and detrusor muscle; composed of interstitial cells, fibroblasts, blood vessels, and afferent/efferent nerves

Lapides Classification System classification system for neurogenic bladder dysfunction based on clinical and cystometric manifestations

Laxative agent that promotes bowel movements through a number of physiologic mechanisms: stool bulking, osmosis, and direct stimulation of peristalsis. Further classified as osmotic and stimulant laxatives

Levator ani primary muscle of pelvic floor; composed of three connected muscles (pubococcygeus, puborectalis, and ileococcygeus)

Lifestyle interventions weight loss, smoking cessation, bowel management, exercise, appropriate fluid intake, and reduced caffeine consumption

Lower urinary tract ureters, bladder, and urethra

Lower motor neuron neurogenic bladder a noncontracting (acontractile or areflexic) detrusor

Nicotinic receptors receptors that react to the neurotransmitter acetylcholine, resulting in contraction of the periurethral and rhabdosphincter muscles and closure of the sphincter mechanism

Lower urinary tract symptoms (LUTS) subjective indicators of lower urinary tract dysfunction. Divided into three (3) categories:

Storage LUTS frequency, urgency, dysuria, nocturnal polyuria, and leakage
Voiding LUTS hesitancy, poor or intermittent stream, straining to void, and terminal dribble
Postvoid LUTS postvoid dribbling and sensation of incomplete emptying

Magnetic artificial sphincter implantation of ring of magnetic titanium beads into anal sphincter, which holds walls of anal canal together in closed position until abdominal muscle contraction overrides the resistance and opens the anal canal

Mass movements series of peristaltic contractions that rapidly propel stool from transverse colon to rectum

Meissner's plexus nerve plexus located in submucosal layer of bowel wall; primary functions are to detect intraluminal substances, control GI blood flow, and regulate epithelial cell function

Mixed urinary incontinence (UI) mixed stress/urge UI; leakage of urine associated with activities that cause increase in intra-abdominal pressure in combination with leakage associated with urgency

Myenteric (Auerbach's) plexus nerve plexus located between longitudinal and circular muscle layers of bowel wall; plays primary role in regulating colonic motility

Neurogenic bladder lower urinary tract dysfunction caused by disturbance of neurologic control mechanisms (most commonly a lesion between the sacral cord and brain)

Neurogenic bowel loss of neural control of defecation; characterized by absent or markedly reduced ability to sense rectal distention and to voluntarily contract the external anal sphincter (EAS)

Neuromodulation therapeutic modality that uses electrical signals to alter involuntary reflexes of lower urinary tract, thus reducing involuntary detrusor contractions

Neurotransmitters chemical messengers that regulate detrusor relaxation and contraction and act at specific receptor sites on the smooth muscle

Nocturia waking at night one or more times to void

Nocturnal polyuria a condition in which the day/night ratio of urine production is reversed

Nonretentive encopresis fecal soiling not associated with stool-withholding behavior

Norepinephrine major sympathetic neurotransmitter; mediates sphincter contraction

Normal transit constipation constipation in individual with normal peristaltic response to stimuli such as colonic distention; caused by dietary/environmental factors leading to reduced peristaltic stimuli (e.g., small-caliber stools)

Obstructed defecation difficult elimination of stool caused by pathology involving the pelvic floor and anorectal junction

OnabotulinumtoxinA a pharmacologic agent to treat neurogenic detrusor overactivity; the neurotoxin is injected directly into the detrusor wall during a cystoscopic procedure

Onuf's nucleus collection of cells in sacral cord that receive input from pontine storage center and mediate contraction of striated sphincter via pudendal nerve

Osmotic diarrhea diarrhea caused by presence of high osmolar substances within the lumen of the bowel that pull fluid into gut

Osmotic laxative agent that "works" by pulling fluid into the lumen of the bowel, thus softening the stool and causing colonic distention and peristalsis

Overactive bladder symptom complex comprised of urinary urgency, with or without urgency incontinence, usually with increased daytime frequency and nocturia, in the absence of UTI or other obvious pathologies

Parasympathetic nervous system branch of autonomic nervous system; mediates detrusor muscle contraction and promotes intestinal peristaltic activity

Partial fecal incontinence (fecal leakage, fecal soiling, fecal seepage, anal leakage) leakage of small amounts of stool into undergarments

Passive fecal incontinence passage of stool or gas without awareness on the part of the individual; usually caused by cognitive impairment or sensorimotor dysfunction and ranges in severity from mild soiling to total evacuation of rectal contents

Pediatric Urinary Incontinence Quality of Life Score (PIN-Q) a questionnaire used to assess the impact the symptoms have on the child's quality of life and to track treatment progress

Pelvic floor network of fascia, ligaments, and muscles that support pelvic organs and oppose downward displacement

Pelvic floor dyssynergia inability to coordinate pelvic floor and sphincter relaxation and abdominal muscle contraction; persistent contraction of anal sphincter and pelvic floor leading to obstructed defecation

Pelvic floor muscle training/exercises program involving routine repetitive contractions of pelvic floor muscles with goal of increasing pelvic floor muscle strength (contractility) and endurance. Patient must learn to isolate and voluntarily contract the pelvic floor muscles while (ideally) keeping the abdominal and gluteal muscles relaxed

Pelvic organ prolapse (POP) the herniation of a pelvic organ toward and through the vaginal introitus

Penile compression device (penile clamps) mechanical devices designed to prevent urine leakage by compressing the penis

Perceived constipation perception of problem with stool elimination when bowel function/stool elimination is actually normal

Periaqueductal gray (PAG) section of midbrain that integrates and forwards signals re: bladder filling to prefrontal cortex. Under inhibitory control by prefrontal cortex; when inhibitory control released, PAG directs pontine micturition center to mediate coordinated voiding

Pessary vaginal device to stabilize and support the bladder neck and to compress the urethra to prevent urine leakage during increased intra-abdominal pressure

Phasic detrusor contractions involuntary detrusor contractions that occur during filling phase of urodynamic study and may or may not result in urinary leakage

Phytotherapeutic Agents (See Plant Extracts)

Plant extracts (phytotherapeutic agents) are commonly used by men with LUTS related to BPH: Saw palmetto (*Serenoa repens*), stinging nettle (*Urtica dioica*), extracts of the African plum tree (*Pygeum africanum*), pumpkin seed (*Cucurbita pepo*), South African star grass (*Hypoxis rooperi*), and rye pollen (*Secale cereale*)

Pontine micturition center (Barrington's nucleus) midbrain structure responsible for assuring that bladder neck and rhabdosphincter are relaxed before the bladder contracts

Pontine storage center midbrain structure responsible for maintaining contraction of striated sphincter during storage phase

Postvoid residual urine (PVR) amount of urine remaining in the bladder after voiding; may be measured by ultrasound or by catheterization

Postvoid symptoms sensation of incomplete emptying and postmicturition dribble, the involuntary loss of urine shortly after voiding

Prefrontal cortex area of cortex that controls decision making regarding when and where to void

Pressure flow study voiding phase of urodynamic study; patient voids into uroflow commode while pressure-sensitive catheter remains in place in the bladder. Provides simultaneous measurement of urine flow and pressures generated by detrusor muscle contraction

Pabd urodynamic measurement of intra-abdominal pressure obtained by pressure-sensitive catheter placed in the rectum

Pdet urodynamic measurement of pressures created by bladder wall stiffness and detrusor muscle contractions; obtained by computer subtraction of Pabd from Pves

Percutaneous tibial nerve stimulation (PTNS) also referred to as posterior tibial nerve stimulation. Form of neuromodulation used to treat overactive bladder (OAB); thought to diminish abnormal reflex arcs associated with overactive bladder by modulating afferent signals from the bladder to the spinal cord; a fine needle electrode is inserted into the lower, inner aspect of the leg, slightly cephalad to the medial malleolus near but not on the tibial nerve

Perineal membrane third layer of pelvic floor; triangular fibrous structure that spans anterior pelvis and limits descent of pelvic organs

Prompted voiding behavioral therapy program in which subjects are prompted to toilet and encouraged with social rewards when they void successfully

PSA velocity rise in PSA value over 1 year; an increase of more than 0.75 ng/mL usually triggers the need for a biopsy

Puborectalis muscle component of levator ani muscle that creates a U-shaped sling around the anorectal junction and the anorectal angle that supports fecal continence

Pves urodynamic measurement of intravesical pressure, obtained by pressure-sensitive catheter placed into the bladder; reflects both intra-abdominal pressures and pressures resulting from bladder wall stiffness or detrusor contractions

Radical prostatectomy removal of the prostate gland and prostatic urethra, with anastomosis of distal urethra to bladder neck

Rectoanal inhibitory reflex (RAIR) reflex relaxation of internal anal sphincter (IAS) in response to rectal distention

"Red flag" bowel symptoms signs and symptoms associated with colorectal cancer (also known as "alarm symptoms")

Retentive encopresis fecal soiling caused by stool-withholding behavior

Sacral nerve stimulation (sacral neuromodulation) stimulation of sacral nerves controlling bladder function and stool elimination using implantable electrodes placed in sacral foramen; used to treat refractory overactive bladder and persistent refractory constipation

Sacral reflex tonic contraction of external anal sphincter (EAS) that is increased during activities that increase intra-abdominal and intrarectal pressures

Sampling reflex differentiation between gaseous, liquid, and solid rectal contents provided by sensory receptors in anal canal; occurs when internal anal sphincter relaxes briefly in response to rectal distention and permits rectal contents to contact receptors in anal canal

Secretory diarrhea diarrhea resulting from damage to epithelial cells in intestinal mucosa; results in abnormal secretion of fluid *into* lumen of bowel and inability to absorb water and electrolytes *from* lumen of bowel

Seminal vesicles store semen; the bulbourethral glands secrete an alkaline fluid prior to ejaculation that neutralizes the acidity of urine to protect sperm.

Simple constipation transient alteration in stool elimination, most often caused by dietary or environmental factors

Slow transit constipation constipation caused by reduced frequency and amplitude of peristaltic contractions in the colon

Slow-twitch muscle fibers muscle fibers that provide sustained tonic contraction; comprise 2/3 of pelvic floor muscle fibers

Sphincteroplasty surgical repair of damaged sphincter; commonly used to repair sphincter damaged by obstetric trauma

Spina bifida congenital neural tube defect involving bony defect in vertebral column; most commonly accompanied by myelomeningocele, herniation of the spinal cord through the bony defect

Spinal cord injury trauma or damage to the spinal cord resulting in loss of motor and/or sensory function

Standardized measurement tools tools that generate robust data that can be used to guide initial treatment decisions and to evaluate changes in symptoms and the efficacy of treatment

Stimulant laxative agent that stimulates peristalsis and stool elimination via activation of ganglion cells in the bowel wall

Stimulated defecation use of peristaltic stimulus to initiate rectal evacuation at time selected by patient; commonly used management approach for patient with neurogenic bowel

Stress urinary incontinence involuntary leakage of urine associated with effort or exertion (activities that cause an increase in intra-abdominal pressure)

Stroke sometimes referred to as cerebrovascular accident or brain attack is as an acute, focal injury of the central nervous system owing to a vascular cause such as cerebral infarction, intracerebral hemorrhage, or subarachnoid hemorrhage

Suprasacral level lesions lesions involving spinal cord above sacral level; correspond with vertebral level injuries of T10 and above

Sympathetic nervous system branch of autonomic nervous system; promotes internal urethral sphincter contraction and bladder wall relaxation; reduces intestinal secretion and motility

Tenesmus persistent sensation of stool in the rectum and the need to defecate

Terminal detrusor contractions involuntary detrusor contractions that occur during filling phase of urodynamic study and typically result in complete bladder emptying

Timed voiding toileting at fixed intervals, such as every 3 hours

Transanal irrigation delivery of water into distal colon to stimulate peristalsis and bowel evacuation; water delivered via balloon-tipped catheter to prevent backflow

Transient fecal incontinence short-term (new onset) incontinence caused by change in stool consistency or sensory awareness

Transit time studies diagnostic tool used to objectively differentiate between normal transit and slow transit constipation; utilizes variety of techniques to determine time required for stool to pass through colon and out of anal canal

Transurethral resection of the prostate (TURP) surgical removal of excess prostatic tissue via a resectoscope inserted through the urethra; the gold standard intervention for the treatment of BPH

Transvaginal electrical stimulation used in treating SUI; causes PFM contraction and increases the number of muscle fibers recruited during rapid contractions

TRUS transrectal biopsy of the prostate; performed with an ultrasound-guided needle

Traveler's diarrhea nonspecific infectious diarrhea, typically bacterial, that occurs when individual travels to area of the world with poor sanitation

Upper motor neuron neurogenic bladder an overactive detrusor that contracts without voluntary control

Upper urinary tract distress impaired function of the upper urinary tracts (kidneys, renal pelves, and ureters), associated with neurogenic bladder dysfunction

Urease enzyme that causes the urea in the urine to hydrolyze to free ammonia, in turn raising the pH and allowing precipitation of minerals such as calcium phosphate and magnesium ammonium phosphate (struvite)

Urethral bulking agents intra- or periurethral injection to plump up the urethral mucosa; this creates artificial urethral cushions that can improve urethral coaptation and restore continence

Urethral caruncle cherry red and abnormally prominent (prolapsed) urethral meatus; caused by estrogen deficiency

Urethral hypermobility distal displacement of urethra in response to increased intra-abdominal pressure

Urethral inserts a sterile disposable, single-use, intraurethral device that can be used by women with stress incontinence to prevent leakage

Urethral pressure profile graphic representation of pressures along length of the urethra; obtained by precise and steady withdrawal of a pressure-sensitive catheter through the urethra

Urethral resistance the detrusor pressure required to overcome the urethral sphincter mechanism and create urinary flow; measured during urodynamic testing

Urethral sphincter mechanism conceptualized as containing two components: elements of compression and muscular elements that promote active urethral closure in response to physical exertion; contains periurethral striated muscle and a rhabdosphincter (formerly called the external sphincter)

Urinary continence voluntary control of voiding; requires anatomic integrity of the urinary system, neurological control of the detrusor muscle, and an intact urethral sphincter mechanism

Urge fecal incontinence fecal incontinence associated with sudden, urgent need to defecate (fecal urgency), usually due to incompetent external anal sphincter (EAS)

Urge inhibition strategies behavioral strategies that patients may be taught to control urgency; include pelvic muscle contractions, controlled breathing, avoidance of sudden activity, and distraction

Urgency sudden overwhelming desire to void that is difficult to delay and often accompanied by fear of leakage

Urge urinary incontinence involuntary leakage of urine accompanied by or immediately preceded by a strong urge to void

Urinary frequency abnormally frequent voiding, typically defined as diurnal frequency >8

Urinary incontinence altered ability to store urine effectively and to control the time and place for voiding; involuntary leakage of urine

Urinary retention incomplete bladder emptying, either due to bladder outlet obstruction or to ineffective bladder contractions

Urodynamic testing several different tests of lower urinary tract function that, taken together, create a picture of its functional status (ability of bladder to store urine at low pressures and to empty effectively and sphincter's ability to maintain closure during filling and to open for voiding)

Uroflowmetry measurement of rate of urine flow (ml/second); noninvasive screening tool for voiding dysfunction. Patient voids into commode equipped to measure rate of urine flow

Urothelium inner lining of bladder, comprised primarily of transitional cell epithelium

Vesicovaginal fistula (VVF) an abnormal tract that forms between the bladder and vagina, allowing urine to continuously drain into the vagina

Video urodynamics urodynamic studies utilizing contrast medium for bladder filling and simultaneous use of fluoroscopic imaging

Voiding dysfunction altered ability to effectively empty the bladder, resulting in some degree of urinary retention

Voiding symptoms slow and/or interrupted stream, the perception of reduced flow; hesitancy, difficulty in initiating voiding; straining, the need to use Valsalva or abdominal muscles to void; terminal dribble, prolongation of the last phase of voiding; hematuria (blood in the urine); and dysuria, a burning sensation or general discomfort during voiding

Watchful waiting conservative approach to management of localized prostate cancer or LUTS. Involves deferral of active treatment

Weighted vaginal cones feedback device to assist women to strengthen their PFMs

Wein classification system classification system for urinary incontinence or voiding dysfunction based on urodynamic findings; classifies lower urinary tract dysfunction as one of the following failure to store because of the bladder: failure to store because of the sphincter, failure to empty because of the bladder, and failure to empty because of the sphincter

Index